Contents

Preface

Four years have passed since the publication of the third edition of this book and sixteen since the first. We are delighted that it remains so popular. In revising the text we have again been surprised, and pleased, by the amount of new knowledge and important changes in management that have become an essential part of the routine care of patients with cancer. Perhaps it is only by writing a book covering all aspects of cancer that these developments can be fully appreciated, though this is hardly an approach that we recommend as a means of keeping up-to-date. A textbook limited to this size and designed to be comprehensible to readers from many backgrounds, requires that only essential information can be presented. We have had to synthesize many differing opinions and summarize interesting controversies which, in a larger text, could have been the subject of more detailed discussion.

This edition is a little shorter than the previous one. To give more information in fewer words is a challenge. We hope the result is an accessible text that avoids being too didactic in tone or synoptic in style.

The aim of the book has not changed. It is to provide an introductory text for doctors, other medical workers, students and scientists interested in the problem of cancer.

Cancer medicine is one of the most rapidly changing of all medical specialities. Not long ago most cancers were treated either by surgery or local radiotherapy, with almost no hope of success if the cancer had spread to involve local lymph nodes, or if distant metastases were present. Recent advances in chemotherapy, hormone therapy, radiotherapy and diagnostic imaging have transformed our clinical practice. Progress in cell biology has led to a far greater understanding of the process of malignant transformation.

We have written this book because we are aware that many busy physicians, surgeons and gynaecologists, who are not themselves cancer specialists, may find it difficult to keep abreast of areas which are of considerable importance to them. General surgeons, for example, spend a substantial portion of their time dealing with gastrointestinal and abdominal tumours, yet have little working knowledge of non-surgical treatment of these conditions. Similarly, gynaecological surgeons need to know more

about what the radiotherapist and medical oncologist can offer.

Many medical schools still do not provide any integrated teaching in cancer medicine, and student knowledge of the management of malignant disease is often acquired from specialists whose main interest may not be related to cancer. Medical students should know more about the disease which is the second largest cause of mortality in the Western world. We hope that trainees in medicine, surgery and gynaecology will also find the book of value, and that it will be of help to postgraduates beginning a career in radiotherapy or medical oncology. Finally, we hope that general practitioners, all of whom look after cancer patients and who have an important role in management and terminal care, will find this book helpful. If specialists in cancer medicine feel it is a useful digest of current thought in cancer management, so much the better. However, this book is not intended primarily for them. There are several very large texts which give specialist advice. Although some of these details necessarily appear in our book, we do not regard it as a handbook of chemotherapy or radiotherapy. To some extent it is a personal view of cancer and its management today and, as such, it will differ in some details from the attitudes and approaches of our colleagues.

We have attempted to give a thorough working knowledge of the principles of diagnosis, staging and treatment of tumours and to do so at a level which brings the reader up to date. We have tried to indicate where the subject is growing, where controversies lie, and from which direction future advances might come. In the first nine chapters we have provided a review of some of the mechanisms of tumour development, cancer treatment and supportive care. In the remaining chapters we have given an account of the principles of management of the major cancers. For each tumour we have given details of the pathology, mode of spread, clinical presentation, and staging and treatment with radiotherapy and chemotherapy. The role of surgery is outlined, but details of surgical procedure are beyond the scope of this book. The references which we have included for further reading have been chosen because they are clear reviews or representative of many similar articles, and sometimes because they are historical landmarks or represent important recent work.

Acknowledgements

We were greatly helped by Maria Khan and her team at Blackwell Publishing. We would like to thank all of them for giving the sustained encouragement that even the most seasoned authors need. Audrey Cadogan and Helen Clements were most helpful editors. We are grateful to our production editors Bridgette Jones and Fiona Pattison who bravely showed no signs of stress at the state of the finished manuscript.

Cover illustration: squamous cell carcinoma. The dividing cell is labelled in red for the actin cytoskeleton and in green for all αv integrins. The authors are indebted to Professor Ian Hart for this image.

R.S., J.T.

Abbreviations

ABCM	doxorubicin, bis-chloroethyl nitrosourea, cyclophosphamide and melphalan
ABVD	doxorubicin, bleomycin, vinblastine and dacarbazine
ACh	acetylcholine
A-COP	A-doxorubicin, cyclophosphamide, O-vincristine, prednisolone
ACTH	adrenocorticotrophic hormone
ADH	antidiuretic hormone
AFP	α-fetoprotein
AHA	autoimmune haemolytic anaemia
AIDS	acquired immune deficiency syndrome
ALL	acute lymphoblastic leukaemia
AML	acute myeloblastic (myelogenous) leukaemia
AMML	acute myelomonocytic leukaemia
ANL	acute non-lymphocytic leukaemia
APC	adenomatous polyposis coli
APUD	amine precursors uptake and decarboxylation
ATRA	all-*trans*-retinoic-acid
BACOP	bleomycin, A-doxorubicin, cyclophosphamide, O-vincristine and prednisone
BCG	bacille Calmette–Guérin
BCNU	bis-chloroethyl nitrosourea
BEP	bleomycin, etoposide and cisplatin
BMT	bone marrow transplantation
BUdR	bromodeoxyuridine
CALLA	common acute lymphoblastic leukaemia antigen
CCNU	*cis*-chloroethyl nitrosourea
CEA	carcinoembryonic antigen
CGL	chronic granulocytic leukaemia
ChlVPP	chlorambucil, vinblastine, procarbazine and prednisone
CHOP	cyclophosphamide, H-doxorubicin, O-vincristine and prednisolone
CIN	cervical intraepithelial neoplasia
CLL	chronic lymphocytic (lymphatic) leukaemia
CMF	cyclophosphamide, methotrexate and 5-FU
CMI	cell-mediated immunity

CML	chronic myeloblastic (myelogenous) leukaemia
CMV	cytomegalovirus
CNS	central nervous system
COMP	cyclophosphamide, vincristine, methotrexate and prednisolone
CR	complete response
CRC	Cancer Research Campaign
CSF	cerebrospinal fluid
CSF	colony-stimulating factor
CT	computerized tomography
CytaBOM	cytarabine, bleomycin, O-vincristine and methotrexate
DIC	disseminated intravascular coagulation
DNCB	dinitrochlorobenzene
DTIC	dimethyltriazenoimidazole carboxamide (dacarbazine)
EBV	Epstein–Barr virus
ECOG	Eastern Co-operative Oncology Group
ED	extensive disease
EF	extended field
EGF	epidermal growth factor
EGFR	epidermal growth factor receptor
EM	electron microscope
EMG	electromyogram
EORTC	European Organization for Research and Treatment of Cancer
EPO	erythropoietin
ER	oestrogen receptor
ERCP	endoscopic retrograde cholangiopancreatography
ESR	erythrocyte sedimentation rate
EVAP	etoposide, vinblastine, doxorubicin and prednisolone
FdUMP	5-fluoro-2-deoxyuridine monophosphate
FIGO	International Federation of Gynaecology and Obstetrics
FPC	familial polyposis coli
FSH	follicle-stimulating hormone
5-FU	5-fluorouracil
G6PD	glucose 6-phosphate dehydrogenase
G-CSF	granulocyte colony-stimulating factors
GH	growth hormone

GM-CSF	granulocyte/macrophage colony-stimulating factors		MMP	matrix metalloproteinase
GSH	glutathione		MOPP	mustine, vincristine (oncovin), prednisone and procarbazine
HBI	hemi-body irradiation		6MP	6-mercaptopurine
HBLV	human B-cell lymphotrophic virus		6MPRP	6-mercaptopurine ribose phosphate
HBV	hepatitis B virus		MRC	Medical Research Council
HCG	human chorionic gonadotrophin		MRI	magnetic resonance imaging
HCL	hairy cell leukaemia		mRNA	messenger ribonucleic acid
HGPRT	hypoxanthine–guanine phosphoribosyltransferase		MSH	melanocyte-stimulating hormone
			MTI	malignant teratoma intermediate
HHM	humoral hypercalcaemia of malignancy		MTT	malignant teratoma trophoblastic
5HIAA	5-hydroxyindoleacetic acid		MTU	malignant teratoma undifferentiated
HIV	human immunodeficiency virus		MVPP	mustine, vinblastine, prednisone and procarbazine
HLA	human leucocyte antigen			
HPV	human papilloma virus		NCAM	neural-cell adhesion molecule
HSV	herpes simplex virus		NHL	non-Hodgkin's lymphomas
5HT	5-hydroxytryptamine		NK	natural killer
HTLV	Human T-cell leukaemia virus		NSABP	National Surgical Adjuvant Breast Project (USA)
HVA	homovanillic acid			
ICRF	Imperial Cancer Research Fund		NSCLC	non-small-cell lung cancer
IF	involved field		NSD	nominal standard dose
IFN	interferon		PCI	prophylactic cranial irradiation
Ig	immunoglobulin		PCR	polymerase chain reaction
IL-2	interleukin-2 (etc.)		PCV	procarbazine, CCNU and vincristine
IPSID	immune proliferative small-intestine disease		PDT	photodynamic therapy
			PET	positron electron tomography
IVU	intravenous urography		PLAP	placental alkaline phosphatase
KS	Kaposi's sarcoma		PNET	primitive neuroectodermal tumour
LAK	lymphokine-activated killer		PR	progesterone receptor
LD	limited disease		ProMACE	Prednisone, methotrexate, A-doxorubicin, cyclophosphamide and etoposide
LET	linear energy transfer			
LH	luteinizing hormone		PSA	prostate-specific antigen
LHRH	luteinizing hormone releasing hormone		PTH	parathyroid hormone
LOPP	chlorambucil, vincristine, procarbazine and prednisolone		PTHrP	parathyroid hormone-related protein
			pUVA	psoralens and ultraviolet light A
LTR	long terminal repeat		PVB	cisplatin, vinblastine and bleomycin
mAb	monoclonal antibody		PVC	polyvinylchloride
MACOP-B	methotrexate, A-doxorubicin, cyclophosphamide, O-vincristine, prednisolone and bleomycin		RS	Reed–Sternberg
			RSV	Rous sarcoma virus
			SCLC	small-cell lung cancer
M-BACOD	methotrexate, bleomycin, A-doxorubicin, cyclophosphamide, O-vincristine and dexamethasone		SVCO	superior vena caval obstruction
			TBI	total-body irradiation
			TCC	transitional cell carcinoma
M-CSF	macrophage colony-stimulating factors		6TG	6-thioguanine
MDR	multi-drug resistance		TGF	transforming growth factor
MDS	myelodysplastic syndromes		TIBC	total iron binding capacity
MEN	multiple endocrine neoplasia		TIMPs	tissue inhibitors of metalloproteinases
MGUS	monoclonal gammopathy of unknown significance		TLI	total lymphoid irradiation
			TNF	tumour necrosis factor
MHC	major histocompatibility complex		TNI	total nodal irradiation

TNM	tumour node metastasis	VAD	vincristine, infused doxorubicin and high-dose dexamethasone
TS	thymidylate synthase		
TSH	thyroid-stimulating hormone	VIN	vulval intraepithelial neoplasia
TSTA	tumour-specific transplantation antigens	VIP	vasoactive intestinal polypeptide
		VMA	vanillyl mandelic acid
UICC	Union Internationale Contre le Cancer	WBC	white blood count

1

The modern management of cancer: an introductory note

Cancer is a vast medical problem. As a cause of mortality it is second only to cardiovascular disease. It is diagnosed each year in one in every 250 men and one in every 300 women. The incidence rises steeply with age so that, over the age of 60, three in every 100 men develop the disease each year (Fig. 1.1). It is often a costly disease to diagnose and investigate, and treatment is time-consuming, labour-intensive and usually requires hospital care. In the Western world the commonest cancers are of the lung, breast, skin, gut and prostate gland (Fig. 1.2). The lifetime risk of developing a cancer is shown in Fig. 1.3.

For many years the main methods of treating cancer were surgery and radiotherapy. The control of the primary tumour is indeed a concern, since it is this which is usually responsible for the patient's symptoms. There may be exceedingly unpleasant symptoms due to local spread, and failure to control the disease locally means certain death. For many tumours—breast cancer, for example—the energies of those treating the disease have been directed towards defining the optimum methods of eradication of the primary tumour. It is perhaps not surprising that these efforts, while improving management, have not greatly improved the prognosis because the most important cause of mortality is metastatic spread. Although prompt and effective treatment of the primary cancer diminishes the likelihood of recurrence, metastases have often developed before diagnosis and treatment have begun. The prognosis is not then altered by treatment of the primary cancer, even though the presenting symptoms may be alleviated. Progress in treatment has been slow but steady. There have been long-running arguments about the degree of success or failure of current treatments. These debates have been fuelled by differing statistical interpretations and by over-optimistic assertions of progress.

Every medical specialty has its own types of cancer which are the concern of the specialist in that area. Cancer is a diagnosis to which all clinicians are alerted whatever their field and, because malignant disease is common, specialists acquire great expertise in diagnosis, often with the aid of techniques such as bronchoscopy and other forms of endoscopy. Conversely, the management of cancer once the diagnosis has been made, especially the non-surgical management, is not part of the training or interest of many specialists. This has meant that radiotherapists and medical oncologists are often asked to see patients who have had a laparotomy at which a tumour such as an ovarian cancer or a lymphoma has been found, but the abdomen has been closed without the surgeon having made an attempt to stage the disease properly, or, where appropriate, to remove the main mass of tumour. This poses considerable problems for the further management of the patient. At a more general level, lack of familiarity with the principles of cancer management and of what treatment can achieve leads to a low level of recruitment into clinical trials. An understanding of the principles of investigation and treatment of cancer has become essential for every physician and surgeon if the best results for their patients are to be achieved.

Recent advances in the chemotherapy and radiotherapy of uncommon tumours such as Hodgkin's disease and teratoma of the testis have led to a more general awareness of the importance of a planned approach to the management of patients. This has been true not only for the problems of individual patients but also in the planning of clinical trials of treatment. It has become clear that for every cancer, an understanding of which patients can be helped or even cured can only come by attention to the details of disease stage and type. Patients in whom these details are unknown are at risk from inappropriate overtreatment or from inadequate treatment, resulting in the chance of cure being missed. Even though chemotherapy has not been of great benefit to patients with diseases such as squamous lung cancer or adenocarcinoma of the pancreas, it is now clearly essential that clinicians with a detailed and specialized knowledge of the risks and dangers of chemotherapy in these and other diseases are part of the staff of every oncology department. Knowing when not to treat is as important as knowing when to do so.

The improvement in chemotherapy of some cancers has greatly increased the complexity of management. Cancer specialists have a particular responsibility to validate the treatment which they give, since the toxicity and dangers of some regimens mean that the indications for treatment have to be established precisely. In a few cases an imaginative step forward has dramatically improved results and the need for controlled comparison with previous treatment is scarcely necessary. Examples are the use of combination chemotherapy in the management of advanced Hodgkin's disease and prevention of central nervous system relapse of leukaemia by prophylactic treatment. However, such clear-cut advances are seldom made. In the main, improvement in treatment is made slowly in a piecemeal fashion and prospective trials of treatment must be undertaken in order to validate each step in management. Modest advances are numerically none the less important for such common diseases. Only large-scale trials can detect these small differences reliably. Collaboration on a national and international scale has become increasingly important, and the result of these studies has had a major impact on management, for example in operable breast cancer. There is always a tendency in dealing with cancer to want to believe good news and for early, uncontrolled, but promising results to be seized upon and overinterpreted. Although understandable, uncritical enthusiasm for a particular form of treatment is greatly to be deplored, since it leads to a clamour for the treatment and the establishment of patterns of treatment which are improperly validated. There have been many instances where treatments have been used before their place has been clearly established—adjuvant chemotherapy in non-small-cell lung cancer, limb perfusion in sarcomas and melanoma, radical surgical techniques for gastric cancer and adjuvant chemotherapy for bladder cancer are examples. The toxicity of cancer treatments is considerable and can only be justified if it is unequivocally clear that the end results are worthwhile either by increasing the cure rate or by improving the quality of life.

The increasing complexity of management has brought with it a recognition that in many areas it is necessary to establish an effective working collaboration between specialists. Joint planning of management in specialized

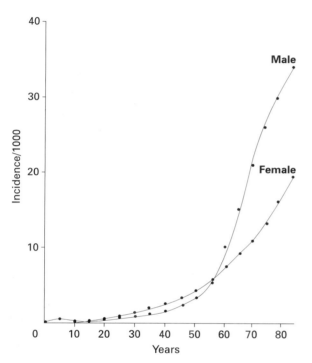

Fig. 1.1 Age-specific cancer incidence in England and Wales.

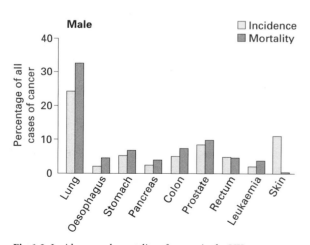

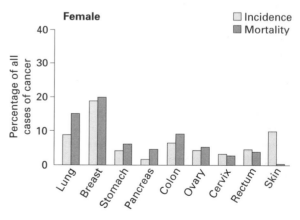

Fig. 1.2 Incidence and mortality of cancer in the UK.

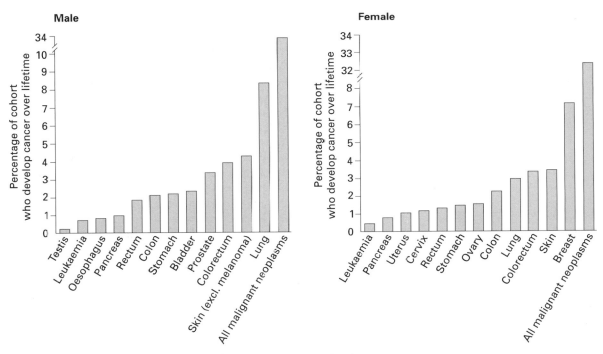

Fig. 1.3 Estimates of the lifetime risk of developing cancer in England and Wales.

clinics is now widely practised for diseases such as lymphomas, head and neck and gynaecological cancer. Surgeons and gynaecologists are now being trained who specialize in the oncological aspects of their specialty. In this way patients can benefit from a co-ordinated and planned approach to their individual problems.

Before a patient can be treated, it must be established that he or she has cancer, the tumour pathology must be defined and the extent of the local and systemic disease determined. For each of these goals to be attained the oncologist must rely on colleagues in departments of histopathology, diagnostic imaging, haematology and chemical pathology. Patients are often referred in whom the diagnosis of cancer has not been definitely made pathologically but is based on a very strong clinical suspicion with suggestive pathological evidence, or where a pathological diagnosis of cancer has been made which, on review, proves to be incorrect. It is essential for the oncologist to be in close contact with histopathologists and cytologists so that diagnoses can be reviewed regularly. Many departments of oncology have regular pathology review meetings so that the clinician can learn of the difficulties which pathologists have with diagnosis and vice versa. Similarly, modern imaging techniques have led

to a previously unattainable accuracy in preoperative and postoperative staging, although many of these techniques are only as reliable as those using them (for example abdominal or pelvic ultrasound). The cancer specialist must be fully conversant with the uses and limitations of imaging methods. The techniques are expensive and the results must be interpreted in the light of other clinical information. The practice of holding regular meetings to review cases with specialists from the imaging departments has much to commend it.

Modern cancer treatment often carries a substantial risk of toxicity. Complex and difficult treatments are best managed in a specialized unit with skilled personnel. The centralization of high-dependency care allows staff to become particularly aware of the physical and emotional problems of patients undergoing treatments of this kind. Additionally, colleagues from other departments such as haematology, biochemistry and bacteriology can more easily help in the investigation and management of some of the very difficult problems which occur, for example in the immunosuppressed patient.

The increasingly intensive investigative and treatment policies which have been adopted in the last 20 years, impose on clinicians the additional responsibility of having to stand back from the treatment of their patients and decide what the aim of treatment is at each stage. Radical and aggressive therapy may be essential if the patient has a reasonable chance of being cured. However, palliative treatment will be used if the situation is clearly beyond any prospect of cure. It is often more difficult to decide when the intention of treatment should move from the radical to the palliative, with avoidance of toxicity as a major priority. For example, while many patients with advanced lymphomas will be cured by intensive combination chemotherapy, there is no prospect of cure in advanced breast cancer by these means, and chemotherapy must in this case be regarded as palliative therapy. In this situation it makes little sense to press treatment to the point of toxicity. The judgement of what is tolerable and acceptable is a major task in cancer management. Such judgements can only come from considerable experience of the treatments in question, of the natural history of individual tumours and an understanding of the patient's needs and wishes.

Modern cancer management often involves highly technological and intensive medical care. It is expensive, time-consuming and sometimes dangerous. Patients should seldom be in ignorance of what is wrong with them or what the treatment involves. The increasingly technical nature of cancer management, and the change in public and professional attitudes towards malignant disease, have altered the way in which doctors who are experienced in cancer treatment approach their patients. There has been a decisive swing towards honest and careful discussion with patients about the disease and its treatment. This does not mean that a bald statement should be made to the patient about the diagnosis and its outcome, since doctors must sustain the patient with hope and encouragement through what is obviously a frightening and depressing period. One of the most difficult and rewarding aspects of the management of malignant disease lies in the judgement of how much information to give to each particular patient, at what speed and how to incorporate the patient's own wishes into a rational treatment plan.

The emotional impact of the diagnosis and treatment can be considerable for both patients and relatives. Above everything else, treating patients with cancer involves an awareness of how patients think and feel. All members of the medical team caring for cancer patients must be pre-

pared to devote time to talking to patients and their families, to answer questions and explain what is happening and what can be achieved. Because many patients will die from their disease, they must learn to cope with the emotional and physical needs of dying patients and the effects of grief and bereavement on their families.

In modern cancer units management is by a team of health-care professionals, each of whom has their own contribution to make. They must work together participating in management as colleagues commanding mutual respect. The care and support of patients with advanced malignant disease and the control of symptoms such as pain and nausea have greatly improved in the last 10 years. This aspect of cancer management has been improved by the collaboration of many medical workers. Nurses who specialize in the control of symptoms of malignancy are now attached to many cancer units, and social workers skilled in dealing with the problems of malignant disease and bereavement are an essential part of the team. The development of hospices has led to a much greater appreciation of the way in which symptoms might be controlled and to a considerable improvement in the standards of care of the dying in general hospitals. Many cancer departments now have a symptom support team based in the hospital but who are able to undertake the care of patients in their own homes, giving advice on control of symptoms such as pain and nausea and providing support to patients' families.

There have been dramatic advances in cell and molecular biology in the last 10 years, with the result that our understanding of the nature of malignant transformation has increased. This trend will continue and places an additional demand on oncologists, namely to keep abreast of both advances in management and the scientific foundations on which they are based. The power of modern techniques to explore some of the fundamental processes in malignant transformation has meant that cancer is at the heart of many aspects of medical research and has led to an increased academic interest in malignancy. This, in turn, has led to a more critical approach to many aspects of cancer treatment. Cancer and its management is now one of the most complex and demanding aspects of medicine. More health-care workers are seeing that cancer medicine is rewarding and interesting, and standards of patient care are improving as a result of these welcome changes.

2 Epidemiology, cure, treatment trials and screening

The epidemiology of cancer, which concerns the study of the frequency of the disease in populations living under different conditions, has been illuminating in several ways. It has allowed the testing of theories about the cause of a cancer by relating a particular characteristic—for example, cigarette smoking—to the occurrence of disease. It has suggested ways in which cancer might be prevented by changing the prevalence of a postulated aetiological agent, as shown by the decline of lung cancer in doctors who have given up smoking. Finally, epidemiological evidence has proved invaluable in planning cancer services.

Terminology and methods in epidemiology

Prevalence means the proportion of a defined group having a condition at a single point in time. *Incidence* means the proportion of a defined population developing the disease within a stated time period. *Crude incidence* or *prevalence rates* refer to a whole population. *Specific rates* refer to selected groups—for example, a higher crude fatality rate from breast cancer in one population might be due to more postmenopausal women being in the population in question. *Standardized populations* should therefore be used when comparing incidence and prevalence.

In trying to find connections between a disease and a postulated causal factor, epidemiologists may construct either *case–control* or *cohort* studies. For example, to determine if there is a connection between dietary fat and breast cancer, a *case–control study* would compare the dietary intake of people with the disease (cases) and those

without (controls). Choosing appropriate controls is vital to the study design. Case–control studies are also suitable for studies of rare tumours in which a group of people who are exposed to the putative aetiological agent are followed and the frequency of the disease is measured. The control group is unexposed, or exposed to a lesser extent. In the case of dietary fat and breast cancer, a *cohort study* would compare the incidence of the disease, over a given period of time, in those with, say, a high-fat and a low-fat diet. If the cancer incidence is low, as it usually is, large numbers of women will be followed over many years before an answer is obtained. Other variables must be allowed for since eating habits, for example, are influenced by social class and ethnic origin and these may in turn be independently linked to the likelihood of developing breast cancer. Cohort studies take a long time, are very expensive and are unsuitable for studies of rare tumours.

There are considerable problems in the interpretation of data obtained from epidemiological studies. A possible relationship between a characteristic and a cancer may be discovered, but there are several considerations which should influence us in deciding whether a causal connection really exists.

1 Is the relationship between the characteristic and the disease specific, or can a similar association be found with other diseases? An association with other diseases does not necessarily invalidate a causal connection but may suggest that both the characteristic and the cancer are themselves associated with another factor. For example, both lung cancer and coronary artery disease are more common in social classes 4 and 5. The problem is then to decide if

these diseases are due to social class itself or to the higher frequency of cigarette smoking in these social groups.

2 Is the relationship a strong one? The likelihood of a causal connection is strengthened if, for example, the risk of cancer in the population showing the characteristic is increased 10-fold rather than doubled.

3 Is there a gradation of risk with differing exposure? This is the situation with lung cancer and cigarette smoking. Such a gradation greatly increases the likelihood of a causal connection.

4 Is the association biologically plausible? For example, it appears intuitively reasonable to accept an association between smoking and lung cancer, but the relationship between smoking and bladder cancer is at first more surprising (see p. 283). It may, however, be difficult to assess the biological basis for an association since often we do not know the explanation for these events until further investigation, perhaps prompted by the discovery of an association, reveals it. Animal models of the disease may help both in suggesting which environmental agents may be causal, and in strengthening the conclusions of epidemiological investigations.

5 Is there an alternative explanation for what has been found and do the findings fit in with other epidemiological data? The nature of epidemiological evidence is such that absolute proof that an association is causal may sometimes be impossible to obtain except by intervention studies in which the suspected factor is altered or removed to see if the incidence of cancer then falls. Such studies are difficult, expensive and time-consuming, especially if randomization is necessary. In some circumstances randomized intervention may be impossible (we cannot randomly allocate people to give up smoking or to continue!) and the epidemiological data derived from studies of the population provide the only possible information.

Geographical distribution of cancer

Clues to the aetiology of cancer have been obtained from studies of the difference in incidence of cancers in different countries, races and cultures. There are obvious difficulties in obtaining reliable data in some countries. Problems of different age distributions can to some extent be overcome by using age-standardized incidence and by restricting the comparison to the mature adult population aged 35–64 years. This age range excludes the ages where the figures are likely to be least reliable. A further difficulty lies in incomplete documentation of histological type. Sometimes the registration refers to the whole organ—bone or lung—without specifying histological type.

Very large differences in incidence of various tumours between countries have been disclosed (Table 2.1). The very high incidence of liver cancer in Mozambique may be related to aflatoxin mould on stored peanuts, and the incidence is now falling since steps have been taken to store the peanuts under different conditions. In the Ghurjev region of Kazakhstan, carcinoma of the oesophagus is 200 times more common than in The Netherlands; and in the Transkei region the incidence of the disease appears to have increased greatly in the last 30 years. The high incidence of carcinoma of the stomach in Japan is in contrast to the UK and the USA where the incidence of the disease is falling [1].

Studies such as these provide strong evidence for environmental factors causing cancer, but there may be an interaction with genetic predisposition.

An analysis of the relative contributions of the environmental and genetic components can be made by studying cancer incidence in people who have settled in a new country and who have taken on a new way of life. Japanese immigrants in the USA, for example, have a similar inci-

Cancer type	Ratio high : low rate	High incidence	Low incidence
Oesophagus	200 : 1	Kazakhstan	Holland
Skin	200 : 1	Queensland	India
Liver	100 : 1	Mozambique	Birmingham
Nasopharynx	100 : 1	China	Uganda
Lung	40 : 1	Birmingham	Ibadan (Nigeria)
Stomach	30 : 1	Japan	Birmingham
Cervix	20 : 1	Hawaii Colombia	Israel
Rectum	20 : 1	Denmark	Nigeria

Table 2.1 Geographical variation in cancer incidence.

Table 2.2 Cancer incidence* in Japanese immigrants compared with country of origin and residents of adopted country.

Cancer	Japanese in Japan	USA (mostly Hawaii)	
		Japanese	White
Stomach	130	40	21
Breast	31	122	187
Colon	8.4	37	37
Ovary	5.2	16	27
Prostate	1.5	15	35

*Incidence: cases per year per 100 000.

dence of colon cancer to native Americans but five times that of Japanese in Japan [2] (Table 2.2) and it is therefore clear that this difference in rates is not mainly genetic.

Temporal distribution of cancer [3]

The incidence of cancer in a given community may change with time, providing further clues to aetiology. With rare tumours, this may be more dramatically apparent when a disease appears as a cluster in a given place at a given time. An example would be several cases of acute leukaemia occurring in close proximity in a town within a short space of time. Such clustering has indeed been observed in acute leukaemia and has been suggested for Hodgkin's disease. Chance effects make analysis difficult. However, in the case of Burkitt's lymphoma, outbreaks in Uganda have been shown to spread from one part of a district to another in a way which cannot be attributed to chance but which fits well with an infective aetiology that is widespread in the community but produces cancer in only a few. More dramatic evidence of environmental factors comes from the change in cancer incidence with time. However, the interpretation of these changes with time may be made difficult by changes in registration methods, by shifts in diagnostic accuracy and by the long latent period of many cancers. The dramatic rise in lung cancer in the Western world can be attributed to smoking but the fall in stomach cancer is of unknown cause.

Causes of cancer suggested by epidemiological studies [4]

The idea that cancer might largely be preventable has gained more widespread acceptance in recent years. Many substances present in the environment or in the diet have

Table 2.3 Some aetiological factors.

Ionizing irradiation	
Atomic bomb and nuclear accidents	Acute leukaemia
	Breast cancer
X-rays	
Diagnostic and therapeutic	Bone cancer
	Acute leukaemia
	Squamous cell carcinoma of skin
Ultraviolet irradiation	Basal and squamous cell skin cancer; melanoma
Background irradiation	?Acute leukaemia
Inhaled or ingested carcinogens	
Cigarette smoking	Cancers of lung, larynx and bladder
Atmospheric pollution with polycyclic hydrocarbons	Lung cancer
Asbestos	Mesothelioma
	Bronchial carcinoma
Nickel	Cancer of the lung and paranasal sinuses
Chromates	Lung cancer
Arsenic	Lung and skin cancer
Aluminium	Bladder cancer
Aromatic amines	Bladder cancer
Benzene	Erythroleukaemia
Polyvinylchloride	Angiosarcoma of the liver
Viral causes	
Papilloma virus	Cancers of the cervix, anus
HHV8	Kaposi's sarcoma
HTLV-1	T-cell lymphoma

been shown to be carcinogenic in animals. The epidemiological approach has been used to investigate the link between human cancers and substances which in animals are known to be carcinogens, and to identify unsuspected carcinogens by observations on human populations without reference to previous animal experiments. Some of the factors which are known or strongly suspected to be carcinogenic in humans are shown in Table 2.3.

Inhaled carcinogens

Cigarette smoking has been the subject of intense epidemiological investigation since the early work of Doll and Hill demonstrated the relationship between smoking and lung cancer. All studies have shown a higher mortality for lung cancer in smokers. This mortality has a dose–response relationship with the numbers of cigarettes smoked and diminishes with time after stopping smoking.

This relationship is discussed further in Chapter 12. Cigarette smoking has also been implicated in the development of carcinoma of the bladder, larynx, pancreas and kidney and may be responsible for 35% of all cancer deaths.

Cigarette smoking is the major known cause of cancer; all other causes are vastly less important. Reversal of this public health hazard will do more to improve health than any other preventative measure.

Atmosphere pollutants such as chimney smoke and exhaust fumes have been widely suspected as a cause of lung cancer. Polycyclic hydrocarbons, such as 3,4-benzpyrene, are present in these fumes and are known to be carcinogenic in humans. The incidence of lung cancer in men in large cities is two or three times greater than in those living in the country. This increase is small compared with the increase in incidence in smokers compared with non-smokers.

Ionizing irradiation

Ionizing irradiation has been well established as a human carcinogen. There has been an increased incidence of leukaemia and breast cancer in the survivors of the Nagasaki and Hiroshima atom bombs. Skin cancer frequently occurred on the hands of radiologists in the days before the significance of radiation exposure was understood. The internal deposition of radium (see Chapter 23, p. 344) was a cause of osteosarcoma as is external beam radiation. There is also an increased incidence of leukaemia in patients treated by irradiation for ankylosing spondylitis. Ultraviolet irradiation is responsible for the increased incidence of skin cancer on sites exposed to intense sunlight.

Background environmental radiation is at a much smaller dose in total, and is received at a much slower rate (less than 10^{-8}) than that of diagnostic X-rays. For most cancers, background radioactivity appears to constitute a small risk at present, with the exception of lung cancer where background radiation from radon is responsible for an increase in incidence [5].

Occupational factors (Table 2.3)

Asbestos inhalation is associated with two types of cancer: mesothelioma of the pleura and peritoneum, and bronchogenic carcinoma. Prolonged and heavy exposure is needed in the case of bronchogenic cancer, and cigarette smoking further increases the risk. In recent years, the incidence of mesothelioma has risen dramatically in both

men and women [6]. This can be related to the widespread use of asbestos in postwar building. There is also an increased risk of lung cancer in workers in nickel refining and the manufacture of chromates, and a possible association with haematite mining and gold mining. Lung cancer has also been described in workers in a sheep-dip factory where there was a very high exposure to inhaled arsenic. These workers had signs of chronic arsenicalism, and the risk of lung cancer with lower levels of exposure is probably very small.

Other human carcinogens have been identified as a result of industrial epidemiological evidence. Aniline dye workers were shown to have a greatly increased incidence of bladder cancer, and this observation led to the demonstration, in animals, of the carcinogenic effect of 2-naphthylamine. Benzidine and 2-naphthylamine have also been implicated in the pathogenesis of bladder cancer in these workers and those in the rubber industry who are also exposed.

Workers in the aluminium industry have been shown to have an increased incidence of bladder cancer. It has been estimated that about 4% of all cancers can be related to occupational factors.

Lifestyle and diet

Some epidemiologists attribute a large proportion of cancers to as yet unspecified industrial poisons and claim that there is an increase in cancer incidence which is unrelated to tobacco consumption. The figures are disputed, however, since there are the confounding variables of improved diagnosis and registration among the poorer sections of society during this period (see below). The issue is intensely political, and the prevention and control of industrial pollution potentially involve large sums of money.

The place of dietary factors in cancer causation is equally poorly understood. Studies have shown that in countries where there is a high average daily fat intake the age-adjusted death rate of postmenopausal breast cancer and colon cancer is also high. The problem is that those countries where dietary fat intake is high also tend to be the most heavily industrialized. Furthermore, the total caloric intake is higher in these nations, and a similar association exists for levels of dietary protein. Overnutrition has been shown to increase the incidence of spontaneous tumours in animals. Obesity appears to be an aetiological factor in cancers of the endometrium and gall bladder. Case–control studies relating dietary fat to cancer incidence have given conflicting results. A recent meta-analysis has attempted to provide an analysis of the risk but the methodological problems and the interpretation of the results present considerable difficulty [7]. Rather than being causally linked to the cancer, it may be that these dietary constituents are associated with other factors which are themselves causal. Other dietary factors which may be associated with the development of cancer are dietary fibre, which may protect against the development of cancer of the large bowel, and vitamin A analogues (retinoids). However, no change in breast cancer risk has been shown in relation to dietary intake of vitamins C, E and A [8]. Two randomized trials of retinoids in patients at high risk of aerodigestive cancer have failed to demonstrate a protective effect of supplementation: indeed lung cancer incidence was slightly higher in the treated group.

Viral causes

Viral infection accounts for 10–15% of human cancer. The importance of viral infection as a cause has increased greatly since the onset of the acquired immune deficiency syndrome (AIDS) epidemic because viral-induced malignancy is a common cause of death.

The mechanisms of viral-induced malignancy are discussed in Chapter 3, p. 23.

Epstein–Barr virus (EBV), Kaposi's sarcoma herpes virus (KSHV) (human herpes virus 8 (HHV8)) are the viruses most clearly associated with cancer [9,10]. EBV causes Burkitt's lymphoma and nasopharyngeal carcinoma in a small proportion of infected patients. The lymphoma occurs in sub-Saharan Africa in the malaria-endemic region. Kaposi's sarcoma has long existed in a similar distribution in sub-Saharan Africa and in the Mediterranean Jewish population. HHV8 is now known to be closely linked with the sarcoma in the endemic and AIDS-related disease as well as in multicentric Castleman's disease and primary effusion lymphoma. The prevalence of antibodies to HHV8 (KSHV) is higher in Italy and Africa than in the UK or the USA.

Papilloma viruses are the major causative factor in the development of cervical cancer. Of over 100 types of virus, types 16, 18, 31 and 33 are particularly high-risk types (6 and 11 being low risk).

Retroviruses are causes of human cancer, the best-defined example being human T-cell leukaemia virus-1 (HTLV-1) which is an endemic infection in southern Japan and the Caribbean, and where the disease in a small proportion of those infected develops. The virus is transmitted from mother to child via the placenta and in breast milk and is also transmitted in semen.

Hepatitis B virus is a DNA virus transmitted by blood and sexual contact. It causes hepatitis and cirrhosis. Hepatocellular carcinoma occurs at 100 times the frequency of non-infected individuals. *Hepatitis C* is an RNA virus that also causes chronic hepatitis with a greatly increased incidence of hepatocellular carcinoma. Both viruses have a worldwide distribution but are especially prevalent in China and Taiwan and intravenous drug takers.

Cancer statistics

Registries have been established in the UK and other countries to record the number of patients developing cancer. The registry is usually notified of new cancer cases by the hospital where the diagnosis is made. In addition, it receives copies of all death certificates of patients within the region, where the diagnosis of cancer appears on a certificate. The quality of the data collected varies greatly between registries and countries. Incomplete information, changing patterns of registration and diagnosis, introduction of screening programmes and improved treatment change the number of patients being registered as dying of the disease in a given area in a given time. Minor fluctuations in incidence should therefore be viewed with caution. Consistent trends over several years require investigation before it can be accepted that a change in the incidence or mortality of a disease is occurring.

Still more caution must be attached to any report which seeks to determine the impact of a treatment by examining cancer registry data. The relative merits of one treatment or another must be determined by prospective randomized trials (see p. 13).

Even the most complete registries may have histological confirmation of the diagnosis in less than 60% of cases, although the completeness of the records with respect to the primary site of the tumour is much greater. The incidence figures for tumours of a defined histological type are therefore usually much less reliable than those which describe their site of origin.

In spite of these reservations, a glance at the age-specific incidence of various tumours is interesting and revealing. For example, the figures for female genital cancer (Fig. 2.1) show that cancers of the ovary and uterus follow a very similar pattern, the incidence rising sharply towards the end of the child-bearing years, reaching a peak postmenopause. An understanding of the causes of these cancers must clearly take into account these dramatic changes. This is not the pattern seen with all adenocarci-

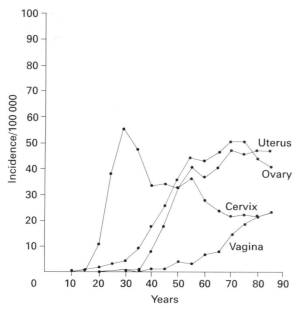

Fig. 2.1 Age-specific incidence of female genital cancer. The figures for cervical cancer include carcinoma *in situ*, diagnosed by screening examination, which accounts for the majority of cases in young patients.

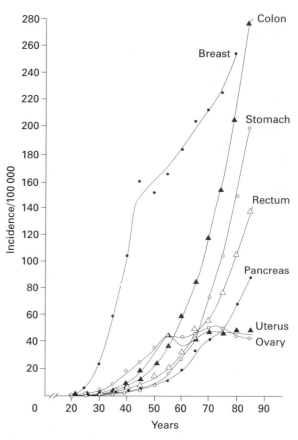

Fig. 2.2 Age-specific incidence of female adenocarcinoma. The incidence of cancer of the breast increases rapidly in pre-menopausal women and then slows. This change is more marked with ovarian and uterine adenocarcinoma. By contrast, the incidence of gastrointestinal cancers shows no relation to menopause but increases markedly over the age of 60.

nomas in women (Fig. 2.2). Indeed, cancer of the ovary and uterus stand out as not showing the typical huge increase in incidence from the age of 60 onwards which characterizes other adenocarcinomas such as bowel, stomach and pancreas.

Cancer of the cervix and of the vagina, chiefly squamous cell cancers, are quite unlike each other in age of onset, that of the cervix being a disease of young and middle-aged women, and that of the vagina a disease of elderly women (Fig. 2.1). The impact of screening programmes for cervical cancer has meant that many of these cases are diagnosed at a very early stage, and study of the histology shows a large percentage of cases diagnosed *in situ*. Should we therefore conclude that the higher incidence of cervical cancer in young women is an artefact of early diagnosis and that these cancers would only have been clinically apparent, if at all, many years later? This problem is discussed in more detail in Chapter 17, but it serves to illustrate how cancer statistics may be dramatically altered by early diagnosis.

The figures for other adenocarcinomas in women (Fig. 2.2) are revealing in another respect. The onset of cancer of the uterus and ovary is earlier than that of the gut and stomach, and does not increase in incidence with old age. Conversely, cancer of the breast rises rapidly in incidence

in early middle age, and then continues to rise in incidence postmenopause but at a slower rate compared to colonic cancer, so that the incidence over 80 years of age is less than that of the colon, while at 40 years of age breast cancer occurs 14 times more frequently. The factors responsible for the origin and growth of breast cancer clearly differ from those giving rise to gastrointestinal malignancy.

Survival data and determination of cure in cancer

When results of cancer treatment are presented, a graph of survival is often shown, or the proportion of patients alive at, say, 5 or 10 years is stated. It is often difficult to decide whether the results mean that some patients are cured. An understanding of how survival figures are derived is therefore essential for judging the effectiveness of treatment.

A *survival curve* is a plot of the proportion of patients surviving as a function of time. An example is shown in Fig. 2.3, where curve A gives the survival up to 20 years for all cases of cancer of the ovary. A disease-free survival curve would be displayed in a similar manner but the *x*-axis would then represent the length of time before the disease reappears. Since some patients may be effectively treated on relapse, the information is not the same as with a survival curve. This is especially true in a condition such as Hodgkin's disease where many patients can be cured on relapse.

Can we judge whether patients are cured by looking at survival curves? The general answer is that cure can be assumed if the group of patients returns to a normal pattern of survival similar to those who have not had the same cancer. In the case of ovarian cancer the comparison would be made with a large population of women with the same age distribution. The survival curve expected in such a population is the *age-adjusted expected survival curve*. In Fig. 2.3 the data for ovarian cancer are shown for a 20-year follow-up period. Curve A is the observed survival of the

patients and curve E is the age-adjusted expected survival curve; it can be seen that A is approximately parallel to E at 15–20 years. The age-adjusted relative survival curve (R) is constructed by dividing the observed survival curve (A) by the expected curve (E). If there is no increased risk of dying due to the cancer, this curve will run parallel to the abscissa. A difficulty might arise if the ability to cure the cancer were dependent on age, for example if young women were more easily cured than elderly women. The age distribution of survivors would then change with time and the age distribution of the control population would therefore have to be adjusted accordingly.

Survival does depend on age for many tumours: Fig. 2.4 shows *age-related survival rates* at 1 and 3 years for a variety of common tumours. For most cancers survival is worse in the elderly population at both 1 and 3 years.

In Fig. 2.3 the survival curves are given for all cases of cancer of the ovary but they could be plotted for individual ages at presentation, or for the *different stages* of the disease. In this way one may investigate whether cure is being achieved only for certain age groups or stages of disease. In practice, however, data on very large groups of patients (thousands) are needed to demonstrate cure with confidence.

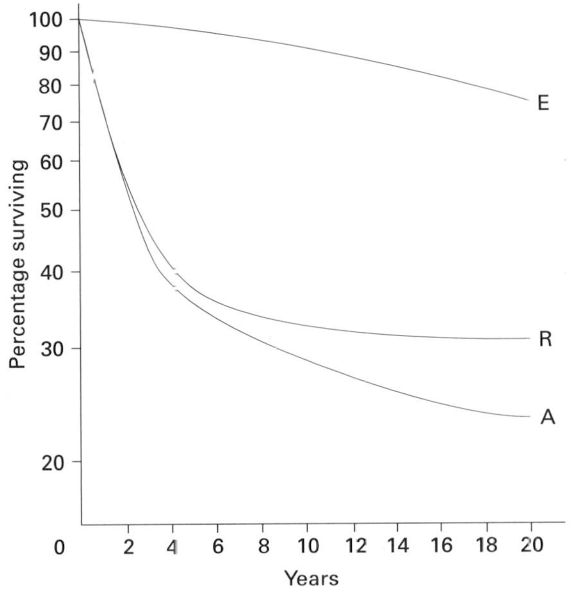

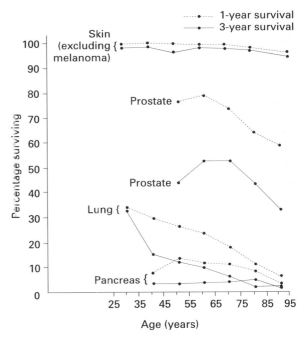

Fig. 2.3 Survival in ovarian cancer. Curve A shows observed survival, curve E shows age-adjusted expected survival and curve R shows relative survival.

Fig. 2.4 Age-related relative survival rates for several cancers. The data for the skin, lung and pancreas are for men, but are similar in both sexes.

A linear-scale plot of survival figures may suggest that a small proportion of patients are going to be long survivors. In Fig. 2.5, for example, the survival figures for a large trial in small-cell bronchogenic cancer are shown on the linear scale. Curve A seems to flatten out at 2 years, which might be interpreted as showing that a proportion of patients are cured. However, on a logarithmic scale, curve B is shown to be a straight line, that is, exponential, indicating that the rate of death has remained constant with time, the slope of the line giving the rate. This shows that up to the 3-year point there is no evidence of cure in the group in question.

Survival in clinical trials is often depicted as an *actuarial survival curve*. This may be thought of as a prediction of how the final survival curve will look if all the cases have similar survival characteristics to those which have been followed longest. In curve A in Fig. 2.6 the survival curve up to 10 years is based on complete 10-year follow-up on all patients. Curve B is an actuarial survival curve. In Fig. 2.7, curve B is a hypothetical survival curve, for similar cases to curve A, of 60 patients where only 50 have been followed for 2 years or more and 10 for 4 years or more. The curve is similar in shape to curve A for the first 2 years (when there are most observations) but appears to show improved survival thereafter. Such a conclusion would be unwise, however, because of the small number of observa-

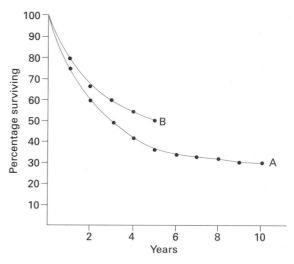

Fig. 2.6 Survival in ovarian cancer (all stages). Curve A represents survival of a group of patients where all patients had been diagnosed at least 10 years previously. Curve B is an actuarial survival curve: none of these patients had been diagnosed more than 5 years previously and some had been diagnosed only 2 years previously (see text).

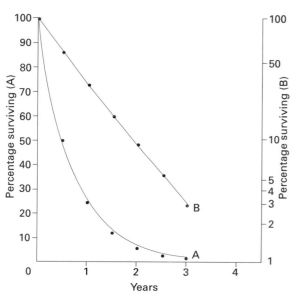

Fig. 2.5 Survival in advanced small-cell carcinoma of the bronchus. There appears to be a flattening of the survival curve (curve A) but the rate of death is in fact exponential (curve B).

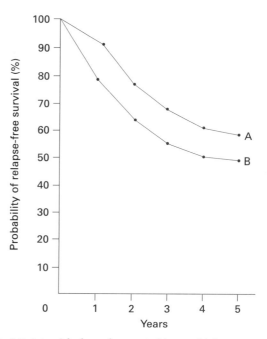

Fig. 2.7 Actuarial relapse-free survival in operable breast cancer. Curve A represents patients who were treated with adjuvant chemotherapy. Curve B represents patients who were given no adjuvant chemotherapy.

tions between 2 and 4 years on which the curve is based. It would not need many deaths to occur to alter the shape of curve B to that of curve A. These curves are less reliable in the 'tails' when the follow-up period for many patients is short and the number of late survivors is correspondingly small.

Assessment of results: trials of treatment

Many of the basic methods and techniques of treatment in cancer have been developed by experienced physicians and surgeons using their common sense. When the treatment has resulted in a clear improvement, as was the case, for example, when mastectomy was first introduced to treat patients with breast cancer, this approach has worked satisfactorily. When differences in treatment results have been less obvious, for example, in the case of simple as opposed to radical mastectomy, the results are harder to evaluate.

The problem of assessment is made more complex by changing criteria for diagnosis and treatment during the period in question. For example, refined methods of detection of metastases at presentation, such as, computed tomography (CT) scanning, may result in patients being rejected for a treatment which in earlier days they would have received. This means survival may alter as a result of a change in selection in the characteristics of the patients being included in the series being analysed. This hidden change might then be falsely attributed to a recently introduced treatment.

Randomized trials

It is now generally accepted that the only way to avoid bias in assessing new treatments is to carry out a randomized prospective comparison of the new treatment with the best standard regimen, or in some cases with no treatment. In this way hidden factors in case selection such as histological subtypes, presence of occult metastases and site of tumour, will be randomly distributed in the two groups. Similarly, factors which are not known to be associated with prognosis at the start of the trial but which are later shown to be so, do not bias the results since these factors should be equally represented in each of the randomly allocated groups, especially if the number of patients is large.

When an analysis of the effect of different treatments is made, the data may be examined for effect on survival or disease-free survival. The results are typically presented as in Fig. 2.7 which illustrates the disease-free survival curves

from a controlled trial of two treatments in breast cancer. Patient group A had received adjuvant chemotherapy and group B had not. There are several points to notice. First, the curves are actuarial curves, that is, not all the patients have been followed for 5 years. If the numbers of long-term survivors are small the tails of the curves may be misleading. Second, a difference in favour of chemotherapy is apparent. The probability of this happening purely by chance can be assessed by statistical methods. The log-rank test is a convenient and commonly used method of comparing survival and disease-free survival curves. The test is especially appropriate for survival curves which separate to reveal a consistent survival difference (that is, where the hazard ratio remains at the same proportion throughout the follow-up period). Other tests are more sensitive to early differences which are less apparent later. Third, if the difference is genuine, it represents a delay in onset of recurrence. This may not be reflected in improved survival. The survival curves for the groups are shown in Fig. 2.8; it can be seen that the difference is much less striking. This apparent discrepancy may be because although there is a delay in onset of metastases in the chemotherapy-treated group leading to an improved

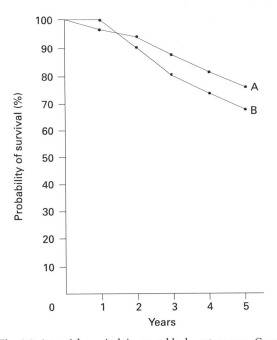

Fig. 2.8 Actuarial survival in operable breast cancer. Curve A represents patients who were treated with adjuvant chemotherapy. Curve B represents patients who were given no adjuvant chemotherapy (see text).

disease-free survival, once metastases have appeared the patients in the control group, who have not received chemotherapy, might benefit from its use so that the overall survival curves are less divergent. Early effects of this type on disease-free survival are often seen in cancer treatment. Delay of recurrence is certainly desirable but, for most treatments, improved survival is the real objective.

A commonly used method of presentation of results is to quote *median* survival, that is, the time from randomization at which 50% of the patients will be alive. These figures are unreliable unless the death rate in the 25–75% range is high and the numbers of patients in the study is large (Fig. 2.9). *Mean* survival times are often misleading because they can be greatly affected by one or two long-term survivors. Analysis of the proportion surviving at a single point in time makes use of only part of the data available. A survival curve analysis is preferred because it makes use of the whole time-span of the study.

It should also be remembered that tests of significance merely provide estimates of the probability that an observed difference (or a more extreme one) could have arisen by chance. There are many considerations besides the probability level which should affect one's judgement about whether the difference is interesting or important, and whether or not it is solely the result of the treatment.

In designing a prospective randomized trial of treatment many factors must be taken into account, some of which may affect the value of the study.

1 *Can a single question be asked?* Wherever possible the hypothesis being tested should be as simple as possible.

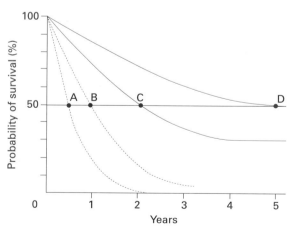

Fig. 2.9 Median survival in cancer trials. Trial 1 (dotted lines) median survival: A, 6 months; B, 1 year. Trial 2 (continuous lines) median survival: C, 2 years; D, 5 years. The differences are reliable in trial 1 but less so in trial 2.

For example, can the study ask the question 'Is treatment A better than no treatment at all?' A simple study design is always preferable but sometimes not possible. Studies in which there is a 'cross-over' from one treatment to another on relapse are sometimes hard to interpret. Studies which include several randomized groups will usually have to be very large if they are to detect realistic differences between the groups.

2 *Which patients will be included?* A precise statement must be made of the type of patient on which the treatments are to be tested.

3 *Are there known prognostic factors?* Patients with 'limited'-stage small-cell lung cancer (SCLC) have a better prognosis than those with 'extensive' disease. In trials of treatment in SCLC it is advisable to randomize limited and extensive category patients separately to ensure balanced numbers of each group in each arm of the study. This is termed stratification. Major prognostic criteria should be stratified, but too many stratifications can cause confusion and are unnecessary in a large trial.

4 *What is the end-point?* Some trials will be concerned with differences in survival, others with disease-free interval, others with local recurrence. In some studies differences in median survival may be shown without any change in the final long-term survival. An example is a trial of the treatment of advanced or metastatic cancer with cytotoxic drugs. Although all patients may die of the disease in both treated and untreated groups, death might be delayed by treatment. Such differences may be clinically worthwhile, especially if associated with symptomatic relief and minimal toxicity.

5 *Is the difference between the treatments in question likely to be large?* This is seldom the case in cancer where, if the effect of the therapy is dramatic, the trial would probably not be considered necessary or justified. To detect absolute differences in survival of 10% with a significance level of 0.05, between 160 and 500 patients will be needed per patient group, the numbers varying with the proportion surviving. It requires fewer patients to show a 10% survival difference between 10 and 20% (a doubling of survival) than between 40 and 50% (an increase of a quarter). Because of the very large numbers of patients necessary to detect even smaller differences with confidence, many cancer trials are collaborative efforts between different centres. Indeed, for rare diseases such as leukaemia or osteosarcoma, treatment trials are almost impossible without such collaboration.

6 *The difficulties of collaboration are considerable.* Investigators participating in the study must agree on what is the most important question to ask: how the treatment should be administered (including details of surgery, radiotherapy and chemotherapy); what the documentation should be and how it should be organized; who will pay for the study; who will analyse the data; and so on. In a disease like breast cancer where the rate of death is low, the answers may not be available for 10 years or more. Physicians are usually, to put it kindly, 'individualistic' in their approach to treatment and large-scale trials sometimes acquire a design which proves an unsatisfactory compromise. Exceptionally intensive treatments cannot be carried out in every hospital and may not be of the same quality as when undertaken by a few specialized units. Such treatments may be 'watered down' in order to include more centres, possibly weakening the intention of the study.

7 *Even if the differences in survival are small they may be clinically worthwhile.* Dramatic advances in treatment are rare. Large randomized studies are usually carried out where it is not clear if one treatment is better than another and differences are therefore likely to be small. A small difference may, however, lead to a change in clinical practice. In breast cancer in postmenopausal women following local therapy, treatment with a drug such as tamoxifen improves survival by 8%; this is a major contribution to management because in 20 000 women 1600 lives can be saved with negligible toxicity. Conversely, some might regard a 7% improvement achieved with cytotoxic chemotherapy as less compelling, due to the greater toxicity of the treatment (although most patients do not take this view). In Europe an 8% improvement in mortality would save 64 000 lives each year. This is a greater saving than that achieved by the successful treatment of diseases such as lymphoma or leukaemia.

There is a growing awareness that our expectations of likely improvements in survival with cancer treatments need to be revised downwards. We cannot expect 20% absolute improvements in survival. We might expect 10–20% improvements in relative survival (from 40% to 44–48%) but such improvements require trials vastly greater than those which we have been accustomed to perform [11]. The reason is shown in Fig. 2.10a. The failure to achieve these numbers leads to false negative results. Figure 2.10b shows the results of treatment trials of adjuvant chemotherapy and/or tamoxifen in breast cancer. The trials were usually small so the 95% confidence intervals overlapped with 'no effect' (see Fig. 13.7, p. 211). The combined dataset shows a clear difference with a reduction of relative risk of 22% (7% increase in 5-year survival) and the confidence intervals are separated from the point where no effect is observed. Trials designed to recruit

thousands of patients need to be of simple design and execution, with flexible entry criteria, and must concern a widely practicable treatment. The organization and execution of these studies is a major task for cancer specialists.

Analysis of the results of randomized trials

Just as it is essential not to be too impressed by dramatic results from uncontrolled studies, it is important not to be intimidated by the authority which randomized clinical trials appear to possess. A critical approach is needed. Some points to watch out for are the following.

1 Is it likely that a false positive result (type I error) or false negative (type II error) has occurred? False positive errors are uncommon. False negative errors are more common, but negative trials are not published as frequently as positive ones because journal editors tend to prefer 'positive' results. Does the trial accord with other studies addressing the same point?

2 *Were the treatments genuinely randomized?* Authors sometimes claim their study was randomized, but a closer inspection of the method reveals it was not. These studies are nearly always misleading.

3 *Did one particular group of patients benefit?* This is an important matter because it allows treatment to be offered selectively and suggests future directions for study. However, it is almost impossible to draw firm conclusions about subgroups from a single study unless it contains thousands of patients.

4 *Have all the patients been included in the analysis, and if not, why not?* Sometimes patients who cannot be evaluated are discarded from the report. One should be aware of this, particularly if it occurs for large numbers of patients. One reason sometimes given is that the patient only completed one part of the treatment before deteriorating. This practice will greatly improve the apparent results because early failures are not included.

5 *Has the trial run for sufficient time to allow enough events (deaths, relapses) to have occurred?* What are the confidence intervals for the treatment difference? A statement of the 95% confidence limits for the treatment difference allows the reader to judge the result being presented and is more informative than a P-value from a significance test. A P-value indicates the level of statistical significance. What the clinician also needs to know is the degree of likely difference. If the confidence interval for the difference in survival between two treatments is from –4% to +15% with a point estimate of 7%, this will be regarded differently from an outcome where the confidence interval

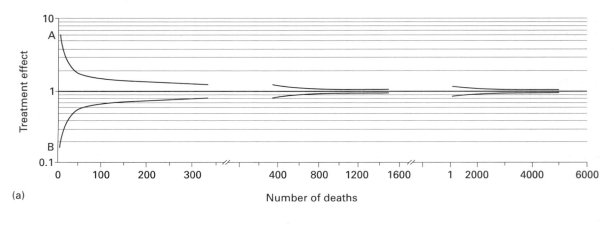

(a)

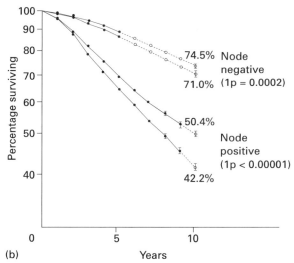

(b)

Fig. 2.10 (a) In a comparison between treatments A and B the darker line at 1 is the line of equivalence between the treatments. The curves represent the 95% confidence intervals for this line. For a result to be significantly different it must lie outside this line. Each horizontal line represents a relative difference of 20% between treatments. A difference of 30% in favour of B will only be seen if there are more than 300 deaths in the study; a difference of 5–10% will require several thousands of deaths to be observed. (b) Results of treatment trials of adjuvant tamoxifen in operable breast cancer. An overview of analysis of many thousands of randomized patients allows a significant survival benefit to be demonstrated in the range of 4–8% with different treatments.

ranges from +4% to +20% with a point estimate of 11%. Although both results may be 'significant', the latter is more compelling because the difference is larger and the certainty of benefit greater.

A problem which has recently become more apparent comes from the use of 'stopping guidelines'. These are statistical methods for the detection of survival differences early in a trial. They were originally introduced to prevent early closure of studies because an effect appeared to be present. Unfortunately, these guidelines are increasingly used rigidly to stop trials leaving the clinician aware that an effect is present but insecure about its size since there are not enough events to make a precise estimate. This practice misses a central point of trials, which is to provide convincing evidence of a clinically worthwhile effect if one is present.

Informed consent

Before starting any treatment most clinicians will want to discuss the benefits and problems of treatment and the possible different approaches which might be used. In a clinical trial doctors also have to discuss the reason for the study, the meaning of randomization and the right of the patient not to be involved. This creates problems for both doctors and patient. Their relationship may be upset by these disclosures, especially the admission that the results of the treatments are not known with certainty. There may have to be discussion of failure rates in the disease. The patient may become confused, and the time necessary for explanation discourages entry into trials. Several studies have shown that patients find the concept of random allocation of treatment, for a disease as serious as cancer, to be a major factor in refusing to take part in trials.

Non-randomized studies of treatment

The difficulties of controlled trials of treatment have led many investigators to perform uncontrolled studies and to report survival with a given treatment in the hope that a clear advantage over the best current methods of treatment will be shown. There is an important role for well-conducted pilot studies, but the results are often misleading or wrong and must be interpreted cautiously.

A compromise has been sought between the cumbersome controlled trial and the unreliable uncontrolled study. This has involved the use of *historical control* which compares present treatment to patients treated in the past. An attempt is normally, but not always, made to match the controls for age, sex, site and stage of tumour and other known prognostic factors such as histological grade and menopausal status. The problems are that staging methods are changing continually, that selection of control cases may not be impartial and that not all prognostic factors will be known.

These studies may sometimes point the way in management and indicate which questions should be asked in large-scale prospective studies. Another variant is the use of 'databases' containing results of treatment of very large numbers of patients. Such analyses have the same problems of selection bias and thus the same unreliability in deciding on the value of a treatment.

Screening for cancer

The aim of screening a population for cancer is to make the diagnosis early and thereby increase the cure rate. When a previously unscreened population undergoes screening a relatively large number of *prevalence* cases are detected. When this same screened population undergoes subsequent screening procedures, the number of new incidence cases is much smaller and the cost per case detected therefore greater. The problem is simply summarized in Fig. 2.11. The objective of screening is simple yet there are many problems and assumptions involved.

1 *What is the sensitivity of the test used?* Highly sensitive tests are essential if the disease is curable early and if the consequences of a false positive test are not physically or psychologically serious for the patients. The Papanicolaou smear is a sensitive test for cervical cancer and the diagnosis can be easily confirmed on biopsy. Screening by ultrasound and serum CA-125 is much less sensitive but may prove to be of value for ovarian cancer. Plasma prostate-specific antigen (PSA) is a sensitive test for prostatic carcinoma but the consequences for management of a positive result are not well defined [12].

2 *Is the disease curable if diagnosed early?* Carcinoma *in situ* or locally invasive carcinoma of the cervix are curable diseases. Earlier diagnosis of colorectal cancer using screening by flexible sigmoidoscopy or faecal occult blood testing may increase cure rate [13]. Tumours such as colorectal cancer present late in their natural history and the limit of detection by screening may be only one or two doublings earlier than when the tumour would be clinically apparent. The question is whether the potential for metastasis is significantly less at the time when such a tumour is detectable by screening methods compared with the stage at which it is clinically apparent.

3 *Is the disease common?* Cancer of the breast, prostate, cervix and lung are so common at certain ages and in certain groups that screening is a practical proposition. Screening a general population for a disease such as gastric carcinoma is less practicable in the UK, but it is in Japan where the disease is much more common. Clearly the incidence of the tumour has to be high enough to justify the screening programme.

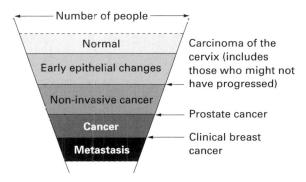

Fig. 2.11 The later in the natural history, the fewer 'false positives', but there is less chance to alter the outcome.

4 *How frequently should the examination be undertaken, and in which population?* In some countries cervical smears are recommended every 3 years in women aged 20–65 years. In the UK, the recommendation is for all sexually active women to be screened every 5 years [14]. It is not clear what recommendations should be made for other investigations such as pelvic examination (for ovarian and uterine cancer) and flexible sigmoidoscopy. The group at greatest risk from ovarian cancer includes nulliparous women over the age of 40 years; and for colorectal cancer, men and women over 50 years. Routine chest X-rays, even in smokers, have failed to show any benefit from early detection of lung cancer. A limited chest CT scan is much more sensitive but its clinical value is unproven. Patients with a greatly increased genetic predisposition to certain cancers—for example, polyposis coli (Chapter 16, p. 25)—should have regular checks by the appropriate specialist (Table 2.4).

5 *What are the disadvantages of screening?* Routine screening examinations can produce anxiety in the mind of the public at large and in certain individuals in particular. If applied to the whole population they would require a great expenditure of time and money. The benefits may be small and achieved at great expense. If the yearly incidence of breast cancer in women aged 50–70 years is taken to be 2 per 1000, by screening 10 000 women every 2 years, 40 new cases may be expected. If this is done by mammography and trained nurses in a clinic the cost might be in the region of £40 per visit. If the cure rate were improved from 40 to 60% by this procedure then eight lives would have been saved at a cost of £200 000. Screening of this type is therefore more expensive than much 'high-technology' medicine.

The longest established screening procedure in the Western world is the cervical smear for carcinoma of the cervix. Breast cancer screening has now been introduced in the UK and other European countries. There remain considerable doubts as to its cost-effectiveness, and difficulties over the treatment to be recommended when early breast cancer is diagnosed (for example, ductal carcinoma *in situ*). Screening procedures which have been proposed, are shown in Table 2.4.

The most important outcome measure in a screening programme is mortality, which may require prolonged follow-up (for example, in the case of breast cancer). The efficacy of the screening programme should also be reflected in a shift towards diagnosis at an earlier stage of the tumour.

Secondary prevention of cancer

Some cancers arise in a 'field' of malignant change in which the tissue adjacent to a cancer has been subject to the same carcinogenic process which gave rise to the initial tumour. The clearest example of this is the squamous carcinoma of the upper aerodigestive tract—mouth, pharynx, oesophagus and bronchi—which have been exposed to cigarette smoke. In the case of head and neck cancer, after successful therapy, 30–50% of patients develop local or regional recurrence and 10–40% a second primary tumour.

In recent years it has been shown that vitamin A analogues are able to modulate the differentiation of epithelial cells, can cause the regression of the lesions of leucoplakia, and diminish the likelihood of developing squamous cancer as long as treatment continues. Isotretinoin (13-*cis*-retinoic acid), given as an adjuvant following treatment of head and neck cancer, greatly diminishes the risk of second cancers developing but does not diminish the likelihood of recurrence. This interesting finding opened the way to other secondary prevention. However, recent trials have shown a deleterious effect in lung cancer. The breast cancer overview [15] has shown a decreased risk of cancer in the contralateral breast in women taking tamoxifen as adjuvant therapy following surgery for breast cancer. This had led to randomized trials of tamoxifen as a primary preventive measure in women at high risk of developing breast cancer.

Table 2.4 Currently used screening methods. Several of these are still under investigation to determine their clinical value.

Cervical cancer (Chapter 17)	Cervical smear
Breast cancer (Chapter 13)	Mammography
Colorectal cancer (Chapter 16)	Occult blood testing Fecal
	Rectal examination
	Flexible sigmoidoscopy
Ovarian and uterine cancer (Chapter 17)	Pelvic examination
	Pelvic ultrasound
	CA-125
Skin cancers (Chapter 22)	Self-examination
Gastric cancer—Japan (Chapter 14)	Radiological and endoscopic examination
Prostate cancer (Chapter 18)	Prostate-specific antigen

References

1 Devesa SS, Silverman DT. Cancer incidence and mortality

trends in the United States: 1935–74. *J Natl Cancer Inst* 1978; 60: 545–71.

2 Haenszel W, Kurihera M. Studies of Japanese migrants: 1: Mortality from cancer and other diseases among Japanese in the United States. *J Natl Cancer Inst* 1968; 40: 43–68.

3 Doll R, Fraumeni J, Muir C. Trends in cancer incidence and mortality. In: *Cancer Surveys*, Vol. 19/20. Cold Spring Harbor Laboratory Press, 1994.

4 Doll R, Peto R. The causes of cancer. *J Natl Cancer Inst* 1981; 66: 1191–208.

5 Darby S, Hill D, Doll R. Radon: a likely carcinogen at all exposures. *Ann Oncol* 2001; 12: 1341–51.

6 Peto J, Hodgson JT, Matthews FE, Jones JR. Continuing increase in mesothelioma mortality in Britain. *Lancet* 1995; 345: 535–9.

7 Boyd NE, Martin LJ, Noffel M *et al.* A meta analysis of studies of dietary fat and breast cancer risk. *Br J Cancer* 1993; 68: 627–36.

8 Hunter DJ, Manson JE, Colditz GA *et al.* A prospective study of the intake of vitamins C, E and A, and the risk of breast cancer. *N Engl J Med* 1993; 329: 234–40.

9 Klein G. Epstein–Barr virus strategy in normal and neoplastic B cells. *Cell* 1994; 77: 791–3.

10 Martin JN, Ganem DE, Osmond DH *et al.* Sexual transmission and the natural history of human herpesvirus 8 infection. *N Engl J Med* 1998; 338: 948–54.

11 Yusuf S, Collins R, Peto R. Why do we need some large, simple randomized trials? *Stat Med* 1984; 3: 409–22.

12 Ganz PA, Litwin MS. Prostate cancer. The price of early detection. *J Clin Oncol* 2001; 19: 1587–8.

13 Hardcastle JO *et al.* Randomised controlled trial of faecal occult blood screening for colorectal cancer. Results of the first 107 349 subjects. *Lancet* 1989; i: 1160–4.

14 Chamberlain J, Moss SM, Kirkpatrick AE *et al.* National Health Service breast cancer screening results for 1991–2. *Br Medl J* 1993; 307: 353–6.

15 Early Breast Cancer Trialist's Collaborative Group. Tamoxifen for early breast cancer. An overview of the randomized trials. *Lancet* 1998; 351: 1451–67.

3 Biology of cancer

The sequence of cellular events that give rise to a metastasising cancer are becoming better understood as a consequence of the advances in cell and molecular biology. Figure 3.1 shows the steps in the development of a cancer. This sequence will be the framework for the brief description of this process.

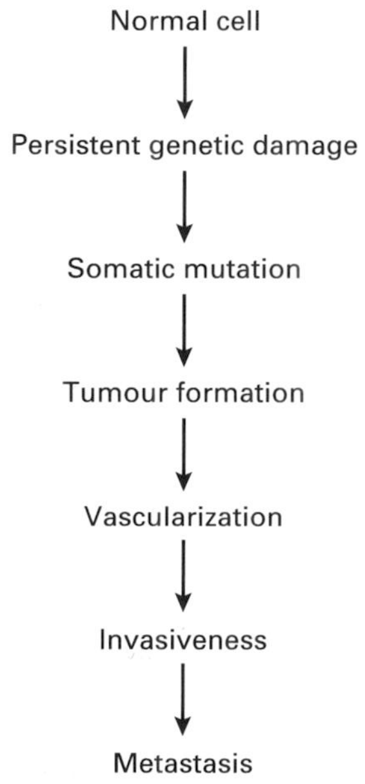

Normal cell
↓
Persistent genetic damage
↓
Somatic mutation
↓
Tumour formation
↓
Vascularization
↓
Invasiveness
↓
Metastasis

Fig. 3.1 Steps in the development of a metastasing cancer.

Carcinogenesis: persistent genetic damage

Chemical carcinogens

It has long been suspected that cancers might have a chemical cause. In 1775 Sir Percival Pott noticed an unusually large number of cases of cancer of the scrotum in chimney-sweeps. In 1895 Rehn pointed out the high frequency of bladder cancer in dye factory workers.

Many carcinogens have been identified in the environment and in food (Table 3.1), but the importance of most of these to human cancer remains uncertain. Some of the mechanisms of chemical carcinogenesis have now been elucidated.

Polycyclic hydrocarbons [1]

These chemicals are among the products of combustion of carbon-containing materials. They are present in coal tar, cigarette smoke, car exhaust fumes and some cooked foods. Following the demonstration that benzanthracene was present in coal tar and was carcinogenic, 3,4-benzpyrene was isolated from coal tar and was also shown to be capable of inducing skin cancers in animals. Not all polycyclic hydrocarbons are carcinogens. It appears that the carcinogenic property resides in one region of the molecule, the K region, to which oxygen is added in a reaction catalysed by cellular enzymes.

This portion of the molecule reacts with cellular DNA, especially with guanine bases. It is this reaction with DNA that is thought to be responsible for its carcinogenic effect.

Nitrosamines

Dimethylnitrosamine was shown to cause liver cancer in animals when added to their food. Nitrites, which are present in many foods, are converted to nitrous acid in the stomach and may then react with amines in food to produce nitrosamines. Thus a mechanism exists for the formation of a potential carcinogen from food. However, there is no definite evidence that the formation of nitrosamines is important in carcinogenesis in humans.

Aromatic amines and azo dyes

Following Rehn's original observation of the increased frequency of bladder cancer in aniline dye workers, the aniline derivatives α-naphthylamine and benzidine were shown to be carcinogens. Later, azo dye derivatives were also found to be carcinogenic including dimethylamino azobenzene (butter yellow) which was used to add colour to margarine. When ingested, these substances produce cancers at sites remote from the gut. They are first metabolized to an active form which is the carcinogen. For example, α-naphthylamine is hydroxylated to a carcinogen which is then glucuronated to an inactive water-soluble form in the liver and excreted in the urine. Glucuronidases in the bladder mucosa liberate the active carcinogen. The cancers develop only in those species which possess this bladder enzyme. The liberated aminophenol reacts directly with guanine bases on DNA and, as with polycyclic hydrocarbons, this is presumed to be the basis of their carcinogenic action. In humans there is a 20-year latent period between exposure and the development of bladder cancer. Cigarette smoke also contains 3-naphthylamine, and bladder cancer is associated with smoking.

Aflatoxin

This toxin is produced by *Aspergillus flavus* which may contaminate staple foods. It may be a carcinogen in hepatic cancer and there is an association between dietary aflatoxin and the high frequency of hepatic cancers, although direct proof is lacking. The hepatitis B virus is involved in the development of a hepatoma, aflatoxin per-

Table 3.1 Some chemical carcinogens.

Polycyclic hydrocarbons	3,4-benzpyrene
Nitrosamines	Dimethylnitrosamine
Aromatic amines and azo dyes	α-naphthylamine
	Dimethylamino azobenzene
	Benzidine
Plant products	Aflatoxin
	Senecis (producing pyrrolozidium)
Alkylating agents	Nitrogen
	Melphalan
	Nitrosourea
	Etoposide
Inorganic chemicals	Arsenic
	Nickel
	Asbestos
	Cadmium

haps acting as a promoter (see below). The toxin is a complex molecule which is metabolized by the same pathway as polycyclic hydrocarbons, and the products react with DNA.

Alkylating agents

Drugs used in the treatment of cancer are also carcinogens. Alkylating agents bind directly to DNA (see Chapter 6, p. 76) and their use has been associated with the development of second malignancies, for example acute leukaemia in patients successfully treated for Hodgkin's disease or ovarian cancer.

Ionizing and ultraviolet irradiation

Irradiation produces breaks in DNA strands and chromosomal abnormalities such as fragmentations, deletions and translocations. These abnormalities lead to cell death in dividing cells. The mechanisms of carcinogenesis are, however, poorly understood. There is no doubt that cancers can be caused by ionizing radiation. Skin cancers and bone cancers are caused by therapeutic radiation. There is a dose-related increase in acute and chronic myeloid leukaemia and in breast and thyroid cancer in the survivors of the atom bomb explosions at Hiroshima and Nagasaki.

It is difficult to extrapolate from the high dose received after the atom bomb explosions, to an assessment of the risks from the much smaller levels of background radiation. The average exposure as a result of toxic waste is

0.001 mSv (millisievert) with a maximum of 0.3 mSv. The average dose from clinical X-rays is 0.3 mSv (the same as from cosmic rays). The average annual total dose in the UK from all sources is about 2.5 mSv. Estimates now place the death rate at about three to five cases per 100 000 per millisievert of prolonged exposure. This would account for perhaps 2000 cancer deaths per year out of 160 000 annually in the UK. Radon gas is one of the most important sources of background radiation. Radiation exposure is a less important cause of cancer than cigarette smoking, and industrial exposure is the least important source of background radiation.

Ultraviolet (UV) light increases the likelihood of development of skin cancer (see Chapter 22). DNA absorbs photons, and alterations in thymine bases occur with the formation of dimers. In normal individuals these pyrimidine dimers are rapidly repaired by nucleotide excision repair. Faulty repair leads to base mismatch mutations. UV damage to the *p53* gene (see p. 28) may be inefficiently repaired and the resulting mutation may lead to an impaired function of the *p53* protein. This, in turn, leads to disordered cell growth. In xeroderma pigmentosum the DNA repair process is faulty, leading to an excess of skin cancers (though not cancers at other sites).

Initiators and promoters in carcinogenesis

Some agents appear to act as 'initiators' (Fig. 3.2): they produce a permanent change in the cells with which they come in contact but do not themselves cause cancer. This contact may result in a gene mutation. Other agents act as 'promoters' producing transient changes and only causing cancer when they are repeatedly in contact with cells which have been 'initiated' by another compound. From a clinical point of view, cancers are more likely to arise as a result of long-continued exposure to an agent, and removal of the agent may result in stabilization or even diminution of the increased risk. Cessation of cigarette smoking is an example of how the risk of developing cancer can be reduced by removal of the stimulus.

Repair of damage to DNA

The action of chemical carcinogens leads to damage to DNA. The production of permanent DNA damage, and the development of the subsequent disorganization of chromosomal DNA that is the characteristic of an estab-

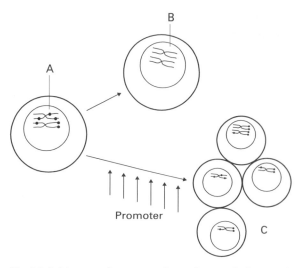

Fig. 3.2 Initiators and promoters in carcinogenesis. In stage A chromosomal damage is caused by an initiator. This might be repaired (as in B) or, under the influence of a promoter, give rise to neoplastic growth (stage C).

lished cancer, depends on the nature of the chemical adduct, the duration of exposure and, importantly, on the efficiency of cellular repair processes. DNA repair is thus central to the process of carcinogenesis. Many of the hereditary cancer syndromes have now been shown to be due to mutation in essential DNA repair genes, resulting in impaired repair over a lifetime. The process of repair is through several mechanisms. These repair processes are essential mechanisms for all living cells. Actively transcribed genes are repaired more efficiently than inactive genes. In *base excision repair* the abnormal DNA base is excised enzymatically, first by endonucleases which cleave the DNA strand, then by exonucleases which remove the abnormal segment, followed by the action of a polymerase which resynthesizes the missing segment which is then joined to the strand by a ligase. More complex lesions, such as those made by alkylating agents and UV light, are repaired by *nucleotide excision repair* [2] in which there is excision of a longer strand of DNA, the strand then being resynthesized by polymerase.

Radiation causes both single and double strand breaks in DNA. Specific processes repair these two types of lesion. While the double strand break is the lethal lesion responsible for the cell-killing effect, the mechanism of radiation-induced carcinogenesis is less well understood.

Inherited defects involving DNA damage or repair processes that predispose to cancer [3]

Genes that regulate the conversion of potentially toxic agents to their active form, and their detoxicification. These are processes that are dependent on enzymes in organs such as the gut, kidney and liver. They are described in more detail in Chapter 6. Common polymorphisms of these genes may account for differences in susceptibility to DNA damage and thus to carcinogenesis.

Genes that repair mismatches of DNA base pairs. Mutation in one of this family of genes causes hereditary non-polyposis colorectal cancer which is an autosomal dominant trait that accounts for 5% of all such cancers.

Genes that maintain the genetic stability of the cell. Genes such as *p53* (see below) regulate cell division so the cell does not divide if there is persistent DNA damage. Several hereditary cancer syndromes are due to defects in these genes (Li–Fraumeni syndrome due to *p53* mutation, retinoblastoma due to *Rb* gene mutation).

Viral causes of cancer

Viruses causing tumours in animals were discovered at the turn of the century. In 1910, Peyton Rous showed that a cell-free filtrate made from avian sarcomas could induce new sarcomas in chickens, and at the same time the disease avian myeloblastosis was shown to be viral in origin. Much later it was realized that viruses might require a long latent period before the tumour appeared. However, it was not until the 1960s that it was appreciated that incorporation of viral DNA into the host genome was usually a prerequisite of malignant transformation, and that the infectious virus might not be isolated from the cancer cell.

Two patterns of viral oncogenesis have been described. In both instances the viral genome is incorporated into the cellular DNA. In the first, the virus has genes, *oncogenes*, which quickly 'transform' the cell in culture and cause tumours *in vivo*. The action of the oncogene dominates the cell. In the second, the virus acts slowly and tumours take longer to appear. These viruses do not transform cells in culture.

RNA viruses

RNA viruses are implicated in the production of a wide variety of tumours in animals, notably lymphomas, leukaemias and sarcomas. In the virus there are two identical RNA molecules within a glycoprotein envelope together with the duplex enzyme reverse transcriptase. Through the action of this enzyme the viruses are able to make the cell synthesize a sequence of DNA, complementary to their RNA, which is incorporated into the host DNA. The action of the DNA leads to the manufacture of new viral proteins, envelope and reverse transcriptase (Fig. 3.3). They are therefore called *retroviruses*. They are of similar appearance on electron microscopy and are the smallest of the tumour viruses.

Some retroviruses (for example, avian leukosis, feline and murine leukaemia) have only three genes and have a long incubation period before producing the tumour in animals. Others rapidly transform cells and are usually isolated from tumours in culture. They produce tumours quickly after inoculation, an example being the Rous sarcoma virus (RSV). RSV has been shown to contain a

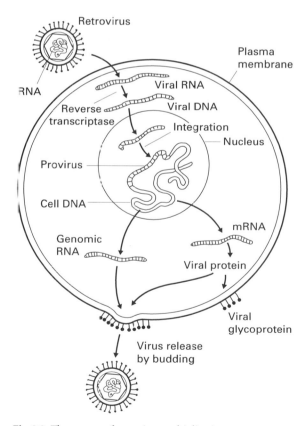

Fig. 3.3 The process of retrovirus multiplication.

gene (v-*src*) which appears to be the gene responsible for transformation of fibroblasts in culture. This gene codes for a protein kinase which phosphorylates tyrosine. Many cellular processes are activated by this means and it is not yet clear how this leads to malignant transformation.

It has become apparent that normal and malignant cells contain DNA sequences which are similar or identical to the oncogenic sequences of RNA tumour viruses. These are known as *cellular proto-oncogenes*, as distinct from viral oncogenes. It is postulated that it is these cellular oncogenes which, when activated by carcinogens, cause the events which lead to malignant transformation (Fig. 3.4). It has been suggested that retroviruses have incorporated these cellular genes into the viral genome during evolution.

The mechanisms of action of the products of gene activation are now better understood. As mentioned above, a phosphokinase is produced by *src* and other viral oncogenes; epidermal growth factor receptor by the v-*erb* B gene; a platelet-derived growth factor (PDGF) fragment by the v-*sis* gene; and a variety of nuclear-binding proteins by the avian leukaemia virus. Viral oncogene products may differ from their cellular counterparts. They lack introns and may have structural differences. For example, the v-*erb* product is the homologue of the cellular receptor for epidermal growth factor (EGF) but lacks part of the extracellular domain including the EGF binding site. Together with loss of a cytoplasmic site for autophosphorylation the receptor is permanently 'switched on'. Normal and malignant cells contain DNA sequences which are similar or identical to the oncogenic sequences of RNA tumour viruses. These cellular oncogenes, when overexpressed or activated by somatic mutation, cause the events which lead to malignant transformation (see Fig. 3.4).

A virus may activate cellular processes by inserting a promoter or enhancer sequence adjacent to a region of a cellular growth-regulating oncogene, disturbing its normal process of control of transcription. This process of insertional mutagenesis may be very complex. An example is the insertion of the viral long terminal repeat (LTR) sequence which may allow transcription of both viral and cellular genes since the LTR may be able to initiate transcription in either direction on the DNA strand. This occurs with the avian leukosis virus which is integrated next to c-*myc*, thereby activating it.

The first retrovirus to be definitely associated with malignancy was the human T-cell leukaemia virus, HTLV-1, isolated from chronic cutaneous T-cell lymphoma. The virus is widely distributed, transmitted sexually, by intravenous drug abuse and perinatally. It is prevalent

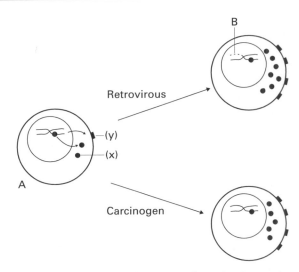

Fig. 3.4 Oncogenes and malignant transformation. In stage A, a normal cell has a low level of proto-oncogene activity producing a growth factor (x), or a differentiation protein or a receptor (y). Carcinogens increase the activity of the proto-oncogene and give rise to neoplastic transformation. Alternatively, infection with a retrovirus leads to insertion of viral promoter sequences or oncogenes (B) and excess oncogene activity, also resulting in neoplastic transformation.

in tropical countries, but in the USA seropositivity is one in 4000. In addition to the association with T-cell leukaemia, it is the cause of tropical spastic paraplegia. The risk of disease over 20 years of seropositivity is about 5%. One of the viral genes *tax*, stimulates the cellular genes to produce IL-2 and IL-2 receptor which stimulate T-cell division.

Retro-viruses may be indirectly carcinogenic as is shown by the human immunodeficiency virus HIV-1, which is the cause of AIDS.

HIV-1 infection is associated with cancers [4]. There are three types that are particularly frequent: intermediate or high-grade B-cell lymphoma, Kaposi's sarcoma (KS) and cervical carcinoma. About 40% of all patients infected will develop a cancer. The relationship between the viral infection and the different cancers is, however, complex and appears to be related to the chronic immune suppression, which allows other carcinogenic viruses to produce cancer. KS, which is associated with a novel herpes virus (KSHV or Human Herpes Virus 8). The lymphomas also have a complex pathogenesis since they are usually tumours of B cells. These are not infected by HIV-1. Other viruses such as Epstein–Barr virus (EBV) may be involved. Similarly, cervical cancer is probably due to a second virus—such as human papilloma virus

(HPV)—in women who are immunosuppressed by HIV-1. The tumour appears particularly aggressive clinically.

Hepatitis C is an RNA virus that is now clearly linked to the occurrence of hepatocellular carcinoma. The risk of the tumour is 100 times greater in infected persons. The mechanism of viral carcinogenesis is not understood. The risk of liver cancer is higher if there is co-infection with HBV. These two viruses infect almost one billion people world wide.

DNA viruses

DNA viruses have also been implicated in the production of cancer. The largest in size is the herpes group, which can cause malignancies in animals. EBV was first demonstrated in cultured cells from a patient with Burkitt's lymphoma and EBV will cause continued proliferation of human B cells *in vitro*. Viral genes maintain the virus in these cells and drive cellular proliferation through activation of cellular growth-regulating genes (oncogenes).

Clinically, in Burkitt's lymphoma antibody titres to viral capsid antigen and membrane antigen are higher in patients than in controls. Nevertheless, many African children are infected with EBV at some time although Burkitt's lymphoma develops in very few, so its role in oncogenesis is not clear. In addition, some non-African cases of Burkitt's lymphoma are not associated with the virus. EBV is also implicated in the pathogenesis of nasopharyngeal carcinoma the tumour cells expressing the viral EBNA-1 antigen.

In 1994 a new herpes virus was found in association with Kaposi's sarcoma occurring in AIDS. This Kaposi's Sarcoma Herpes Virus (KSHV) is now designated HHV8 and is found in the spindle cells of the tumour in all cases of Kaposi's sarcoma. HHV8 is also found in the cells of primary effusion lymphoma and in multicentric Castleman's disease. The virus encodes a cyclin that promotes cell cycle progression. This may be essential in producing cellular proliferation.

Human papilloma viruses are a very large family of viruses. They are the cause of cutaneous warts and some benign papillomas. Most viral types produce a limited proliferation. Other types have a much greater propensity to cause malignant transformation [5]. These high risk types are 16, 18, 31 and 33. Over 90% of cases of *in situ* carcinoma of the cervix contain HPV genome sequences. The virus plays a causative role in the invasive and multiple squamous cancers of the skin that frequently occur in patients on long term immunosuppressive therapy. The mechanism of oncogenesis is still not fully understood. There are eight early and two late viral genes. There is random integration of viral DNA into the cells of the basal epithelium. The early genes E6 and E7 drive the cellular proliferation.

Hepatitis B is associated with the development of hepatocellular carcinoma (see Chapter 15). The risk is 200 times greater than in non-infected persons. Although the mechanism of production of the cancer is not clear, it seems likely that the virus provokes continued cellular proliferation as viral infected cells are removed by immune attack. Possibly the proliferating cells are then susceptible to other carcinogens, for example, aflatoxin. HBV gene products such as HBx activate growth-signalling pathways and these may have a more direct role in tumour production.

This brief summary shows that an essential mechanism of carcinogenesis is damage to DNA and the efficiency of its repair. The initial damage if not repaired is followed at a variable interval by increasing chromosomal instability and somatic mutation. Although many of these mutations will be lethal, others will not, and the malignant phenotype emerges. Our understanding of how this process works has greatly improved in recent years with increased knowledge of the control of the cell cycle and the discovery of key proteins that can halt cell division if the genome is damaged.

An initial mutation in a growth-regulating gene may not be sufficient to produce tumour progression, but a succession of such events will be. The important mutations will be in activating mutations in genes that promote cell growth—*oncogenes*, disabling mutations in those genes that suppress growth—*tumour suppressor genes*, and mutations in those genes that produce proteins that are responsible for ensuring that cell division does not take place if DNA is damaged. Successive mutations in several of these genes leads to increasing cellular disorganization and loss of control of cell growth. The next section describes the action of oncogenes and the essential features of the control of the cell cycle.

Cellular oncogenes

The discovery of the sequence homologies between viral oncogenes and DNA found in normal and cancer cells has led to a greater understanding of growth regulatory mechanisms which may be abnormal in malignant cells. The term 'oncogene' may perhaps be a misnomer since, in malignancy, there may be abnormal activation of a normal gene or an abnormality in the gene leading to abnormal expression. In this sense these are not cancer genes but proliferation-inducing genes whose regulation may be disturbed in cancer.

Genes have been identified by homology with retroviral genes by DNA transfer and by gene rearrangements. The mechanisms of activation of the genes are varied.

In Burkitt's lymphoma there is reciprocal translocation of part of chromosome 8 with chromosomes 2, 14 or 22. The 8;14 translocation is commonest. The c-*myc* oncogene is adjacent to the part of chromosome 8 which is translocated, and the translocation is accompanied by reorganization of the c-*myc* gene. In chronic granulocytic leukaemia the c-*abl* oncogene with its translocation partner *bcr* forms a fusion protein resulting in permanent expression of growth-inducing tyrosine kinase. Activation of a single proto-oncogene in this way does not often lead to malignancy. Increased expression of cellular oncogenes has been found in many human cancer cell lines, for example, c-*myc* in small-cell lung cancer and Burkitt's lymphoma, and N-*myc* in neuroblastoma.

Figure 3.5 shows a simplified scheme of the events which occur following binding of a growth factor to a membrane-associated receptor [6]. The receptor activates a signal-transducing protein which may in turn bind other molecules such as guanine nucleotides (when the signal transducer is then called a G protein). These molecules in turn may stimulate the activity of a second messenger such as cyclic adenosine 3′-5′-phosphate. Alternatively, the internal component of the receptor may have tyrosine kinase activity leading to phosphorylation of tyrosines on intracellular proteins which results in activation.

Some oncogenes and their products are shown in Table 3.2. The oncoprotein c-*erb* B1 is the receptor for EGF. Binding of EGF (the ligand) to the receptor activates its tyrosine kinase activity which leads to protein phosphorylation in the cell. Altered expression or mutation of c-*erb* B1 in cancer (or by viral homologue v-*erb*) may lead to overactivation of receptor activity.

Membrane proteins bind guanosine 5′-triphosphate (GTP) and also have GTPase activity which terminates the signal. Abnormal G proteins may be produced by mutated *ras* oncogenes, which have deficient GTPase activity and consequently lead to defective signal termination. The *ras* family consists of three members (H-*ras*-1, K-*ras*-2, N-*ras*) and other proteins which show partial homology (*rho*, R-*ras*, *ras*, *rab*). Activating *ras* mutations have been found in 40% of human colon cancers, and 95% of pancreatic cancers. Excess production of the *ras* protein has

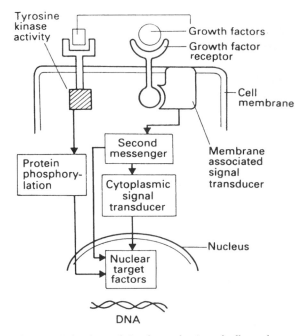

Fig. 3.5 Mechanisms of signal transduction of cell membrane-associated receptors for a growth factor. The normal events are shown in this simplified diagram. Abnormal activation may contribute to tumour growth.

Table 3.2 Some oncogenes and their products associated with cancer in humans.

Oncogene	Activity	Association with human tumour
abl	Membrane tyrosine kinase	Chronic myeloid leukaemia, acute leukaemias
erb B1	EGF receptor	Breast cancer
erb B2	EGF receptor activity	Increased oppression in breast cancer (comedo and *in situ*)
sis	Platelet-derived growth factor	? Breast cancer
ras	G protein	Adenocarcinoma of lung, prostate, large bowel

been found in these cancers. The *ras* protein is capable of transforming fibroblasts in tissue culture, and its expression is associated with various stages of differentiation in embryonic life.

Tumour suppressor genetic mechanisms in cancer development [7]

Some genes result in abnormal growth regulation when they are deleted, that is they act in a recessive manner with its translocation partner *bcr* forms a fusion protein resulting in permanent expression of a growth-inducing tyrosine kinase. Usually both alleles must be affected and for this reason these recessive mechanisms have been most clearly defined in inherited cancer syndromes where there is a germline mutation or deletion of one allele and the tumour is associated with deletion or mutation of the remaining allele in childhood or adult life. Chromosome loss has been studied by using cell–cell hybrids, and it has been shown that introduction of single chromosomes can suppress the tumorigenicity of cultured cells which lack a particular chromosome. Table 3.3 lists some of the features distinguishing oncogenes and in this way probably does not often lead to malignancy.

Retinoblastoma (p. 377), Li–Fraumeni syndrome (p. 344) and Wilms' tumour (p. 370) are among the best-studied tumours where recessive mechanisms have been shown. Knudson suggested that retinoblastoma would arise as a two-step process in which a germline allele loss would be followed by loss of the other allele. It seems that loss of the second allele is usually by recombination or mitotic non-disjunction. Survivors of retinoblastoma have a 300 times greater risk of osteosarcoma. It is not known why the tumours are restricted to these sites (bone and eye). The *Rb* gene is located at chromosome 13q14.

The Wilms' tumour gene is located at 11p13 and, like retinoblastoma, loss of this region of the gene is found sporadically in non-inherited cancers such as osteosarcoma. Hereditary forms of Wilms' tumour are rare, and 50% of people with the abnormal gene do not develop the

tumour. The non-inherited tumour does, however, sometimes show a deleted 11p13 band and polymorphism studies have shown chromosome loss at this site in almost 50% of tumours.

In the Li–Fraumeni syndrome there is a germline mutation in the *p53* gene. Affected families are characterized by the proband having sarcoma in childhood, early onset of breast cancer in the mother or female siblings, and increased likelihood of cancer of the brain, adrenal gland or of leukaemia in other members. The *p53* protein is a cell cycle regulatory nuclear phosphoprotein. It is frequently mutated in sporadic cancers of many types.

Cell division [8,9]

When a cell is going to divide there is a phase of cell growth (G1) following which the cell moves to a phase of DNA synthesis (S phase) resulting in two genetically identical copies of the chromosomal DNA. The duplicate chromosomes are termed sister chromatids. They appear as condensed chromosomes in the cell until mitosis begins. A phase of cell growth occurs (G2) before entry into mitosis, which is initiated by proteins known as cyclin-dependent kinases (Fig. 3.6). At the onset of mitosis, prometaphase, each member of the pairs attaches at its centromere to proteins that will form part of the mitotic spindle. Unattached chromatids issue a delaying signal until all are attached and the spindle formed (metaphase). The nuclear membrane disappears while this process is occurring. A second set of proteins assembles—the anaphase-promoting complex—that degrade proteins that prevent anaphase from beginning. In anaphase there is enzymic cleavage of the ties (cohesins) that bind the two sister chromatids and the two sets of chromosomes separate to opposite poles of the cell. The cell divides and the daughter cells pass into a prolonged resting phase (G0) or into a first growth phase (G1) that leads to a further cycle of DNA replication.

At each stage there are checks to ensure the fidelity of the process before it continues. Mitosis does not begin

Table 3.3 The distinguishing features of tumour suppressor genes and oncogenes.

Tumour suppressor genes	Oncogenes
Recessive in effect	Dominant in effect
Often tissue-specific tumours, e.g. retinoblastoma	Tendency to broad specificity
Deletions promote cancer	Translocations increase activity
Germline inheritance in some cases	Both hereditary and non-hereditary forms

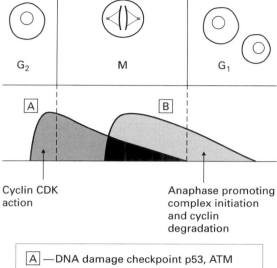

Fig. 3.6 Diagrammatic representation of the process of mitosis and the checkpoints. The terms are explained in the text.

until the presence of DNA damage has been detected by proteins such as p53 (see below), ATM and CHK2. The integrity of the mitotic spindle phase is checked by BUB1 and MAD proteins (see Fig. 3.6). If these proteins are inactive the chromosomes fail to segregate correctly.

Chromosomal instability is a hallmark of cancer where cells are often aneuploid. There are many ways in which such instability can be produced bearing in mind the complexity of the mitotic process. Mutations in many of the genes maintaining normal mitosis have been described in cancer. For example, *p53* mutations are frequent in established cancers. The lack of functional p53 protein that results allows cell division to occur in the presence of DNA damage leading to further genetic changes and tumour progression. Some of the protective proteins are targets for viral carcinogenesis. HTLV-1 produces a protein (*TAX*) that degrades MAD1 and results in chromosomal instability. Numerous other proteins are involved in the regulation of mitosis, such as APC (which is mutated in adenomatous polyposis).

The instability of chromosomal structure, apart from contributing to the malignant phenotype (mobility, invasion and metastasis), also confers a susceptibility to genotoxic damage that accounts for the response of cancers to cytotoxic drugs. Screening for new anti-cancer drugs will exploit this susceptibility of cancer cells.

Inheritance of cancer [10]

There are numerous inherited genetic abnormalities which predispose to the development of malignancy. The major syndromes are shown in Table 3.4. There has been great progress in the isolation and cloning of some of the genes involved in familial cancer syndromes. This is leading to an understanding of the molecular mechanisms of oncogenesis which has a wider significance than the inherited disorder itself. As discussed on p. 23, several inherited cancer syndromes are due to mutations in genes that are important in DNA repair or in detecting damage to DNA. For example, in xeroderma pigmentosum and ataxia telaniectasia the inherited abnormality is in a DNA-repair proteins. The genetic defects in cancers of the breast, ovary and colon also involve DNA repair pathways.

In addition to single gene defects that carry a high risk of cancer, there are probably numerous polymorphisms that increase the cancer risk to a small degree. These may code for enzymes or proteins involved in detoxification of carcinogens, in DNA repair, or in growth factor signalling. Common polymorphisms, each carrying only a small increase in cancer risk may nevertheless be of great quantitative importance in contributing to the total inherited cancer susceptibility of an individual. Screening for genes predicting for an increased likelihood of developing cancer will have major implications for cancer screening and for counselling services.

Clonal origin, progression and growth of a cancer

There are three major characteristics of cancer. First, that growth is not fully responsive to the normal constraints in the parent tissue. Second, that cancers always show a degree of anaplasia, which is a loss of cellular differentiation. This is associated with a lack of some of the functions of the normal, differentiated, parent tissue. Third, that cancers have the property of metastasis, that is the ability to spread from the site of origin to distant tissues.

While these features are present in most human cancers, some of these properties are not absolutely distinct from normal tissues. Thus it is true that the normal regulatory mechanisms controlling growth are defective in cancer, but there often remains a check or constraint on the pattern of growth of human neoplasms (see below). Similarly, although we regard the most anaplastic of cancers as 'undifferentiated' in the sense that they seem to have arisen from the more primitive precursors of the differentiated

Table 3.4 Constitutional (inherited) genetic factors in cancer.

Abnormality	Cancer
Chromosomal abnormalities	
Trisomy 21 (Down's syndrome)	Acute leukaemia
47 XXY (Klinefelter's syndrome)	Breast cancer
Mosaicism (45X0/46XY)	Gonadoblastoma
11p– (aniridia–Wilms' syndrome)	Wilms' tumour
13q– (multiple malformations)	Retinoblastoma
Inherited bowel disorders	
Polyposis coli (AD)	Carcinoma of colon
Gardner's syndrome (AD)	Carcinoma of colon
Peutz–Jeghers syndrome (AD)	Duodenal cancer
Tylosis palmaris (AD)	Oesophageal cancer
Neurological-cutaneous disorders	
Von Recklinghausen's	Sarcomas, glioma
neurofibromatosis (AD)	Acoustic neuroma
Retinal/cerebellar angiomatosis	Medullary thyroid cancer
(Von-Hippel–Lindau	Phaeochromocytoma
syndrome) (AD)	Hypernephroma
Tuberous sclerosis (AD)	Ependymoma
	Gliomas
Skin disorders (see Chapter 9, Table 9.2)	
Breast and ovary	
BRCA1, BRCA2	Breast and ovary
Paediatric cancers (see Chapter 24)	
Immune deficiency disorders	
X–linked lymphoproliferative	Lymphoma
syndrome (XLR)	
Ataxia telangiectasia (AR)	Lymphoma
	Gastric cancer
Sex-linked agammaglobulinaemia	Lymphoma
(Bruton) (MR)	
Wiskott–Aldrich syndrome (XLR)	Lymphoma
IgA deficiency (S, AD, AR)	Adenocarcinomas
Miscellaneous syndromes	
Hemihypertrophy (AR)	Wilms' tumour
	Hepatoblastoma
Beckwith's syndrome (gigantism,	Wilms' tumour
macroglossia, mental retardation,	
visceromegaly) (S)	Hepatoblastoma
Multiple enchondromas (Oller's	Chondrosarcoma
syndrome) (S)	
Bloom's syndrome (telangiectasia,	Leukaemias
short stature, chromosome	
fragility) (AR)	Numerous other cancers
Fanconi's anaemia (skeletal	Acute leukaemia
abnormalities, mental retardation,	
pigmented patches)	

AD, autosomal dominant; AR, autosomal recessive; S, sporadic; XLR, X-linked recessive.

tissue, many cancers none the less do retain some of the functions of the mature tissues. Metastasis is, however, a property unique to cancer. Furthermore, it is metastasis which in most instances kills the patient, and understanding the biology of metastasis is one of the central problems of cancer research.

The following section is concerned with the events which follow the carcinogenic event and which lead to the development of an invasive, metastasizing malignancy.

Monoclonality and heterogeneity in cancer

There is now a considerable body of evidence that most human neoplasms are monoclonal in origin. This means that the original oncogenic event affected a single cell, and that the tumour is the result of growth from that one cell. There are two major lines of evidence which have led to this conclusion. First, certain women are heterozygotes for two forms of the enzyme glucose-6-phosphate dehydrogenase (G6PD). The gene for the enzyme is carried on the X chromosome and, in female heterozygotes, either the maternal or paternal form is present on either one of the X chromosomes. In a female, each cell loses activity of one or other X chromosome and therefore, in a heterozygote for this enzyme, every cell in the body will have either one form of the enzyme or the other. In studies on haematological malignancies arising in heterozygotes for G6PD, the cancers are found to contain either the maternal or the paternal form of the enzyme, implying that the original cancer arose from one cell which either had one form of the enzyme or the other.

In chronic granulocytic leukaemia the restriction of the enzyme expression is found in cells of the granulocyte series and, importantly, in red cells and platelets, as well as implying that a stem cell is affected by the malignant process.

The technique is more difficult to apply to carcinomas. It is still possible that some carcinomas arise from a 'field of change' in a tissue with many clones arising at the same time. An interesting analysis of bladder cancer in women has shown that in cells arising in different areas of the bladder there was the same pattern of suppression of the X chromosome in all cells from a given tumour, while the normal bladder cells showed random suppression of one or other of the two chromosomes. This strongly suggests a single clonal origin. In addition, there was the same pattern of allele deletion on 9q, while losses on 17p and 18q were variable, suggesting these were later events in the evolution of the tumour.

The second line of evidence pointing towards the

monoclonal origin of cancer comes from lymphomas and other lymphoid malignancies in which it can be shown that the immunoglobulin produced by the lymphoid neoplasm (on its surface, or exported into the blood in the case of myeloma) is nearly always monoclonal, being of a single class and showing restriction of light chain expression (see Chapter 27).

The concept of monoclonality has sometimes led investigators to believe that there is a far greater uniformity of behaviour of cancer than is in fact the case. In spite of the monoclonal origin of neoplasms, heterogeneity appears to arise during the course of development of the tumours. This has important implications for treatment and for understanding the nature of metastases.

How does heterogeneity arise if cancer is monoclonal? Malignant transformation is accompanied by genetic instability that causes phenotypic differences in clonogenic cells. Some cells with mutations survive and undergo still further changes, while others, depending on their ability to survive hormonal, biochemical or immunological adversity, die. The mature tumour can therefore be envisaged as being composed of cells that are monoclonal in origin, but diverse in capacity to metastasize and to resist cytotoxic drugs and immune attack.

A sequence of chromosomal alteration during the progression from colonic polyp to colonic cancer is illustrated in Fig. 16.2. As the tumour progresses increasing genetic instability occurs with different cells within the same tumour showing a wide variety of chromosome breaks, deletions and reduplications [11]. Morphologically, this is accompanied by change in nuclear appearance and increasingly bizarre and pleomorphic cytological forms.

Many cancers acquire mutations in the *p53* gene. This gene encodes a nuclear phosphoprotein which appears to act as a check to the cell cycle, arresting the cell in G_1 as a result of DNA damage. Ultraviolet light and cytotoxic drugs induce a rapid increase in *p53* in normal cells due to a stabilization of the protein after translation. Loss of *p53* function by mutation allows mitosis to begin with damaged DNA. The mutations in the *p53* gene that occur in cancer result in a conformational change in the protein making it inactive. Mutant forms of the protein may be unable to bind to DNA. *p53* mutation may thus be an important step on the pathway of tumour progression where an already malignant cell is permitted to move into cell cycle without time to repair damaged DNA. Further mutations can then occur.

Diversity within the cell population of a single tumour therefore occurs with regard to growth rate, cytoplasmic constituents, hormone receptor status, radiosensitivity and susceptibility to killing by cytotoxic agents. For example, in the case of small-cell carcinoma of the bronchus, different levels of cytoplasmic calcitonin, histaminase and L-dopa decarboxylase have been found in the primary tumour compared with a metastasis. Primary and secondary tumours may also show karyotypic differences.

Heterogeneity of neoplasms presents a formidable problem for the cancer therapist. If a single tumour shows diversity in cell phenotype and antigenic expression, it becomes hard to imagine how immunological attack can be successful. Likewise, a single tumour may contain cells with a wide variation in susceptibility to cytotoxic agents, thus providing the means for drug resistance to become clinically evident with repeated drug treatment.

The growth of cancer

Normal tissues vary greatly in both the rate of cell division and the numbers of cells which are actively proliferating. Examples of rapidly proliferating cells are the intestinal mucosa, the bone marrow, the hair follicle cells and normal tissue regenerating after injury, for example after surgical resection or infections.

An idealized representation of the way in which proliferation occurs in a normal tissue is shown in Fig. 3.7. This figure shows the stem or progenitor cell supplying a proliferating pool of cells which follow a particular differentiation pathway. These become mature cells which are held

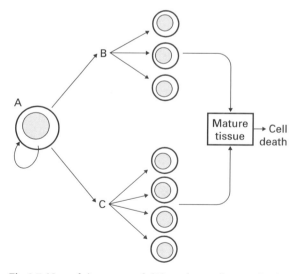

Fig. 3.7 Normal tissue renewal. (A) produces cells committed to differentiation path B or C. Cellular proliferation leads to mature tissue and then to cell death.

to be incapable of further division and subsequently die. While this model may apply also to human cancers, it is possibly an oversimplification. Tumours probably do contain progenitor and mature cells but it is not clear whether cell renewal in a tumour comes from a small progenitor fraction. Nevertheless, the model is useful in explaining many aspects of tumour growth. While the progeny of stem cell division go through successive divisions their number increases, but the number of further divisions they are 'programmed' to make declines concomitantly. The stimulus to death, and its mechanism, is a programmed process under genetic control. Programmed cell death has been termed *apoptosis*. The morphological changes are condensation of the nucleus followed by pitting and explosion of the cytoplasm. The cell density rises, there is endonuclease activation and the DNA is cleaved. The process involves the release of caspase enzymes from mitochondria and is shown in Fig. 3.7. The cell may thus be switched to growth arrest, cell death or division by active processes. The *bcl*-2, *ras* and *LMP*-1 genes permit population expansion, while *p53* may prevent this.

When a tumour is treated with radiation or cytotoxic drugs it may shrink in size. This response may be entirely at the expense of later, non-self-renewing cells, in which

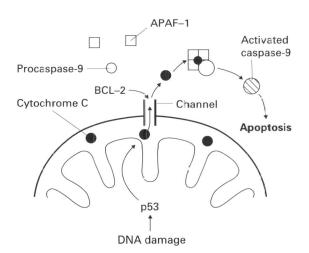

Fig. 3.8 Apoptosis induced by DNA damage.
• DNA damage and p53 activation triggers cytochrome C release from mitochondria through a voltage-regulated anion channel in the outer mitochondrial membrane.
• Cytochrome C causes an oligomer of apoptosis activating factor-1 (APAF-1), which binds procaspase-9 and activates it.
• Activated procaspase-9 initiates apoptosis.
• BCL-2 blocks the voltage channel and is therefore anti-apoptotic. BAX enhances cytochrome release and is anti-apoptotic.

case the tumour will regrow. To prevent regrowth it is probably essential to kill the progenitor or stem cells. The growth fraction of a tumour is the proportion of cells in active proliferation. Many cancer cells have long cycle times and calculations of the growth fraction may underestimate the proliferative capacity of the tumour. These slow-growing cells are probably less susceptible to chemotherapy, particularly using cycle active agents. It is possible that the cell cycle time in these cells may shorten as a result of cytoreductive treatment.

A normal tissue grows and develops to a point when cell proliferation is balanced by cell loss and the tissue remains static in size, unless subjected to a changing environment, for example the normal breast ductular tissue during the menstrual cycle or during pregnancy. In a cancer, on the other hand, the regulatory mechanisms are defective and the tumour gradually increases in size.

Normal cell somatic cell division is accompanied by loss of a repeating DNA sequence found at the tip of chromosomes called telomeres. When telomeres are lost all cell division ceases. Telomerase is an enzyme with reverse transcriptase properties which catalyses telomere formation. It is overexpressed in many cancers and may be one mechanism for sustaining tumour growth [12].

Nevertheless, it must be emphasized that sustained growth does not necessarily mean rapid growth. Figure 3.9 shows the volume doubling time of an almost spherical squamous carcinoma. Slow exponential growth can be seen with a volume doubling time of 1 year. During their growth, tumours undergo cell loss as well as cell renewal. This cell loss is partly due to the vascularization of tumours being defective. There is often inadequate nutrition when cells are more than 150μ from a nutrient capillary. Sometimes the centres of human cancers are grossly necrotic where the tumour has clearly outstripped its blood supply. Other possible causes of cell loss are unsuccessful mitosis (possibly due to chromosomal aberrations), and death of tumours by immune or inflammatory attack as a result of both specific immunity and nonspecific processes excited by the tumour.

In tissue culture doubling times of human tumours are variable. It is not clear whether tumours exhibit a consistent rate of growth from the origin of the cancer to the time when the patient has a massive tumour and is about to die. Exponential growth can be observed in some human malignancies. In the case shown in Fig. 3.9, if one were to extrapolate back to the origin of the tumour, it would prove to have arisen some 30 doublings (30 years) before the clinical presentation—if the growth had been exponential at the same rate throughout this time. We

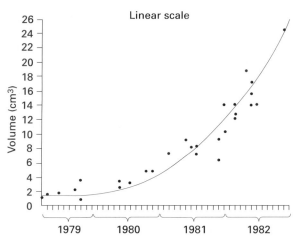

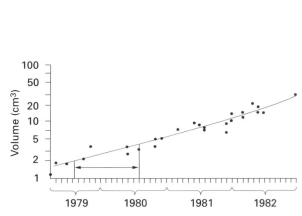

Fig. 3.9 Growth of a squamous carcinoma. The patient had a peripheral squamous carcinoma, untreated because of dementia and hypertension. Over 4 years this almost spherical tumour increased slowly in size exhibiting exponential growth with a doubling time of just over 1 year (horizontal arrows).

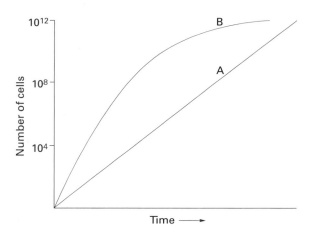

Fig. 3.10 Two models of kinetics of tumour growth. In curve A the growth is exponential. In curve B there is progressive slowing of growth rate with increasing size, termed Gompertzian growth.

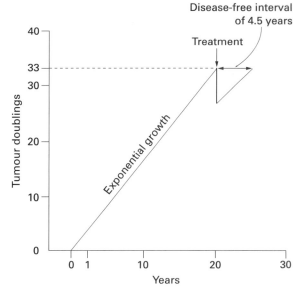

Fig. 3.11 The lifespan of a tumour. The tumour is clinically apparent after 33 doublings. Treatment reduces the tumour mass, but the disease is again clinically detectable after 4.5 years.

have no way of knowing whether spontaneously arising tumours grow faster when they are small and then slow down. For *visible* tumours, there is some evidence that a progressive slowing of the rate of growth may sometimes occur—a type of growth pattern known as Gompertzian (Fig. 3.10). It is clear that a clinical cancer is late in its natural history by the time it presents (Fig. 3.11), and this has implications for the possible success or failure of screening programmes to detect cancer early. Similarly, in a tumour with a volume doubling time of 70 days, a treatment which caused a reduction of 10 doublings would delay its reappearance for over 2 years if the growth rate was unchanged. This might lead to erroneous claims for the treatment if the follow-up time was short. These over-simplifications make the point that, in the treatment of clinically apparent tumours, the disease is already late in its natural history.

Differentiation in cancer

In a normal tissue the progeny of stem cells develop into the mature cells. During this process the cells acquire specialized structures, functions and biochemical properties; a process known as differentiation. Cellular differentiation continues progressively for several cell divisions after the stem cell.

Although cancer cells differ from their normal tissue counterparts in many respects, these differences are often ones of degree. When pathologists talk of an *undifferentiated* tumour, they mean one which does not look morphologically like the normal tissue. Some of the histological features will be present but the arrangement of cells appears chaotic and disorganized, with variation in nuclear size and shape. An *anaplastic* carcinoma is one in which all the characteristic morphological appearances have disappeared to the extent that the primary tissue of origin cannot be determined.

The term 'undifferentiated' often carries the implication that the neoplasm has somehow reverted to a more primitive state. It is, however, possible that the oncogenic event has occurred early in the cell's differentiation pathway (for example, in the stem cell) and that the neoplastic proliferation is occurring in a phase of cell development at which the cell has not yet acquired the mature functional characteristics of the final tissue. The neoplastic counterpart might therefore be morphologically and functionally similar to the stage of cellular differentiation at the point where the malignant proliferation occurred.

Changes in cell surface properties are associated with the structural and functional alterations, with the acquisition of markers for various stages in the cell's differentiation pathway. Numerous cell surface proteins and glycolipids have been identified, some of which are differentiation-linked, and others which are expressed on the cell surface in increased amounts when the cell is undergoing division but are not detectable in the resting phase.

Invasion, angiogenesis and metastasis [13,14]

The malignant cell is able to escape from normal control of growth. When normal tissues proliferate, they do so to the point where cell–cell contact exerts an inhibiting role on further mitosis. This inhibition is lost in malignancy. Tumours will grow and increase in size when planted subcutaneously in immunosuppressed mice, while normal tissues will not. The nature of the cell surface glycoproteins differs from normal cells with an increase in sialic acid content, and alterations in the surface charge. The locomotor apparatus of cells (microfilaments and microtubules) becomes disorganized and the cells alter their shape and show membrane movement at sites of contact with normal cells.

At the same time the tumour cells become locally invasive, although the biochemical basis of this property is ill understood. Tumour cells may show decreased adhesiveness and attachment compared with normal cells. Secretion of enzymes is part of the mechanism of invasion. Several enzymes play a part in the proteolysis of the intracellular matrix which accompanies invasion by tumour cells. Among these is the family of matrix metalloproteinase (MMP) enzymes, which includes collagenases, gelatinases and stromelysins. They are secreted as inactive enzymes and are activated by disruption of the sulphydryl group which holds the metal atom (often zinc). This leads to a conformational change and activation of the enzyme. Tissue inhibitors of metalloproteinases (TIMPs) terminate the activity. Certain tissues are characteristically resistant to invasion, for example compact bone, large blood vessels and cartilage. Presumably some of these properties of cancer cells relate to normal processes of tissue remodelling and repair. However, the relation of the invasive phenotype to patterns of known genetic change in cancer is not understood.

As the tumour grows, tumour blood vessels proliferate under the influence of tumour angiogenesis factors which stimulate capillary formation. The tumour vasculature offers a potential approach to treatment. Tumour cells stimulate endothelial cell proliferation by production of angiogenic cytokines such as vascular endothelial growth factor (VEGF), PDGF and basic fibroblast growth factor. Endothelial cells can, in turn, stimulate tumour cell growth. A gram of tumour may contain 10–20 million endothelial cells that are not themselves neoplastic.

Antigens of normal endothelial cells may be upregulated in proliferating tumour endothelium including procoagulant factors. Apart from cytokines, hypoxia in the tumour circulation may also regulate production of VEGF and other factors. During angiogenesis, endothelial cells invade the stroma and divide to produce a capillary sprout, which later takes on a tubular form. As with cancer

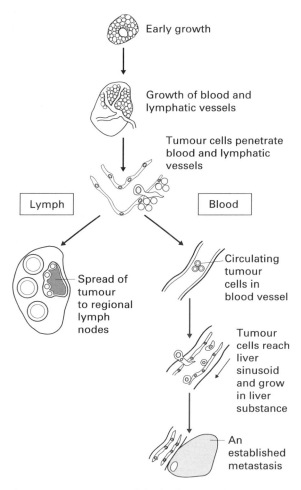

Early growth

Growth of blood and lymphatic vessels

Tumour cells penetrate blood and lymphatic vessels

Lymph

Blood

Spread of tumour to regional lymph nodes

Circulating tumour cells in blood vessel

Tumour cells reach liver sinusoid and grow in liver substance

An established metastasis

Fig. 3.12 Tissue invasion and the development of metastasis.

anatomy is often important, for example, gastrointestinal cancers typically spread via the portal venous system to the liver. Tumours may also metastasize via a tissue space; for example, those arising in the peritoneal cavity may seed widely over the peritoneal space, and lung cancer may spread over the pleura. Certain tumours characteristically spread to some structures while others do not; for example, sarcomas typically metastasize to lungs, and breast cancer to the axial skeleton. The biological mechanisms for these preferences are not known.

Regional lymph nodes may form a barrier to further metastases from the primary site. It is not clear whether lymph nodes create a barrier to spread of tumour by virtue of specific immune mechanisms.

Having penetrated the vascular compartment, tumour cells must withstand the process of arrest in the capillary bed of an organ and then start to divide. At this site the tumour cell must leave the capillary bed of the new tissue. To do this the tumour cell must pass through the capillary endothelium and survive attack by host defence mechanisms such as phagocytic cells and so-called *natural killer* (NK) cells.

The capacity for invasion and colonization of distant tissues varies with different tumour types, presumably related to the pattern of gene expression associated with the tumour. With time most cancers acquire enough genetic change to become invasive and metastasizing, but this may take several years even after the tumour is clinically apparent. An example is low-grade lymphoma. Similarly a tumour of the same type and degree of differentiation has a different tendency to metastasize in different individuals. This has led to a search for molecular markers that might relate to outcome more precisely than histopathological appearances alone (although this is by far the best single determinant). Within a single tumour there is heterogeneity in the metastatic potential of its constituent cells. Cloned sublines from a single tumour differ markedly in their ability to metastasize. The basis of this variability is not known.

It is apparent that the problems of tissue invasion, metastatic spread and tumour heterogeneity are among the most fundamental in cancer research and clinical management of cancer patients. The lack of homogeneity of tumours, the similarities between tumours and their parent tissue and the lack of a single identifiable lesion in cancer cells which distinguishes them from normal, together mean that many of our simple assumptions about tumour immunity and the mode of action of cytotoxic drugs must be looked at critically, particularly if

cells, this invasion may involve a complex interplay between MMPs, produced by the endothelial cells, and their natural inhibitors (see below).

One of the results of local invasion is that tumour cells can enter vascular and other channels of the body and metastasize. The sequence of events is shown in Fig. 3.12. Lymphatic spread, which is particularly common with carcinomas, follows invasion of lymphatic channels, and the tumour cells grow in cords and clumps in the lymphatic vessels and lymph nodes. From there, spread to distal lymph nodes readily occurs. Haematogenous spread occurs after tumour cells have entered the vessels near the primary tumour or have been shed into the blood from the thoracic duct. Tumour cells are then trapped in the next capillary network, that is, in the lung or liver. Local

they are derived from experiments using homogeneous tumours.

Tumour immunology

The idea that human tumours might be recognized as foreign to the host has obvious attractions because, if an immune response to the tumour occurred as part of the disease, or could be provoked artificially, there would be opportunities for using such an immune response diagnostically or therapeutically.

Immune responses to cancer

T-lymphocyte reactivity against human tumours is being reinvestigated now that it is possible to identify types of lymphocyte reliably, using antibodies (usually monoclonal — see below) to lymphocyte surface antigens which relate to function. Thus subpopulations of T cell with cytotoxic, helper and suppressor function can be identified in blood, lymph nodes and the infiltrates in tumours. T cells can be separated from NK cells in cytotoxicity experiments. It has now become clear that, in many cytotoxic systems, T-cell killing will only take place if there is genetic identity between the effector T cells and the targets. This leads to difficulty in demonstrating specific T-cell antitumour cytotoxicity in humans, because the effector and target cells need to be derived from either the same individual, or one identical with respect to histocompatibility antigens.

This problem can be surmounted by techniques whereby antigen-specific T cells can be grown and multiplied in culture. This allows T cells with both specific and defined functions to be propagated *in vitro*. T cells from blood, draining lymph nodes or, better still, from tumours, can now be isolated, expanded in number and cloned, allowing a more precise definition of their properties and target specificity. Carcinoma cells usually express class I major histocompatibility (MHC) antigens on their surface, but not class II. Cellular proteins are degraded in the cell to peptides which can bind to class I MHC. These are potential recognition targets for specialized antigen presenting cells to stimulate a T cell response. The questions are therefore the nature of the peptides which are tumour-derived, whether they differ from cellular peptides of normal cells and whether they can be presented in such a way as to provoke an anti-tumour response.

Until tumour antigens are defined and the nature of the immune response to them, if any, is elucidated, active specific immunity to cancer remains an elusive goal. However, recent identification of melanoma-associated peptides has led to the first trials of tumour vaccines based on a defined antigen. The evidence from melanoma is tantalizing but it is still unclear how generally applicable this approach might be. In other tumours, in the absence of knowledge of the antigens to which a specific and effective immune response could be generated, attempts have been made to provoke immunity by altered, widely distributed, epithelial membrane antigens. A related approach is to generate antibodies to the idiotype (the specific binding region) of other antibodies which recognize cell surface antigens. The anti-idiotype antibodies act as if they were the 'tumour antigen' itself and may be more effective in provoking an immune response in which the actual tumour is damaged. This approach has so far not proved to be clinically useful. Nevertheless, immunization to protect against recurrence is an attractive therapeutic strategy if it can be realised.

Vaccines to viral antigens of hepatitis B, EBV or HPV may prove to be a practical approach for immunization to prevent cancer in high-risk groups, but tumour-associated antigens are not sufficiently defined for this to be a practical proposition.

Monoclonal antibodies

The development of monoclonal antibody technology has allowed a serological definition of the tumour cell surface with a hitherto unattainable precision. Some of the potential uses of monoclonal antibodies are listed in Table 3.5.

So far, monoclonal antibodies to human tumours have not been shown to define an antigen exclusively associated with malignant proliferation. Other antigens may be expressed as a result of rapid cell division, and while they may be demonstrable in some cancers, using monoclonal reagents, they may also be present on some normal tissues. The 'anticancer' monoclonals thus far produced appear to be identifying antigens which are expressed at a particular stage of differentiation of the cell type.

It is already clear that monoclonal reagents will be very useful in the classification of cancer and in the diagnosis of undifferentiated tumours (Fig. 3.13) and possibly of therapeutic value in clearing sites such as the bone marrow of unwanted cells as part of the technique of autologous or allogeneic bone marrow. Coupling radio-

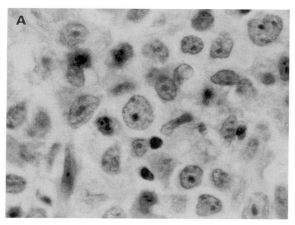

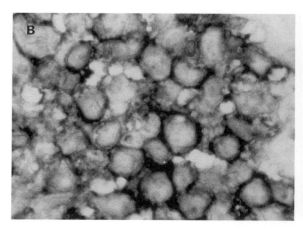

Fig. 3.13 Use of monoclonal antibodies for immunocytochemical diagnosis. (A) Undifferentiated nasopharyngeal tumour. Differential diagnosis would include anaplastic carcinoma, lymphoma and melanoma. (B) Same tumour as in (A), stained for common leucocyte antigen using a monoclonal antibody. The tumour cells show dark membrane staining, indicating that the tumour is a lymphoma.

Table 3.5 Potential uses of monoclonal antibodies in cancer*.

Classification of tumours in tissue sections
Identification of 'undifferentiated' tumours in tissue sections
Diagnosis and classification of leukaemias
Diagnosis of metastatic tumour cells in low frequency, e.g. in bone marrow
Elimination of unwanted cells from bone marrow, e.g. metastatic tumour cells, residual leukaemic cells
Tumour localization by isotopically labelled antibody
Measurement of tumour products and 'markers', e.g. α-fetoprotein, CEA, peptide hormones
Coupling with cytotoxic agents or isotopes to kill tumour cells

CEA, carcinoembryonic antigen.
* See p. 95.

isotopes to these antibodies may be of value in tumour localization and treatment, while coupling of a cytotoxic agent to the monoclonal may provide a means of specific therapy if the antibody can be shown not to identify vital host cells such as gut or marrow stem cells.

Treatment with non-specific immune or inflammatory mediators has not been generally effective (Table 3.5). These cytokine treatments are discussed in Chapter 6 (p. 95). Expansion of autologous lymphokine-activated killer (LAK) cells *in vitro*, by using IL-2, followed by reinfusion of the expanded and activated cell population has been extensively investigated. The aim is to divert a large number of activated non-specific cytotoxic lymphocytes to the tumour. There is little evidence that there is an increase in response over that achieved by the lymphokine (IL-2) alone. Curiously, with most of these immunologically non-specific approaches to cancer treatment (BCG, IL-2, interferon, LAK cells) responses are confined to the same tumour types, namely mela-noma and renal cell carcinoma. It is clear that there is something exceptional about these two tumours which renders them occasionally responsive to mediators of inflammation.

References

1 Hecht SS. Tobacco smoke and lung cancer. *J Natl Cancer Inst* 1999; 91: 1194–210.

2 Friedberg EC. How nucleotide excision repair protects against cancer. *Nature Reviews (Cancer)* 2001; 1: 22–33.

3 Shields PG, Harris CC. Cancer risk and low-penetrance susceptibility genes in gene-environment interactions. *J Clin Oncol* 2000; 18: 2309–15.

4 Beral B, Newton R. Overview of the epidemiology of immunodeficiency-associated cancers. *Mongr Natl Cancer Inst* 1998; 23: 1–6.

5 Lowy DR, Schiller JT. Papillomaviruses and cervical cancer: pathogenesis and vaccine development. *Mongr Natl Cancer Inst* 1998; 23: 27–30.

6 Downward J. The ins and outs of signalling. *Nature* 2001; 411: 759–62.

7 Haber DA, Fearon ER. The promise of cancer genetics. *Lancet* 1998; 351 (Suppl. 11): 1–8.

8 Hagan IM, Bridge AJ, Morphew M, Bartlett R. Cell cycle control and the mitotic spindle. *Brit J Cancer* 1999; 80 (Suppl. 1): 6–13.

9 Malumbres M, Barbacid M. To cycle or not to cycle: a critical decision in cancer. *Nature Reviews (Cancer)* 2001; 1: 222–31.

10 Landor NM, Greene MH. The concise handbook of cancer family syndromes. *J Natl Cancer Inst* 1998; 90: 1039–71.

11 Ilyas M, Straub J, Tomlinson IPM, Bodmer WF. Genetic pathways in colorectal and other cancers. *Eur J Cancer* 1999; 35: 335–51.

12 Meyerson M. Role of telomerase in normal and malignant cells. *J Clin Oncol* 2000; 18: 2626–34.

13 Folkman J. Clinical applications of research on angiogenesis. *New Engl J Med* 1995; 333: 1757–62.

14 Fox SB, Gasparini G, Harris AL. Angiogenesis: pathological, prognostic, and growth-factor pathways and their link to trial design and anticancer drugs. *Lancet Oncol* 2001; 2: 278–89.

4 Staging of tumours

Although the overall prognosis of malignant tumours is often summarized by stating the proportion of patients alive at 5 or 10 years, such figures usually conceal a wide variation in survival, ranging from cure to death within a few months of diagnosis. The search for indicators of prognosis has occupied the attention of oncologists for many years. The object is to identify those patients for whom a treatment strategy (for example, surgery alone) is likely to be successful and conversely, those in whom it is bound to fail—generally because of tumour extension beyond the obvious or visible primary site. For these patients, a different approach must be adopted.

Staging the extent of the disease at presentation is one aspect of the identification of factors which will influence prognosis in any individual patient. The purposes of careful staging of tumour spread are as follows.

1 To impose discipline in the accurate documentation of the initial tumour.

2 To assist our understanding of tumour biology.

3 To give appropriately planned treatment to the individual patient.

4 To be able to give the best estimate of prognosis.

5 To compare similar cases in assessing and designing trials of treatment (see Chapter 2).

Staging notation

For many tumours a useful staging notation is the TNM system developed by the American Joint Committee on Cancer Staging and End Result Reporting [1]. This system has the virtue of simplicity, drawing attention to the prognostic relevance of the size or local invasiveness of the primary tumour (T), lymph node spread (N) and the presence of distant metastases (M). It is widely used for solid tumours including cancers of the breast, head and neck, non-small-cell lung cancer and genitourinary cancers. It has obvious limitations, for example in disorders such as diffuse lymphoma where the disease is often generalized, and is clearly inappropriate for leukaemias. Even in some solid tumours, such as small-cell carcinoma of the bronchus and ovarian cancer, the practicality and usefulness of the system is limited. In these diseases different approaches must be used for staging, which are described in the appropriate chapters. For many gynaecological tumours the FIGO system (International Federation of Gynaecology and Obstetrics) is often preferred (see, for example, p. 264).

The primary tumour (T)

In some cancers the size of the primary tumour relates to prognosis. This is well illustrated by many cancers of the head and neck, for example in the oropharynx and oral cavity (see Chapter 10). In other tumours the T stage relates not to size but to depth of invasion, for example in melanoma, colon and bladder cancer (Fig. 4.1a). In squamous lung cancer the size and site of the primary tumour are both factors of prognostic importance (Fig. 4.1b). In some diseases the mode of spread makes T status largely

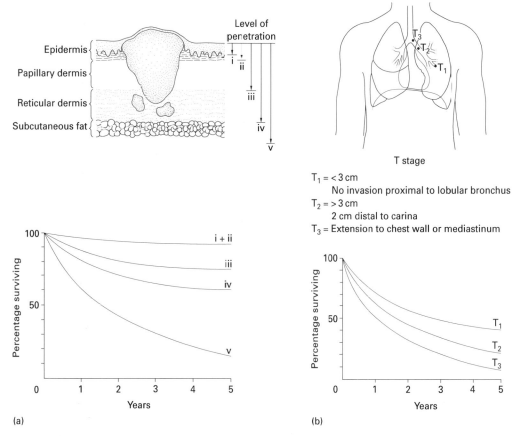

Fig. 4.1 Prognosis related to local extent of primary tumour: (a) melanoma; (b) squamous carcinoma of the lung.

irrelevant. Examples include ovarian cancer, soft-tissue sarcoma and small-cell carcinoma of the lung. In such tumours 'stages' or stage groupings are used which are often composites of tumour size and local or distant invasion. In melanoma, the depth of involvement in millimetres is the best predictor of prognosis of the primary tumour. In squamous lung cancer local invasiveness and tumour site are as important as tumour size (pp. 183–5).

Lymph node involvement (N)

Nodal involvement has profoundly important prognostic influence in many solid tumours (Fig. 4.2). In head and neck, bladder and large bowel cancers, for example, it is probably the most important determinant of survival. In most types of cancer, fixed (N_3) lymph nodes, which are surgically inaccessible, carry a far worse prognosis than mobile ipsilateral (N_1) nodes. Nodal involvement often

reflects a high probability of haematogenous metastases, as for example in breast carcinoma. In other diseases, particularly cancers of the head and neck, it has considerable prognostic importance because of the higher local failure rate, often with fatal results.

Presence of metastases (M)

This clearly defines a group of patients who are surgically incurable. With few exceptions (notably testicular tumours) the presence of distant metastatic disease has grave prognostic implications, usually proving fatal within months or a few years of diagnosis. Metastases may have been detected by clinical examination alone, or may have been found by investigation using specialized techniques.

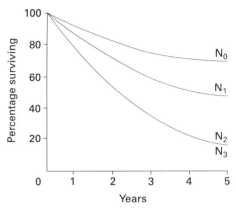

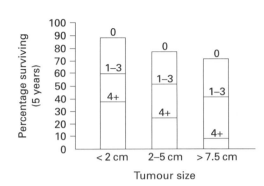

Prognosis related to N stage (all cases)
N_0 = no palpable nodes
N_1 = mobile ipsilateral nodes
N_2 = fixed ipsilateral nodes
N_3 = supra- and infra-clavicular nodes

Prognosis related to tumour size and number of involved nodes

Fig. 4.2 Breast cancer. Prognosis related to N stage and to number of involved nodes and tumour size.

Staging techniques

Many techniques are available for determining the extent of spread of a tumour at the time when a patient first presents. Much information can be obtained by investigations such as chest X-ray, full blood count and liver enzyme tests. These investigations are performed routinely in a patient who has been diagnosed as having cancer or where the diagnosis is suspected.

A chest X-ray may show metastases in the lungs or the bones or extension of a bronchogenic carcinoma into the pleura or overlying ribs. Hilar or paratracheal lymph node enlargement may also be present. These findings indicate that the tumour has spread beyond its site of origin, and will considerably alter the approach to management.

A full blood count may show anaemia of an iron-deficient type, or a normochromic anaemia typical of the anaemia of chronic diseases. Occasionally, the blood film may show leucoerythroblastic anaemia with immature white and red cell precursors present. This is typical of widespread bone marrow infiltration and is most frequently caused by adenocarcinomas, particularly adenocarcinoma of the breast. Bone marrow examination may be performed if infiltration is suspected. In some tumours, for example small-cell carcinoma of the bronchus, marrow examination is sometimes part of the routine staging and when localized treatment with radiotherapy is considered in addition to chemotherapy. Occult marrow involvement is detected in 5–10% of cases but in 20–30% with immunostaining (p. 187). Bone marrow examination is usually performed in patients with newly diagnosed non-Hodgkin's lymphoma, in which the probability of marrow involvement is higher.

In recent years diagnostic imaging has been revolutionized by technical advances and has led to a previously unattainable degree of precision in staging of the extent of the primary tumour and in assessing whether there has been metastatic spread. Many of these investigations are time-consuming, expensive, and very much dependent on the skill and enthusiasm of the radiologist. It is important to maintain a degree of scepticism about equivocal findings, especially if these are not in accordance with the clinical circumstances.

Ultrasound

Diagnostic ultrasound has been greatly refined in the last 15 years [2]. It was first introduced into clinical practice in the 1950s and relies on the differing echo patterns which tissues create when bombarded by sound from an ultrasonic transducer. These echoes are generated at interfaces of tissues whose density differs, then recorded, interpreted and presented as a two-dimensional display. The orientation of the slice or 'cut' is determined by the operator, who places the probe in the position most appropriate for demonstrating the organ and abnormality suspected (Fig. 4.3). This flexibility allows images to be obtained in many planes. Ultrasound echoes cannot be obtained if the organ is shielded by an area of bone or gas since these reflect all the sound from the beam and no echoes can be obtained from beyond these structures. For this reason ultrasound has its main diagnostic use in the abdomen and soft tissues. A great advantage of ultrasound is that it is cheap, quick and non-invasive (though invasive techniques have also been developed—see below). It can therefore be used to monitor responses to treatment, with measurements being made between chemotherapy cycles. Other techniques, such as computed tomography (CT) scanning, which are more accurate, are too expensive to be used in this way and the dose of radiation is too high.

Ultrasound is particularly useful for diagnosis of liver metastases (Fig. 4.3). The type of echo obtained varies depending on the kind of metastases which are present. Thus echo-poor areas are often associated with lymphomas and

sarcomas, while gastrointestinal metastases produce a more echo-dense appearance. In colorectal cancer the accuracy of ultrasound approaches that of CT scanning. It is also of value for assessment of obstructive jaundice, and is often used in conjunction with CT scanning.

In the kidney, ultrasound examination is frequently able to detect a renal carcinoma and distinguish this from cysts. The accuracy in this differential diagnosis is of the order of 90% and the resolving power is approximately 2–3 cm. Ultrasound of the thyroid is useful in making the distinction between solid and cystic lesions, and in the testis it can sometimes demonstrate an occult or doubtfully palpable tumour. It is also often used in distinguishing solid and cystic masses within the breast. Endoscopic ultrasound is increasingly used, for example by the transrectal route—particularly valuable for the assessment of prostatic carcinomas. Endoscopic ultrasound

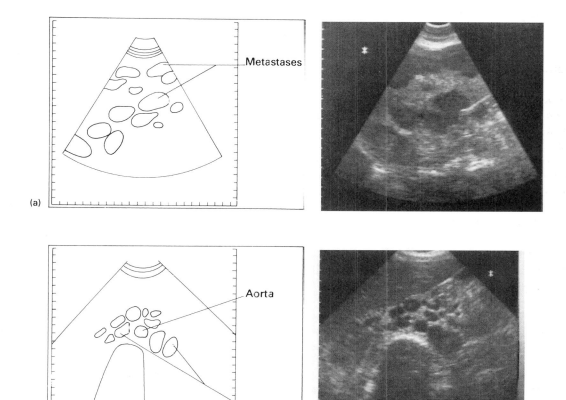

Fig. 4.3 Diagnosis of hepatic metastases and lymph node enlargement by ultrasound. (a) Hepatic metastases. Several large metastases are shown in this transverse scan of the liver.

(b) Para-aortic lymph nodes. These are demonstrated lying in front of and behind the aorta.

of the oesophagus is proving valuable in the staging of distal tumours or those at the gastro-oesophageal junction since these may be potentially operable. These are otherwise difficult to assess prior to attempting a hazardous surgical procedure. For pelvic tumours, transvaginal ultrasonography has also proven valuable — for example, to assess the thickness or extent of a vulval or vaginal carcinoma.

Computed tomography

Modern CT scanners are able to demonstrate normal anatomy in detail which would have been thought impossible in the early 1970s. The accuracy of the technique has been greatly improved and its use in staging continues to be defined. There are, however, many limitations to its use, with both false positive and false negative results. For example, in the abdomen, false positives are usually due to confusion with non-specified bowel loops and false negatives to the inability of CT to detect malignant infiltration of normal-sized nodes. Clarity of the CT scan image depends partly on the presence of the normal fat planes which surround anatomical structures. If these are lost, alteration of the anatomy is less easily detected. The tomographic technique can demonstrate a tumour by showing distortion or enlargement of an organ, or a change in its density. In cancer, the CT scan is of use both in demonstrating the extent of infiltration of the primary tumour (T staging) and in delineating metastatic spread to adjacent lymph nodes and to other structures such as liver or lung (N and M staging).

Computed tomography scanning is of great importance in the definition of the spread of tumours within the chest [3]. Several studies have shown that chest X-ray and conventional tomography greatly underestimate the extent of infiltration of lung cancer within the chest, particularly in the mediastinum (Fig. 4.4). The CT scan has also been valuable in demonstrating the true extent of infiltration of tumours arising in the head and neck, particularly in the paranasal sinuses (Fig. 4.5). For retroperitoneal structures, CT scanning remains the most reliable preoperative investigation and is particularly useful in demonstrating both lymph node enlargement and abnormalities of the adrenal and pancreas. Using fine flexible needles, CT-guided aspiration may help in the distinction between a benign and malignant neoplasm (Fig. 4.6), or between an inflammatory mass and a carcinoma, for example in the pancreas. The extent of retroperitoneal tumours such as sarcomas and lymphomas can be assessed with CT scanning, as can the size of malignant tumours of the kidney. In the pelvis, CT scanning frequently demonstrates the extent of advanced carcinomas of the cervix, bladder, prostate and rectum (Fig. 4.7).

However, interpretation requires considerable expertise. Computed tomography scanning is also used to determine the degree of lymph node involvement. In the chest, the CT scan is much more reliable than chest X-ray

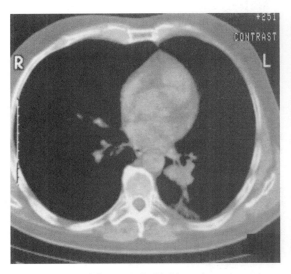

Fig. 4.4 CT scan of thorax. Left-sided bronchogenic carcinoma behind the heart. The tumour extends to the pleura. The chest X-ray was normal.

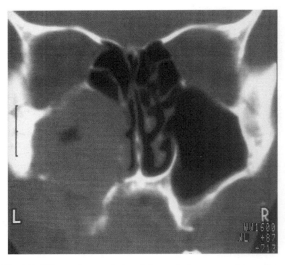

Fig. 4.5 CT scan (coronal plane) through the nose and maxillary antrum. A large tumour fills the left maxillary antrum, destroying its walls and extending medially into the nasal fossa.

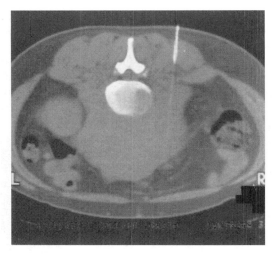

Fig. 4.6 CT scan of the abdomen, showing a large para-aortic mass. The track of a CT-guided biopsy needle is shown.

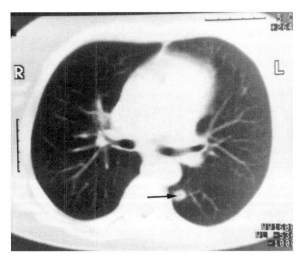

Fig. 4.8 CT scan of thorax, showing a solitary metastasis (arrowed) behind the heart. In this patient with osteosarcoma, the chest X-ray was normal.

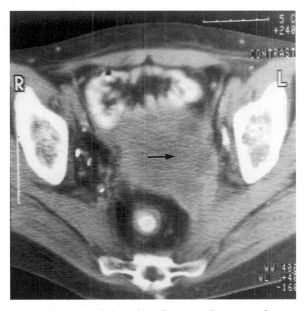

Fig. 4.7 CT scan of the pelvis, showing a large central mass (arrowed) anterior to the rectum. This was an advanced carcinoma of the cervix.

or lung tomography in demonstrating mediastinal and hilar node involvement. In the abdomen, CT scanning delineates pelvic and abdominal lymph nodes, though with lesser clarity than in the chest. Lymph nodes must usually be enlarged to more than twice their normal size before they can be confidently assessed as pathological.

Of the widely available methods, CT remains the most sensitive for assessing pulmonary metastases [4]. It is used for this purpose in testicular germ cell tumours and osteosarcomas, where occult pulmonary metastases are frequently demonstrated in patients whose chest X-ray is normal (Fig. 4.8). The technique is particularly valuable in demonstrating metastases which lie in front of and behind the heart or subpleurally, which are not visible on plain X-ray. In the liver, CT scanning is now more sensitive than ultrasound examination, though much more expensive. The technique is made more accurate by using intravenous contrast, which may also clearly distinguish benign from malignant hepatic lesions. Computed tomography scanning is also the most widely used method of demonstrating brain metastases (see p. 44) (Fig. 4.9).

Magnetic resonance imaging (MRI)

Magnetic resonance imaging has provided important additional detail in imaging particular areas of the body, especially the brain and spinal cord and in sarcomas [5]. In this technique the patient lies within an intense magnetic field which produces magnetization of atomic nuclei in the patient, in the direction of the field. Electromagnetic pulses are then applied to the patient to change the direction of this nuclear magnetization. Following the cessation of the pulse, the nuclei return to their orientation within the static field. This recovery time, which is measured by the scanner, depends on exchange of energy between protons and surrounding atoms and molecules. The recovery time is different in tumours compared with normal tissues. The technique has proved particularly valuable in the brain, where deep-seated primary tumours can be visualized (Fig. 4.10). Magnetic resonance imaging has been able to detect tumours in the brainstem, cerebellum and deep midline structures when CT scanning has been inconclusive. The use of gadolinium contrast techniques has refined the role of MR scanning still further.

In the spine, MRI has largely replaced myelography since it often demonstrates secondary deposits without the need for lumbar puncture. Use of gadolinium contrast further increases the diagnostic range. In bone and soft-tissue sarcomas, MRI provides unsurpassed detail of the extent of the primary site, which greatly assists the surgeon and radiotherapist in operative and planning technique (Fig. 4.11a). Abdominopelvic MRI scanning is also superior to CT, at least in definition of cervical anatomy and pelvic node assessment (Fig. 4.11b).

For imaging of tumours of the pancreaticobiliary tree, magnetic resonance cholangiopancreatography (MRCP) is now increasingly used as an alternative to the more invasive endoscopic procedure (ERCP). It was originally described in 1991 and has the advantage of not requiring administration of exogenous contrast materials [6], making it ideal for patients with allergy to iodine-containing compounds. Its accuracy is generally considered to be as good as ERCP in many clinical situations and it is less expensive.

Isotope scanning

Scanning with radioactive isotopes is a simple and widely available technique for assessing metastatic spread. In certain sites it has rather poor accuracy, that is, a low percentage of correct results. This is due both to a poor sensitivity of detection (the percentage of positive tests in abnormal tissues) and poor specificity (percentage of negative tests in normal tissues). However, the dose of radiation is small, the technique is safe and reproducible and it is relatively inexpensive.

Skeletal metastases are best demonstrated by isotope scanning, and bone scans are now the most frequent test requested in most service departments [3]. Technetium-

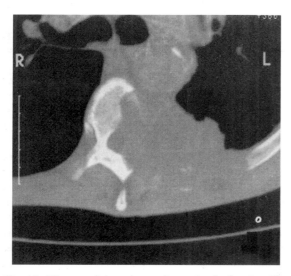

Fig. 4.9 CT scan of thoracic vertebra at level of carina. The vertebra and rib are largely destroyed by local extension of a bronchogenic carcinoma.

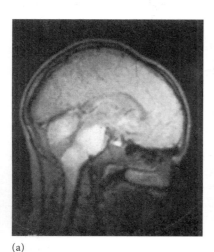
(a)

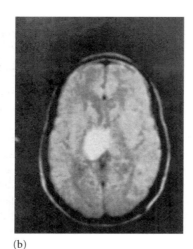
(b)

Fig. 4.10 (a) MRI scan (sagittal view) showing large brainstem tumour. The CT scan was normal. (b) MRI scan of brain showing deep-seated thalamic tumour which was not clearly shown on the CT scan.

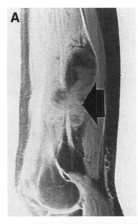

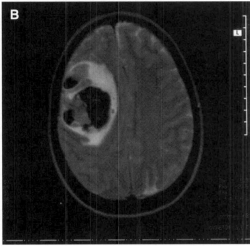

Fig. 4.11 (A) MRI scan of soft-tissue sarcoma in the lower half of the femur. The tumour mass (arrowed) is seen to be closely applied to the femur, and the femoral artery is clearly seen passing through the substance of the tumour. (B) MRI scan of the brain showing a very large metastasis. An area of haemorrhage is shown as a dense, black, central opacity. The midline structures are displaced from right to left.

labelled phosphate compounds are usually used. The isotope is rapidly taken up into bone, rate of uptake being related to both blood flow through the bone and the amount of new bone formation. Metastases cause increase in blood flow and an increase in osteoblastic activity, usually sufficient to be demonstrable as areas of increased uptake of isotope (Fig. 4.12). An exception to this is in multiple myeloma where osteoblastic activity is minimal.

Because of the non-specific nature of the uptake, a variety of other conditions will cause increased uptake. Rib fractures, arthritis and vertebral collapse from osteoporosis may all give rise to increased uptake and be misinterpreted as due to metastases in a patient with a malignancy. Single areas of increased uptake in an otherwise fit patient should therefore be interpreted with extreme caution. X-rays of the affected region should be taken and, if necessary, a CT scan should be obtained if the presence of a metastasis would materially alter the therapeutic decision. This is especially important if the single site is in the vertebral column, since degenerative disease is common at this site. In spite of these problems an area of increased uptake in a patient with cancer is likely to be due to a secondary deposit and should be carefully evaluated. Multiple areas of increased uptake are almost certainly due to disseminated tumour. An isotope bone scan is generally regarded as an important staging investigation in all patients with newly diagnosed carcinoma of the breast.

In the liver, scanning is performed with ^{99m}Tc-labelled sulphur colloid. Metastases appear as areas of diminished uptake. Isotope liver scanning is less accurate than ultrasound or CT scanning, and hepatic isotope scanning has now been largely eclipsed.

New techniques of scintigraphy employ tracer doses of labelled monoclonal antibodies to detect metastases from colorectal cancer. In breast cancer and malignant melanoma, the technique of sentinel node staging is becoming established as a likely competitor to formal regional lymphadenectomy. Sentinel node surgery has the potential to eliminate the need for axillary lymph node clearance, for example, in many breast cancer patients, since it provides an excellent predictive power of the order of 95%, without axillary disturbance [7]. The technique relies on lymphoscyntigraphy for localization of the node and minimally invasive surgery to remove it. Unexpected patterns of drainage may be revealed, of considerable value in surgery.

Drugs such as octreotide (a somatostatin analogue) can be labelled and will bind to neuroendocrine tumours bearing somatostatin receptors, and can be used to detect metastases.

Positron emission tomography (PET) scanning

In recent years, PET scanners have become more widely available. The technique relies on computer-assisted image reconstruction using signal-emitting tracers such as radiolabelled sugars. Fluorodeoxyglucose is the most commonly used. The tracer is injected intravenously, with preferential uptake in sites of tumour activity. Positron emission tomography is able to give information on the

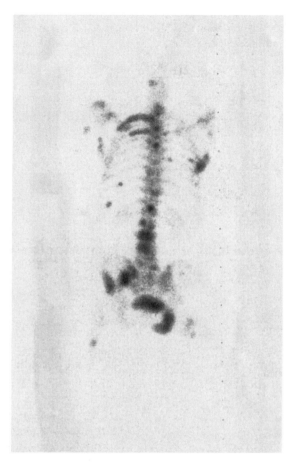

Fig. 4.12 Isotope bone scan, showing multiple bone metastases. This patient had a carcinoma of the prostate.

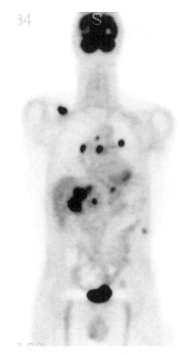

Fig. 4.13 PET scan using 18-fluorodeoxy-glucose in non-small cell lung cancer (NSCLC) showing widespread metastases (clinically undetectable) including both hilae, right supraclavicular fossa and porta hepatis.

Table 4.1 Indications for FDG PET imaging in oncology.

Main indications
Preoperative staging of non-small-cell lung cancer [8]
Staging of recurrent disease in lymphoma and colorectal cancer
Assessment of melanoma greater than stage II
Investigation of a solitary pulmonary nodule

Secondary indications
Preoperative staging of head and neck cancer
Staging of recurrent breast cancer
Distinction between scar or recurrence or tissue necrosis or
   recurrence
Brain tumour grading

Emerging indications
Assessment of tumour response to therapy
In vivo imaging of drug action

FDG, fluorodeoxy-glucose.

location, size and nature of tumour deposits, to a level sometimes unobtainable by other techniques. Most malignant tumours show an increase in glucose metabolism allowing differentiation from benign lesions with PET scanning using 18-fluorodeoxy-glucose (FDG). The technique can also distinguish between tumour recurrence and radiation necrosis, a distinct advantage, at least in some situations, over CT or MRI scanning (Table 4.1). Detection and localization of metastases may also be more readily accomplished (Fig. 4.13). Because of the quality of high-resolution MRI or CT imaging for cancer diagnosis, but a lesser power of discrimination of residual activity following treatment, PET scanning may find its most valuable role in the future in tumour monitoring post-treatment [9,10].

Diagnosis of specific metastatic sites

Pulmonary metastases

A chest X-ray is the most widely used method of screening. Computed tomography scanning greatly increases diagnostic accuracy with an overall sensitivity up to 60–65%. Doubtful lesions such as subpleural deposits and isolated opacities can be examined by percutaneous needle aspiration. Small pleural effusions, not apparent on chest X-ray, may also be demonstrated.

Bone metastases

Bone scanning is the most accurate and rapid means of screening for bone metastases. Skeletal X-rays are used to demonstrate the degree of bone erosion at a site of metastasis if an alternative explanation for increased isotope uptake, such as trauma or infection, is possible. Percutaneous needle aspiration of bone can be undertaken safely at many sites and is helpful when the diagnosis is uncertain. Magnetic resonance scanning is useful to demonstrate intramedullary metastasis.

Hepatic metastases

Biochemical tests of liver function are the most widely used screening procedure. For imaging the liver, ultrasound and CT scanning are useful for diagnosis of not only hepatic metastases but also adrenal, mesenteric and other sites of abdominal disease [11]. These investigations may confirm metastatic liver disease even if the liver function tests are normal. In lymphomas (particularly Hodgkin's disease), abdominal CT scanning is now the most widely performed staging procedure, useful both for hepatic deposits and also (more commonly) to demonstrate intra-abdominal lymph node involvement.

Brain metastases

Computed tomography scanning is widely available and is the usual preliminary investigation, although it is seldom positive in neurologically normal patients. Magnetic resonance scanning is more sensitive and can show leptomeningeal spread when CT scans are normal.

The role of surgery in diagnosis and staging

With the increasing precision of simpler diagnostic techniques, such as aspiration cytology, percutaneous needle biopsy and CT-guided fine-needle biopsy, major surgical procedures are sometimes unnecessary simply to establish the diagnosis. In carcinoma of the pancreas, for example, it has previously been difficult to obtain histological confirmation without laparotomy. The increasing use of non-surgical techniques (or fine-needle inspiration biopsy) often leads to a preoperative tissue diagnosis. This may allow new therapeutic approaches to be considered in the future, in which planned surgery might be undertaken following preoperative radiotherapy or chemotherapy. With the emphasis on tailoring of treatment to the extent of the disease, the cancer surgeon sometimes performs staging procedures which are not in themselves therapeutic but are intended to assist radiotherapists and medical oncologists in deciding their therapeutic strategy.

Based on these findings, it may sometimes be appropriate to proceed to laparotomy and resection of residual tumour deposits (Table 4.2). Increasingly sophisticated methods of staging may lead to a spurious improvement in outcome, simply because of the 'stage-shift' effect. Accurate staging is not itself directly therapeutic.

Table 4.2 Effects of staging on survival ('stage-shift' effect).

	(a) Tumour diagnosed in 1950s, but with only clinical staging carefully treated with surgery for stages I and II		(b) Same tumour diagnosed and staged in 1980s; treated with surgery for stages I and II as in 1950s	
	All cases (%)	5-year survival (%)	All cases (%)	5-year survival (%)
Stage I: local disease	40	50	10	80
Stage II: local nodules involved	40	20	40	40
Stage III: distant metastasis	20	2	50	10
Overall 5-year survival (%)		28.5		29

Tumour markers

Some malignant tumours produce proteins which can be detected in the blood and which may serve as a marker both of the presence of the tumour and sometimes of its size. Specific tumour markers are generally fusion protein products associated with the malignancy in which an oncogene is translocated and fused to an active promoter of a separate gene [12]. Measurement of these tumour markers has become an important part of the management of testicular and ovarian germ cell tumours, choriocarcinoma and hepatoma. The ideal requirements for a tumour marker are as follows.

1 *The markers should always be produced by the tumour type.* This is not the case for the great majority of markers

Table 4.3 Tumour markers in malignant disease. (a) Serum markers. (b) Molecular markers for diagnosis.

Disease	Marker	Marker in use				Marker still at experimental stage
		Screening	Detection and diagnosis	Staging and prognosis	Follow up	
(a) Serum markers						
Colon cancer	Carcinoembryonic antigen			(X)	X	
Breast cancer	CA-15-3			X	X	X
	CA-27-29					X
Prostate cancer	Prostate-specific antigen	X			X	
Ovarian cancer	CA-125		X		X	
	CA-19-9					X
Thyroid cancer	Thyroglobulin		X		X	
(medullary carcinoma)	Calcitonin		X		X	
Testicular cancer	Human chorionic gonadotrophin		X		X	
	α-Fetoprotein		X		X	
(b) Molecular markers						
Sarcoma:						
Synovial sarcoma	t(X;18)				X	
Ewing's sarcoma	t(11;22)					
Alveolar rhabdomyosarcoma	t(2;13)					
Granulocytic sarcoma	t(9;11)					
Myxoid liposarcoma	t(12;16)					
Round cell liposarcoma	t(12;16)					
Clear cell sarcoma	t(12;22)					
Dermatofibrosarcoma protuberans	t(17;22)					
Melanoma	Tyrosinase					
Adrenal cortical carcinoma	Steroids					
Adrenal medullary carcinoma	Catecholamines					
Lymphoma	t(8;14), t(11;14) t(2;5), t(3;14) CD25 CD44					

(X), occasional use (prostate-specific antigen) or possible future use (carcinoembryonic antigen).

(Table 4.3). In teratoma, α-fetoprotein (AFP) and human chorionic gonadotrophin (HCG) are present in serum in 75% of cases and HCG is present in almost all choriocarcinomas. Apart from carcinoembryonic antigen (CEA) and acid phosphatase, most other markers are of little value in diagnosis or staging.

2 *The marker should give an accurate and sensitive indication of tumour mass.* This is the case with the α-subunit of HCG and AFP in germ cell tumours and prostate-specific antigen (PSA) (to a lesser extent) in prostate cancer. CEA-producing colorectal cancer and CA-125-producing ovarian cancer can also be monitored by serum levels. In many other tumours the marker is inconsistently produced or is too insensitive to be a useful guide to treatment.

3 *The marker should be produced by recurrent and metastatic disease.* One of the major uses of markers is to diagnose recurrence early. Occasionally in teratomas recurrent disease is associated with a rise in either HCG or AFP, even though the original tumour produced both. Marker-negative recurrences (from a previously positive tumour) are rare. Similarly a rise in CEA, PSA or CA-125 may precede clinical evidence of recurrence in bowel, prostate or ovarian cancer, respectively.

4 *The tumour should be amenable to therapy.* There is little value in detecting recurrence early if no treatment is available or should be withheld until symptoms develop. For example, recurrence of pancreatic cancer is seldom curable and early diagnosis of metastasis may serve only to alarm the patient. Conversely, in teratoma a rise in AFP or HCG is a firm indication for full investigation since curative treatment is available.

5 *The marker should be specific for the disease and easy to measure.* Some markers, for example AFP and HCG (α-subunit), are seldom present unless there is a tumour. However, AFP may be raised in pregnancy and with liver disease. CEA can be produced in inflammatory bowel disease as well as in colorectal and pancreatic cancer, and raised levels are found in smokers. The advent of sensitive radioimmunoassay techniques has led to the measurement of AFP and HCG as a routine in germ cell tumours and hepatoma. Some peptide hormones, for example antidiuretic hormone (ADH), are extremely difficult to measure accurately.

6 *The marker should ideally be inexpensive and sensitive enough for population screening.* In ovarian cancer for example, most cases are diagnosed at an advanced and incurable stage so the mortality from this condition is now greater than for cervix and uterus combined. Use of CA-125 is one of the more promising techniques for population screening for this condition.

Examples of tumour markers are given in Table 4.3. Some of these are in daily clinical use and justify more detailed consideration.

Human chorionic gonadotrophin (β-HCG)

The β-subunit is measured to avoid cross-reactivity with luteinizing hormone. Human chorionic gonadotrophin is measured by radioimmunoassay. It is used to detect and monitor therapy in choriocarcinoma and testicular and other germ cell tumours. The half-life ($t_{1/2}$) is 24–36 h, and it is measurable in both blood and urine (where it gives a positive pregnancy test). In addition to its value in monitoring response and relapse, it has been shown that values over 10 000 IU/l are indicative of a poor prognosis in germ cell tumours [12]. A β-core fragment has recently been described which is of low molecular weight and is found in the urine. It seems to be produced by a wide variety of non-trophoblastic tumours. Its role as a marker is not yet defined.

α-Fetoprotein

This protein is similar in size to albumin and is a major serum component before birth. It may cross the placenta and be detected in maternal blood. It is produced during liver regeneration and is elevated in viral hepatitis and cirrhosis. α-Fetoprotein is produced by malignant yolk-sac elements in germ cell tumours (see Chapter 19) and by the malignant hepatocytes in hepatomas. Occasionally, after successful treatment with chemotherapy, a persistent rise in AFP occurs, presumed to be a drug effect on the liver. This can be a source of confusion in assessing response. It is also present in small amounts in some patients with pancreatic carcinoma and occasionally in gastric carcinoma. The plasma half-life is 5–7 days.

Placental alkaline phosphatase (PLAP)

This is an isoenzyme of alkaline phosphatase which is found in the serum in patients with seminoma. It is associated with bulky disease and disappears quickly on treatment and is thus of marginal value in monitoring response.

Carcinoembryonic antigen

Carcinoembryonic antigen refers to one of a family of glycoproteins produced by many epithelial tumours, the molecule usually being demonstrable at the cell surface rather than at the cytoplasm. It is produced by normal colonic epithelium but is not usually present in the blood unless there is inflammation or neoplasia involving the epithelium. It is present in 25% of cases of Dukes B colonic cancer, 45% of Dukes C and 70% of metastatic cases. Its low incidence in early stages makes it of no value in screening. It is also found in plasma in pancreatitis, heavy smokers, ulcerative colitis and gastritis, thus limiting its usefulness in diagnosis. Its value in early diagnosis of recurrent disease is limited by the lack of successful therapy in the majority of patients. Conversely, early surgical exploration of potential local anastomotic recurrences are increasingly undertaken in patients in whom CT scanning coupled with a rise in CEA level has aided the diagnosis while the patient is still asymptomatic. The increasing use of surgical resection, radiation and chemotherapy in patients with advanced colorectal cancer has led to an increased use of this tumour marker. Carcinoembryonic antigen is elevated in approximately 60% of cases of advanced ovarian cancer and 40–70% of advanced breast cancers. It is therefore of little value in diagnosis of metastasis from an unknown primary site.

CA-125

This is a complex antigen which is a glycoprotein of high molecular weight produced in coelomic epithelium and re-expressed in epithelial ovarian, pancreatic and breast cancer. Four-fifths of ovarian cancers are associated with antigenaemia and rising or falling levels correlate with disease in 93%. Levels above the upper limit of normal (35 U/ml) are not specific for ovarian cancer (being found in endometriosis, hepatitis and benign ovarian lesions) and are thus of limited value for screening. During treatment, CA-125 levels fall, but persistent disease is often found even when plasma levels are normal. However, elevated or rising levels can be used to detect early relapse after treatment. A rising level during chemotherapy indicates treatment failure.

CA-19-9

This is a mucin-like antigen which is a polysialated Lewis blood group antigen. Elevated levels are found in 80% of cases of pancreatic cancer and 75% of cases of advanced colorectal cancer. However, it may also be present in serum in benign hepatic and biliary tract disease [13]. Its value is limited by non-specificity and the lack of effective treatment of pancreatic cancer.

Molecular staging of cancer

Occult locoregional spread of cancer is a common cause of local recurrence, and an early indicator of subclinical dissemination [14]. Since malignancies develop from the progressive accumulation of mutations in genes of somatic cells, these mutations can be used as powerful molecular markers. Useful examples would include the detection of mutations in the urine of patients with bladder cancer and in the stools of patients with colorectal cancer—identical to those present in the primary tumour [15]. Genetic changes can be detected in metastatic tumour cells by fluorescent *in situ* hybridization [16]. Molecular assays can detect small clusters of cancer cells that would otherwise have been missed in routine histopathological staining. Molecular staging of cancer may soon have improved clinical implications. In node-negative breast cancer, for instance, molecular staging might demonstrate a small number of cancer cells thereby identifying cases in which systemic therapy is clearly indicated.

References

1 Union Internationale Contre le Cancer. Sobin LH, Wittekind Ch, eds. *TNM Atlas: Classification of Malignant Tumours*, 5th edn. New York: Wiley-Liss, 1997.
2 Bragg DG, Rubin P, Youker JE, eds. *Oncologic Imaging*. New York: Pergamon Press, 1985.
3 Epstein DM, Stephenson LW, Gefter WB *et al.* The value of CT in the preoperative assessment of lung cancer. *Radiology* 1986; 161: 423–7.
4 Siegelman SS, Zerhouni EA, Leo FP *et al.* CT of the solitary pulmonary nodule. *Am J Roentgenol* 1980; 135: 1–13.
5 Brant-Zawadski M, Norman D, eds. *Magnetic Resonance Imaging of the Central Nervous System*. New York: Raven Press, 1987.
6 Barish MA, Yucel EK, Ferrucci JT. Magnetic resonance cholangiopancreatography. *N Engl J Med* 1999; 341: 258–64.
7 Krag D, Moffat F. Nuclear medicine and the surgeon. *Lancet* 1999; 354: 1019–22.
8 van Tinteren H, Hoekstra OS, Smit EF *et al.* Effectiveness of positron-emission tomography in the preoperative assessment of patients with suspected non-small-cell lung cancer. *Lancet* 2002; 359: 1388–92.
9 Eary JF. Nuclear medicine in cancer diagnosis. *Lancet* 1999; 354: 853–7.
10 Bomanji JB, Costa DC, Ell PJ. Clinical role of positron emission tomography in oncology. *Lancet Oncol* 2001; 2(3): 157–64.
11 Zeman RK, Paushter DM, Schiebler ML *et al.* Hepatic imaging: current status. *Radiol Clin N Am* 1985; 23: 473–87.

12 Lindblom A, Liljegren A. Tumour markers in malignancies. *Br Med J* 2000; 320: 424–7.

13 Begent RHJ, Rustin GJR. Tumour markers: from carcino-embryonic antigen to products of hybridoma technology. *Cancer Surv* 1989; 8: 108–21.

14 Caldas C. Molecular staging of cancer: is it time? *Lancet* 1997; 350: 231.

15 Sidransky D, Tokino T, Hamilton SR *et al.* Identification of *ras* oncogene mutations in the stool of patients with curable colorectal cancer. *Science* 1992; 256: 102–5.

16 Pack S, Vortmeyer AO, Pak E, Liotta LA, Zhuang Z. Detection of gene deletion in single metastatic tumour cells in lymph node tissue by fluorescent in-situ hybridization. *Lancet* 1997; 350: 264–5.

Radiotherapy

Ever since the discovery of X-rays by Roentgen in 1895, attempts have been made not only to understand their physical nature but also to use them both in the biological sciences and in a variety of human illnesses. The development of the X-ray tube rapidly led to clinical applications, first as a diagnostic tool and later for therapy in patients with malignant disease. The discovery of radium by Marie and Pierre Curie in 1898 also resulted in the use of radioactive materials for the approach to cancer, since surgery was the only alternative approach available at that time. Over the past 80 years our understanding of the physical characteristics, biological effects and clinical roles of ionizing radiation has greatly increased.

To understand the nature of radioactivity and radioactive decay, it is important to grasp the concept of a natural spectrum of electromagnetic waves whose energy varies widely, in inverse proportion to the length of the wave itself. This spectrum (Fig. 5.1) includes X-rays (very high energy and very short wavelength), visible light rays (of intermediate wavelength and energy) and also radiowaves (of generally longer wavelength and lower energy) which are responsible for modern telecommunications and include the transmission signals for radio and television. Of these various types of electromagnetic wave, only X-rays and gamma rays (the terms are almost interchangeable) are of sufficiently high energy to produce the ionization of atoms which occurs when a beam of radiation passes through biological tissue.

In the process of ionization, the essential event is the displacement of an electron from its orbital path around the nucleus of the atom. This creates an unstable or ionized atom, and a free electron which is normally 'captured' by a neighbouring atom, which then becomes equally unstable because of its possession of an extra negative electric charge. When radiation beams pass through living tissue, the intensity, duration and site of these ionization events can be controlled by varying the characteristics of the radiation source. This permits a deliberate and controlled cellular destruction in the case of therapeutic radiation (radiotherapy), whereas with diagnostic radiation, trivial and short-lived alterations occur which usually have no permanent biological effect. The creation of the radiographic image is due to the differential alteration of the X-ray beam by biological tissues containing atoms of differing atomic weights.

Sources and production of ionizing radiation

Radioactive isotopes

Radioactivity is an unalterable property of many naturally occurring atoms which exist in a relatively unstable state. Although the identity of any given atom is defined by the number of protons and electrons it possesses, the atoms of any one element may contain differing numbers of nuclear neutrons, so that their atomic weights (as determined by the proton and neutron component) differ. Such atoms or *isotopes* occur naturally in fixed proportions, and most pure substances (particularly metals such

Table 5.1 Therapeutically useful isotopes.

Isotope	Type of radiation	Energy (MeV)	Half-life
^{60}Co	β,γ	0.31(β), 1.17 and 1.33 (γ)	5.3 years
^{137}Cs	β,γ	0.51 (β) and 0.66 (γ)	30 years
^{131}I	β,γ	0.61 (β) and 0.36 (γ)	8 days
^{198}Au	β,γ	0.96 (β) and 0.41 (γ)	2.7 days
^{32}P	β	1.71 (β)	14 days
^{192}Ir	γ	0.36–0.6 (γ)	74 days
^{226}Ra (decays to radon, then Ra A,B,C)	α then β,γ	1.0 (γ)	1620 years for radium but 3–27 min for Ra A,B,C

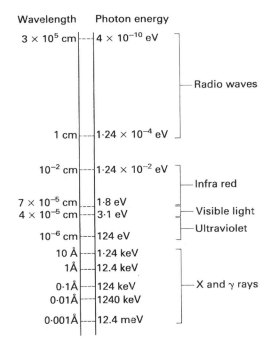

Fig. 5.1 The electromagnetic spectrum.

as iron, manganese and cobalt) consist of mixtures of these isotopes. Emission of radioactivity is one of the consequences of physical decay of unstable atoms resulting in a final and more stable state. The rate and intensity of these emissions varies with each element.

There is a wide variety of naturally occurring radioactive materials, whose chief characteristic is the emission of electromagnetic waves of a frequency which can produce ionization within biological materials. Historically, these emissions have been divided into α, β and γ waves, depending on the characteristics of the emission. Alpha particles are no more than helium nuclei, emitted from unstable or decaying radionuclides. It is worth remember-

ing that although many of the properties of radioactive emission are better understood in terms of their characteristic waveforms, the 'wave' also has features of a particle. Alpha and beta emissions are best understood in terms of these features since α particles are positively charged helium nuclei, with a substantial mass, and β particles are no more than electrons, with a negative charge but almost no mass. Gamma rays, on the other hand, carry no charge.

Although α, β and γ rays can all produce ionization in tissues, it is the gamma rays which have the greatest application in radiation therapy. For example, in a reaction of great clinical importance, the unstable isotope of cobalt, with an atomic number of 60, disintegrates to a more stable isotope (atomic number 59) by discharging one of its nuclear neutrons, together with gamma rays. The characteristics of the emitted gamma radiation are constant for this particular reaction, and the rate of the nuclear disintegration is unalterable, such that after 5.33 years, exactly half of the original radioactive material still remains, thus defining the radioactive half-life of ^{60}Co. The half-life is an important concept in theoretical and clinical work, and varies between a fraction of a second, and hundreds or thousands of years (Table 5.1). Radium, widely used before the introduction of more suitable radioactive materials, has a half-life of 1620 years, which meant that radioactive sources for therapeutic use never needed replacing. Beta particles, or electrons, however, are now increasingly used as their characteristics are generally more suitable. Other atomic fragments are being studied since they have theoretical advantages as a result of their different biological effects. These include neutrons, protons and pi-mesons.

Although the early radioactive substances discovered by the Curies and others were all naturally occurring, modern high-energy physics has provided ready access to many new materials, or artificially manufactured isotopes. These substances, *radionuclides*, are generally manufactured in nuclear reactors by heavy particle bombardment of natural materials. The chief advantage is that their properties more closely resemble the theoretical ideal for radioactive half-life, gamma-ray characteristics and intensity, than any natural substance. The changing demands of both diagnosis, for example in radioisotope imaging, and therapy have led to ever-increasing attempts at producing new radioactive isotopes with differing radiation characteristics. For therapeutic work, this includes the production of both sealed and unsealed sources. For sealed sources, the radioactive material is physically enclosed by an impenetrable barrier such as the platinum casing of a typical radium or caesium needle, so that the radioactive material can be inserted into the tissue to be irradiated, and then removed at some predetermined time. With unsealed sources, such as ^{131}I, the isotope is physically ingested either by mouth or by injection, passing via the bloodstream to the end organ and taken up (in this case, by the thyroid), where the effects of the radioactive emission cause local damage to both the normal thyroid gland and the cancer within it. The isotope cannot then be recovered.

Unsealed sources are widely used in diagnostic work such as the radioactive technetium bone or brain scan. In therapeutic work, the most specific and ideal application is for carcinoma of the thyroid, where radioactive isotopes of iodine (usually ^{131}I) are given by mouth, and selectively taken up by the thyroid gland and thyroid cancer cells providing 'internal' irradiation to a high intensity without compromising other organs by the delivery of an unacceptable dose of radiation at an unwanted site. Use of injectable radioactive phosphorus (^{32}P) for bone marrow irradiation in polycythaemia rubra vera is another well-known example. Radionuclide therapy provides specificity, efficiency and low toxicity, together with excellent palliation and the prospect of repeated treatment. However, limitations include the unavoidable patient isolation, storage of radioactive waste and the high cost—particularly of some of the newer forms of treatments. Nonetheless, the current therapeutic indications of unsealed radionuclide treatment for malignant disease have expanded in recent years.

For use in clinical work, the choice of either naturally occurring or artificially produced radioactive isotopes will depend on the clinical requirement. For example, in interstitial implantation work, where radioactive needles are directly placed adjacent to or even within the malignant tissue, caesium needles have increasingly been employed in preference to radium, because of the more suitable characteristics of the emitted radiation from this material. This is because the specific activity (number of radioactive

disintegrations per second) is so high with radium that protection for doctors, radiographers, nurses and other staff has always been a major problem. With caesium, however, the specific activity is substantially lower, making protection easier.

Radioactive isotopes are also used as a source of external radiation (teletherapy). All clinical departments place a heavy clinical reliance on their external therapy techniques since the majority of tumours are deeply situated and inaccessible to irradiation by direct implantation (brachytherapy). Nowadays, when gamma irradiation from a major radioactive source is employed, the most common choice of material is ^{60}Co, a material which emits a high-energy gamma ray (mean energy 1.2 MeV) of sufficient penetration to allow for treatment of deeply situated tumours. Cobalt-60 has a reasonably satisfactory half-life of 5.3 years, so that major source replacement will not be required more than every 3–4 years.

A traditional cobalt unit is in essence no more than a cylindrical source of ^{60}Co produced artificially within a nuclear fission pile, placed in a protective shell made of lead, and supplied with a simple mechanism for moving the source into the treatment position when required. This type of equipment, though largely rendered obselete because of replacement by linear accelerators (see below), has advantages of reliability and longevity, as well as being relatively inexpensive to purchase and maintain. Its disadvantages are that there is a substantial 'penumbra' of scattered radiation, which forms a significant part of the edge of the beam, and that treatment times can be lengthy—particularly when the source has started to age, since radioactive decay results in a loss of residual radioactive material and treatment time increases proportionately.

Artificial production of X-rays and particles

Shortly after the discovery of radium by the Curies, Roentgen constructed the first X-ray apparatus, consisting of a sealed glass vacuum tube containing an electrode at one end and a target at the other. Heating the electrode resulted in a discharge of electrons which travelled relatively easily through the vacuum, to bombard the target at the other end of the tube. This produced characteristic rays which, like those of radium, could create an image on a photographic plate. The nature of these rays was uncertain; *X-rays* therefore seemed the most suitable title. It gradually became clear that X-rays and gamma rays were fundamentally similar although their method of production is quite different. Unlike the gamma irradiation from radioactive materials whose characteristics cannot be changed other than by altering either the choice or the purity of the material, X-rays of quite different properties can be produced simply by varying the voltage input to the cathode of the X-ray tube.

X-rays used for diagnostic radiology are generated in a low-voltage machine (for example, 50 kV) and have a longer wavelength and less penetrating power. By contrast, therapeutic X-rays are much more powerful, varying from 50 kV up to 30 MeV, a 600-fold increase. As voltage is increased, X-rays of shorter wavelength are produced, which have far greater penetration within human tissue.

For therapeutic use, one of the chief criteria for successful treatment is the availability of X-rays of sufficient penetrating power, or depth dose, to deal effectively with deep-seated tumours. For this reason, departments of radiotherapy need a range of equipment with a wide spectrum of clinically useful X-ray beams available to deal with both superficial tumours such as skin cancers and those more deeply situated, such as tumours of the mediastinum or pelvis. With conventional or *orthovoltage* X-ray equipment, the maximum deposition of radiation energy is in the superficial tissues, with a steep fall-off (Fig. 5.2), such that the dosage received by a deep tumour

which may be 10 cm or more below the skin surface is low, and limited by the skin reaction that this treatment will inevitably cause. The physical and electromagnetic problems of safely applying a very high tension (voltage) input had to be overcome before further progress could be made.

Fortunately, most of these technical difficulties were solved in the 1960s with the advent of an entirely fresh approach to the generation of high-energy megavoltage beams and the development of the modern linear accelerator. The principal feature is the acceleration of electrons down a cylindrical 'waveguide' terminating in the deliberate bombardment of a fixed target by electrons travelling almost at the speed of light, thus producing a beam of much higher intensity (Fig. 5.3). As well as possessing much greater depth dose, these beams typically have far less in the way of scattered radiation, leading to a much cleaner, higher quality and more precise beam with a narrower penumbra than with traditional cobalt apparatus. In addition, the output (or dose rate) is considerably greater, leading to shorter treatment times. The linear accelerator has now become the standard workhorse of modern radiotherapy departments in the developed world. A further important advantage of this equipment is that the target can be moved out of position, yielding a beam of high-velocity electrons (instead of X-rays) of 30 MeV energy or more which can be useful therapeutically in certain clinical situations (see below).

To the clinician, the fundamental difference between X-ray and electron therapy lies in their entirely different depth-dose characteristics (Fig. 5.2). With X-ray or gamma-ray therapy, the amount of radiation energy deposited at any given depth of tissue (the depth dose) falls

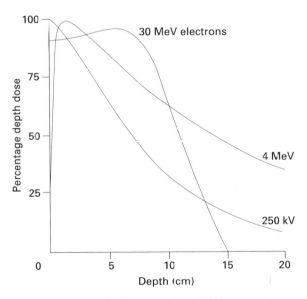

Fig. 5.2 Typical depth–dose curves for radiotherapy equipment (kilovoltage, megavoltage and 30 MeV electron beam). There is skin 'build-up' over the first centimetre for megavoltage therapy but not for kilovoltage or electron treatment. Depth dose for both megavoltage and electron beam therapy is much superior to kilovoltage treatment and the 'skin-sparing' effect has great clinical benefit.

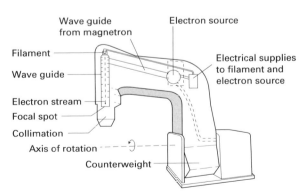

Fig. 5.3 Schematic representation of an isocentrically mounted 4–8 MeV linear accelerator. From Meredith & Massey (1972) with permission.

off exponentially, which means that however powerful the source and whatever the distance, unwanted areas of tissue will be irradiated, both superficial to the tumour area and also beyond it. The entrance and exit dose will irradiate a substantial volume of normal host tissue, and this unavoidable characteristic is usually the limiting factor in a course of treatment. With electron therapy this disadvantage is at least partly overcome, since the beam decays completely at a depth entirely dependent on the energy of the electron beam.

With low- and medium-voltage X-rays, the energy deposited in the tissues is critically dependent on the mean atomic number of the tissue in which this deposition is occurring. With high-voltage X-rays, gamma rays and electrons, the energy absorbed by the tissue is much less dependent on the atomic number, so that the drawbacks of very high bone absorption (with its twin problems of dosage inhomogeneity and radionecrosis) are largely avoided. Radiotherapists are therefore very careful when irradiating superficial lesions situated over bone or cartilage, which require treatment with low-voltage (superficial) beams. For this reason, electron therapy is often preferred in these cases, particularly for skin tumours which overlie an area of cartilage. Common examples include basal cell carcinomas on the nose or pinna of the ear.

A further intriguing possibility under active clinical trial at present is the use of heavy charged and uncharged particles, including neutrons, protons and pi-mesons. All of these beams have theoretical advantages, although the capital expenditure required for the development and building of neutron and charged particle generators is substantially greater than the cost of more conventional equipment. Only a few centres throughout the world have these resources available at present.

Biological properties of ionizing radiation

Tumour sensitivity

Since the beginning of the twentieth century, clinical scientists have been fascinated (and puzzled) by the extraordinary cellular events which occur when living tissue is exposed to a beam of ionizing radiation. It is now clear that radiation-induced damage may be lethal, resulting in cell death, or sublethal, in which case the cellular damage can be partially or completely repaired. In general, the degree of radiosensitivity of any given tumour type will depend not only on the immediate damage sustained by the cell (a measure of its true 'intrinsic' sensitivity) but also on

its ability to repair the sublethal damage that has been caused. Although a high degree of radiosensitivity is generally required if there is to be any hope of a radiation cure, other factors may prevent the realization of this aim; radiosensitivity is not in itself sufficient. Acute lymphoblastic leukaemia (ALL), for instance, is highly radiosensitive, since small malignant lymphoblasts are permanently damaged by a relatively low dose of radiation. However, the widespread nature of this disease, which by definition affects the whole of the bone marrow and therefore every organ supplied by the peripheral bloodstream, made it impossible until recently to deliver curative radiotherapy without fatal overirradiation. The modern technique of allogeneic bone marrow transplantation (BMT) has resulted in safe delivery of total-body irradiation to a sufficiently high dosage for total irreversible ablation of the malignant marrow elements. It is not the bone marrow transplant itself which is the therapeutic event, but the lethal radiation damage inflicted on the leukaemic cell population.

The physicochemical events which take place within the radiation-damaged cells are far from understood. Although there is little doubt that the important target site is the nuclear DNA, it is less common for the damage to be inflicted as a result of a 'direct hit', though this mechanism will certainly produce irreversible cleavage of the DNA strands. More commonly the effects are indirect, resulting in the production of unstable, highly reactive and short-lived free radicals which in turn produce destruction of the normal DNA molecule with which they rapidly react. The probability of a lethal cell injury varies not only with the quantity of radiation energy deposited in the tissues (a function of the output of the radiation beam) but also with the intensity of the beam and with its 'type', that is, whether the radiation is produced by gamma rays, electrons, neutrons or other particles. These differences give rise to the concept of linear energy transfer (LET) which refers to the amount of radiation energy transferred to the tissue per unit track length by the particular beam. In general, kilovoltage beams of X-rays have a higher LET than megavoltage beams, and neutron beams have a very much higher LET than X-rays or gamma rays. Thus appropriate adjustments in total doses will have to be made if neutron therapy, for example, is offered as an alternative to conventional treatment. Another important principle is that the relatively protective effect of hypoxia (on tumour cells) is particularly apparent with beams of relatively low LET. This is one of the reasons why neutron therapy was long thought to be more effective regardless of the state of oxygenation of the malignant tissues.

Experimental studies have shown that human tumour cells have markedly different intrinsic radiosensitivities which closely parallel clinical experience. Our present understanding of this correlation postulates two components to cell kill: the α component which is log-linear (exponential) and therefore appears as a straight line in dose–survival curves (Fig. 5.4); and a bending or β-component which occurs over a shorter dose range and at low dose levels. Intrinsic differences in sensitivity are most marked in the low-dose region (clinically of greatest importance) below 2 Gy (200 rad) per treatment fraction, and low-dose-rate irradiation is likely to exaggerate these differences. Indeed, at low dose rates, less sensitive cells become relatively more resistant. This is often forwarded as an argument for larger fractions in less sensitive tumours. In the linear quadratic mathematical model, using an α component which is the linear dose function and β the square of the dose, cell survival is the common end-point. Fractionation tends to spare late-responding tissues more than early-responding tissues and tumours.

In other clinical circumstances, failure of radiation therapy may occur because of the recurrence of disease after apparently successful radiation treatment. This is a frequent event, for example in squamous cell carcinoma of the bronchus, where careful assessment by chest X-ray and even bronchoscopy may well demonstrate an apparently satisfactory response to treatment. When relapse occurs,

often 1–2 years after primary treatment, what can we suggest by way of explanation? One widely held view, for which there is a good deal of experimental evidence, is that at the time of the initial treatment, there is a spectrum of cellular sensitivity to the radiation, and that the degree of oxygenation of each cell is the key determining factor. A great deal of radiobiological work has gone into defining and characterizing this phenomenon, and almost all studies (both with experimental animals and *in vitro* tissue culture systems) have shown that well-oxygenated cells are substantially more radiosensitive than those which are anoxic.

This difference in sensitivity may be reflected in a two- or three-fold increase in the dosage required for tumour eradication in an anoxic environment (Fig. 5.4), and the clinical importance of this observation is thought by many to be critical, since cells far removed from a good arterial supply will inevitably be relatively anoxic. In large tumours with a relatively rapid growth rate and in areas of necrosis where vascularization is poor, anoxia may be a major cause of radioresistance, and experiments using microelectrodes for measurement of oxygen tension have confirmed these theoretical predictions.

Quite apart from the oxygen effect, the progenitor cells will not be equally radiosensitive, so that recurrence after apparently successful treatment may be due to repopulation through regeneration of the radioresistant stem cells within the tumour. This can take place either after a complete course of radiotherapy, or rapidly, even between fractions given, say, on a daily basis. There is at least some evidence that regrowth through repopulation may be more delayed with malignant tissues than with normal host cells, and that this may be an important basis for the difference between the relatively adequate regenerative capability of many normal tissues, in contrast to the more permanent destructive effects on malignant tumours. This is analogous to the effects of chemotherapy on normal and malignant tissue (see Chapter 6).

Fractionation and cell death

Fractionation, the use of repeated dosage of radiation within a course of treatment, has long been the subject of considerable interest. Early radiation workers rapidly realized that repeated use of modest radiation doses seemed to be the best method of safely delivering a higher total dose of radiation than would be possible with a single large treatment, and that, in general, led to a greater likelihood of cure. Interest in fractionation has developed because of a natural desire not only to understand the

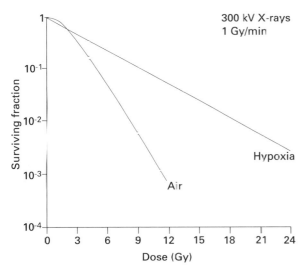

Fig. 5.4 Fractionation: the effect of repeated doses of radiation. Fractionation increases the differential cytotoxic effect on normal and malignant tissue.

mechanisms of radiation-induced cell damage, but also to learn how best to exploit this phenomenon and to advise the clinician as to the optimal choice of fraction size and overall treatment time. These are important details which might make the difference between success and failure. In most single-dose experiments, the degree of damage to the malignant cell (usually measured by inhibition of cell division) is directly proportional, in a log-linear fashion, to the radiation dose (Fig. 5.4). The important additional feature is that at low dosage, the steep curve is flattened to form a characteristic 'shoulder'. With relatively more radioresistant cells (such as malignant melanoma) the shoulder will be broader, and the rest of the curve less steep.

Most theorists agree that the shoulder region represents an area of sublethal damage, from which repair is possible. With repeated or fractionated treatment, further radiation damage can be inflicted before completion of this repair, although naturally the degree of cell recovery between fractions will depend on the interval and intensity of each fraction of treatment (Fig. 5.5).

In addition, fractionation of treatment encourages early improvement in tissue oxygenation which, by reduction of the tumour bulk, leads to relief of vascular obstruction, a more effective blood supply and greater sensitivity to subsequent doses of irradiation, again due to the oxygen effect. In addition to these theoretical advantages, fractionated treatment has other practical benefits since the earlier fractions often produce a significant improvement in clinical well-being, allowing better tolerance of the total course. This allows much greater flexibility

from a course rather than a single treatment, permitting, for example, for a change in radiation volume and/or dose rate, which may well be called for as the tumour begins to resolve.

Conversely, lengthy periods of fractionated treatment—often up to 6 weeks in current practice—carry the potential disadvantage of tumour cell repopulation during the course of therapy, with acceleration of repopulating clonogenic cells as little as 1 week after initiation of treatment. For this and other reasons there is increasing interest in the concept of continuous hyperfractionated treatment, using two or three treatment fractions in a single day and treating the patient within a much shorter period of time, even including weekends, for (say) 2–3 weeks rather than the conventional 6-week period.

Despite these general comments, there have been few satisfactory studies comparing different fractionation regimens. Most radiotherapists rely on approaches which have been empirically tested and found acceptable in terms of both effectiveness and toxicity. For example, lengthy fractionation regimens of 6 weeks of daily treatment are often used for squamous carcinomas, while other radiotherapists offer treatment which takes no more than 3 or 4 weeks. Very careful estimates of dose equivalence have to be employed when comparing treatment regimens since all radiotherapists know that, for example, the radiobiological effect of a single dose of 10 Gy is greatly in excess of the effect produced by 10 daily doses of 1 Gy. A yardstick for measurement of dose equivalence is therefore essential, not only for prospective trials of fractionation regimens but also for the radiotherapist who may sometimes need to deviate from the standard regimen for a whole host of reasons. Unexpected machine breakdown, pressures on equipment and staff shortages can all occur unpredictably from time to time.

Response of biological tissues to radiation

Normal tissues

In clinical practice, successful eradication of malignant cells depends on the difference between the sensitivity (and/or repair capacity) of these cells compared with those of normal surrounding tissues also subjected to radiation therapy. However precise our tumour imaging with isotope scanning, computed tomography or magnetic resonance imaging technology, this will always remain a limiting factor. Figure 5.6 demonstrates the relatively narrow gap within which the radiotherapist has

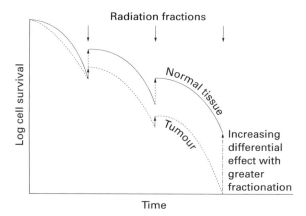

Fig. 5.5 Effect of oxygen concentration on cytotoxicity of X-rays. The survival of Hela cells are shown under conditions of hypoxia and in air.

to operate, between tumour and host tissues. The more radiosensitive the tumour, the wider is this therapeutic 'window' and the lower is the dose required—allowing a greater chance of cure with few, if any, side-effects. Since the adverse effects of radiation limit the clinician in choice of dosage, an understanding of the radiation tolerance of normal host tissues is an important facet of the radiotherapist's training and practice. Very wide discrepancies of the radiation tolerance of different organs have been demonstrated (Table 5.2); in general, the most radiosensi-

tive (and easily damaged) tissues are those with rapid cell division—the bone marrow, the stem cells of the gonads and the epithelial lining of the alimentary tract.

A particularly tragic and clear-cut illustration of the critical importance of radiation dose for long-term damage was provided by the unintended overirradiation of over 200 cancer patients treated in the UK at a single centre in 1988 (Tobias 2000). Due to the miscalibration of a radiocobalt source, most of these patients received doses of 25% above the recommended prescribed level, with varying effects dependent upon the site. Many patients treated for breast carcinoma suffered profound local effects in the breast itself, together with local chest wall damage (including rib fracture) and in some cases a brachial plexus radioneuropathy. It seems clear that relatively small dose excesses ('small' at least in comparison with current drug therapy) can, for the radiotherapist, result in disastrous and in many cases irreversible consequences.

Clinically, there is an important distinction to be drawn between early, *acute*, effects and later, *chronic*, damage. It is not necessarily the intensity of the acute reaction which determines the probability and duration of the long-term effects. Even where recovery from acute irradiation appears complete, the 'reserve' of stem cells in these organs is often permanently depleted, so that further treatment with either radiation therapy or cytotoxic drugs may well produce a surprising degree of tissue damage including, for example, marrow suppression. Understanding of this long-term but latent (invisible) damage is of great importance since increasing numbers of cancer patients are likely to be offered both these forms of therapy.

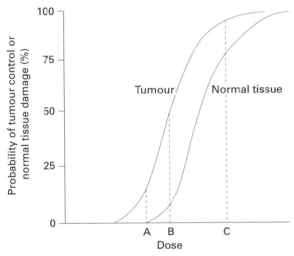

Fig. 5.6 The relation between X-ray dose and outcome of radiotherapy. From Withers (1992) with permission.

Table 5.2 Radiosensitivity of normal and malignant tissue.

Radiosensitivity	Normal	Malignant
Highly sensitive	Marrow	Lymphoma
	Gonad	Leukaemia
	Gut (mucosa)	Seminoma
	Lymphatic tissue	Ewing's sarcoma
	Eye (lens)	Many embryonal tumours
Moderately sensitive	Liver	Small-cell lung cancer
	Kidney	Breast cancer
	Lung	Squamous carcinomas (including
	Skin	gynaecological, head and neck, and
	Breast	skin tumours)
	Gut wall	Adenocarcinomas of the bowel
	Nervous tissue	Glioma
Relatively insensitive	Bone	Sarcoma of bone and connective tissue
	Connective tissue	Muscle
	Melanoma	

Highly radiosensitive tissues

Haemopoietic tissues

The bone marrow is exceedingly sensitive to irradiation. In humans, a single total-body dose of 4 Gy would prove lethal to about half of all patients, the majority of these deaths due to early myelosuppression producing anaemia, neutropenia and thrombocytopenia. With localized treatment at high dose (a much more common clinical situation), long-lasting inhibition of myelopoiesis occurs, but usually without appreciable effect on the blood count. Lymphopenia is a well-recognized complication of localized radiotherapy at any site, resulting from irradiation of the blood as it passes through the beam — a consequence of the extreme radiosensitivity of the small lymphocyte. Allogeneic BMT has permitted whole-body irradiation to a higher dose (often up to 10 Gy) as part of the therapy for acute leukaemia and other diseases, including non-Hodgkin's lymphoma and myeloma. In addition, large areas of the body can now be treated with therapeutic irradiation for widespread and painful bony metastases (for example, from myeloma or carcinoma of the prostate) without recourse to marrow transplantation techniques, since the unirradiated marrow is able to compensate by increased production. This is the basis of so-called 'hemibody irradiation', an increasingly used method of simple palliation for patients with widespread metastatic disease, which can be repeated to the opposite half of the body providing a suitable gap of 6–8 weeks is allowed between the two fractions of treatment.

The gonads

In the testes and ovary, small single doses of radiotherapy can permanently damage reproductive function, although the testis is undoubtedly more sensitive. It is likely that some of the primitive spermatogonia (the precursors of the spermatocytes) may be sensitive to a dose of as little as 1 Gy, although a dose as low as this would be unlikely to reduce the human sperm count to zero. The radiation sensitivity of the hormone-producing testicular Leydig cell is very much less, so that large doses of radiotherapy to the human testis do not result in loss of secondary sexual characteristics. In the female, single doses of 4–5 Gy have been used to induce artificial menopause, although some 30% of women appear to continue regular menstruation following this single fraction of radiation. Fractionated treatment to 10–12 Gy results in complete cessation of menses in virtually every patient.

Moderately radiosensitive tissues

This group is characterized by relatively low cell turnover rates which are paralleled by a relative — but by no means complete — insensitivity to radiation; these include nerve cells, including the brain itself, as well as the spinal cord and peripheral nervous system, skin, kidney, gut and other sites (Table 5.2).

Nervous tissue

The nervous system is of great concern partly because the sequelae of damage to the central nervous system can be both profound and irreversible, and also because, for the large majority of malignant brain tumours, radiation therapy is much the most valuable non-surgical modality available (see Chapter 11). During the early acute phase of radiation response, the blood vessels, nerve cells and supporting glial structures are all injured directly; sufficiently large doses may result in acute cerebral oedema and a sudden rise in intracranial pressure. These changes will gradually subside, but chronic effects include demyelination, vascular damage with proliferation of subendothelial fibrous tissue and, eventually, brain necrosis if the dose is sufficiently high. It is generally accepted that the hypothalamus, brainstem and upper cervical spine are rather more sensitive to radiation than other parts of the brain, and it is also thought that concurrent administration of chemotherapy (chiefly methotrexate and vincristine) may also reduce radiation tolerance.

Irradiation of the spinal cord may pose even more problems, particularly since this may be unavoidable in, for example, the palliation of painful bony metastases of the spine. The radiation tolerance of the spinal cord is governed by a variety of important details such as the length of cord irradiated, the fractionation employed and the total dose given. It is widely held that for a 10 cm length of cord, a total dose of 40 Gy in 4 weeks is safe although many clinicians err on the side of great caution since radiation myelitis, leading to irreversible paraparesis, is such an appalling complication. Recent work with total-body irradiation has shown that a single dose of about 10 Gy delivered to the whole length of the spinal cord very rarely produces significant neurological sequelae, although the mildest (reversible) late complication, that of Lhermitte's syndrome of paraesthesiae in the extremities on flexion of the neck, is often encountered. Moreover, with prophylactic spinal cord irradiation in children with medulloblastoma, the risk of clinically significant neurological sequelae, after doses as high as 30 Gy applied over 5–6 weeks to the whole of the spinal cord, seems acceptably low. In general, careful fractionation should be employed wherever a significant length of cord is likely to be irradiated in a patient whose survival may be prolonged. For palliative radiation treatment it seems prudent to recommend the lowest effective dose which is compatible with durable pain relief, particularly since further treatment may well be required, inevitably adding to the possibility of cord damage.

The skin

A portion of skin will be irradiated in all patients treated by external methods of X-ray therapy. Historically, the skin reaction was the chief guide in determining the total radiation dose. With modern high-energy (megavoltage) equipment, far fewer severe skin reactions are seen, since the scattered radiation component of these beams is almost exclusively in the forward direction so that maximum energy deposition takes place well beneath the skin surface (Fig. 5.2). None the less, clinically important skin reactions can still pose major problems both with orthovoltage and even with megavoltage beams (Table 5.3). Typically, the changes consist of an erythema of increasing severity, leading to dry and then moist desquamation, followed (if the radiation therapy is discontinued) by a repair process associated with progressive fibrosis, hyperplasia of vascular elements (sometimes resulting in telangiectasia much later on) and also by excessive pigmentation which may be permanent, although depigmentation can also occur. If the skin is further irradiated at a time when moist desquamation is evident, then extensive skin and subcutaneous necrosis may occur; this takes place when the treatment is separated by months or even years. It is therefore unwise to attempt re-irradiation of recurrent skin carcinomas, since the risk of necrosis is ever present and such cases are usually better treated by surgery. Skin 'appendages' such as sweat glands, sebaceous glands and hair follicles are also damaged directly by radiation. Radiation-induced epilation of the scalp is an in-

evitable drawback of whole-brain irradiation for cerebral metastases, which is in other respects an effective technique with few side-effects. Hair regrowth will usually occur, given time, even when a radical dose has been used as, for example, in children with medulloblastoma.

The eye

The eye is frequently irradiated, particularly during the treatment of carcinomas of the maxillary antrum and paranasal sinuses and in the definitive radiation therapy of orbital lymphomas, rhabdomyosarcomas, retinoblastomas and other orbital tumours. It is often not appreciated that for the most part, the eye is relatively radioresistant, particularly its more posterior structures. Careful attention to detail can result in a healthy eye with very adequate vision even after whole orbital irradiation. However, there are two important points to remember. First, the greatest danger to the eye is posed by dryness of the cornea, leading to keratoconjunctivitis sicca. This generally results from lack of tear formation following irradiation of the lacrymal gland, which can be avoided in most instances by the use of a small lead shield. Second, the most radiosensitive structure of the eye is the lens, which is particularly sensitive to large single fractions of irradiation. Cataract formation can often be prevented by the use of a pencil-shaped corneal shield, although there is always the danger of underirradiation of important structures deep to the protected cornea and lens.

The kidney

The kidney is frequently irradiated during treatment of abdominal or retroperitoneal tumours, and is a relatively radiosensitive structure. Both glomerular filtration rate and renal plasma flow are reduced after modest radiation doses, and it is often a year or more before recovery begins. Acute radiation nephritis can occur when the dose to both kidneys is no greater than about 25 Gy in 5 weeks. The acute clinical syndrome includes proteinuria, uraemia and hypertension which can be irreversible and even fatal. More chronic changes include persistent albuminuria and poor glomerular and tubular function, which may be lifelong even in patients who recover from the acute syndrome. These complications are particularly likely to occur after whole abdominal irradiation.

The gut

Although both small and large bowel tissues are sensitive

Table 5.3 Skin reactions to radiotherapy.

Early changes	Later changes
Erythema	Fibrosis
Dry and moist desquamation	Loss of pigment
Pigmentation	Telangiectasia
Epilation	Loss of skin appendages
Loss of sweat gland function	Loss of connective tissue
Tissue oedema	

to radiation, the rectum deserves special mention since this is frequently the organ of limiting tolerance when treating carcinomas of the cervix and other pelvic tumours. Acute radiation reactions, accompanied by diarrhoea, tenesmus and occasional rectal haemorrhage, are encountered both with external irradiation of the pelvis and with intracavitary treatment. The later radiation effects are of even greater importance, and include oedema and fibrosis of the bowel, which once again may be responsible for diarrhoea, painful proctitis and rectal bleeding, sometimes progressing to stricture, abscess or fistula formation. Occasionally these complications are severe enough to warrant temporary or even permanent colostomy or may cause difficult diagnostic problems by mimicking symptoms of recurrence of the cancer. Radiation damage to the small bowel is pathologically similar to that of the rectum and may limit treatment of intra-abdominal tumours. Late sequelae include stricture formation which may cause intestinal obstruction.

Less radiosensitive tissues

Bone

Therapeutic radiation of bone is a particular problem in children since normal growth may be interrupted, especially when the epiphyseal plate is included in volumes taken to radical dosage, as this area is responsible for the increase in length of any growing long bone. Direct irradiation of the epiphysis interferes with the high mitotic rate of the cartilaginous cells adjacent to the shaft. Radiation damage to the metaphysis may also be severe, though apparently fully reversible provided that the radiation dose is moderate.

The severity of radiation-induced deformity and/or growth disturbance is much greater with high dosage, most particularly with large radiation volumes. The advent of megavoltage irradiation has been particularly helpful in this respect. Nevertheless, in children treated for medulloblastoma, where the whole spine is irradiated to a minimum dose of 30 Gy in 5–6 weeks, the majority of survivors have some deficit in the sitting height. As many as one-third remain persistently below the third centile for height. Younger children are at particular risk but this has to be accepted when radiotherapy is essential for cure, as in medulloblastoma. The late sequelae of radiotherapy and chemotherapy following treatment of childhood cancer are discussed in Chapter 24. Modern treatment with growth hormone replacement has greatly reduced the severity of these problems.

Other connective tissues

Muscle, tendon and connective tissue are all relatively insensitive to radiation and do not usually limit dosage. Fibrosis may occur when high or repeated doses are used, sometimes leading to loss of joint mobility and contractures.

Late sequelae of radiation

In addition to the specific effects on the various organs described above, there are a number of important long-term hazards following the use of radiotherapy. These include carcinogenicity, mutagenicity and teratogenicity, and are all attributable to a fundamental property of ionizing radiation, namely its biological effect on nuclear DNA with consequent permanent damage to genetic material.

Carcinogenesis

This is a well-documented phenomenon. Survivors from Hiroshima have an increased incidence of neoplasia, particularly leukaemia. Recently an increased incidence of breast cancer has been reported, 35 years after the acute radiation damage was inflicted. Analysis of a large series of patients with ankylosing spondylitis treated by low doses of radiotherapy has demonstrated a 10-fold increase in the incidence of leukaemia. Occasionally malignant change develops at the site of previous localized irradiation, for example osteosarcoma of the scapula following radiation for carcinoma of the breast. In children treated for retinoblastoma, late orbital neoplasms may occur (see Chapter 24).

These studies illustrate the general points that neoplasia tends to occur within an organ directly affected by the radiation beam, that there is usually a latent period of at least 10 years before neoplasia develops, and that even moderate doses of irradiation, such as those that used to be employed for benign disease during childhood or young adult life, may lead to a radiation-induced malignancy later on. Much higher doses of radiation are usually given to patients with cancer, but the patients are usually older and have a far smaller likelihood of long survival, so that the true risk of late radiation carcinogenesis is much less amenable to study. Patients with cancer also have a higher probability of developing a second neoplasm. This is sometimes due to common risk factors—for example, patients cured of early laryngeal carcinomas who continue to smoke and then succumb to carcinoma of the bronchus. Patients with cancer also have an inherent increased probability of developing a second malignancy for reasons which are currently unclear. Increasingly, patients are treated with radiation and cytotoxic chemotherapy, the latter adding to the risk of carcinogenesis. This is well demonstrated by the higher risk of acute leukaemia and breast cancer following treatment of Hodgkin's disease (see Chapters 6 and 25). As more patients are treated with, and cured by, the combination of radiation and chemotherapy, we must expect the incidence of second neoplasms to rise. Although the risk of radiation carcinogenesis is low, it should deter radiotherapists from treating benign skin and other disorders, particularly in children, which could be more safely dealt with by other means.

Teratogenicity

Minimal exposure, even to 'soft' X-rays in pregnant women is extremely hazardous because of the risk of growth retardation and serious malformation in the developing embryo. Irradiation during the last trimester, well after organogenesis is complete, is safer although growth retardation may still occur. Radiation treatment of pregnant women must be avoided wherever possible. This may well lead to difficult clinical decisions, especially when the diagnosis of malignancy is made early in the pregnancy. For example, in patients with pelvic tumours there is general agreement that during the first trimester of pregnancy, treatment should be given as if the patient were not pregnant (unless it can be safely delayed). Spontaneous abortion will always occur but few would feel justified in delaying therapy for perhaps 6 months until the pregnancy is over.

Mutagenicity

This refers to genetic alteration in somatic or germ cells resulting from their direct irradiation. In somatic cells these mutations may be the basis of radiation-induced carcinogenesis. In germ cells mutation may lead to fetal death or abnormality, although in humans most germ cell mutations are thought to be non-viable. For these reasons abnormal births following scattered irradiation to the testis are very uncommon.

Technical aspects of radiotherapy

In order to deal adequately with both surface and deep-seated tumours, departments of radiotherapy must possess a suitable range of equipment, comprising superficial (low-energy), orthovoltage (medium-energy) and supervoltage (high-energy) machines. In general, a department will need to draw on a population of at least half a million in order to have a sufficient throughput of new cases. At least 40% of cancer patients require treatment with radiotherapy at some point. Important additional features of the modern department include facilities for planning the radiation treatment, closely liaising with departments of medical physics. For many patients, multi-field techniques are used and the physics staff, in conjunction with the radiotherapist, will decide (usually with the aid of a planning computer) on the most appropriate field arrangement. Modern computing techniques aid us in the generation of isodose curves (similar to contour lines on an ordnance survey map) defining points of equal radiation depth dose and making suitable corrections for tissues of unusual density such as lung or bone (Fig. 5.7). A treatment simulator is essential in order to reproduce the characteristics of the radiation therapy apparatus in its geometry, capability and limitations, without delivering any treatment. This allows an accurate pretreatment appraisal of both the tumour volume to be irradiated and the best alternative techniques. In addition, a mould room will be necessary to produce treatment immobilization devices such as individually manufactured perspex head

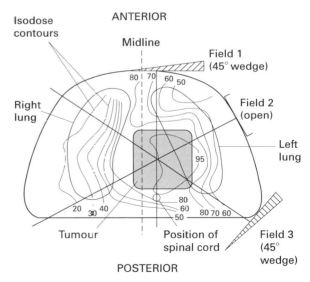

Fig. 5.7 Typical plan for multi-field irradiation of carcinoma of left main bronchus, showing site of tumour, position of lungs and isodose contours.

shells for use in head and neck or brain tumour work. Templates for superficial irradiation of irregularly shaped skin cancers, or for individualized shaped fields (such as the 'mantle' or 'inverted-Y' fields for irradiation of patients with Hodgkin's disease) are also produced in the mould room.

As pointed out by Horwich, 'since the birth of radiotherapy at the beginning of this century it has been apparent that the radiotherapist must be fully conversant with the physics of ionizing radiation and with technical aspects of radiation delivery systems, including machine design, dosimetry, treatment planning and simulation, fixation and beam alignment' (Horwich 1990). Clearly, it is the radiotherapist's responsibility not only to judge whether radiotherapeutic treatment is indicated but also to decide upon the best technique, field arrangement, choice of therapy unit, total dose and fractionation. Although these technical aspects of radiotherapy are often thought to be synonymous with the total workload of the radiotherapist, they in fact form a limited part of the task. Perhaps even more important is his or her continuing and ever-present role as the clinician responsible for diagnosis, management and follow-up of patients with cancer. In the UK, where the division of radiotherapy from diagnostic radiology occurred early, departments of radiotherapy have been entirely clinical (that is, non-diagnostic) for well over 30 years.

Radiotherapy planning and treatment techniques

Non-radiotherapists are often puzzled by the technical vocabulary which radiotherapists use, making it difficult for them to understand the intentions, achievements and limitations of the techniques employed. A short glossary follows.

Treatment prescription

The total dose and treatment time are normally prescribed at the outset of treatment, though in certain circumstances the radiotherapist may prefer to prescribe, say, the first week's treatment and then make a further decision as to whether or not to continue. Total absorbed dose is given in rad (the cgs unit) or Gray, Gy (the increasingly preferred SI unit)—note that $1\,rad = 100\,erg/g$ and $1\,Gy = 1$ J/kg of absorber, and that $1\,Gy = 100\,rad$. Some radiotherapists prefer the centigray to the Gray, since the centigray and the rad are identical. For most treatments, the total dose is split into a number of equal fractions given either on a daily basis or intermittently. The number of fractions of treatment is also prescribed by the radiotherapist. The treatment volume, that is the volume of tissue to be covered by the prescribed radiation dose, is determined by the radiotherapist using whatever radiological and imaging aids he or she feels to be necessary.

Maximum, minimum and modal dose

Since it is impossible to achieve homogeneous irradiation of the desired volume without irradiation of surrounding normal tissue, the radiotherapist must decide on the appropriate compromise. One traditional approach was to prescribe to a *maximum* dose, that is, a dose which would not be exceeded, even if this particular dose level was reached only in a small part of the tumour. The opposite approach, to prescribe to a *minimum* dose, which represented the lowest possible dose level, was also commonly used. The problem with prescriptions of this kind is that neither maximum nor minimum dosage is necessarily representative as a reference dose. A more satisfactory recommendation is to the *modal* dose, that is, the particular dose level occurring with the greatest frequency in the prescribed volume—by definition a more representative dose level. The *applied* dose is used where the radiotherapist wishes to prescribe the dose at the surface of the skin. If he or she wishes to state more precisely what the dose at a certain depth should be (for example, when treating spinal metastases where the dosage at a certain depth is of greater interest than the surface dose) a *depth-dose* prescription may be preferable. The radiotherapist may specify a certain dose at, say, 4 cm depth for metastases in the upper spine, but at 7 cm depth for those in the lower spine, following the expected normal anatomy.

Open (direct) and wedged fields

An open or direct field is usually applied perpendicular to the patient's skin surface and the beam emerging from the treatment machine is not modified in any way. In treatments using several fields (multi-field techniques), a number of fields, usually two to four, are used and, by inserting wedges of various dimensions into the beam and using radiation fields applied obliquely, the tumour volume can be irradiated to a more homogeneous level (Fig. 5.7). The use of multi-field arrangements, often employing wedged fields, has permitted safer megavoltage irradiation of deep-seated tumours to a high dose level.

Parallel opposed fields

The simplest type of multi-field technique is provided by a two-field arrangement where the fields are applied in opposite directions, usually to the anterior and posterior skin surface (Fig. 5.8), and the block of tissue in between irradiated. This technique is widely used and, if necessary, the fields can be shaped so that important structures are avoided, for example, the use of the 'mantle' irradiation technique for patients with supradiaphragmatic Hodgkin's disease where the lungs are protected from overirradiation (see p. 393). For parallel opposed pairs of fields, the dose normally prescribed is the *midplane* dose since this will define the dose achieved at a point midway between the two fields and indeed midway between the anterior and posterior skin surface of the patient.

Shrinking field technique

During a course of treatment it is sometimes desirable to reduce the treatment volume so that part of the initial treatment volume is treated to a certain dose level and a smaller area then taken to a higher dose. This is often done, for example, in pelvic tumours such as carcinomas of the bladder or prostate, where the original treatment volume might include pelvic lymph nodes with the intention to treat these to a 'prophylactic' dose of irradiation to

deal with microscopic disease, while the primary site requires a higher dosage. A further good example is the irradiation technique often employed in a primary bone sarcoma such as Ewing's tumour, where the whole of the long bone might be irradiated to a moderate dose, the field being reduced during treatment so that the primary tumour site receives the full total dose.

Systemic irradiation

This refers to radiotherapy not as traditionally used for specific local sites but throughout the whole body or substantial parts of it. Whole-body irradiation is well established as a means of eradicating leukaemia or lymphoma cells prior to allogeneic or autologous BMT (it is this irradiation which kills the tumour cells—not the transplant itself!). Hemi-body irradiation, usually to the upper or lower half of the body, is increasingly used as an excellent palliative technique for multiple painful bone metastases and in multiple myeloma (see Chapter 27).

Immobilization devices

For precision work, particularly treatment of head and neck cancers, it is essential that the patient be absolutely still and in a reproducible position throughout the whole of the lengthy treatment period. The best means of achieving this is to use an immobilization device such as a perspex headcast (Fig. 5.9), individually made by obtaining a plaster-of-Paris impression, which is then used to produce a perspex shell which fits the patient snugly and can be screwed to the treatment couch. Use of these devices also carries the advantage that field markings can be made on the cast rather than the patient, thereby avoiding unsightly ink marks or tattoos, and ensuring accurate reproduction for each day's treatment.

There have been numerous attempts to enhance the local and regional control of cancer by means of novel approaches using particle beams (see above), stereotactic external beam radiation therapy, radiosensitivity drugs, photodynamic therapy (PDT) and other techniques. Few of these approaches are yet established as standard therapy, indeed most, after promising theoretical preclinical data, have failed to withstand the rigours of the prospectively randomized clinical trial—nitroimidazole radiosensitizers are perhaps the best example. Hyperfractionation, already referred to, and hypofractionation are also areas of major research efforts at present. PDT has been increasingly used in oral and gastrointestinal tumours, and is a form of treatment dependent on the

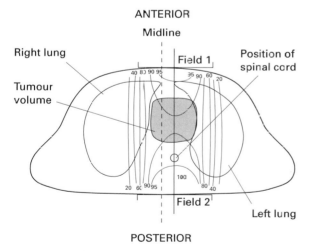

Fig. 5.8 Typical anteroposterior parallel pair field arrangement. This is often used for treating thoracic or pelvic tumours. In this instance the patient had an inoperable carcinoma of the bronchus, and the tumour position and size were determined by CT scanning. The spinal cord is also shown since irradiation of this structure is often dose-limiting with this set-up.

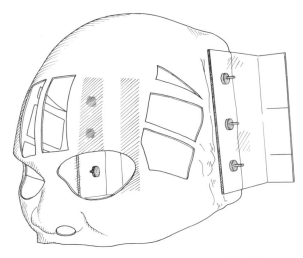

Fig. 5.9 Perspex head shell. Shells are individually made to ensure accurate positioning. These are widely used in treatment of tumours of the head and neck, and for pituitary tumours.

excitation of a number of photoactive compounds by laser-generated light of the appropriate wavelength. Haematoporphyrin derivatives are synthetic haemoglobulin compounds which, when administered systematically, may localize in human tumour tissue. When exposed to laser light of the correct wavelength, dose derivatives react with oxygen to form a highly reactive fragment which appears to be locally cytotoxic.

Conformational therapy

This is a promising new technique in which the high-dose volume is designed to conform more closely with the target volume. The prime intention is to use external beam therapy to better effect by excluding more normal tissue than was previously possible, thereby increasing the dose which can safely be applied to the tumour volume. Evaluation of these techniques is under active study at present, increasingly using customized field shaping designed from three-dimensional 'beam's-eye view' planning. Clear-cut disease-free survival benefits are increasingly being reported, particularly for irradiation of high-grade prostatic cancers. These and other novel aspects of radiotherapy are well reviewed by Ruckdeschel (1989) and by Lichter and Lawrence (1995).

Integration of radiotherapy and chemotherapy

Remarkable changes in the therapy of cancer have occurred over the past 25 years. Whereas it was once unusual for patients to be treated with both radiotherapy and cytotoxic chemotherapy, it has now become commonplace. This trend is certain to continue for at least two reasons. First, radiation therapy is now increasingly used as an alternative to surgery for treatment of the primary tumour, particularly with carcinoma of the larynx and other head and neck sites, carcinoma of the cervix, anus and, over the past few years, with many carcinomas of the breast, bladder and prostate. Second, there is increasing use of chemotherapy both for palliation and, in some tumours, as adjuvant therapy immediately preceding or succeeding the initial local treatment.

There are important disadvantages and even risks in the simultaneous use of both treatments. Some cytotoxic agents act as radiation sensitizers, increasing the local reactions from radiotherapy and occasionally producing 'recall' of previous skin reactions. The most important example is actinomycin D, although there is evidence that other drugs such as doxorubicin may also interact with radiotherapy in this way. For example, oesophageal stricture has been documented in patients undergoing mediastinal irradiation and concurrent treatment with this drug. The danger of doxorubicin-induced cardiomyopathy occurs at a lower dosage in patients who have undergone mediastinal or chest wall radiation, if a significant volume of cardiac muscle has been included. For patients undergoing wide-field irradiation, particularly if a substantial volume of bone marrow is involved (such as in children with medulloblastoma), the use of adjuvant chemotherapy may lead to more troublesome myelosuppression than with the radiation alone. In general, it is true that the synchronous use of chemotherapy and radiotherapy (particularly with radiation-sensitizing drugs) leads to greater toxicity. The combination should be avoided particularly when treatment is palliative or large areas of mucosa are being irradiated. There is, however, increasing interest in the use of concurrent chemoradiation regimens in order to improve local control (in tumours such as Ewing's sarcoma or small-cell lung cancer), and at the same time to treat micrometastatic disease.

Despite the theoretical drawback of increased toxicity, there are many advantages to combined use of radiotherapy and chemotherapy as initial treatment, especially when administered synchronously. Radiotherapy, as a powerful local tool, is often able to produce tumour control with minimal physiological disturbance, though without effect on occult metastases. It may not be possible to ensure satisfactory irradiation of the primary tumour and its lymph node drainage area if nodal metastases are known to be present, for example, in gynaecological, testicular or bladder tumours with known para-aortic involvement. Conversely, chemotherapy can seldom be relied upon to deal adequately with the primary tumour, though it does at least offer hope in dealing with occult metastatic disease. Combined therapy should then represent a logical approach, indeed it is clear that in a number of major squamous cell primary sites, synchromous chemoradiotherapy now represents the gold standard of treatment with radical intent (cervix, anus, vulva, oesophagous, head and neck: see specific chapters).

Use of chemotherapy with curative intent after radiation failure represents a different form of combined therapy, since the treatments are separated in time. This approach is only likely to be successful in highly chemosensitive tumours such as Hodgkin's disease, in which chemotherapy for radiation failure is probably as successful as it is for primary therapy. A newer concept, as yet relatively unexplored, is the use of 'adjuvant' radiotherapy in patients treated primarily by chemotherapy. In small-cell carcinoma of the bronchus, for example, chemotherapy is now widely employed as the mainstay of treatment. We now have to ask whether mediastinal irradiation, formerly the most widely used method of treatment, still has a role to play (see Chapter 12). Radiotherapy may also be valuable in a slightly different adjuvant fashion as, for example, in the use of cranial irradiation as prophylaxis for children with ALL in whom meningeal relapse is substantially reduced by routine irradiation, since the cerebrospinal fluid is poorly penetrated by the drugs used for systemic control.

Further reading

Abulafi AM, Williams NS. Photodynamic therapy for cancer. *Br Med J* 1992; 304: 589–90.

Adams GE. The clinical relevance of tumour hypoxia. *Eur J Cancer* 1990; 26: 420–1.

Benson RJ, Burnet NG. Altered radiotherapy fractionation: an opportunity not to be missed. *Clin Oncol* 1998; 10: 150–4.

Bentzen SM. Towards evidence based radiation oncology: improving the design, analysis and reporting of clinical outcome studies in radiotherapy. *Radiation Oncol* 1998; 47: 5–18.

Burnet NG. Three-dimensional treatment planning for radiotherapy. *Clin Oncol* 1993; 10: 1–2.

Chatal J-F, Hoefnagel CA. Radionuclide therapy. *Lancet* 1999; 354: 931–5.

Coleman CN. Beneficial liaisons: radiology meets cellular and molecular biology. *Radiother Oncol* 1993; 28: 1–15.

Dasu A, Denekamp J. New insights into factors influencing the clinically relevant oxygen enhancement ratio. *Radiation Oncol* 1998; 46: 269–77.

Dewey WC, Ling CC, Meyn RE. Radiation-induced apoptosis: relevance to radiotherapy. *Int J Radiation Oncol Biol Physics* 1995; 33: 781–96.

Dische S, Saunders MI. The rationale for continuous, hyperfractionated accelerated radiotherapy. *Int J Radiation Oncol Biol Physics* 1990; 19: 1317–20.

Dobbs J, Barren A, Ash DV *Practical Radiotherapy Planning*, 3rd edn. London: Edward Arnold, 1999.

Fowler J. The linear quadratic formula and progress in fractionated radiotherapy. *Br J Radiotherapy* 1989; 62: 679–94.

Gilbert HA, Kagan AR. *Modern Radiation Oncology: Classic Literature and Current Management*, Vol. 1 (1978); Vol. 2 (1983). New York: Harper & Row.

Hall EJ. *Radiobiology for the Radiologist*, 3rd edn. Philadelphia: J.B. Lippincott, 1988.

Höckel M, Schlenger K, Mitze M *et al.* Hypoxia and radiation response in human tumors. *Semin Radiation Oncol* 1996; 6: 3–9.

Hopper C. Oncological Applications of Photodynamic Therapy. In: *Current Radiation Oncology*, Vol. II (Tobias JS, Thomas PRM, eds). London: Edward Arnold, 1996: 107–20.

Horwich A. *Combined Radiotherapy and Chemotherapy in Clinical Oncology*. London: Edward Arnold, 1992.

Horwich A. The future of radiotherapy. *Radiotherapy Oncol* 1990; 19: 353–6.

Illidge TM. Radiation-induced apoptosis. *Clin Oncol* 1998; 10: 3–13.

Lichter AS, Lawrence TS. Recent advances in radiation oncology. *N Engl J Med* 1995; 332: 371–9.

Meredith WJ, Massey JB. *Fundamental Physics of Radiology*. Baltimore: Williams & Wilkins, 1972.

Moss WT, Cox JD, eds. *Radiation Oncology: Rationale, Technique, Results*, 6th edn. St Louis, MO: Mosby, 1989.

Moysich KB, Menezes RJ, Michalek AM. Chernobyl-related ionising radiation exposure and cancer risk: an epidemiological review. *Lancet Oncol* 2002; 3: 269–79.

Nielsen OS, Bentzen SM, Sandburgh E *et al.* Randomised trial of single dose versus fractionated palliative radiotherapy of bone metastases. *Radiotherapy Oncol* 1998; 47: 223–40.

Perez CA, Brady LW. *Principles and Practice of Radiation Oncology*. Philadelphia: J.B. Lippincott, 1992.

Ruckdeschel JC. Attempts to enhance locoregional control of cancer by radiotherapy, phototherapy and combined modality therapy. *Curr Opin Oncol* 1989; 1: 231–5.

Saunders M, Dische S, Barren A, Harvey A, Gibson D, Parmer M. Continuous hyperfractionated accelerated radiotherapy (CHART) versus conventional radiotherapy in non-small cell lung cancer: a randomised multicentre trial. *Lancet* 1997; 350: 161–5.

Shatal JF, Hoefangel CA. Radionuclide therapy. *Lancet* 1999; 354: 931–35.

Symonds RP. Recent advances: radiotherapy. *Br Med J* 2001; 323: 1107–10.

Tannock IE. Treatment of cancer with radiation and drugs. *J Clin Oncol* 1996; 14: 3156–74.

Tobias JS. Clinical practice of radiotherapy. *Lancet* 1992; 339: 159–63.

Tobias JS. Risk management and radiotherapy for cancer. *Clin Risk* 2000; 6: 13–16.

Tobias JS, Ball D. Synchronous chemoradiation for squamous carainomas. *Br Med J* 2001; 322: 876–8.

Tobias JS, Thomas PRM, eds. *Current Radiation Oncology*, Vols 1–3. London: Edward Arnold, 1994, 1995, 1998.

Withers HR. Biological basis of radiation therapy for cancer. *Lancet* 1992; 339: 156–9.

Zelefsky MJ, Leibel SA, Kutcher GJ, Fuks Z. Three-dimensional conformal radiotherapy and dose escalation: where do we stand? *Semin Radiation Oncol* 1998; 8: 107–14.

6 Systemic treatment for cancer

For many years there has been little change in the 5-year survival rate for some common cancers. There has been a modest improvement in some tumours, for example in bladder cancer and cancer of the rectum, which is related in part to earlier diagnosis, but other tumours such as lung and pancreatic carcinoma have nearly as bad a prognosis now as in 1980. Failure to improve survival is largely due to the fact that the major cause of death is lymphatic and blood-borne metastasis. Better methods of control of the primary site have a modest effect on metastatic spread, which has often occurred by the time of surgery. Hopes of improvement in survival lie mainly in the development of better methods of treatment of metastases. The systemic treatment of cancer has, in the last 20 years, become an important part of cancer management. In some uncommon tumours such as childhood cancers, lymphomas and teratomas, great progress has been made with the use of cytotoxic drugs. In other more common cancers the results have been less impressive, although modest improvements in survival have been obtained with chemotherapy and endocrine therapy in breast and colorectal cancer.

Since the treatments are sometimes toxic, a clear understanding of the uses and limitations of chemotherapy and other forms of medical treatment is essential. If there is a reasonable chance of cure, toxicity and expense can usually be accepted. If there is not, then the potential benefits of palliative treatment with cytotoxic agents must be carefully weighed against unwanted effects.

Chemotherapy

Nitrogen mustard was introduced into clincal practice in 1946. The effectiveness of this class of compound in producing regression in lymphomas was rapidly established, as was the gastrointestinal and haematological toxicity they produced. In 1947 Farber showed that aminopterin could produce remissions in acute leukaemia. This was followed by the production of the closely related drug methotrexate in 1949. Development of other drugs followed swiftly: 6-mercaptopurine in 1952, and the antitumour antibiotic actinomycin D in 1954. Since 1965, numerous new antimetabolites, alkylating agents and antibiotics with significant activity have been developed, many of which are related to the parent molecules. Examples of important drugs introduced into clinical practice in the last 20 years are epipodophyllotoxins, platinum analogues and taxoids. These agents have a direct effect on DNA or cell division. Recently drugs with new methods of action have excited much interest, for example signal transduction inhibitors. The process of discovery, preclinical testing and clinical evaluation is slow. The final realization of the value of a new drug may take 10 years or more following its original discovery.

The development of an anticancer drug

Before an agent is introduced into practice it undergoes evaluation on human tumour cells in culture, on animals and then in early clinical trials. Preclinical screening is now largely using panels of human tumour cell lines. Evidence is sought for efficacy and, in particular, efficiency of killing against particular tumour types.

Animal toxicological studies are then performed, together with assessment of responsiveness of human cancers grown as xenografts in nude mice. Using larger animals, data on pharmacokinetics, optimum schedule and toxicity are obtained, including dose, absorption, tissue distribution, plasma half-life and pathways of metabolism and excretion. Drugs showing activity are then taken forward to early (phase 1) clinical studies. The patients selected have cancers which are widespread and usually resistant to a wide variety of cytotoxic agents. The aims are to determine optimum dosage, schedule, pharmacokinetics and metabolism. Any tumour response or toxicity is noted. Previously treated patients have a much lower tumour response rate than patients whose tumours have not previously been treated. Phase 1 studies are therefore not optimal for determining efficacy. In the next phase (phase 2) a more detailed study is made on patients with tumours of defined categories, both previously treated and untreated. Here an assessment of tumour responsiveness is made. In subsequent studies the drug will be assessed in combination with other agents active in a particular disease. This process usually consists of several different types of study. The simplest is a non-randomized, single-agent study in which a more precise definition of response and toxicity is made in a single tumour type. Occasionally such studies are a randomized comparison against another single, well-established agent.

When evidence of activity has been confirmed the new agent is combined with other established drugs and again used in a chosen tumour type and stage. Here the aim is to assess efficacy and tolerability of the combination regimen. Such studies carry more weight if a randomized comparison is made with a standard regimen of generally accepted value. The combination may then be assessed in very large-scale studies in which the value of chemotherapy in improving survival in a given tumour is assessed as precisely as possible.

Principles of cancer chemotherapy

The cell cycle

After cell division cells may enter a growth phase, G_1, in preparation for a subsequent division. This lasts for a variable period of time in different tissues. Alternatively cells

may rest in G_0 phase. After G_1 the cells move into the phase of DNA synthesis, S phase, in which the amount of chromosomal material is doubled. The cell then passes through a premitotic phase, G_2, and then into mitosis, M, in which the pairs of chromosomes separate and the cell divides.

As with other tissues, tumours are heterogeneous with respect to cell division—some cells proliferating, others dying or dormant. The tumours probably contain progenitor or 'stem' cells which are capable of cell division, continuously renewing and increasing the tumour mass (see Chapter 3). The tumour growth rate also depends on the proportion of cells dividing at any given time, called the growth fraction. In experimental tumours the *growth fraction* falls as the tumour becomes larger; however, in humans, direct proof that small tumours have a higher growth fraction is lacking. Increase in size of a cancer is a balance between cell division and cell loss. It appears that self renewal in cancers is often slower than in the normal tissue counterpart. Vascularization of large tumour masses is often defective and the rate of cell death is high in those areas of tumour more than 150 μm from a capillary.

Cytotoxic drugs produce their effect by damaging the reproductive integrity of cells. The more rapidly growing tumours with a high growth fraction are more likely to respond to drug treatment. This, however, is a generalization. The explanation of why some types of cancer (lymphoma, testicular cancer, leukaemia) are sensitive to cytotoxic drugs and other types (pancreatic, colonic cancer) are not, is almost certainly not solely a matter of cell kinetics. It may also be related to mechanisms by which the cell death (apoptotic) response is invoked and on the efficiency of repair of damaged DNA.

Most cytotoxic regimens have been derived empirically, not on the basis of cell kinetics. Some drugs (for example, methotrexate) are only effective at a particular phase of the cell cycle such as DNA synthesis, while others, such as alkylating agents, exhibit some action even against resting cells. Table 6.1 shows the phase specificity of some anticancer drugs.

The relationship between cell cycle and cell death is modified by repair mechanisms. In a resting cell, DNA damage by an alkylating agent may be repaired before the cell moves into cycle, if the repair mechanisms are efficient and the interval between drug exposure and onset of DNA synthesis is long.

Attempts have been made to time drug administration in such a way that the cells are synchronized into a phase of the cell cycle which renders them especially sensitive to the cytotoxic agent. For example, in experimental systems,

Table 6.1 Phase specificity of anticancer drugs.

Phase of cell cycle	Effective agents
S phase	Cytosine arabinoside, methotrexate, 6-MP, hydroxyurea
Mitosis	Vinca alkaloids, taxoids
Phase non-specific	Alkylating agents, nitrosoureas, antibiotics, procarbazine, cisplatin

vinblastine can be used to arrest cells in mitosis. These 'synchronized' cells enter cycle together and can be killed by a cycle active S phase specific agent, such as cytosine arabinoside. Other mechanisms of synergy between drugs may be important; for example, cyclophosphamide depletes intracellular glutathione, which may lead to increased sensitivity to agents normally detoxified by glutathione such as other alkylating agents. However, most drug schedules are not devised on the basis of cell kinetics or synergy but on the knowledge of toxicity and practicability.

Kinetics of cell killing by cytotoxic drugs

In experimental systems a given dose of a cytotoxic drug kills a given proportion of cells and not a given number. This *fractional cell kill hypothesis* is shown diagrammatically in Fig. 6.1. A single dose of a drug might, for example, kill 99% of cells and will do so whether 10^{12} cells are treated (leaving 10^{10} cells) or 10^4 cells (leaving 10^2 cells). If true for solid human cancers, the implications are that a small tumour will be killed by fewer chemotherapy cycles than a large one. Because fewer exposures to drugs will be needed there will be less chance of resistance emerging. Drugs should then be scheduled in such a way as to produce maximum killing. This will depend on the rate of regrowth of the tumour and on the rate of recovery of the normal tissues which have been most damaged by the drug. In humans these tissues are usually the gut and marrow which regenerate quickly in comparison with most cancer tissue (Fig. 6.1). For this reason pulsed intermittent therapy, with time for normal tissues to recover, is the usual method of drug administration.

This approach has both theoretical and practical limitations. First, the fractional cell kill hypothesis was validated in homogeneous rapidly growing experimental tumours. Extrapolation of data to slowly growing human cancers has obvious weakness. Second, experimental tumours grown as ascites or in body fluids (such as leukaemias) can

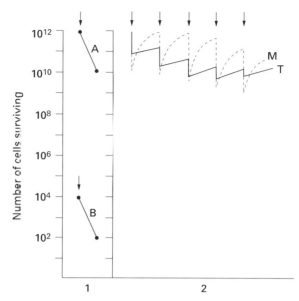

Fig. 6.1 Fractional cell kill. In section 1 of the figure a given dose of a drug is shown killing 99% of cells in both case A and case B. In case A the tumour is reduced from 10^{12} cells to 10^{10} cells and in case B from 10^4 to 10^2 cells. In part 2 of the figure, T shows the effect of repeated drug administration (arrowed) on tumour growth. With repeated doses there is less killing of tumour, indicating the emergence of drug resistance. M shows the effect of drug administration on marrow progenitor cells. The marrow recovers quickly, but with repeated doses this is less complete and myelosuppression becomes clinically evident.

be assumed to have uniform exposure to a drug. This is obviously not the case for poorly vascularized solid neoplasms, so that the kinetics of killing will be a much more complex function than the first-order kinetics of experimental systems. Third, the proportion of inherently insensitive tumour cells may be a function of size of the tumour (see drug resistance, below), being greater with large tumours. Fourth, the rate of regrowth of the tumour may change with repeated chemotherapy. Although this does not appear to occur with experimental ascitic tumours, the situation may be different for solid tumours. Fifth, the recovery of normal tissues—as judged, for example, by blood count—may appear complete after the first few cycles, but becomes less so as treatment proceeds (Fig. 6.1), which limits dosage in successive cycles. Finally, there are very few clinical data on the dose–response relationship for a given cytotoxic drug in a particular tumour. The clinical pharmacology of cytotoxic drugs is extremely complex and varies from drug to drug. There is clinical evidence that an antitumour effect of a drug will only be seen if a maximum dose is given, and in practice the range from ineffective to maximum tolerated dose may be quite small.

These considerations notwithstanding, pulsed intermittent therapy is the schedule of drug administration most widely employed in cancer chemotherapy, and this has been derived from both experimental and clinical findings.

The use of drugs in combination

Even in sensitive tumours, such as Hodgkin's disease, single-agent chemotherapy is rarely curative. It is therefore logical to try and improve response rate and duration by the use of drugs in combination. The intention behind the combined therapy is to circumvent as many resistance mechanisms as possible. This approach soon proved effective in childhood leukaemia and adult lymphomas and has been adopted for a wide variety of other tumours.

The development of a combination chemotherapy schedule should follow a number of general principles.
1 Only drugs which are known to be effective as single agents should be used.
2 Wherever possible, it is preferable to use drugs of non-overlapping toxicity.
3 Pulsed intermittent treatment should be used, to allow gut and marrow recovery.
4 Ideally, each drug should be used in its optimal dose and schedule.
5 Where possible, drugs with synergistic killing effects should be used (normally not known in practice).
6 Drugs which work at different phases of the cell cycle are used if practicable.
7 Most schedules are derived from an informed empiricism.
The improved efficacy of these combination regimens has several possible explanations:
1 The tumour is exposed to a wider variety of agents, and the chances of complete resistance are smaller.
2 A maximal killing effect is achieved without undue toxicity.
3 There may be less opportunity for the early emergence of a resistant cell population.

Resistance to cancer chemotherapy

The rate of conversion of a drug to its active form, and its rate of elimination are determinants of efficacy. The determinants of this process in the body are *constitutional*, the result of the genetic make-up of the individual. With the tumour there are, in addition to the constitutional susceptibility, *tumour-related* mechanisms, determined by factors in the tumour itself. The latter include over- or under-expression of mechanisms of metabolism within the tumour which have arisen as a result of somatic mutation, and the delivery of the drug to the tumour as determined by the properties of the tumour vasculature.

Some of the mechanisms of tumour resistance will therefore be an expression of host metabolism and resistance, while others will be tumour related.

Drug metabolism [1]

The degree of response in an individual to a drug depends on constitutional factors that control drug absorption, distribution and metabolism of the drug before it reaches the tumour. The efficiency of these processes is affected by genetic differences in individuals, which lead to changes in structure of proteins that are responsible for these functions. This inherited basics of variation in response is known as *pharmacogenetics*. For some anticancer drugs the molecular basis for variation is understood and genetic differences in drug metabolism have been linked to important outcomes such as tumour response or, conversely, toxicity. Various genetic changes may be responsible.

Mutations may eliminate activity of enzymes responsible for metabolism of the drug to an active form or that lead to degradation of the agent.

Polymorphisms of genetic structure such as single nucleotide alterations or minor amino acid changes are common and usually cause minor changes in function.

The tumour cells will also contain these inherited genes but will also show somatic genetic changes that influence the effect of the drug on the tumour itself.

EXAMPLES

1 *Mercaptopurine* is converted by an enzyme TPMT (thiopurine methyl transferase) to an inactive form. Of the population, 10% are heterozygous for a mutant allele and 0.3% are homozygous. The mutant allele confers an inability to degrade the drug (severe in the case of homozygotes) with resulting drug toxicity but increased antitumour effect.
2 *Irinotecan* is a topoisomerase I inhibitor. It is converted by CYP3A (a hepatic cytochrome) to an inactive form, and by an enzyme CE (carboxylesterase) to an active form called SN38. SN38 is inactivated in the liver by glucuronyl transferase (UGT1). Polymorphisms in the promoter

region of UGT1 lead to less drug metabolism and more toxicity. Less activity of CYP3A has the same effect.

These examples show the potential of this approach in cancer treatment. With the advent of simple genotyping techniques it will become possible to determine polymorphisms that relate to outcome of cytotoxic treatment either in terms of cure rate, susceptibility to acute toxicity or long-term drug complications such as second malignancy. The aim will be to individualize treatment for patients to a greater extent than currently.

Tumour-related resistance

The cells in a solid tumour are not uniformly sensitive to a cytotoxic drug before treatment starts. Genetic instability develops as cancers grow and somatic mutation causes heterogeneity with respect to resistance to drugs. This provides a partial explanation for greater drug resistance in large tumours where this process has progressed further.

As the tumour grows the frequency of development of resistant cells increases so that large tumours have a greater number of intrinsically resistant cells. This resistance is produced by one or more of the mechanisms shown in Table 6.2 and discussed below. Its cause is genetic instability leading to diversity in concentration and function of enzyme or transport proteins. Host defence mechanisms and the use of cytotoxic drugs exert a selection pressure encouraging the survival of the resistant cells, which grow and multiply.

In addition to this type of cellular resistance at least two other mechanisms are important. The first is diminished vascularity of parts of the tumour as it becomes larger, resulting in hypoxia and decreased drug penetration. There is also evidence to suggest that, as with radiotherapy (see Chapter 5) cellular hypoxia may be a determinant of resistance to cytotoxic agents. The second is that only a small proportion of cells may be in cycle, allowing time for repair from cytotoxic damage before cell division.

Cellular mechanisms of resistance to cytotoxic drugs [2]

Somatic mutation and the survival advantage of resistant cells mean that a distinction between 'intrinsic' and 'acquired' cannot be made. The cellular mechanisms are a combination of genetic alteration and selection of cells which have the resistance mechanisms found in normal cells. These resistance mechanisms may be found singly in some cells, or more than one mechanism may coexist in a

Table 6.2 Cellular mechanisms of resistance to anticancer drugs.

Mechanism	Drug (examples)
Efficient repair to damaged DNA	Alkylating agents
Decreased uptake by cell	Methotrexate
	Doxorubicin
Increased drug efflux (*p*-glycoprotein)	Epipodophyllotoxin
	Vinca alkaloids
	Anthracyclines
Decreased intracellular activation	6-MP, 5-FU
Increased intracellular breakdown	Cytosine arabinoside
Bypass biochemical pathways	Methotrexate
	6-MP
	Asparaginase
Gene amplification or over-production of blocked enzyme	Methotrexate
	Nitrosoureas

cell. In the entire tumour we can expect that numerous mechanisms will be present, unevenly distributed in the cellular population.

One of the unexplained phenomena of cancer chemotherapy is that some tumours are generally sensitive to drugs while others are resistant. This inherent sensitivity or resistance extends to drugs of many different classes and mechanisms of action. Thus lymphomas and germ cell tumours show extreme sensitivity (and chemocurability) while pancreatic cancer and melanoma are highly resistant. This general susceptibility is not easily explained by any of the individual mechanisms detailed below, except possibly in the induction of cell death (apoptosis) more easily in some cell types.

Some of the mechanisms of resistance are summarized in Table 6.2 and are outlined briefly below. It must be emphasized that these mechanisms are the properties of normal as well as malignant cells.

MULTIDRUG RESISTANCE (MDR) [3]

This is a membrane of glycoprotein (*p*-glycoprotein, pgp, gp170), of molecular weight 170 kDa, which acts as a drug efflux pump reducing the intracellular concentration of some, but not all, cytotoxic agents. This protein has an homology with a bacterial cell wall transport protein and is widely distributed in nature. In normal tissues it is found in the endothelium of the upper gastrointestinal tract, in the adrenal and kidney. It may act as a detoxifying mechanism. Its presence confers relative resistance to a series of cytotoxic agents such as vinca alkaloids, anthracyclines and epipodophyllotoxin. There is some clinical evidence that pgp expression in tumours correlates with worse prognosis (for example, in childhood soft-tissue sarcoma) but it is not clear whether this is directly due to an adverse response to cytotoxic agents. The effect of pgp can be reversed *in vitro* by calcium channel-blocking drugs (such as verapamil), but with this drug it is difficult to attain appropriate plasma concentrations clinically and, thus far, there has been little clinical success in reversing the MDR mechanism. Other drugs are being evaluated [4]. The MDR genes are part of a family of genes which produce proteins important in drug efflux.

MULTIDRUG RESISTANCE ASSOCIATED PROTEIN

This protein acts as transporter to the exterior of the conjugate formed between a drug and glutathione (GSH, see below). The importance of this mechanism is not yet well established but high levels of expression of the protein have been found in several cancer cell lines.

GLUTATHIONE

This small tripeptide is an -SH containing reducing agent which also acts as a general intracellular detoxifying agent. In the cytosol it is kept in the highly reduced -SH form by gluthathione reductase and serves to prevent unwanted S–S linkages in proteins which might result in incorrect folding. These are a series of transferases which facilitate the reaction of GSH with a toxin. The transferase specificity of many cytotoxic agents is not yet clear. Polymorphism in the transferases relates to outcome in childhood acute myeloid leukaemia [5].

For alkylating agents in particular, the GSH concentration and glutathione transferase activity appear to be important determinants of cellular sensitivity. Concentrations vary widely in different normal tissues and in tumours and do not, in general, correlate with drug sensitivity. It may be possible to alter cellular sensitivity by agents which deplete intracellular glutathione, or by agents which inhibit transferases, such as ethacrynic acid. In cells made resistant to nitrogen mustard the increase in transferase activity is due to gene amplification (see below), but it is not clear if this mechanism is important in spontaneous tumours.

GENE AMPLIFICATION

In tumour cell cultures, cells showing resistance to some cytotoxic agents exhibit amplification of genes responsible for mediating resistance. Gene amplification appears to be hereditable during successive cell divisions. An example is amplification of the dihydrofolate reductase gene, leading to increased intracellular levels of this enzyme which confers relative resistance to methotrexate (see p. 79). Other examples include amplification of

glutathione *S*-transferase isozymes (important in resistance to alkylating agents) and O_6 alkyltransferase (which confers resistance to nitrosoureas).

INCREASE IN DNA REPAIR (see Chapter 3)

Covalent adducts between alkylating agents (and other drugs) and DNA bases are excised by enzymes. The reactions are complex, involving DNA glycosylases and polymerases. Repair mechanisms include *base excision repair* in which glycosylases excise the damaged base from the sugar, and *nucleotide excision repair* in which larger portions of the DNA strand are excised and religated. We know very little both about DNA repair in cancer cells, compared with normal cells, and whether drug resistance is related to increased efficiency of repair of cytotoxic drug-induced DNA damage. The repair mechanisms differ with lesions at chemically distinct sites on the bases, and may vary in efficiency at different sites in the gene and depending on whether the gene is being transcribed.

DECREASED DRUG ACTIVATION

Agents such as cytosine arabinoside and 5-fluorouracil (5-FU) are converted in the cell to an active form before exerting antitumour effect. Low levels of converting enzymes or competing enzyme pathways may decrease intracellular concentrations of active drug.

Drugs such as cyclophosphamide are converted to the active form in normal tissues (in this case the liver). Heritable differences in efficiency of activation will lead to variation in the amount, and rate of formation, of active drug. These are not intracellular mechanisms in the tumour but may account for diminished drug efficacy. The cellular concentration of a reducing enzyme such as DT-diaphorase may be critical in conversion of bioreductive drugs, such as quinones, to their active form.

OTHER MECHANISMS

Increased intracellular drug breakdown (for example, deamination of cytosine arabinoside, inefficient membrane transport (methotrexate), and competing enzyme pathways such as asparagine production by asparagine synthetase decreasing the efficacy of asparaginase) are among the numerous biochemical pathways subverting drug effect. Many of these are discussed in relation to individual drugs (see below).

Remission induction and maintenance

Clinical complete 'remission' or 'complete response' of a tumour is a clinical description which is compatible with up to 10^{10} cells still being present. If treatment stops, the relapse-free interval is dependent on the size of the residual tumour and the growth rate of the surviving cells. These two variables account for the shape of the curves of remission duration. The aim of initial chemotherapy is to induce clinical complete response, if possible.

'Maintenance' therapy was a term introduced in treatment of acute leukaemia where, following the induction of a remission, chemotherapy of a less intensive type is used to 'maintain' the remission. In acute lymphoblastic leukaemia (ALL) this has been shown to contribute to survival. The improvement is due to continued cytotoxic effect on the tumour when the induction therapy has not completely eradicated the disease. The treatment is therefore not 'maintenance' but continued treatment.

In most tumours 'maintenance' therapy has not been shown to improve the results of cyclical combination chemotherapy given over a period of several months. In Hodgkin's disease, for example, survival is not improved by continuing to treat the patient after six cycles have been given. A similar lack of effect has been found in small-cell lung cancer (SCLC) and testicular tumours. In these diseases the patient is cured (or not) during the early phase of treatment. There are strong arguments (discussed above) for ensuring that initial treatment is as intense as possible.

Adjuvant chemotherapy

Following resection of an operable cancer (for example, of the breast or colon) many patients will develop local or distant recurrence. Chemotherapy can be used as an adjuvant to surgery to eradicate micrometastases at this early stage. Chemotherapy may be more effective on small tumours than when they have become clinically detectable. There is little doubt that this approach has been very effective in sensitive paediatric tumours such as Wilms' tumour, Ewing's sarcoma and rhabdomyosarcoma. It is now apparent that modest benefits may be obtained, but that the degree of benefit can only be determined in trials of considerable size to exclude moderate biases which influence results of smaller trials (discussed in Chapter 2, p. 15). Adjuvant chemotherapy is of proven value in premenopausal women with breast cancer, may be of value in colorectal cancer, and is under investigation in locoregional inoperable non-small-cell lung cancer (NSCLC), inoperable head and neck cancer, and advanced bladder cancer. These important uses of chemotherapy (and hormone and biological therapy) will be better defined over the next decade as the necessary studies are completed. It is highly probable that adjuvant chemotherapy

will improve survival to a small degree in many common cancers.

Predicting sensitivity to anticancer drugs

Several techniques have been used to attempt to assess the activity of a drug against the patient's own tumour. These have included: measurement of inhibition of cell growth or metabolism in cell suspension or short-term culture; inhibition of the formation of clones of cells grown in soft agar; and growth inhibition in longer-term cell cultures.

The problems, both technical and in interpretation, are formidable. Cell suspensions may not be representative of the whole tumour; not all tumours will form clones in soft agar; longer-term cultures often cannot be established; and the pharmacology and exposure of the drug are different in culture than *in vivo*. These difficulties are increased by the methodological problems of proving that there is a benefit in selecting drugs for an individual patient rather than using a standard combination. Drug combinations usually contain many or most of the active drugs so that selection in the assay may be only to predict which drugs to leave out. It will be difficult to show survival benefit by this means, although toxicity may be reduced. It seems probable that the current *in vitro* tests can predict clinical resistance fairly reliably. They are less accurate in predicting sensitivity. At present they do not have a place as a routine procedure in cancer chemotherapy.

What cancer chemotherapy has achieved

The majority of curable cancers are uncommon tumours such as childhood cancers, leukaemias, lymphomas and testicular tumours. Other cancers are partially responsive but the impact of chemotherapy on survival is relatively small. These other cancers include cancer of the breast, SCLC, ovarian cancer and cancer of the colon. Figure 6.2 shows that the overall contribution of chemotherapy to *cure* is relatively small. However, in advanced cancer, even if survival is not improved, individual patients may gain symptomatic relief.

Classes of cytotoxic drugs, mode of action and toxicity
Alkylating agents and nitrosoureas [6]

These very reactive compounds produce their effect by covalently linking an alkyl group ($R-CH_2^+$) to chemical

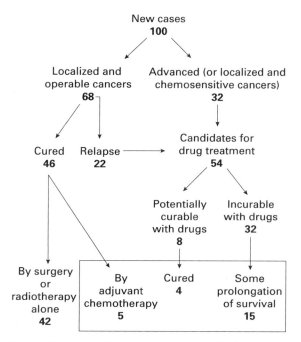

Fig. 6.2 The impact of cancer chemotherapy. The flow diagram gives the proportion of new cancer cases which might be expected to benefit from drug treatment (skin and *in situ* cervical cancer are excluded). One in four patients with cancer benefit from chemotherapy.

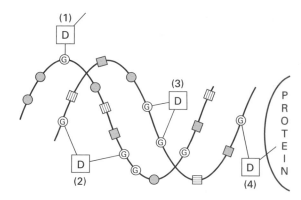

Fig. 6.3 The two strands of DNA are shown with the four bases represented by symbols (○ⓖ▢▥). Most alkylating agents react at the N_7 position of guanine (ⓖ). The drug (▢) forms either a mono-adduct (1) or an *inter-strand* crosslink (2), or an *intra-strand* crosslink (3) or a DNA-protein crosslink (4). The strands of DNA are shown with the major (wide) groove and the minor (narrow) groove. Most commonly used alkylating agents bind to guanine in the major groove, but minor groove agents are under development. The toxic lesions are *inter-* and *intra-strand crosslinks*. The formation of crosslinks between guanine is not random but depends on the base sequence which determines the 'fit' of the agent into the major groove. Mono-adducts are more frequent but more easily repaired than crosslinks. The toxicity of DNA–protein crosslinks is not known.

moieties in nucleic acids and proteins. The principles are shown in Fig. 6.3. Nitrogen mustard, for example, has two chloroethyl side-chains and one of these binds to the 7-nitrogen group of guanine. After forming this bond, for drugs with another side-chain (as with nitrogen mustard), another link can be formed which results in DNA strands being cross-linked, either within a strand or between strands. The commonly used alkylating drugs bind in the major groove of DNA. There is selectivity in the nucleotide sequence in which the drug forms the guanine N7 bond. The cross-link is also dependent an the chemical structure of the drug—the length of DNA over which it can span and the nature of the chemical reaction on the opposite strand. Alkylating agent damage is therefore selective. This may account for some of the observed differences in response of different tumour types since some genes may contain regulatory sequences more vulnerable to alkylation than others or can repair these lesions more efficiently. There is good evidence that the cross-link is the lesion determining cellular cytotoxicity.

Impairment of DNA replication is the major mechanism of cytotoxicity. Alkylating agents which are bifunc-

tional (with two alkylation products) are more cytotoxic than monofunctional compounds by virtue of the cross-linking they produce. The cell can repair itself against this damage by excision of the damaged segment of DNA, with the formation of a new segment of DNA which is then linked to the strand. Although DNA alkylation occurs at any stage in the cell cycle, it seems to have more lethal consequences if it occurs during the S phase, possibly because the cellular checkpoints (such as *p53*) can initiate apoptosis if repair of damage has not occurred before mitosis is due to begin.

CYCLOPHOSPHAMIDE (ENDOXANA, CYTOXAN) (Fig. 6.4)
This is a stable inactive compound which is well absorbed when given orally. It is activated in the liver by the cytochrome P450 system to 4-hydroxycyclophosphamide and thence to phosphoramide mustard and acrolein (Fig. 6.4). The latter is responsible for the haemorrhagic cystitis which is a complication of prolonged or high-dose administration. 2-Mercaptoethane sulphonate (mesna), which binds acrolein in the urine, prevents this complication. After oral administration maximal plasma concen-

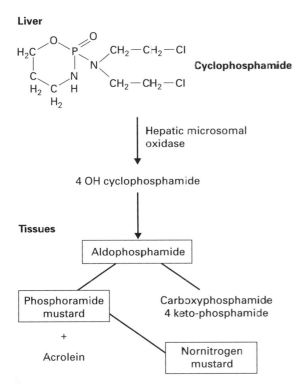

Fig. 6.4 The metabolism of cyclophosphamide. The boxed compounds are alkylating agents. Acrolein is the major cause of haemorrhagic cystitis.

trations are reached in 1 h, and the plasma half-life of the drug is 5–6 h. Little unchanged drug is excreted. The dosage, route and schedules of administration are very variable. In solid tumours such as SCLC, a single intravenous dose of around 1 g/m² is often used, but in breast or ovarian cancer and some lymphomas it is often given orally in lower dose (for example, 100 mg/m² daily). There are numerous tumours in which the drug has been found to be useful, and it is the most versatile alkylating agent in terms of activity and method of administration.

Very high-dose cyclophosphamide (5–10 g/m²) has been used in solid tumour chemotherapy and in allogeneic marrow transplantation for leukaemia and aplastic anaemia. Because the drug must be converted to an active form in the liver, it is not suitable for local use. Haematological toxicity is common, but thrombocytopenia is less marked than with other alkylating agents. Nausea and vomiting accompany intravenous administration, and nausea may also occur when it is given orally. The drug is not vesicant if extravasation occurs. Haemorrhagic cystitis and bladder fibrosis commonly occur, and alope-

cia is frequent with higher doses. Pulmonary fibrosis occurs, as it does with other alkylating agents. High doses may be complicated by inappropriate secretion of antidiuretic hormone (ADH), leading to hyponatraemia. As with most alkylating agents, male infertility is usual. Haemorrhagic carditis has been reported with very high doses.

IFOSFAMIDE

This compound is structurally closely related to cyclophosphamide but one of the two chloroethyl groups is sited on the nitrogen atom and the other on the oxazophosphorine ring nitrogen. Like cyclophosphamide, it is activated by hepatic P450 oxidases. Acrolein, liberated during its metabolism, causes haemorrhagic cystitis, but this is prevented by mesna. Toxicity also includes a neurological syndrome with somnolence, confusion and fits. It is more frequent when given in high dose and if there is impaired liver function. The cause is unknown. The half-life is about 6 h. It is given by short or long infusion and schedules vary greatly. Hydration is necessary. Renal tubular and glomerular dysfunction are frequent and are especially severe in children. The drug is moderately myelosuppressive. It may be more active than cyclophosphamide in squamous carcinomas and sarcomas. The schedules of administration are varied, ranging from 1 h to continuous infusions. There appears to be no pharmacological reason for preferring one over another. Very high dose administration may increase response in sarcomas.

MELPHALAN (ALKERAN) (Fig. 6.5)

This is a stable alkylating agent in which the two chloroethyl groups are linked to phenylalanine. It was originally hoped that this would result in selective activity against melanoma, but in conventional doses this has not proved to be the case. It is usually given orally (for example, 10 mg daily to an adult for 7 days every 4–6 weeks). It is well absorbed, not vesicant and has a half-life of 90 min. Delayed leucopenia and thrombocytopenia occur, but nausea, vomiting and alopecia are infrequent. The drug is used in myeloma, less frequently in ovarian and breast cancer, and has a similar activity to cyclophosphamide in these tumours. With prolonged continuous use there is an appreciable risk of the development of myeloid dysplastic states, leading to acute leukaemia. It is used intravenously as part of high-dose chemotherapy regimens in solid tumours using peripheral blood stem cell transplantation.

CHLORAMBUCIL (LEUKERAN) (Fig. 6.5)

In this compound the two chloroethyl groups are linked to

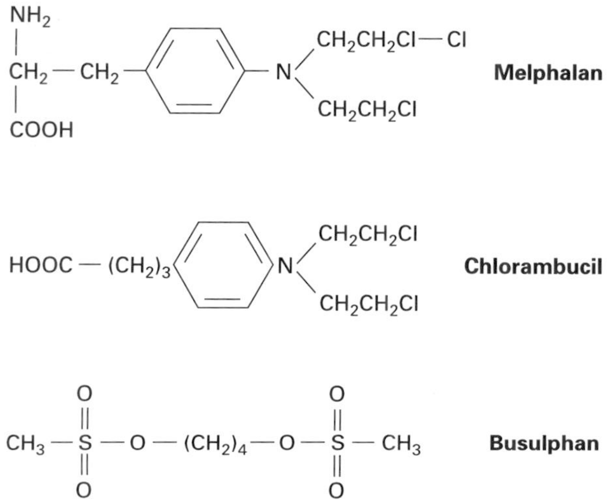

Fig. 6.5 The structures of other commonly used alkylating agents.

a phenyl group. It is a stable compound, well absorbed orally, with a plasma half-life of 90 min. The drug is usually given in low continuous dose (for example, 4 mg daily) or as a higher intermittent dose (for example, 10 mg daily for 2 weeks). It produces its antitumour effects slowly, and its myelosuppressive effect is gradual in onset but persistent. Thrombocytopenia is frequent but haemorrhagic cystitis rarely occurs. It is generally well tolerated and is widely used in the treatment of low-grade lymphomas, particularly in the elderly, and as part of combination chemotherapy regimens in Hodgkin's disease.

BUSULPHAN (MYLERAN) (Fig. 6.5)
This compound differs in structure from other alkylating agents, being an alkyl sulphonate. It is exceptional in that it has very little action apart from bone marrow depression. Thrombocytopenia is frequent, and pancytopenia develops, which may be irreversible. Pulmonary fibrosis is a complication of long-term administration, which occurs with other alkylating agents but is especially frequent with this drug. Other side-effects include skin pigmentation, glossitis, gynaecomastia and anhidrosis. It is used in the treatment of chronic granulocytic leukaemia and in some very high-dose regimens.

MECHLORETHAMINE (MUSTINE, HN₂)
Mustine is now seldom used except, in some centres, as part of the chemotherapy regimen in Hodgkin's disease. It is given by intravenous injection and undergoes rapid

transformation so that within minutes it is no longer in active form. It must be given immediately into a fast-flowing intravenous drip and is an intense irritant outside a vein. The usual dose is 6 mg/m². The toxic effects are nausea and vomiting, leucopenia, thrombocytopenia, thrombophlebitis and tissue necrosis if extravasated.

BCNU (CARMUSTINE)
Bis-chloroethyl nitrosourea (BCNU) was the first nitrosourea to be used clinically. It has a wide spectrum of activity similar to the alkylating agents. It is lipid-soluble and penetrates the blood–brain barrier which is assumed to exist for primary brain tumours. However, the response rates are low in primary tumours and the effect usually transient.

It is usually given intravenously and the half-life is very short—less than 5 min. The major toxic effect is bone marrow depression, which is characteristically delayed for 5–6 weeks. Nausea and vomiting are frequent and renal and hepatic drainage may occur, as do oesophagitis and flushing. It is not vesicant. Long-term follow-up of children treated for brain tumours reveals a high incidence of asymptomatic pulmonary fibrosis which may become symptomatic at any time [7].

BCNU and *cis*-chloroethyl nitrosourea (CCNU, see below) bind to the O_6 position of guanine and the cross-link is formed with the opposite cytosine. Adducts formed by BCNU and CCNU with the O_6 position of guanine are repaired by the enzyme O_6 alkyl transferase. High levels of this enzyme are associated with resistance to nitrosoureas. The enzyme removes the adduct and is itself then inactivated.

CCNU (LOMUSTINE)
Cis-chloroethyl nitrosourea is rapidly absorbed and metabolized, and is usually given by mouth. The products of metabolism have a plasma half-life of 1–2 days, and the metabolites can be detected in the cerebrospinal fluid (CSF). As with BCNU, the major toxic effects are nausea, vomiting and delayed bone marrow depression. For this reason the drug is given at 6-week intervals. Nausea and vomiting can be reduced by spreading the dose over 2 or 3 days.

DIMETHYLTRIAZENOIMIDAZOLE CARBOXAMIDE (DTIC)
This drug probably produces its cytotoxic effect by functioning as an alkylating agent. It is administered intravenously and is vesicant if extravasated. It was initially introduced as a treatment for melanoma, but the results have proved disappointing. It is sometimes used in

combination chemotherapy for soft-tissue sarcoma, but evidence for its value is meagre. It is also included in some regimens for Hodgkin's disease. It causes severe nausea and vomiting, and myelosuppression is frequent. Damage to liver and peripheral nerves occurs, as do flushing and myalgia.

Antimetabolites: drugs blocking formation or action of pyrimidines

METHOTREXATE (Figs 6.6 and 6.7)

Several folic acid antagonists have been developed but only one, methotrexate, is now widely used. The antifolate action is complex and includes inhibition of the enzyme dihydrofolate reductase. This enzyme is essential for reducing dihydrofolate (FH_2) to tetrahydrofolate (FH_4), which in turn is converted to a variety of coenzymes that are essential in reactions where one carbon atom is transferred in the synthesis of thymidylate, purines, methionine and glycine. Methotrexate, and other antifolates, are polyglutamated inside the cell. This process increases the efficiency of binding to dihydrofolate reductase. The critical effect in preventing cell replication appears to be the blocking of synthesis of thymidine monophosphate as shown in Fig. 6.6. The block of thymidine monophosphate synthesis results in inhibition of DNA and RNA synthesis and the drug is therefore S phase specific. The block in activity of dihydrofolate reductase can be bypassed by supplying an alternative intermediary metabolite. This is N_5-formyl-FH_4, variously termed leucovorin, citrovorum factor or, more commonly, folinic acid. It is converted to the FH_4 coenzymes, needed for thymidylate synthetase to function.

The most important mechanism of methotrexate resistance appears to be the production of large amounts of dihydrofolate reductase. In methotrexate-resistant cells there may be an increase in the number of copies of the gene coding for dihydrofolate reductase. This may appear as dense homogeneous staining regions on chromosomes or in small chromosome fragments called double minute chromosomes. These regions appear stable and may be responsible for the continuation of methotrexate resistance in subsequent cell divisions. Other resistance mechanisms are the production of enzyme with decreased affinity for methotrexate, and impaired transport into cells.

The mechanisms of excretion distribution and metabolism make it one of the most dangerous cytotoxic drugs in routine practice. The drug is completely absorbed from the gut at low dosages, but incompletely at higher doses. After intravenous injection there is an initial rapid distribution phase (half-life 45 min), then a slower phase of renal excretion (half-life 2–3 h) followed by a very slow phase when the drug concentration is low. It is this latter, prolonged, phase of clearance that is responsible for toxicity to marrow, gut and mucous membranes. If there is ascites or a pleural effusion the drug may accumulate in these sites and then be slowly released from the 'reservoir' (or third space), causing unexpected toxicity even from a low dose. The drug is 50% bound to albumin from which it can be displaced by drugs such as salicylates, sulphonamides, tetracycline and phenytoin. It is not metabolized significantly but is mainly excreted unchanged in the urine, especially in the first 8 h, by both glomerular filtration and tubular secretion. Drugs which compete for tubular secretion, or the presence of renal

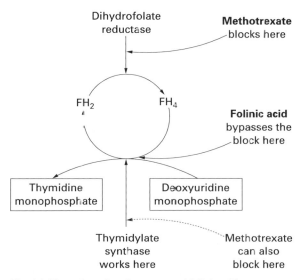

Fig. 6.6 The action of methotrexate and folinic acid.

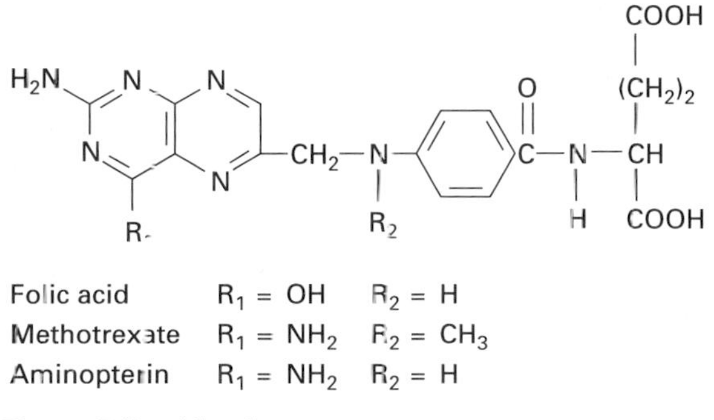

Folic acid R_1 = OH R_2 = H
Methotrexate R_1 = NH_2 R_2 = CH_3
Aminopterin R_1 = NH_2 R_2 = H

Fig. 6.7 Folic acid analogues.

failure, may greatly delay the excretion of the drug and thereby increase toxicity.

When given at high doses the CSF concentrations can achieve cytotoxic levels of up to 10% of the plasma concentration. The drug can also be administered intrathecally, usually at a dose of $10 \, mg/m^2$, and high CSF levels are thereby achieved, especially in the spinal CSF.

The toxicity is mainly haematological and to epithelial surfaces. Pancytopenia develops rapidly after a large dose. After 4–6 days oral ulceration, diarrhoea (which may be bloody) and erythematous skin rashes will occur. Other toxic effects include alopecia; renal failure with high doses; hepatic toxicity (occasionally leading to cirrhosis); pneumonitis; and osteoporosis after long-term therapy.

Methotrexate is part of the established treatment of ALL. It is also used in non-Hodgkin's lymphomas, breast cancer, osteosarcoma and choriocarcinoma. To overcome methotrexate resistance the drug is often used in high dose followed by folinic acid rescue. Doses of methotrexate can be increased over 100-fold provided the effect of the drug is reversed at 24 h. Meticulous attention to hydration is essential. Urinary alkalinization is needed to prevent methotrexate deposition in the renal tubule. This is accomplished by sodium bicarbonate or acetazolamide. Plasma levels of methotrexate must be measured at 24 and 48 h. Correctly monitored there is little toxicity but the approach is potentially very dangerous. It is expensive and the value of the procedure uncertain, although improved response rates have been claimed in osteosarcoma (see Chapter 23). Newer antifolates include edatrexate and trimetrexate. Their advantage over methotrexate is uncertain.

THYMIDYLATE SYNTHASE (TS) INHIBITORS [8]
Thymidylate synthase is also an attractive target for selective inhibition of thymidine monophosphate formation from dioxyuridine monophosphate (Fig. 6.8). Raltitrexed has been shown to be effective in advanced colorectal cancer, with activity also in breast and ovarian cancer. The drug is given at $3 \, mg/m^2$ as bolus infusion every 3 weeks. Its side-effects are nausea, diarrhoea and leucopenia, but these are relatively infrequent and the drug is generally well tolerated. Other TS inhibitors are in development.

5-FLUOROURACIL (Fig. 6.8)
A fluorine atom is substituted for hydrogen on the uracil molecule. The 5-FU molecule can enter into many reactions where uracil would be the normal participant. 5-Fluorouracil has to be activated to 5-fluoro-2-deoxyuridine monophosphate (FdUMP). The conversion of 5-FU to

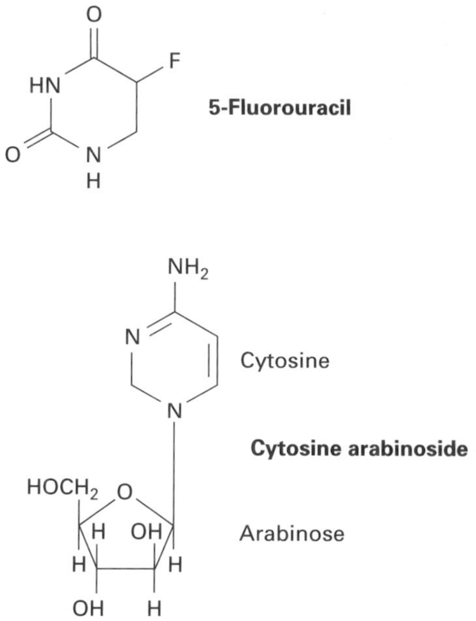

Fig. 6.8 The structure of the pyrimidine analogues.

FdUMP can proceed through a variety of pathways, and resistance to the drug is associated with decreased activity of the enzymes necessary for this conversion. FdUMP interferes with DNA synthesis by binding to the enzyme TS and inactivating it (Fig. 6.8). The effect of the block can to some extent be overcome if thymidine is given (similar to the effect of folinic acid rescue for methotrexate). Conversely, folinic acid enhances 5-FU activity by stabilizing the binding of FdUMP to TS. Folinic acid is used as a means of increasing the effectiveness of 5-FU, although the degree to which this is selective for the tumours is not clear and the therapeutic ratio may not change greatly. Nevertheless, response rates of colorectal cancer metastases are increased with the combination. 5-Fluorouracil is also incorporated into RNA, but the importance of this for its antineoplastic effect is not certain. 5-Fluorouracil is more toxic to proliferating cells, that is, it is cycle specific, but it does not seem to have an effect at a particular phase of the cycle. Recovery from 5-FU involves the synthesis of both TS and the normal substrate deoxyuridine monophosphate.

The intestinal absorption of 5-FU is erratic, so the drug is usually given intravenously. Plasma clearance is rapid (half-life 15 min). Much higher plasma concentrations are achieved by rapid intravenous injection than by continuous infusion, and the toxicity of the drug is greater when given by bolus injection. The drug penetrates the CSF well. There are many schedules of administration using 5-FU alone, or with leucovorin, in intermediate dose or in very high dose. Myelosuppression is commonest between 10 and 15 days. Care is necessary in the presence of hepatic dysfunction. Hepatic arterial or portal vein infusion of 5-FU has been used to treat hepatic metastases from colon cancer. The drug has activity against adenocarcinoma of the gut, breast and ovary, but responses are infrequent and tend to be transient. 5-Fluorouracil is used as adjuvant therapy in colorectal cancer. In this situation, it has been given alone, or with folinic acid (see p. 25).

The drug is generally well tolerated but toxic effects include nausea, diarrhoea, stomatitis, alopecia, myelosuppression, cardiac disturbances and a cerebellar syndrome.

CYTOSINE ARABINOSIDE (CYTARABINE, ARA-C) (Fig. 6.8)
In this analogue of cytidine the pyrimidine base is unchanged but the sugar moiety differs by an alteration in the position of a hydroxyl group. The drug is converted by a series of enzymic steps to its active form known as ara-CTP. This is an inhibitor of DNA polymerize but it is not clear if this is the mechanism of its cytotoxic action. It would explain why the drug is markedly cell cycle, S phase, specific. Resistance to the effect of the drug could either be due to low levels of one of the converting enzymes (deoxycytidine kinase) or to increased rates of deamination. The former seems to be the major mechanism.

The drug is very poorly absorbed from the intestine. After intravenous injection there is a fast phase of clearance (half-life 20 min) followed by a slower phase (half-life 2 h) and the clearance is largely determined by the speed of deamination in the liver and other tissues. The drug penetrates well into the CSF and deamination occurs slowly at this site. Because it is S phase specific it is usually given as multiple intravenous injections or as a continuous intravenous or subcutaneous infusion.

The agent is mainly of use against acute myeloblastic leukaemia (AML) but is also used in ALL and poor-prognosis lymphomas. It is of little value in solid tumours, which usually have a low growth fraction.

The toxic effects include marrow suppression, oral ulceration, diarrhoea, nausea and vomiting and, uncommonly, central nervous system (CNS) toxicity. It is particularly toxic in the presence of hepatic dysfunction since the liver is the chief site of deamination.

GEMCITABINE
This is a recently introduced fluorinated derivative of deoxycytidine nucleotide. It has multiple intracellular tar-

gets, but its chief action is as a substrate for deoxycytidine kinase which converts the drug to a triphosphate and allows its incorporation into DNA in place of cytosine. The synthesis of DNA is blocked after the next base pair is incorporated in the chain. The drug has linear pharmacokinetics and is excreted in urine in the form of its chief metabolite. It is usually administered as a 30-min infusion once a week. Its dose-limiting toxicity is myelosuppression (especially thrombocytopenia). Fever, rash, abnormal liver function tests and fatigue are other toxicities which depend on schedule of administration. The drug has significant single-agent activity against NSCLC, and also has activity in breast and ovarian cancer. Its role in combination therapy is being evaluated.

Antimetabolites: drugs blocking formation or action of purines

There are several cytotoxic agents which are analogues of the natural purine bases and nucleotides. They are in wide use as cytotoxic and immunosuppressive agents. 6-Mercaptopurine (6-MP) and thioguanine are derivatives of hypoxanthine and guanine, respectively, but with the keto group on carbon-6 replaced by a sulphur atom. Drugs of this class usually undergo enzymatic conversion to the active form.

6-MERCAPTOPURINE (Fig. 6.9)
6-Mercaptopurine must be converted to the nucleotide to become active. This is done by the enzyme hypoxanthine–guanine phosphoribosyltransferase (HGPRT). The resultant nucleotide is 6-MP ribose phosphate (6-MPRP). This accumulates in the cell and inhibits several important metabolic reactions in the formation of normal nucleotides. The cytotoxicity of the drug cannot be ascribed to disruption of a single metabolic pathway and cell death probably results from multiple biochemical abnormalities. However, inhibition of purine nucleotide biosynthesis is a major action of the drug. 6-Mercaptopurine is also incorporated into DNA as 6-thioguanine (6-TG) but the contribution of this reaction to cytotoxicity is not clear.

Resistance to the action of 6-MP is often due to low levels of the converting enzyme HGPRT, and such cells also show resistance to 6-TG and azaguanine. Increased rates of drug breakdown may also be important. Dephosphorylation may also be a mechanism of resistance to 6-thiopurines generally.

6-Mercaptopurine is readily absorbed from the gut, and about half of an oral dose is excreted as antimetabolites in 24 h. After intravenous injection the drug is rapidly

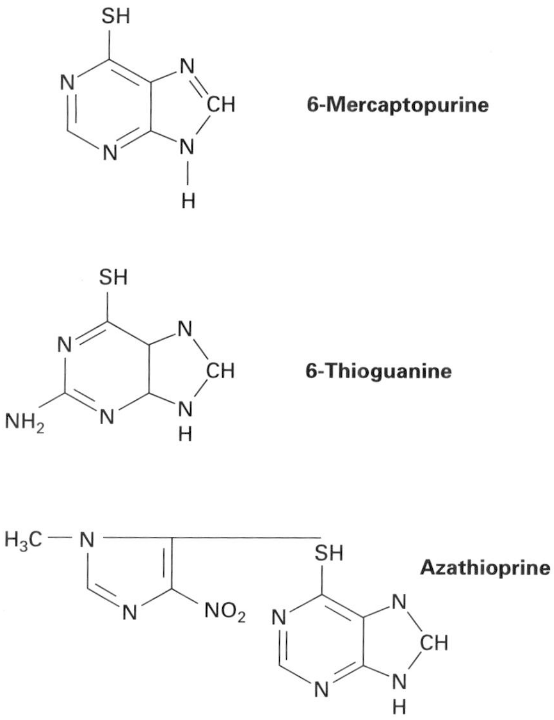

Fig. 6.9 The structures of commonly used purine analogues.

cleared from the plasma (half-life 90 min) due to distribution and metabolism. A major site of metabolism is the liver, where xanthine-oxidase rapidly converts the drug to an inactive form. The xanthine-oxidase inhibitor allopurinol blocks this conversion, but this increases toxicity as well as effectiveness and the therapeutic ratio is unchanged. If allopurinol is used in the early stages to prevent hyperuricaemia it will increase the toxicity of 6-MP. 6-Mercaptopurine is widely used in remission maintenance in ALL. Its use as an immunosuppressive agent has largely been superseded by azathioprine. The frequent occurrence of cholestatic jaundice with 6-MP has made it less satisfactory for long-term administration. Its other toxicities are nausea and vomiting with gradual and reversible bone marrow suppression. The usual maintenance dose in ALL is 50–100 mg/day.

AZATHIOPRINE (IMURAN) (Fig. 6.9)

This drug was developed in an attempt to decrease the rate of inactivation of 6-MP. The drug acts as a 'prodrug' whereby 6-MP is slowly formed in the tissues. It is degraded in the liver by xanthine-oxidase, and allopurinol increases its toxicity. The drug is well absorbed orally and is partly excreted by the kidneys, so that its toxicity is greater if renal failure is present. Reversible bone marrow depression is the major toxicity. It is most widely used as an 'immunosuppressive' agent in connective tissue diseases and renal allograft recipients. The usual dose is 1–2 mg/kg/day.

6-THIOGUANINE (Fig. 6.9)

This purine analogue has a mode of action similar to that of 6-MP. It is well absorbed orally and peak concentrations are achieved in 6–8 h. About half the dose is excreted in the urine as metabolites within 24 h. Degradation by xanthine-oxidase does not appear to be an important aspect of detoxification and the drug can be used safely with allopurinol. The drug is widely used as part of remission induction and maintenance in AML. It has also been used as an immunosuppressive. The average oral daily dose is 2 mg/kg. Reversible bone marrow depression is the major toxicity, but nausea and diarrhoea may also occur.

FLUDARABINE

This drug is closely related to cytosine arabinoside. The purine is fluorinated and competes for incorporation into DNA, inhibiting cell replication by acting as a chain terminator when incorporated into the newly synthesized DNA. It also inhibits RNA synthesis. It is active in low-grade lymphomas and chronic lymphocytic leukaemia, even in tumours resistant to conventional agents. Its toxic effects include myelosuppression and immunosuppression.

2-DEOXYCOFORMYCIN (PENTOSTATIN)

This increasingly used drug is closely related to adenosine and is a potent inhibitor of adenosine deaminase. The drug has proved to be active both as an immunosuppressive and in treatment of lymphomas (see Chapter 26).

VINCA ALKALOIDS AND TAXANES

Vinca alkaloids are extracted from the periwinkle, *Catharanthus roseus*, and were observed to cause granulocytopenia in animals. Subsequently they were shown to be mitotic spindle poisons, and their mode of action is related to other agents such as colchicine.

The stages of mitosis are described in Chapter 3, p. 30. The vinca alkaloids and other mitotic inhibitors act by binding to tubulin, which is the constituent protein of the microtubules. The assembly and function of the microtubules during metaphase is shown in Fig. 6.10. Exposure of the cell to vinca alkaloids leads to rapid disappearance of the microtubules because no further assembly can take place (Fig. 6.10). Conversely, the taxane drugs

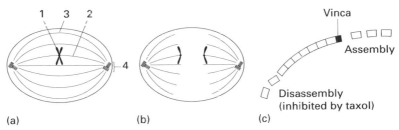

Fig. 6.10 The assembly and function of microtubules during metaphase. (a) The chromosome pair (1) is attached to a microtubule (2) which is assembled at the equatorial region (3) and disassembled at the centriole (4). (b) In the anaphase the chromosome pair is divided and pulled to opposite ends of the cell. (c) A microtubule is a polymer of the protein tubulin which is made up of α and β subunits. Vinca alkaloids bind to tubulin, blocking further assembly, but disassembly continues. Taxol prevents disassembly.

promote assembly of microtubules and inhibit their disassembly.

In cell lines vinca resistance is associated with both the appearance of the 180 kDa membrane glycoprotein and resistance to many other agents (MDR, p. 74). There is often cross-resistance from one vinca alkaloid to another and between vinca alkaloids and podophyllotoxins. Taxane resistance may also be mediated by decreased binding to tublin.

VINCRISTINE

Vincristine is administered intravenously usually in a dose of 1.5 mg/m^2 (maximum 2 mg) and can be repeated weekly when used in the young. It is poorly and unpredictably absorbed from the gut. It is vesicant if it escapes from the vein into the tissues. The pharmacokinetics are similar to those of vinblastine (see below).

The drug is useful in treatment of lymphatic malignancies such as Hodgkin's disease, non-Hodgkin's lymphoma and ALL. In these diseases it is usually used in combination with other drugs such as steroids and alkylating agents. It also has a place in treatment of other cancers such as breast cancers, small-cell carcinoma of the bronchus and brain tumours.

The toxicity of the drug is mainly neurological, and peripheral neuropathy is an almost invariable sequel to long-term administration. It is especially likely to occur in the elderly and those with liver disease, and may be severe and incapacitating. Loss of reflexes and paraesthesia occur early and are not usually regarded as indications for cessation of treatment, but severe myalgic and neuritic pain and motor weakness and/or peripheral sensory loss are signs that treatment should be stopped. Nerve conduction is usually preserved even with severe neuropathy, but electromyography shows a pattern of denervation. Cranial nerve palsies occasionally occur. It is probable that vincristine blocks the passage of tubulin from proximal to distal axonal sites. Autonomic neuropathy often occurs, with constipation and ileus; symptoms can be partially alleviated with bulk laxatives. Myelosuppression is mild, increasing the usefulness of the drug when used in combination. Alopecia occurs in 20% of patients and a syndrome of inappropriate release of ADH occurs. The drug sometimes causes thrombocytosis.

VINBLASTINE (VELBE)

After intravenous injection the drug disappears from the plasma in three phases, with half-lives of 4 min, 1 h and 16 h. Much of the drug remains tissue-bound for many days. In the blood it binds to platelets, red cells and plasma proteins. All vinca alkaloids behave in a similar manner and clinical differences cannot be explained on pharmacokinetic grounds. Indications for the use of vinblastine are similar to those for vincristine. In addition, vinblastine is often used in high dose for the treatment of testicular teratoma in combination with cisplatin and bleomycin (see below and Chapter 19). In these high doses neutropenia and ileus are common. Vinblastine causes more myelosuppression but less neurotoxicity than vincristine. The usual intravenous dose is 6 mg/m^2 weekly. Extravasation leads to cellulitis. Alopecia and mucositis are infrequent side-effects.

VINDESINE

This semisynthetic addition to the vinca alkaloids has a similar spectrum of activity but appears to have additional activity in NSCLC. The toxicity of the drug is intermediate between that of vinblastine and vincristine. Myelosuppression and neurotoxicity both occur.

VINORELBINE

This is a vinca alkaloid which has shown significant activity in advanced NSCLC and breast cancer, with a response rate of about 25%. Its toxicity is myelosuppression but peripheral retinopathy is less marked.

PACLITAXEL (TAXOL) [9]

This drug is an extract from the bark of the Pacific yew *Taxus brevifolia*. It promotes assembly of microtubules and inhibits their disassembly. It is poorly water-soluble and is formulated in cremophor oil. When infused, the dose-limiting toxicity is neutropenia. Other side-effects are neuropathy, alopecia and myalgia. It is active in advanced ovarian cancer, with a response rate of 30%, and is also effective for breast cancer; responses have been reported in NSCLC and melanoma. When combined with anthracyclines, mucositis has been dose-limiting. It is currently given as a 3-h infusion.

Docetaxel (Taxotere) is a novel semisynthetic taxoid. It has significant activity against breast cancer and NSCLC, and some activity in a number of other tumours, including cancers of the head and neck, ovary and pancreas. The dose-limiting toxicity is neutropenia, but other side-effects are hypersensitivity, skin reactions, fluid retention, neuropathy and alopecia. The current treatment schedule is usually a 1-h infusion every 3 weeks.

TOPOISOMERASE INHIBITORS

Topoisomerases are nuclear enzymes that alter the three-dimensional structure of DNA. They cause breaks in the strands which allow the DNA to unwind during cell division. Two broad classes of enzyme are described (topoisomerase I and II).

Epipodophyllotoxin derivatives: etoposide (VP16-213) and vepesid (VM26) These substances are semisynthetic derivatives of extracts of *Podophyllum peltatum*, the American mandrake. Topoisomerase II is an enzyme involved in reversibly cleaving DNA so that it can unwind during cell division. The drug stabilizes the enzyme–DNA 'cleavable complex' and results in DNA strand breaks. The drugs have an early rapid phase of clearance followed by a slower phase (half-life 11–39 h for vepesid and 2–13 h for etoposide). They enter the CSF in low concentration. Etoposide is the drug most widely used. It is absorbed erratically from the gut with a plasma availability of about 50% of the intravenous dose. The drug can be infused at high dose. However, mucositis then becomes dose-limiting. At conventional doses bone marrow suppression is the major toxicity. Etoposide is highly protein-bound

and about half the drug is excreted in the urine in 72 h. After dilution it is stable for about 24 h, depending on the concentration. Etoposide activity is highly schedule-dependent. In SCLC the response rate is greatly increased by repeated daily administration compared with the same total dose as a single infusion.

TOPOISOMERASE I INHIBITORS (CAMPTOTHECIN, IRINOTECAN, TOPOTECAN) [10]

The prototype drug is camptothecin, derived from *Camptotheca acuminata* (a Chinese tree). It binds to the enzyme–DNA complex, stabilizing it, preventing DNA replication and provoking breaks of the DNA double strand.

Irinotecan has now been extensively evaluated. It is active in a wide range of carcinomas, especially of the gut and lung. The main toxicities are myelosuppression and diarrhoea. The drug is excreted in bile and urine and has a long half-life. It is a prodrug which is converted to an active metabolite. Topotecan is a similar agent whose major toxicity is bone marrow suppression; it has not yet been fully evaluated.

Drug resistance depends on altered topoisomerase I function, *p*-glycoprotein and poor conversion of irinotecan to its active metabolite (see p. 74).

The drugs are useful in treatment of lymphomas, acute leukaemias, SCLC, testicular and brain tumours. The toxic effects are alopecia, leucopenia, nausea and vomiting, febrile reactions and peripheral neuropathy.

Antitumour antibiotics

Many antitumour antibiotics have now been produced from bacterial and fungal cultures. They produce their effect by binding to DNA, intercalating between base pairs.

ACTINOMYCIN D (DACTINOMYCIN)

This antibiotic was first isolated from *Streptomyces* in 1940. At low concentrations it blocks DNA-directed RNA synthesis and at higher concentration also blocks DNA synthesis. The drug does not react directly with RNA. The molecule intercalates between guanine–cytosine base pairs and the transcription of DNA is blocked. The drug inhibits the division of all rapidly dividing cells. Resistance appears to be associated with both impaired drug entry and increased drug efflux.

It is given intravenously and is cleared within a few minutes. The usual daily dose is 15 µg/kg, and this can be repeated daily for 4–5 days. A further course of injections can be given 3–4 weeks later. It is, however, more usual to give the drug as a single injection of 15 μg/kg in combination with other agents (such as vincristine and cyclophosphamide).

Its main use has been in the treatment of childhood cancers, such as rhabdomyosarcoma, Wilms' tumour and Ewing's sarcoma. It is of less value in adult tumours. The toxicities are nausea and vomiting, myelosuppression, mucositis and diarrhoea. It sensitizes tissue to radiation.

DOXORUBICIN AND DAUNORUBICIN

These are anthracycline antibiotics produced from a species of *Streptomyces* fungus. Doxorubicin is a useful agent with a wide spectrum of activity against many tumours and differs from daunorubicin only in the substitution of an -CH group for a hydrogen atom.

Both drugs bind tightly to DNA, deforming the helical structure. The drugs intercalate between base pairs, but there appears to be no base specificity in the binding. Breaks in DNA strands have also been shown to occur. The drugs also produce highly active intracellular free radicals which may be important in producing some of the toxic effects, for example cardiac toxicity. Drug resistance is mediated, at least in part, through the MDR drug-efflux protein (p. 74). There appears to be complete cross-resistance between these two drugs as well as some degree of cross-resistance with vinca alkaloids and actinomycin, probably due to the MDR mechanism. The drugs are effective mainly against cells in S phase.

Both drugs are injected intravenously into a fast-running drip, and are highly vesicant. They are cleared rapidly from the plasma, but there is a slow terminal clearance of doxorubicin. There is rapid uptake into spleen, kidney, lungs, liver and heart, but not into the brain. The drugs are metabolized in the liver, and severe toxicity may result if they are given to patients with impaired liver function. With doxorubicin, 40% is excreted in the bile as free drug, adriamycinol and other metabolites. With both drugs the major and acute side-effects are bone marrow depression, nausea and vomiting, mucositis, alopecia and gastrointestinal disturbance. Alopecia can perhaps be lessened by cooling the scalp with ice packs for 25 min before and after drug administration. The most important chronic and dose-limiting side-effect is cardiotoxicity causing arrhythmias and heart failure. It is related to the total dose administered and is a major risk above a total dose of 500 mg/m^2. However, cardiac damage may occasionally occur with total dose of as little as 300 mg/m^2. In addition to total dose, the drug schedule may be important. High peak plasma concentrations may be associated with more toxicity. Subclinical cardiac toxicity may be

more frequent than suspected previously, which may be of great importance in the treatment of childhood tumours. Cardioprotective agents are currently under evaluation [11]. Doxorubicin has a wide spectrum of activity in childhood and adult tumours including lymphomas, small-cell bronchogenic carcinoma, adenocarcinomas of ovary, breast and stomach, bone and soft-tissue sarcomas, liver and bladder cancer.

Daunorubicin is of value in the treatment of ALL and AML. Dosage schedules vary but 50 mg/m^2 once weekly is often given.

MITOXANTRONE

This is an anthraquinone related to doxorubicin which binds to DNA. When injected intravenously it has a terminal half-life of 36 h. It is vesicant and has a spectrum of activity similar to doxorubicin, with useful effects in metastatic breast cancer, lymphoma and leukaemia. The main toxicity is myelosuppression. It causes less alopecia than doxorubicin and possibly less cardiotoxicity. The usual single dose schedule is 12–15 mg/m^2 repeated every 3 weeks.

MITHRAMYCIN

This antibiotic is derived from *Streptomyces plicatus*. It had some clinical use in the treatment of hypercalcaemia because it inhibits osteoclast action. It has activity against embryonal carcinoma of the testis. It inhibits RNA synthesis, possibly in a manner similar to actinomycin D. It crosses the blood–brain barrier and penetrates into brain tumours. It is locally irritant, is inactive orally, and is therefore given intravenously. In full doses (25 μg/kg) it causes nausea, stomatitis, thrombocytopenia, a haemorrhagic tendency and impaired renal and liver function.

BLEOMYCIN

This antibiotic was derived from a mixture of glycopeptides isolated from *Streptomyces verticillus* but is now chemically synthesized. The drug inhibits DNA synthesis and causes breaks in the DNA chain. It arrests cells in G$_2$.

The drug can be given parenterally by any route. It disappears from the plasma with an initial half-life of 1 h and then more slowly (half-life 9 h). It is excreted in the urine, and caution is needed with impaired renal function. The drug concentration is very low in the brain and CSF, and it appears to be concentrated mainly in skin and lung. Many tissues contain an inactivating enzyme which hydrolyses the drug, and the levels of this enzyme appear to correlate with resistance. It is active in squamous carcinomas of the head and neck, skin and cervix and against lymphomas and testicular tumours.

The drug is valuable in combination with other agents because it causes little bone marrow toxicity. Skin toxicity is characterized by pigmentation, erythema and vesiculation. It also causes mucosal ulceration, pulmonary infiltrates and fibrosis. These toxic effects are serious, sometimes disabling. and are related to total dose, with a high risk when the dose exceeds $300\,mg/m^2$. Acute pyrexial reactions commonly occur, and can be relieved or prevented by hydrocortisone. In rare cases, cardio-respiratory collapse occurs. A small subcutaneous test dose at the start of treatment is a wise precaution.

The dosage schedule varies considerably but is usually of the order of $15\,mg/m^2$ as a single dose which can be repeated weekly.

Miscellaneous agents

CIS-DIAMMINE DICHLOROPLATINUM (CISPLATIN)

The drug is only active in the *cis* form. It acts as an alkylating agent. It diffuses into cells, and the chloride ions are then lost from the molecule. The compound then binds to DNA, producing inter- and intrastrand cross-links. The binding appears to be mainly to guanine groups. The drug is administered intravenously. The early half-life is about 40 min and the later phase of clearance is slow (half-life 60 h). It is 90% bound to plasma protein, and is taken up in the kidney, gut, liver, ovary and testis but not in the CNS.

The drug is highly nephrotoxic, and when administered in high dose a high urine flow is essential, with intra-venous fluids being administered before the drug and for 24 h after. Renal function may worsen during repeated cycles and the plasma creatinine level and clearance should be checked regularly. With some high-dose regimens mannitol is used to maintain urine flow. Loss of K^+ and Mg^{2+}/Ca^{2+} in the urine may require electrolyte supplementation in both the short and long term. Nausea and vomiting are severe with higher doses, and ototoxicity may be irreversible so that pretreatment audiometry should be carried out. Myelosuppression is not severe, but peripheral neuropathy is frequent and often subclinical.

Cisplatin is very effective in the treatment of testicular tumours and, in combination with vinblastine and bleomycin, has revolutionized the outlook in advanced disease (see Chapter 19). It is also effective in cancer of the ovary and bladder as well as in lymphomas and small-cell carcinoma of the bronchus. It is active in osteosarcoma and squamous cancer of the head and neck.

CARBOPLATIN (PARAPLATIN)

This analogue of cisplatin has a different spectrum of toxicity from cisplatin but is active in the same tumours. It is given intravenously and the area under the concentration–time curve (AUC) is given by the formula $AUC = (GFR\,(ml/min) + (25)n$ where n is the desired multiple. Thus dose required for AUC 5 in a patient with a glomerular filtration rate (GFR) of 120 is $(120 + 25) \times 5 = 725\,mg$. Some drug regimens are given according to this formula, others on a conventional dose per square metre basis. The main toxicity is myelosuppression, which may be profound. Typically its onset is at 14–21 days and for this reason intervals between treatments may need to be 28 days. It causes less nausea and vomiting than cisplatin and is not as nephrotoxic or neurotoxic. The drug is given by intravenous injection in saline or dextrose/saline. Pre-hydration and posthydration are not necessary unless there is vomiting. In testicular cancer the drug is less effective than cisplatin since dose reduction is necessary due to myelosuppression. It is active in SCLC and ovarian cancer. In the latter its ease of administration makes it valuable for palliative treatment.

L-ASPARAGINASE (CRASNITINE, ELSPAR)

When L-asparaginase was first shown to have antitumour effects, it was hoped that it might prove to be an agent acting exclusively on malignant cells. The enzyme is produced by *Escherichia coli* and *Erwinia carotovora* and its action is based on the observation that while most normal tissues synthesize asparagine, some tumour cells need an exogenous source which the enzyme removes. Resistance may be related to the appearance of asparagine synthetase in the tumour cells.

The drug is initially eliminated rapidly from the circulation, but the later half-life is 6–30 h. It does not penetrate into the CSF. There is no marrow, gut or hair follicle toxicity, but anaphylaxis, pancreatitis, hyperglycaemia, raised liver enzymes with fatty change in the liver, confusion, somnolence, coma and hypofibrinogenaemia all occur and the drug is extremely nauseating.

The main use of the drug is in remission induction in ALL. The dosage schedules vary considerably with different combinations of drugs.

PROCARBAZINE (NATULAN)

This drug is the most useful of the hydrazine derivatives which were originally synthesized as monoamine oxidase inhibitors and found to have antitumour activity. The mode of action is, however, unclear. Metabolic activation is needed and the active product may be a methyldiazonium ion which acts as an alkylating agent. The drug oxidizes at 37°C and hydrogen peroxide is formed but does not appear to be responsible for the cytotoxic effect. Interphase is prolonged and mitosis is suppressed with breakage of chromatin strands.

The drug is very well absorbed from the gut, and rapidly equilibrates with blood and CSF. After intravenous injection the half-life is 7 min and the drug is rapidly metabolized. The toxic effects are nausea and vomiting, leucopenia, CNS disturbances (especially psychological upsets), flushing with alcohol, and hypertensive reactions to foods rich in tyramine.

The drug is usually given in a dose of 100 mg/m² daily for 1–2 weeks. It is especially useful in Hodgkin's disease and in brain tumours.

HYDROXYUREA (HYDREA)

This drug was synthesized over 100 years ago, but was only found to have antineoplastic activity much later. It blocks the action of ribonucleoside diphosphate reductase and thereby interferes with DNA synthesis. It causes leucopenia and megaloblastic changes in the bone marrow. It is S phase specific, and has been used in attempts to produce cell synchronization.

The drug is well absorbed orally and enters the CSF. It is excreted in the urine. The usual dose is 20–30 mg/kg/day, or 80 mg/kg every 3 days. Toxic effects are mainly marrow suppression and gut disturbances. Its main use is in chronic granulocytic leukaemia.

HEXAMETHYLMELAMINE (HEXALAN)

Although this drug has a similar structure to the alkylating agent triethylene melamine, it does not act as an alkylating agent itself. Indeed, its mechanism of action remains largely unknown. It is well absorbed orally and is rapidly metabolized.

The drug is administered in 2–3-week cycles of 12 mg/kg/day and is active in ovarian and cervical cancer. Nausea, vomiting and neurotoxicity are major problems with its use. Abdominal cramps and diarrhoea occur and leucopenia may develop. Central nervous system toxicity includes altered mental state, extrapyramidal effects and convulsions.

New targets in drug development

Drugs acting on signalling pathways

The pathways that transmit external signals into the cell have formed targets for new drug development. The aim is to block the subsequent processes of protein production and cell division. These processes are essential for normal cells. There may be many alternative pathways for each signalling event. The therapeutic action in cancer will therefore depend on the degree to which the tumour relies on the pathway concerned.

RECEPTOR TYROSINE KINASES (RTK)

The action of RTKs is shown in very simplified form in Fig. 6.11. Ligands activating the pathway include epithelial growth factors (EGF), transforming growth factor-α (TGF-α), vascular endothelial growth factor (VEGF) and

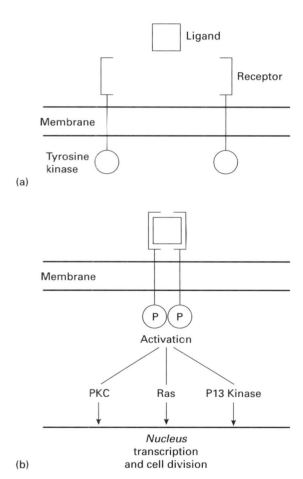

Fig. 6.11 The receptor tyrosine kinase action. (a) The receptor is external and tyrosine kinase internal to the cell membrane. (b) The ligand causes dimerization and the kinase is activated by phosphorylation (P). This results in activation of protein kinase C, Ras and PI3 kinase to produce transcription and DNA synthesis.

their receptors HER 1–4. Overexpression of HER-2 is present in 30% of breast cancers. Herceptin is a humanized monoclonal antibody that blocks HER-2 and has been shown to increase response and prolong survival in advanced disease. Drug equivalents are being developed as are inhibitors of VEGFr.

C-*abl* is a cytoplasmic tyrosine kinase which forms a fusion protein with *bcr* as a result of the 9;22 translocation in chronic myeloid leukaemia (see Chapter 28, p. 450). The action of the *bcr*/*abl* protein appears critical for chronic myeloblastic leukaemia (CML) growth. STI 571 is a drug that blocks this action and which produces a high and prolonged response rate in CML.

RAS INHIBITORS

Activation of *ras* is important in malignant growth. The *Ras* family of proteins must be modified biochemically by the enzyme farnesyl transferase before they are activated. Inhibitors of this enzyme have shown activity in model systems.

INHIBITORS OF PROTEIN KINASE C (PKC)

There are many isoforms of PKC. Bryostatin is the first agent to be tested clinically and has shown some activity, with myalgia as the main toxicity. It is now being tested in combination. Staurosporine acts at the catalytic site of PKC and has shown antitumour activity in phase 1 studies. This drug and its derivatives bind to an acid glycoprotein in plasma and this prolongs the half-life. They are now being tested in combination with conventional cytotoxic drugs.

Cyclin-dependent kinases (CDKs)

Cyclin-dependent kinases are essential components of the cell cycle regulatory mechanism. Various inhibitors have now entered phase 1 studies. The best studied of these is flavopiridol which has shown activity against a variety of tumours. Diarrhoea and myalgia are the main toxicities. Other compounds are in development.

Metalloprotease inhibitors

Matrix metalloproteases are secreted enzymes involved in tumour cell movement through connective tissue. They are secreted in an inactive form and are cleaved to become active. Tissue inhibitors of metalloproteases (TIMPs) regulate their action. They appear to be important in local invasion and in metastasis. The most studied inhibitor is marimistat. It slowed the rise of tumour markers in phase 2 studies but larger studies have not confirmed its clinical value. The main toxicity is myalgia.

Inhibitors of angiogenesis

Approaches to the inhibition of angiogenesis have been: to target the tumour endothelium by toxins—combrestatins are the most promising drugs at present. Inhibition of angiogenetic cytokines, such as VEGF, and those of the endogenous angiogenesis inhibitor angiostatin are other approaches that hold promise for the future.

The administration of cytotoxic agents

There is much to be said against the occasional chemotherapist. Most surgeons, gynaecologists and physicians are quite unfamiliar with cytotoxic agents and, when they attempt to use them, often run into difficulty because of lack of either experience or an appropriate organization to give drugs, check on blood counts and enquire into side-effects. For best results, chemotherapy should be in the hands of those expert in its administration.

Patients on outpatient regimens

The majority of patients can receive their drugs in this way, especially if the person giving them is the same each time and gets to know the best antiemetic or sedative regimen for *that patient.* Some patients are not sick at all, others vomit several hours later and prefer to get home quickly and take a 5-hydroxytryptamine-3 (5-HT$_3$) antagonist, others vomit at the sight of the needle and require premedication with diazepam or prochlorperazine. There is little doubt that trained nurses are the best people to give the drugs. They become very expert in putting up intravenous infusions and noting side-effects from previous drug treatment, and there are seldom difficulties with extravasation. Newly qualified house staff are not nearly as capable or as accessible to the patient during the day. Patients undergoing cytotoxic chemotherapy should be aware of the nature of the treatment and its possible hazards. It is easier to make sure that patients receive adequate information if the treatment is the responsibility of a single department. The patient should be told of the nature of the drugs, what the possible side-effects might be and which of these effects should lead the patient to contact the hospital. For example, he or she should be told to report fever or sore throat so that a blood count can be taken. It is worthwhile to give explanatory leaflets about chemotherapy, and drug cards giving the names, dosage and purposes of the drugs are very useful (Fig. 6.12).

Patients staying overnight

Some regimens such as those containing high-dose platinum, or a methotrexate infusion, require an overnight stay. It is convenient and efficient to have designated overnight-stay beds for this kind of chemotherapy where the admission is planned in advance and is relatively informal. The ward chemotherapy nurse gives the drugs after the patient has been seen by a doctor. The nurse arranges the next admission and ensures that the patient knows when to come back for interim blood counts.

Patients on lengthy regimens

These patients, many of whom are on treatments where there is a serious possibility of prolonged myelosuppres-

sion, are admitted to hospital. They are under the care of a single team, experienced in the use of intensive cytotoxic regimens and in mitigating the side-effects of the drugs, and familiar with the supportive techniques required (see Chapter 7).

Chemotherapy-induced vomiting [12]

The mechanisms by which chemotherapy induces vomiting are not well understood. Both peripheral (gastric and intestinal) and central stimuli may be important. A schematic representation is shown in Fig. 6.12. Studies on high-dose metoclopramide (see below) have shown that blockage of 5-HT$_3$ receptors is part of its action and have led to the introduction of 5-HT$_3$ antagonists as a new class of antiemetic.

Intravenous alkylating agents, doxorubicin and cisplatin typically produce nausea and vomiting 2–8 h after injection, and the symptoms persist for 8–36 h. Other drugs do not cause vomiting so frequently. After one or two cycles of chemotherapy some patients suffer from anticipatory nausea and vomiting at the sight of the nurse, doctor, intravenous infusion or hospital or even on setting out on the journey to hospital. In these patients prophylactic antiemetic therapy must be given a considerable time before chemotherapy.

Several different types of drug can be used to prevent or treat vomiting (Table 6.3). None is satisfactory in all patients and most are only partially effective. Antiemetic therapy should be started prophylactically, and often a satisfactory regimen can be established in each individual patient by trial and error.

5-HT$_3$ antagonists

This class of compound represents a major step forward in the control of vomiting. Control of cisplatin-induced emesis is achieved in 60% of patients—similar to optimum results obtained with combinations of metoclopramide, maxolon and dexamethasone. Ondansetron, tropisetron and graniseteron are selective 5-HT$_3$ antagonists. The main site of action (central or peripheral) is still unclear. Ondansetron has good oral bioavailability. Both are safe and well tolerated. The terminal plasma half-life of ondansetron is approximately 3 h. Side-effects include headache, flushing and constipation. Hepatic dysfunction decreases metabolism. The usual dose of ondansetron is 8 mg by slow intravenous infusion, then two further doses 4 h apart followed by 8 mg twice daily to prevent delayed emesis, for 3 days.

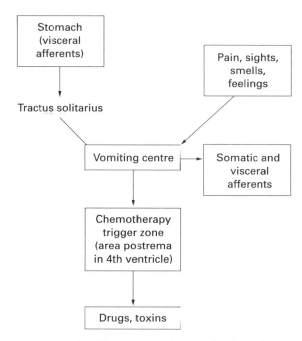

Fig. 6.12 A simplified scheme of events in chemotherapy-induced vomiting. The site of action of antiemetics is not shown since the details are not clearly established. 5-HT$_3$ receptors are assumed to play a role in the central and peripheral mechanisms. Chemotherapy may damage cells of the intestinal lumen, liberating 5-HT from enterochromaffin cells.

Table 6.3 Antiemetic agents.

Agent	Dose	Action	Toxicity
Ondansetron	0.15 mg/kg 4-hourly	5-HT$_3$ antagonist	Constipation, headache
Granisetron	3 mg i.v. over 5–10min	5-HT$_3$ antagonist	Constipation, headache
Metoclopramide	10 mg p.o. or i.v. or 1–2 mg/kg i.v. repeated 3-hourly	Dopamine and 5-HT$_3$ antagonist (central and peripheral)	Extrapyramidal symptoms, diarrhoea
Dexamethasone	8–16 mg i.v. before treatment	Unclear	Restlessness, mood changes
Benzodiazepines, e.g. lorazepam	1–2 mg p.o. or i.v. every 4–6 h	Cerebral cortex, ? histamine receptor blocking agent	Sedation, hypotension, hallucinations, dysphoria, dizziness, ataxia
Phenothiazines, e.g. prochlorperazine	12.5 mg i.m. or 25 mg suppository	Dopamine antagonist	Extrapyramidal symptoms, drowsiness
Butyrophenones, e.g. haloperidol	0.5–1 mg p.o. or i.v. repeated 4–8 h	? Dopamine antagonist	Extrapyramidal symptoms, akasthesia

i.m., intramuscularly; i.v., intravenously; p.o., by mouth.

PIPERAZINE PHENOTHIAZINES

These include prochlorperazine and perphenazine. They are effective antiemetics in some patients but must be used near the maximum dose, at which point extrapyramidal reactions are common, particularly with intravenous administration.

ALIPHATIC PHENOTHIAZINES

The most commonly used agents are chlorpromazine and promazine. They have more sedative and less antiemetic properties and are more liable to produce hypotension.

METOCLOPRAMIDE

This drug appears to act on the trigger area, possibly through blocking dopamine receptors. It increases gastric emptying. The drug can be given intramuscularly or intravenously and may cause extrapyramidal side-effects, restlessness and diarrhoea. In low dose (10 mg orally or intravenously) it has little activity.

Metoclopramide is often used in high dose in the prevention of vomiting. It is probable that it is more effective at high dose, and some studies have shown that it is more effective than phenothiazines and may act as a 5-HT$_3$ receptor antagonist. The incidence of extrapyramidal side-effects does not appear to be greater in high dose. Randomized trials have shown high-dose metoclopramide to be superior to phenothiazines.

BENZODIAZEPINES

Although these drugs have no antiemetic properties they may make the vomiting more tolerable by inducing a somnolent state in which the patient cannot remember the period of nausea clearly. Intravenous lorazepam is useful for this purpose.

BUTYROPHENONE DERIVATIVES

These drugs are dopamine receptor blocking agents which work centrally. Haloperidol is the most widely used and is partially effective against cisplatin-induced vomiting.

Long-term complications of cancer chemotherapy

More children and young adults are now surviving diseases such as acute leukaemia, lymphoma and testicular cancer which were formerly incurable. Survival has been achieved by intensive combination chemotherapy. It has become apparent that chemotherapy of this type is associated with long-term complications in some patients. The recognition of these sequelae has emphasized that treatment of great intensity must be justified by a clear benefit in survival and that such drug and radiation therapies must be restricted to those categories of patient in which they are essential for survival. Long-term follow-up of patients is essential since some of the complications may develop many years after treatment is discontinued.

Impaired gonadal function

Suppression of spermatogenesis occurs in the majority of

men being treated with combination chemotherapy. Procarbazine and alkylating agents seem to have the greatest adverse effect, methotrexate and doxorubicin less so. The degree of infertility and its permanence vary with different regimens [13]. With MOPP therapy (mustine, vincristine, prednisone and procarbazine) for Hodgkin's disease (see Chapter 25) 95% of men will have long-lasting infertility. With the doxorubicin, bleomycin, vinblastine and dacarbazine regimen this is less, and with the cisplatin, vinblastine and bleomycin regimen for teratoma there is frequent recovery of fertility. Damage to the germinal epithelium is associated with a rise in serum follicle-stimulating hormone (FSH), which normally stimulates spermatogenesis. While prepubertal boys do not appear to experience long-lasting endocrine changes from chemotherapy, intensive chemotherapy during puberty damages Leydig cells and is accompanied by a rise in both FSH and luteinizing hormone (LH), low testosterone levels and gynaecomastia.

The likely effects of chemotherapy must be discussed with all postpubertal males. Sperm-storage facilities must be available for all such patients. Three semen samples should be collected over a week before treatment. This can be reduced to two if treatment is urgent. It is essential that the likely outcome of the storage procedure is discussed in full. The samples should be kept, with the documentation, for at least 10 years together with instructions about destruction of the samples in the event of death. Successful pregnancy by artificial insemination is still infrequent using stored samples. When the quality and number are low the technique of intracytoplasmic sperm injection (ICSI) is increasingly being used with success.

Ovarian failure is often produced by combination chemotherapy and is more frequent the nearer the patient is to her natural menopause. Even if menstruation does not cease, subfertility is common and the duration of the reproductive years of life is shortened, with earlier menopause. Temporary oligomenorrhoea is common with the onset of chemotherapy. The onset of the true menopause can be determined by a rise in FSH that is not suppressed by hormone replacement therapy (HRT). HRT should be offered to all women with a premature menopause induced by chemotherapy. There is no effective method of cyropreserving oocytes.

Pulmonary fibrosis [14]

Pulmonary damage is produced by many cytotoxic drugs (Table 6.4). Most alkylating agents will produce pulmonary fibrosis with long-term impairment of diffus-

ing capacity. Busulphan is, however, more likely to do so than other drugs. Bleomycin causes pulmonary infiltrates, a phenomenon related to total dose which is very common over $300\,mg/m^2$. These infiltrates may diminish when the drug is stopped but permanent fibrosis often follows.

Liver disease

Many drugs cause a transient rise in plasma enzymes (nitrosoureas, methotrexate, cytosine arabinoside) but permanent hepatic dysfunction is rare. Permanent liver damage can occasionally occur with antimetabolites (Table 6.4).

Second cancers after chemotherapy

Second malignancies have been noted after long-term administration of alkylating agents, particularly melphalan and chlorambucil, typically given to patients with ovarian cancer and myeloma. In both cases there is an increased risk of AML. Almost all alkylating agents are leukaemogenic, and there is increasing evidence that second cancers are also induced by anthracyclines and epipodophyllotoxins.

Studies have clearly demonstrated the increased risk of leukaemia in Hodgkin's disease and ovarian cancer. In Hodgkin's disease [15] the relative risk is higher in young patients and is greatly outweighed by the survival advantage of treatment. In ovarian cancer the survival benefit of chemotherapy is less marked. Chemotherapy-induced leukaemia is associated with non-random chromosomal deletions (for example, on chromosomes 5 and 7), and the leukaemia tends to be refractory to treatment. Bladder

Table 6.4 Pulmonary and hepatic toxicity of cytotoxic drugs.

Drug	Effect
Pulmonary	
Busulphan and nitrosoureas (and other alkylating agents)	Fibrosis
Bleomycin	Pulmonary infiltrates and
Mitomycin C	fibrosis
Hepatic	
Methotrexate	Fibrosis
6-MP and azathioprine	Cholestatic jaundice and necrosis
Asparaginase	Fatty infiltration

cancer is a reported complication of cyclophosphamide therapy but the risk appears to be very small.

Long-term immunosuppressive therapy in renal allograft recipients (and the immune suppression in acquired immune deficiency syndrome) also predisposes to the development of cancer. Lymphomas are the commonest malignancy, particularly large-cell lymphoma of the brain. The average time of onset is 2 years but the risk persists indefinitely.

Postulated mechanisms are a direct carcinogenic effect of the drugs, diminished 'immune surveillance' and activation of oncogenic viruses in immunosuppressed individuals. In radiation-induced cancers of bone there appears to be an added risk if chemotherapy has been used as well.

Principles of hormone therapy

The demonstration by Beatson in 1896 that inoperable breast cancer sometimes regressed after oophorectomy was one of the most remarkable discoveries in the history of cancer treatment. Many years later, Huggins demonstrated that metastatic prostatic cancer would regress with orchidectomy or the administration of oestrogens. In recent years, there has been a transformation in our understanding. In at least one tumour, breast cancer, knowledge of the hormone receptor status of the tumour has become clinically important.

Steroid hormone receptors

There are receptor proteins for steroid hormones in both the cytoplasm and the nucleus. Interaction between the hormone and its receptor modifies DNA activity and hence cell growth and replication. These events are depicted diagrammatically in Fig. 6.13.

The steroid hormone, unbound to plasma protein, crosses the cell membrane by a mechanism which is not well understood. The hormone then links to the cytoplasmic receptor protein and the complex undergoes a conformational change in either the cytoplasm or the nucleus. This hormone–receptor complex binds to a nuclear protein which in turn exerts a controlling activity on DNA. There then follows an increase in RNA polymerase activity which results in the synthesis, first of messenger RNA, and then of cytoplasmic protein. After 24 h DNA synthesis occurs, followed by cell division.

This model appears to be generally applicable to a variety of steroid hormones. The synthesis of the receptor

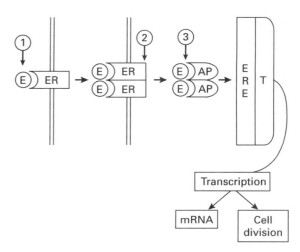

Fig. 6.13 Oestrogen (E) binds to the oestrogen receptor (ER) which dimerizes. The complex becomes active (AP) and binds to oestrogen-response elements (ERE) in the nucleus. Other proteins (T) involved in transcription, such as RNA polymerase II, are activated leading to protein synthesis and cell division. Goserelin lowers the plama oestrogen (1); Fulvestrant, (2) prevents receptor dimerization and activation; Tamoxyfen binds to the active complex inactivating its role in initiating transcription.

proteins is promoted by the hormone to which they bind and that other hormones can reduce the synthesis of receptor proteins; for example, progesterone inhibits the synthesis of oestrogen receptor (ER).

Using these concepts of hormone action, several strategies for modifying tumour growth can be developed: the plasma concentration of the stimulating hormone might be lowered by ablative therapy, either surgical, radiotherapeutic or chemical. Once the hormone has entered the cell it may be prevented from binding to the receptor by either competitive inhibitors or reduction of receptor synthesis. It might also be possible to block the binding of the complex to the nuclear 'acceptor' protein.

In practice it is often difficult to determine the site of action of agents used in hormone therapy. Tamoxifen, for example, appears to bind to the ER but may also affect its synthesis, and the tamoxifen–receptor complex may also block the acceptor site in the nucleus.

The situation may become clearer when it is possible to measure the concentration of receptor molecules independently of their hormone binding properties. It may then be possible to say whether lack of oestrogen binding, for example, is due to lack of receptor protein or to lack of free binding sites.

Hormone receptor assays

Attempts to use the presence of a hormone receptor to predict the responsiveness of an individual tumour to hormone manipulation have been only partially successful. The usual assay is a measure of uptake of isotopically labelled hormone by homogenized tumour cells. The degree of binding varies, and an arbitrary cut-off point has to be made in what is in fact a gradation from negative to positive. In studies on tissue sections it can be shown that in breast cancer some cells are ER-positive and others ER-negative. The overall expression of ER status is thus an oversimplification of the position. Furthermore, the presence of hormone receptors does not prove that they are functionally active. Oestrogen promotes the synthesis of progesterone receptor (PR) in breast cancer cells, and measurement of PR may thus provide a better measure of functionally active ER than measurement of ER itself. At present it is clear that in breast cancer, for example, the absence (or very low values) of an ER strongly predicts a lack of response to hormone manipulation, and that high levels of receptor are indicative of probable response. Intermediate values are associated with a variable response rate.

The role of hormone therapy in individual tumours is discussed in detail in the appropriate chapters.

Approaches to hormone therapy

Lowering the plasma hormone concentration

This may be done by medical or surgical means.

MEDICAL

In premenopausal women the main source of oestrogens is the ovary, but some oestrogens are formed as a result of the peripheral conversion of androgens, formed in the adrenal. This conversion takes place in muscle, liver and fat, and is mediated by aromatase enzymes. After the menopause the adrenal becomes the main source of oestrogens by production of androgen (δ-4-androstenedione), which is converted in the peripheral tissues. However, the adrenal is not the only source of oestrogen precursors, and breast tissue itself can synthesize oestrogens. Aromatase inhibitors block the action of aromatase enzymes and also depress synthesis of androgens and cortisol in the adrenal itself. In premenopausal women the major source of oestrogen synthesis is the ovary, which is not dependent on aromatase enzymes. Inhibition of aromatase prevents the conversion of androgens to oestrogen—the only source of the hormone in postmenopausal women. The new aromatase inhibitors have increased effectiveness and greater tolerability than the precursors such as aminogluthethimide. Anastrozole (Arimidex) suppresses plasma oestrogen to undetectable levels without affecting the cortisol response to adrenocorticotrophic hormone (ACTH). It may replace tamoxifen as the hormone treatment of choice in postmenopausal women with breast cancer (see Chapter 13).

Luteinizing hormone releasing hormone (LHRH) is a decapeptide released from the hypothalamus to act on the pituitary (Fig. 6.14). Analogues of LHRH such as goserelin and leuprorelin cause an initial pituitary stimulation, followed by an inhibition of gonadotrophin release which causes a profound fall in plasma testosterone in men and in circulating oestradiol in women. Goserelin (Zoldex) may prove to be the treatment of choice in producing ovarian ablation in premenopausal women with breast cancer. Goserelin is given by subcutaneous injection once a month. If combined with an antiandrogen such as flutamide (see below) more profound suppression of androgen effect is achieved, which may have some extra benefit in prostate cancer.

Blocking the action of circulating hormones Antioestrogens, of which the most notable example is tamoxifen, have been a major advance in the treatment of metastatic breast cancer. The action of tamoxifen is not fully understood. The drug appears to exert its effect by bind-

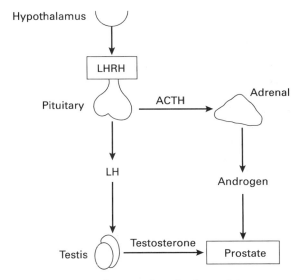

Fig. 6.14 LHRH analogues at first stimulate and then suppress LH release, resulting in a fall in testosterone release from the testis. This results in regression in hormone-dependent prostate cancer.

ing with the cytoplasmic ER, but its affinity for the ER is much less than that of oestrogen itself. Possibly the drug–receptor complex undergoes a conformational change which blocks its entry to nuclear sites of activity. Other receptor sites which bind tamoxifen but not oestrogen have also been described; however, the balance of evidence at present suggests that tamoxifen exerts its effect by competitively binding with ER, thus displacing oestradiol. Tamoxifen does not increase plasma oestradiol levels in postmenopausal women but does do so in premenopausal women. Tamoxifen has a prolonged terminal half-life in plasma and after 1 month of treatment the plasma concentration exceeds that of oestradiol by as much as 1000-fold. It is for this reason that a dose–response effect is not usually observed clinically. Toxic effects are uncommon, the most frequent being mild nausea and hot flushes. Occasionally a flare-up of the breast cancer may be seen which is then sometimes followed by a response. The long-term use of tamoxifen is associated with a small increase in uterine cancer, and a possibly beneficial alteration in plasma lipid concentrations.

The mechanism of acquired resistance to tamoxifen is unclear since the cancer cells still contain ER. It is possible that the cell's dependence on oestrogen is bypassed by other mechanisms such as growth factor stimulation.

A new class of antioestrogens binds to the oestrogen receptor and inactivates it. The lead molecule in this class of drugs in Fulvestrant (ICI 182 780). The drug binds to the receptor but impairs the dimerization necessary for the active form of the receptor to be formed (Fig. 6.13). The drug–receptor complex is degraded and ER-mediated gene transcription is prevented.

Megestrol acetate is a synthetic antiandrogen. It blocks the synthesis of testosterone, reducing plasma testosterone levels. Adrenal androgens (androstenedione) are also reduced. The drug also blocks the action of testosterone on prostatic carcinoma cells, and this is a further mechanism for its action in the disease. Cyproterone acetate and flutamide have an antiandrogen effect which may be valuable in prostatic cancer. Flutamide does not inhibit pituitary LH release and blocks the negative feedback which testosterone produces, resulting in a rise in serum testosterone. Flutamide has no progestogen activity.

SURGICAL

Oophorectomy (surgical or radiotherapeutic) will abolish oestrogen secretion by the ovary in premenopausal women and was widely used as a first step in hormone treatment of advanced breast cancer. Knowledge of the ER status is useful because the likelihood of response in ER-positive tumours is 50%, compared with only 5% in ER-negative tumours in which the procedure may not be worthwhile.

Adrenalectomy sometimes produces further responses in premenopausal patients with advanced breast cancer responding to oophorectomy. This is probably due to residual sex hormone synthesis by the adrenal. The tumour response occurs despite adequate glucocorticoid replacement. Hypophysectomy produces a similar effect. Both of these operations have been rendered almost obsolete since the advent of aromatase inhibitors (see below). Orchidectomy is effective in reducing plasma testosterone levels and has been widely used as treatment for metastatic prostatic carcinoma.

Additive hormone therapies

In breast cancer these include oestrogens, androgens, glucocorticoids and progestogens. Oestrogen receptor-positive breast cancers will sometimes regress with exogenous oestrogen, which indicates that we still have gaps in our knowledge of the mechanism of action of hormone therapies. Medroxyprogesterone acetate and megestrol acetate produce responses in about 20% of patients. They possibly do this by lowering the cytoplasmic ER content and responses are usually only seen in ER-positive tumours but appear independent of PR status. Progesterone derivatives produce responses in about 30% of uterine carcinomas, usually in cases which are ER-positive or PR-positive.

Cytokines in cancer treatment

Cytokines are a group of proteins, some of which regulate the growth of cells while others modulate the immune response and inflammation. They are usually glycosylated and of low molecular weight. They are produced by cells of various types and usually act over short distances (as autocrine or paracrine stimuli) (Table 6.5). In cancer therapy they may regulate tumour cell growth, be directly cytotoxic, excite an inflammatory or immune response in the tumour, or speed normal tissue recovery from the effect of cytotoxic drugs. Cytokine treatment has an established role in only one or two, rather uncommon, tumours.

Interferons

Three classes of interferon (IFN) have been defined: α, β

Table 6.5 Clinical activity of cytokines.

Interferons	
Hairy cell leukaemia	90% response. Improved prognosis
Chronic myeloid leukaemia	70% response often with Philadelphia –ve marrow in chronic phase
Follicular lymphoma	60% response
Myeloma	Decreased relapse rate
Essential thrombocythaemia	50% response
Melanoma	20% response
Renal cell carcinoma	20% response
Kaposi's sarcoma	30% response
Interleukins	
IL-2	
Renal cell carcinoma	15–30% response
Melanoma	15–30% response

and γ. At first they were of interest because of their antiviral properties, but it is now clear they have a wide spectrum of activity. Their antitumour activity is complex. They may have a direct antiproliferative effect on normal and neoplastic cells, they induce differentiation in some leukaemic cell lines, and they enhance the cytotoxicity of T, natural killer and lymphokine-activated killer (LAK) cells (see below). Expression of major histocompatibility class I and II is increased on tumour cells.

The clinical activity of IFNs is summarized in Table 6.5. Side-effects include an influenza-like illness with rigors, headache, muscle pains and fever; leucopenia may occur. These symptoms are dose-related. Most patients can tolerate 3×10^6 units of α daily for many weeks. Neutralizing antibodies may develop.

Interleukins

Interleukins (ILs) are a family of peptides which act as modulators of immune and inflammatory responses. Interleukin-2 has received most clinical attention.

Interleukin-2

This is a glycoprotein (molecular weight 15 kDa) produced by activated T cells. It binds to a cell surface receptor on T cells This receptor has two subunits, each of which can bind IL-2 with low affinity but together bind with high affinity. Interleukin-2 stimulates production of IFN-α, and tumour necrosis factor (TNF, see below) and activates cytotoxic lymphocytes. These kill cells without

the need for antigen recognition or histocompatibility specificity.

As a single agent IL-2 produces responses in 15–30% of patients with metastatic renal carcinoma and melanoma. Some of these responses are very durable. Continuous infusion may have some advantages over bolus injection (continuous activation, fewer side-effects). The combination of LAK cells (where the patient's own lymphocytes are activated and expanded *in vitro* and then returned to the patient) and IL-2 may produce more complete responses, but overall response rates are similar. Side-effects of IL-2 are considerable: fever, lethargy, hypotension, adult respiratory distress syndrome, nausea, vomiting, anaemia, neutropenia, disorientation and somnolence. These effects are dose-related.

Interleukin 6 (IL-6)

This cytokine is produced in the bone marrow and by human osteoblasts. It appears to act as a paracrine growth factor in myeloma and is overproduced in this disease. The reason for the overproduction is unclear. Its production is dependent on IL-1. Interleukin-6 stimulates osteoclast activity and appears to stimulate platelet production.

Monoclonal antibodies (mAb) in cancer therapy

After many years of development mAbs now have an established place in cancer treatment. The technical advances that have made this possible are as follows.

1 Humanization of mouse antibodies avoiding formation of antiantibodies.

2 Development of high-affinity antibodies by techniques using bacterial phages.

3 Production of antibodies of varying size and affinity with different degrees of tissue penetration.

Antibodies may be altered to produce an antitumour effect by many means. The most commonly employed techniques are shown in Fig. 6.15 and are described in the accompanying legend. For each of these approaches there are limitations and possibilities.

1 *Direct killing by complement or by antibody-dependent cell cytotoxicity.* In this approach the Fc portion of the antibody must bind to the Fc receptor (I and II) on the effector cell and avoid binding to Fc RIII which is inhibitory. This mechanism of cell killing is the mode of action of Herceptin which binds to the ERB B2 receptor in breast cancer, and Rituximab—an anti-CD20 mAb used to treat B-cell lymphoma.

2 *Examples of a mAb carrying a toxin or radioactivity or an*

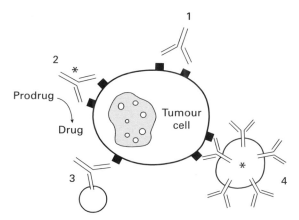

Fig 6.15 Methods of tumour killing by mAbs. **1** The mAb binds to the tumour antigen and results in cell killing by direct compliment mediated cell killing or by antibody-dependent cell killing by macrophage. **2** The mAb carries radioactivity, or a toxin, or a cytokine which mediates the tumour cell killing, or the mAb may carry an enzyme that converts a prodrug to an active drug. **3** The mAb is bispecific. One binding site attaches to tumour, the other to an antitumour effector cell. **4** the mAb may be attached to a liposome that contains drugs or toxins.

activating enzyme are humanized anti-CD33 conjugated to the DNA minor-groove binding agent calicheamicin (gemtuzumab). CD33 is expressed on acute myeloid leukaemia blasts. Gemtuzumab induces remission in drug-resistant relapse. The approach using toxins such as ricin coupled to mAbs has not proved practicable due to unacceptable vascular toxicity. Coupled radioisotopes such as 90-yttrium or 131-iodine are attractive strategies because of the possibility of bystander killing. 90-Yttrium labelled anti-CD20 and 1311-labelled anti-CEA are in clinical trial. Antibodies armed with an enzyme that cleaves a prodrug (ADEPT—antibody-dependent enzyme prodrug therapy) are showing clinical promise in metastatic colorectal cancer. The enzymes have proved immunogenic limiting the dosage regimen.

3 *The approach using bispecific antibodies are still in the early phase of development.* Attachment to effector T cells has led to extensive toxic cytokine release, limiting the use.

4 *Immunoliposomes are an effective means of increasing delivery of a toxin or radioactivity, but are difficult to produce.* They have considerable promise in approaches where the target is the tumour vasculature.

Future approaches

Future approaches are likely to include the following.

1 Targeting tumour vasculature using targets such as VEGF and VEGF receptor.
2 Obtaining the optimal antibody size and affinity for maximum tissue penetration and target binding.
3 Developing mAbs capable of delivering more than one killing mechanism.
There are still considerable problems to overcome relating to gene delivery (whatever the vector), of distribution and uptake in normal tissue, of specificity of activation, of the effectiveness of bystander killing and of formation of antiviral antibodies.

Gene therapy

The possibility of changing the genetic structure of cancer cells to kill the tumour, or change its growth rate, has become more of a reality now that so much is known about the genetic changes that accompany malignant transformation. To exert its effect the gene must gain access to the cell. The delivery is via a *vector*. This may be a virus that is defective in replication and into which the gene has been inserted usually with a promoter that becomes active in the cell. An alternative strategy is to package the gene in a liposome.

Gene therapy for cancer may have one of several aims.
1 To restore function of a defective tumour suppressor gene.
2 To block the action of a mutated or overexpressed oncogene.
3 To insert a gene that can activate a prodrug or produce other cell-killing effects.
4 To modify susceptibility to immune attack.
The restoration of function of a defective suppressor gene such as *p53* or *APC* (adenomatous polyposis coli) has been shown to inhibit tumour cell growth in model systems. This is perhaps a surprising result in view of the multiplicity of genetic defects in cancer cells. The mechanism of the observed effects is not necessarily through the predicted function. For example the antitumour effect of expressing *p53* may be related to antiangiogenic effects.

Viral gene vectors have been used to insert factors (oligonucleotides or ribozymes) that block the action of dominant oncogenes and thereby inhibit tumour growth. However the most successful example has been the use of small molecules (that is, drugs) that block oncogene action (for example STI571, see p. 450). It is surprising that this approach would work in view of the multiplicity of oncogenes that may be overexpressed in a complex tumour. The effect is probably most valuable where a single overexpressed gene dominates in driving tumour growth as in the case with the *BCR–ABL* tyrosine kinase in CML.

The advantage of the approach using genes that convert an inert prodrug into an active drug is that the active agent can kill cancer cells near the cell into which the gene has penetrated—the so-called *bystander* effect. A bystander effect on the vascular system occurs when antiangiogenesis genes are inserted into tumour cells. Another approach is to use viruses that replicate selectively in cancer cells. Such selectivity may be based on the necessity for cell division for the gene to be active, or on the absence of an active *p53* or *RB* (retinoblastoma) gene. A related approach is to use a replication-deficient virus that will only divide if a normal tissue gene promoter is expressed, for example the promoter for prostate-specific antigen in prostate cancer.

References

1 Relling MV, Dervieux T. Pharmacogenetics and cancer therapy. *Nature Rev Oncol* 2001; 1: 99–108.

2 Simon SM, Schindler M. Cell biological mechanisms of multidrug resistance in tumors. *Proc Natl Acad Sci* 1994; 91: 3497–504.

3 Moscow JA, Cowan KH. Multidrug resistance. *J Natl Cancer Inst* 1988; 80: 14–20.

4 Ford J, Hait W. Pharmacology of drugs that alter multidrug resistance in cancer. *Pharmacol Rev* 1990; 42: 155–99.

5 Davies SM, Robison LL, Buckley JD *et al*. Glutathione *S*-transferase polymorphisms and outcome of chemotherapy in childhood acute myeloid leukaemia. *J Clin Oncol* 2001; 19: 1279–87.

6 Hartley JA. Alkylating agents. In: Souhami RL, Tannock I, Hohenberger P, Horist J-C, eds. *Oxford Textbook of Medicine*. Oxford: Oxford University Press, 2001: 639–54.

7 O'Driscoll BR, Hasleton PS, Taylor PM *et al*. Active lung fibrosis up to 17 years after chemotherapy with carmustine (BCNU) in childhood. *N Engl J Med* 1990; 323: 378–82.

8 Jackman AL, Calvert AH. Folate-based thymidylate synthase inhibitors as anticancer drugs. *Ann Oncol* 1995; 6: 871–81.

9 Huizing MT, Misser VH, Pieters RC *et al*. Taxanes: a new class of antitumour agents. *Cancer Invest* 1995; 13: 381–404.

10 Dancey J, Eisenhower EA. Current perspectives on camptothecins in cancer treatment. *Br J Cancer* 1996; 74: 327–38.

11 Dorr RT. Cytoprotective agents for anthracyclins. *Semin Oncol* 1996; 23: 23–34.

12 Fauser AA, Fellhauer M, Hoffman M *et al*. Guidelines for anti-emetic therapy: acute emesis. *Eur J Cancer* 1999; 35: 361–70.

13 Clark ST, Radford JA, Crowther D *et al*. Gonadal function following chemotherapy for Hodgkin's disease: a comparative study of MVPP and a seven-drug regimen. *J Clin Oncol* 1991; 13: 134–9.

14 Weiss RB, Muggia FM. Cytotoxic drug-induced pulmonary disease. *Am J Med* 1980; 68: 259–66.

15 Kaldor JM, Day NE, Clarke EA *et al*. Leukemia following Hodgkin's disease. *N Engl J Med* 1990; 322 (7–13): 1–6 for study of ovarian cancer.

7 Supportive care and symptom relief

Talking about the diagnosis and treatment

Major disease brings anxiety and worry, but few diseases are associated with such dread as cancer, with its imagined inevitable sequel of certain death, pain, lingering and suffering. One of the most difficult and rewarding tasks for the physician is to set the disease in its right context, to explain the treatment, to give enough information at the correct rate and time, to sustain hope, and to be accessible, supportive, competent, open-minded and, above all, kind.

The patient has a life outside the consulting room. He or she will interpret what is said in the light of his or her own experience and apprehensions. Cancer is commonest in the elderly. In the course of a long life many patients will have had friends or relatives who have died of the disease. They may perhaps have cared for a member of the family with cancer. These experiences will have an important influence on a patient's expectations. Cancer and its treatment are widely discussed in the media. Although patients are better informed now, their knowledge is often fragmentary and disorganized. Some patients may have recognized the seriousness of a symptom—haemoptysis, unexplained weight loss, a lump or backache—but be too anxious (or too afraid of surgery) to voice their suspicions. Other patients may have no idea of the possible diagnosis.

As with patients, the attitude of physicians is influenced by their experience and training. Frequently the first diagnosis of cancer is made by a specialist in another area such as general surgery, gynaecology or chest medicine. Some of these doctors may themselves have a very pessimistic view of cancer and what can be achieved by treatment. Furthermore, the specialist has often had little opportunity to get to know the patient before the diagnosis has been made. A lack of familiarity, both with what can be achieved by treatment and with the patient, combined sometimes with fear of the disease, may lead the physician or surgeon into euphemisms and half-truths. Words may be used such as 'growth' or 'ulcer' to soften or obscure the diagnosis, while the doctor often betrays his real meaning by appearing evasive or unclear.

This attitude means that, unless the patient is bold and asks for a more frank statement of the diagnosis, the doctor may be unable to assess what impact his or her words have had. Because the meaning of the diagnosis is being avoided it becomes difficult to allow the patient to express his or her fears or ask the appropriate questions. The patient may in fact be under the impression that the diagnosis is worse than it actually is, that he or she has only a short time to live or that treatment will be to no avail. The doctor's evasions may then strengthen this opinion. An ill-informed patient may learn of the diagnosis by other means—from a pathology request form, a hospital porter, a well-meaning friend or an overheard remark. If the diagnosis is discovered accidentally the patient may realize that the intention behind concealment was to spare him or her anxiety, but may feel let down by the doctor and be cautious in accepting any further reassurance.

The attitude of cancer specialists has now moved towards a fuller discussion of the diagnosis and treatment. What is said to the patient must, however, be well judged and carefully delivered. All physicians make errors of judgement which shake their confidence with the next patient they see, but it is essential not to retreat from these discussions when difficulties have occurred. It is important to learn from one's mistakes.

If possible, it is useful to assess the attitude of the patient before the diagnosis is made. Questions such as 'What do you feel is wrong with you?' or 'Have you any particular anxieties about what might be wrong?' are often very revealing since the patient will sometimes admit, for example, to a fear of malignancy. Such information allows the physician to ask the patient whether, if this proves to be the diagnosis, he or she would want to know the details of what is found.

It is sometimes possible to make the diagnosis before major surgery is undertaken—by bronchoscopy for lung cancer, needle biopsy in breast cancer or endoscopy for gastrointestinal disease. When the diagnosis has been established preoperatively and treatment by surgery is necessary, it is hardly possible, still less desirable, that the diagnosis is not discussed and the probable operative procedure described. Often the diagnosis only becomes apparent after an operation and the patient will be waiting to hear the result. In either case when talking to patients about their diagnosis, doctors need to have a clear idea of what they are going to say and the words they will use, although they must be prepared to modify their approach if the situation demands it.

In explaining the diagnosis, the word 'cancer' is the only word which unequivocally conveys the nature of the complaint. Many physicians use the words 'malignancy', 'tumour' or 'growth' with the best of intentions, but this carries the risk that the patient will fail to realize the true nature of the disease (indeed, this is often what is intended). It is true that in the elderly or very anxious, the word 'cancer' may occasionally be very frightening and there are some patients for whom other terms may be necessary. Many patients have only a vague idea of what cancer means and are surprised that the disease is nearly always treatable and sometimes curable. The explanation of the diagnosis must be combined with a realistic but hopeful account of what can be done. Few patients can exist without hope of any kind. This does not mean that a cure is promised but the patient must feel confident that every attempt will be made to cure him or her and know that there is a possibility of success, if that is the case. If a cure is likely this must be stressed and a much more optimistic account of the disease can be given. Even when the prognosis is

poor, the doctor must show how treatment may help to achieve a reasonable period of healthy and enjoyable life.

The manner in which the explanation is given is critical. The doctor should be unhurried, speak clearly and not technically, look at the patient's face while speaking, show that he or she is not frightened or discomfited by the diagnosis and indicate by look and gesture that he or she is competent and prepared to discuss the problem calmly. There is a limit to the number of facts which a patient can assimilate during one conversation, particularly under stressful circumstances. Too much information may progressively extinguish the understanding which a short account would achieve. Not infrequently the patient may seem to understand, but in fact be too anxious to take in anything of what is being said. This failure of understanding is not 'denial' but is due to confusion and anxiety. It is a good policy to stop frequently and enquire if what is being said is clear or if there are questions which the patient wants to ask. Simple drawings often clarify the site of the illness or what radiotherapy or surgery are attempting to achieve. When the patient is able to ask questions it implies that he or she has understood at least part of the explanation. The doctor should make it quite clear that members of the team will always be pleased to answer questions and that there will be an opportunity to talk again in a day or two. One discussion is seldom enough. It may take a few days for the patient to start to understand and to take a realistic view of the situation and at that stage want to know more. It is usually advisable therefore to impart the details of the diagnosis and treatment over a period of time. The facts of the diagnosis are given first with a brief outline of treatment, gradually giving more information as the patient begins to come to terms with his or her position.

Some physicians ask relatives for advice on how much to tell the patient, particularly when they are in doubt about the correct approach. This can be helpful, but there is a risk that the relatives may misjudge the patient and, out of love and sympathy, suggest that the truth is withheld when the patient would have wished otherwise. It is, of course, essential that relatives have a clear understanding of what has been said, and why, and that the medical team do not give contradictory accounts. For this reason, the doctor should explain to the rest of the medical and nursing team exactly what has been said, with an idea of the words that have been used and what the reaction has been. The same information should be conveyed to the relatives, but the discussion about prognosis may have to be more pessimistic with relatives than with the patient. It is unwise to give patients a prognosis measured in a finite time because they tend to remember the stated number of months or years, however many qualifications are made, and such predictions are often incorrect.

The patient's reaction may be a mixture of acceptance, anxiety, anger and grief. It is essential to be understanding and not to be irritated by unjustified hostility if it occurs. This demands a lot from the doctor, who must have enough self-confidence and maturity to realize that, in the end, the patient will come to trust his or her honesty and support.

At a later stage the physician, while discussing the details of investigation and treatment, may wish to explain that an illness such as cancer will alter the patient's self-perception. That is, the patient will tend for a while to view himself or herself as 'ill', and minor aches and pains which would previously have been ignored may be magnified in the patient's mind and be interpreted as symptoms of relapse. In explaining that this is an understandable but usually temporary phase, the physician should make it clear that he or she will be seeing the patient regularly and, if symptoms occur which cause anxiety, the patient should get in touch. The best cancer departments operate an 'open-door' policy of this type, eliminating a lot of bureaucratic difficulty for the patient who may otherwise be given an appointment weeks ahead for a problem which is immediate. The ideal arrangement is where the hospital specialist works in close collaboration with the family doctor in providing support and reassurance. The family practitioner may have long and invaluable experience of the patient and his or her family.

Whenever a patient visits, either for a regular review or because of a symptom, the physician should give as much time to discussion as to the technical aspects of examination and investigation. It is greatly to be regretted that some doctors, and most health administrators, regard heavily booked clinics as a sign of efficiency. A five-minute consultation with a cancer patient is nearly always bad medicine.

Many cancer treatments have a bad reputation. Fear of being burnt or scarred by radiotherapy is very common and a careful explanation of modern advances is sometimes needed. Alopecia, nausea and vomiting are unpleasant side-effects of chemotherapy. Patients have heard of these and, understandably, fear them. If chemotherapy is judged necessary, then the reasons should be explained. Patients will easily grasp the idea that cancer may not be localized and that a systemic treatment is being given to prevent or treat any recurrence from cancer cells which may have spread to other sites. Indeed, they often find the idea of a systemic as well as a local treatment reassuring.

The ways in which the side-effects can be mitigated should be clearly explained.

Although patients will usually accept the need for radiotherapy or chemotherapy, they may find the reality worse than they had imagined. This is particularly true for chemotherapy, which often goes on for many months. There can be few things more miserable than repeated, predictable episodes of severe nausea and vomiting. Patients may begin to feel that they cannot go through with treatment and then find themselves in a frightening dilemma. On the one hand, they are fearful of jeopardizing their chance of cure and of disappointing the doctor; but on the other, the side-effects may produce progressive demoralization. In the case of a potentially curative treatment—for example, for Hodgkin's disease, testicular tumours or acute lymphoblastic leukaemia—the doctor must try to sustain the patient through the treatment and do all he or she can to see it completed. For many cancers of adult life the benefits of chemotherapy are, however, much less clear. In these cases the worst outcome is that a patient is made to feel wretched by the treatment and guilty at stopping, and is then frightened at the prospect that he or she has jeopardized the chance of survival. If relapse occurs there may be self-blame and depression. The responsibility for this situation is as much the doctor's as the patient's. When chemotherapy is being given without a reasonable prospect of cure and the patient cannot continue, the physician should be sympathetic and reassuring, and explain that he or she does not feel let down by the patient and that the prognosis has not been materially worsened.

There are few other branches of medicine which demand simultaneously such technical expertise and kindly understanding as cancer medicine. The strains on doctors are considerable, especially if they take the human aspect of their work seriously. It is a great failing in doctors if they talk to patients only about the physical and technical aspects of their illness, rely heavily on investigation in making treatment decisions and find it difficult to give up intensive measures and accept that patients cannot be cured. Technical prowess has then replaced a thoughtful analysis of patients' feelings and what is in their best interests.

Sustaining and counselling a patient and his or her relatives is a matter of teamwork, and the psychological aspects of the disease are as important as the physical. The special problems of dealing with children with cancer are discussed in Chapter 24. Treating patients with cancer demands great resources of emotional energy on the part of doctors and others in the medical team. In some units, part of the work of talking to patients is taken over by psychiatrists, psychologists, social workers or other counsellors. Invaluable though this help may be, we do not think it desirable that some members of the medical team should see themselves as technical experts and that, when human feelings intrude into the medical situation, patients should be sent to talk to someone else about their problems.

Support, counselling and rehabilitation

With any disease it is important to put oneself in the patient's position and try to anticipate the problems which are likely to arise. For example, it may seem obvious that mastectomy is a mutilating operation and that some pre- and postoperative psychological support will be necessary. Nevertheless, many women do not receive adequate advice from their doctors. What may be less obvious (until one thinks of it) is that partners of women with mastectomy may be in need of explanation too. Indeed, the reaction of a partner to the operation may be of fundamental importance in helping the patient to recover from her illness. Such advice is seldom offered.

In addition, many patients with cancer face specific problems of rehabilitation as a result of surgical and other treatments. Rehabilitation and counselling are an essential part of the general care of cancer patients. In recent years specialized support services have developed to help patients overcome the effects of the illness and its treatment, and to return as far as possible to a normal life.

Stoma care

Successful treatment of cancer of the bowel or bladder will sometimes require permanent colostomy or ileostomy. Similarly, in the treatment of gynaecological cancers, there will be a few patients in whom a permanent colostomy, resulting from radiation damage to the large bowel, is the price of a radiotherapy cure (see Chapter 17). Although some patients manage their stoma without difficulty, others require a great deal of education and help, and the role of the stoma therapist has now become established. Patients must learn not only how to keep the stoma clean and healthy, but also how to recognize the complications that might demand further surgical review, such as prolapse or stricture. Although a left-sided colostomy is relatively easy to manage, there are considerable difficulties with an ileostomy because of the fluid loss of 400–

500 ml/day which can lead to electrolyte disturbance, dehydration (especially if gastrointestinal infection occurs) and greater aesthetic difficulties. Advances in surgery may lead to continent ileostomies, but at present most patients need to wear an appliance. The British Colostomy Association and Ileostomy and Internal Pouch Support Group offer support and practical help.

Breast prostheses

Most large hospitals should now have some form of mastectomy counselling service, not only to provide psychological support for patients who have undergone mastectomy, but also to offer expert advice regarding external prostheses. Almost all patients, including those with very radical operations, can now, when clothed, disguise their defects since a wide variety of prostheses, brassieres and swimsuits are available. A nurse or counsellor specializing in the problems of mastectomy is of great help and many patients will benefit from the advice available from the Mastectomy Association. Nevertheless, an increasing number of women are unhappy with any form of external prosthesis and request prosthetic implantation surgery, which they hope will give them a more normal contour and the opportunity for more adventurous dress. Part of the mastectomy counsellor's job is to advise such patients that, contrary to their expectation, following surgery they cannot expect to look completely normal.

Laryngectomy rehabilitation

Following total laryngectomy, the patient has to be taught how to create an oesophageal voice, using techniques of air swallowing and careful phonation which can only be acquired with the help of an experienced speech therapist. Although some patients find this straightforward, the majority require careful tuition, and some never achieve a satisfactory voice. For these patients, a vibrating device or 'artificial larynx' should be available. The vibrating device is held against the neck, and permits a vibrating column of air to be produced which, with careful phonation by the patient, gives monotonous, barely acceptable but comprehensible speech. In a few centres, permanent valves are now being implanted which increase the power and durability of speech. Although these experimental techniques may well have a place in the future rehabilitation of laryngectomy patients, it should be stressed that well taught oesophageal speech can be very acceptable indeed. The National Association of Laryngectomy Clubs may provide further helpful advice.

Limb prostheses

The regional limb-fitting centres are responsible for providing both temporary and permanent external prostheses for those who have lost limbs, whether through trauma or surgery. Traditionally, amputation has been the mainstay of treatment for bone and soft-tissue sarcoma. Most patients, including children, adapt remarkably well to the loss of a limb, and many are able to drive a car, participate in sport, and lead a full and active life. In children, the limb must be replaced as the child grows and care must be taken with the details of weight, length, construction and fitting in order to avoid unequal pressure on the spine which might lead to scoliosis.

Other prostheses

Other sophisticated prostheses may also be necessary, particularly for patients with facial defects following radical surgery of the head and neck region. In particular, radical surgery for tumours of the maxillary antrum, orbit and nasal fossa, though curative, may result in substantial disfigurement which can only be covered by external prostheses. Remarkable results can be obtained, but the work is highly specialized.

Home support

Learning how to use a colostomy bag or walk with an artificial limb is the start of a much more complex process of rehabilitation, in which the development of self-reliance and self-esteem needs encouragement. While many patients achieve this with the help of their family, some are more isolated and require more professional help. The importance, for example, of a modified bathroom with supporting rails and wheelchair access may well be underestimated compared with the surgical and oncological challenge that the patient represented, but may help to make possible an independent existence at home. Community nursing help may allow patients to leave hospital relatively early after major operations, improving morale and reducing both the cost of the operation and also its morbidity from postoperative complications.

National counselling organizations

In a general hospital the work of counselling patients and their families is made easier if much of the inpatient treatment is in a specialized unit. In such a unit the nursing staff become very skilled in anticipating the problems of the disease and its treatment. When frequent admissions are necessary, for example for chemotherapy, it is of great help to the patient to see familiar faces. There is also a considerable benefit to be gained by having medical social workers who are especially skilled and interested in the problems of cancer. They not only provide another source of advice and reassurance but also will be knowledgeable about the local availability of counselling groups, nursing support, bereavement organizations and facilities for the care of the dying.

Self-help groups have arisen in many counties, organizing themselves nationally. Such groups have an enormous amount to offer, provided that they take care to give well-balanced and sensible advice. Many patients find it very helpful to talk about their problems with fellow sufferers, and much detailed practical advice may be given which few doctors are in a position to match.

Cancer treatment and the quality of life

Most cancer treatments are unpleasant, producing short- and long-term side-effects which interfere with the patient's quality of life. Assessment of this quality of life is not straightforward. Important criteria include the length of time spent in hospital, the ability to return to work, or at least to an independent life after treatment, and the degree of relief from troublesome symptoms, particularly pain. Other aspects of morbidity, such as nausea, fatigue, depression and anorexia are more difficult to measure.

Wherever possible, the distinction between *radical* and *palliative* treatment intent should be kept in mind. For example, patients with widely metastatic breast cancer are often treated with combination chemotherapy, and remissions, often lasting several months, are frequently seen. However, since cure is never achieved, such treatment is palliative and offered to patients with symptomatic deposits which are likely to respond. Frequently this approach is not followed and patients with widely disseminated cancers (including far less sensitive tumours than carcinoma of the breast) are treated routinely with combination chemotherapy.

Where two types of treatment appear to give similar results, one should choose the less toxic. For example, chemotherapy for Hodgkin's disease has been made much more acceptable by the substitution of chlorambucil and vinblastine for mustine and vincristine (see Chapter 25). In certain situations, where there is a slight possible advantage to a more toxic treatment, the greater toxicity might outweigh the slight improvement in results. For example, in infiltrating carcinoma of the urinary bladder, there may be a slight survival advantage in a combination of irradiation and radical cystectomy, compared with treatment by radiotherapy alone. However, the extra few months of median survival are obtained at the cost of both a permanent ileostomy and a high risk of impotence. Given a choice, many of us might opt for radiotherapy alone, despite the slightly greater risk, particularly since surgery is still possible if there is local recurrence.

The treatment of some tumours by radiotherapy can give local control rates which are the equal of surgery. This is reflected by the increasing use of radiotherapy for carcinoma of the cervix, of the head and neck, bladder, prostate and breast. In each of these sites, there are important physiological and psychological advantages to treatment with radiotherapy. Radical surgery can usually be performed if relapse occurs. Finally, one should remember that there are some patients with malignant disease in whom treatment may not be immediately necessary. For many patients with follicular lymphoma the course is so indolent that treatment is unnecessary, often for several years. In patients with asymptomatic but inoperable squamous carcinoma of the bronchus, there is often no advantage to early treatment with radiotherapy or chemotherapy, since such treatment does not prolong life and may cause side-effects (see Chapter 12). Treatment may be better withheld until a troublesome symptom such as haemoptysis, dyspnoea or pain from a secondary deposit becomes apparent.

For these reasons, when trials of cancer treatments are undertaken it may be important to include some assessment of quality of life, especially if there is unlikely to be a substantial difference in cure rate. In this way, any advantage in terms of survival or local control can be set against the morbidity which the treatment has induced.

Symptom control [1,2]

Pain

Relief of pain is a particularly important aspect of the management of cancer. Cancer pain may arise from viscera when it is often poorly localized and variable; from the bones and limbs (e.g. bone metastasis) when it is persistent and localized; and often worse at night or 'shooting', when neuropathic. Patients often have more than one cause of pain.

The first step in management is to make an accurate clinical assessment of the pains that the patient is experiencing, their site, severity and duration. The use of a pain assessment chart is helpful in defining the main problem and in monitoring the progress with time.

Analgesics

There is no single ideal analgesic and most patients will require drugs of different strength and dosage during the course of their illness. It is convenient to group analgesics into three classes according to their strength, as shown in Table 7.1.

1 *Mild analgesics.* This group includes aspirin, paracetamol and non-steroidal anti-inflammatory agents. These can be valuable for considerable periods of time. Aspirin and the non-steroidal anti-inflammatory agents (indomethacin, ibuprofen and the like) are particularly helpful in bone pain. Side-effects include dyspepsia and gastrointestinal bleeding. They can be combined with agents from a more powerful class (for example, aspirin and papaveretum tablets).

2 *Moderate analgesics.* This group includes codeine, dextropropoxyphene, oxycodone, pentazocine and dipipanone. These agents are more effective than those in the mild analgesic group but at the cost of greater side-effects, particularly constipation. Dextropropoxyphene is sometimes combined with paracetamol, and many patients prefer this to paracetamol alone. Oxycodone is particularly valuable as it is available in the form of suppositories. Pentazocine should be avoided because it commonly produces hallucinations. It has a partial antagonist action to morphine and should not be used in combination with opiates.

3 *Powerful analgesics.* These drugs, which include morphine and related compounds (synthetic and semisynthetic derivatives), are powerful in their pain-relieving effects and are the mainstay of analgesic therapy for patients with unremitting pain. Almost all patients with severe cancer pain require regular medication with analgesics of this type. Useful agents include morphine, diamorphine, methadone, pethidine, dextromoramide, papaveretum (often combined with aspirin as effervescent compound tablets) and buprenorphine. Ordinary morphine and diamorphine are active for only 4 h and should be given 4-hourly, but long-acting oral tablets of morphine sulphate are now available.

The choice of opiate analgesic and dosages should be determined by the patient's need [3]. For example, many patients are comfortable and pain-free with small regular dosage (10–20 mg every 4 h) of morphine or diamorphine, while others require 20 times this dose. There are

Table 7.1 Analgesics for pain relief in cancer.

Drug	Duration of action (h)	Toxicity
Mild analgesics		
Aspirin	4–6	Gastrointestinal bleeding and abdominal pain
Paracetamol	2–4	Skin rash; hepatic damage with overdose
Propionic acid derivatives (e.g. ibuprofen)	2–6	As aspirin
Indole derivatives (e.g. indomethacin)	8	As aspirin
Moderate analgesics		
Codeine and dihydrocodeine	4–6	Constipation, excitement
Oxycodone	8–10	Constipation, hypotension, nausea, dysphasia
Pentazocine	3–4	Nausea, dizziness, palpitations, hypertension, dysphasia
Dipipanone	6	Constipation, mental confusion, respiratory depression
[Paracetamol with codeine or dextropropoxyphene (longer with sustained-release preparations)]		
Powerful analgesics		
Morphine sulphate	4–6 (longer with sustained-release preparations)	Constipation, hypotension, nausea, dysphasia
Diamorphine	4–6	As morphine sulphate
Methadone	15–30	As morphine sulphate, more nausea, cumulative
Hydromorphone	4–6	Useful in patients with morphine intolerance
Dextromoramide	6	Dizziness, sweating, constipation, respiratory depression
Pethidine	3	Nausea, dry mouth, respiratory depression

few other drugs with as wide a dose range. In most patients, oral medication is appropriate and effective, though in those with, for example, complete obstruction from pharyngeal or oesophageal cancer an alternative route will have to be found. Sublingual buprenorphine can be a useful alternative but it antagonizes the effect of morphine and should therefore neither be abruptly substituted for morphine nor given with it concurrently. Treatment by rectal suppositories of oxycodone or morphine can be extremely effective. In very occasional cases, where both the oral and rectal routes are unavailable, suppositories can be given vaginally.

Regular intramuscular or intravenous treatment with opiates is almost never required, though subcutaneous or intravenous infusions of diamorphine can be valuable if treatment by other routes proves unsatisfactory. Diamorphine is preferable because of its very high solubility, allowing volumes for injection to be small. Very rarely, regular administration of epidural morphine may be necessary for relief of severe, localized pain, but this should never be considered as a long-term solution unless other

methods of regular opiate administration have been tried.

An important addition to the family of useful opiates is the long-acting morphine now available in oral tablets. Since both morphine and diamorphine must be given frequently throughout the day, the availability of long-acting morphine is of real value, particularly to the active patient. When changing the treatment from diamorphine to long-acting morphine, that the dose ratio of diamorphine to morphine is 2:3, so that a patient on, say, diamorphine 20 mg 4-hourly (total daily dosage 120 mg), will require 180 mg of morphine daily, or long-acting morphine 90 mg twice daily. Hydromorphone HCl, a semisynthetic opioid derivative, can be useful in morphine-intolerant patients and is available in sustained-release preparations (given 12-hourly). Transdermal patches of fentanyl (a semisynthetic opioid) at an initial dose of 25 mg/h (in patients not previously exposed to opioids) or by appropriate dose transfer in patients taking morphine may offer good pain control with less constipation, nausea and daytime drowsiness and is useful for nauseated patients.

All patients taking regular opiate medication will require advice regarding constipation. Regular laxatives are usually (but not always) necessary, and may need to be given in above normal doses. Regular danthron–poloxamer mixture (or capsules) are effective. The standard daily dose of 10–15 ml (or one to three capsules) in divided daily doses may be insufficient for patients on large doses of morphine and a stronger suspension is available. Nausea, vomiting and sedation are the other important side-effects of opiate analgesics but are less consistent. Although sedation usually disappears with time, nausea may persist and require treatment. Haloperidol is effective as is cyclizine, although phenothiazines are more sedating (Table 7.2).

Guidelines for pain control in terminal cancer patients (Fig. 7.1)

1 *Use enough analgesia to be effective.* Regular aspirin, or compound paracetamol–dextropropoxyphene tablets can be effective for many weeks especially in musculoskeletal pain. A change to dihydrocodeine will then usually give further pain relief. Use of morphine or related agents should be considered when drugs of lesser effect are inadequate for the patient's pain. At this stage less powerful agents such as dipipanone, aspirin or non-steroidal anti-inflammatory agents may be useful to supplement the regular morphine dose. A common useful starting dose of diamorphine elixir is 10 or 20 mg every 4 h, but some patients need more than 1 g of diamorphine daily for adequate pain relief. Addiction is not a problem and opiates should not be withheld for fear of producing it. Dysphoria and loss of lucidity may occur and can be distressing. In such cases a lower dose may have to be accepted, even if pain relief is incomplete, and additional analgesia attempted by other means (see below) (Fig. 7.2).

2 *Give analgesics regularly rather than on a 'when required' basis.* Patients should not have to 'earn' their analgesia. Morphine and diamorphine need to be given every 4 h to be effective, but most patients can manage on slow-release morphine tablets (see above).

3 *Warn patients about side-effects.* This particularly applies to constipation. High-fibre diet and regular laxatives are sufficient to deal with this important and painful problem in most cases. Metoclopramide, prochlorperazine or cyclizine can be useful if nausea is a persistent problem.

4 *Keep drug prescriptions as simple as possible.* Some opiates antagonize each other and should never be given together (for example, sublingual buprenorphine and oral diamorphine).

Table 7.2 Classification of drugs used to control nausea and vomiting. From [4].

Putative site of action	Class	Example
Central nervous system		
Vomiting centre	Antimuscarinic	Hyoscine hydrobromide, prochloperazine
	H_1 receptor antagonist	Cyclizine, dimenhydrinate,
	Antimuscarinic*	Prochlorperazine
	5-HT$_2$ receptor antagonist	Methotrimeprazine
	D_2 receptor antagonist	Metaclopramiole, domperidone
	5-HT$_3$ receptor antagonist	Granisetron, ondasetron, tropisetron
Cerebral cortex	Benzodiazepine	Lorazepam
	Cannabinoid	Nabilone
	Corticosteroid	Dexamethasone
Gastrointestinal tract		
Prokinetic	5-HT$_4$ receptor antagonist	Metoclopramide, cisapride
	D_2 receptor antagonist	Metoclopramide, domperidone
Antisecretory	Antimuscarinic	Hyoscine, glycopyrrolate
	Somatostatin analogue	Octreotide, vapreotide
	Vagal 5-HT$_3$ receptor	5-HT$_3$ receptor antagonist, Granisetron, ondansetron, blockade tropisetron
Anti-inflammatory	Corticosteroid	Dexamethasone

*Antihistamines and phenothiazines both have H1 receptor antagonistic and antimuscarinic properties.

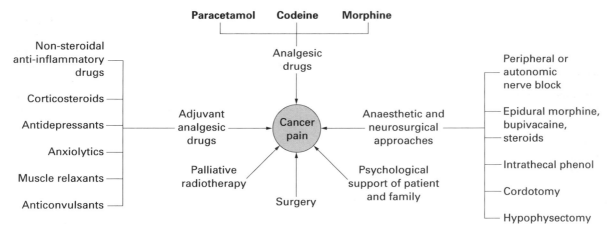

Fig. 7.1 Treatment of cancer pain. From [5] with permission.

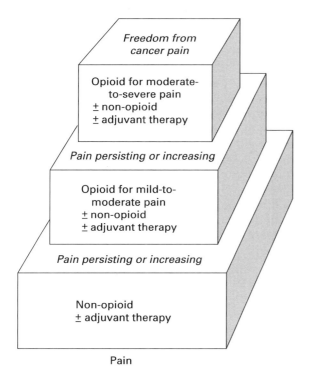

Fig. 7.2 Three-step analgesic ladder of the World Health Organization. Reproduced from a report of the World Health Organization with permission of the publisher.

5 *Consider alternative methods of pain control.*
   (a) Alternative routes of analgesic administration: oral, sublingual, rectal, vaginal or even (rarely) via colostomy; subcutaneous, intramuscular, intravenous, percutaneous using fentanyl. The past 5 years have seen an increase in familiarity with subcutaneously administered morphine infusions, using a simple, constant-rate syringe driver which the patient can usually manage very effectively at home, with a boost facility for additional flexibility.
   (b) Alternative approaches. Consider radiotherapy for painful bone metastases, surgical internal fixation for pathological fractures and other procedures such as nerve block and neurosurgical approaches.

Nerve blocks, surgical procedures and other approaches

Some patients with cancer have intractable pain at a particular site, which responds poorly even to high doses of opiates. Radiation is often a highly effective treatment for localized pain, particularly when it arises in bone. If this is ineffective an alternative technique is a nerve block which destroys pain and other sensations in the affected part of the body. The technique requires great skill and is usually performed by an anaesthetist with special training. Local dorsal root block using fine-needle insertions of phenol or absolute alcohol is the commonest method (Fig. 7.2). A similar technique can be used to produce coeliac or brachial plexus block.

Surgical destructive procedures are rarely necessary but may have to be considered if all else fails. Spinothalamic tractotomy is an operation performed on the spinal cord in which the fibres carrying pain are divided. Anatomical specificity is often possible since the pain fibres are arranged in the lateral spinothalamic tract in an orderly fashion. Pain relief may, however, not be complete since other spinal pathways may also subserve pain sensation.

Operations can also be considered at higher levels (for example, thalamotomy) if tractotomy is ineffective.

Epidural infusions

Epidural infusions of local anaesthetic or opiates can sometimes be used to control pain when the oral route proves difficult due to nausea. The infusions are intermittent or continuous and use an infusion pump (such as that used for subcutaneous infusion) which is connected to a catheter in the epidural space. Tolerance to local anaesthetics occurs quickly so that the effect lasts only a few weeks. Infection may occur. Pain relief may be obtained without paralysis or autonomic disturbance.

Other procedures

These include transcutaneous nerve stimulation and acupuncture analgesia, both of which can be valuable even in patients taking large doses of opiates. The mechanisms of these methods may involve a stimulation of endogenous endorphins at a central level.

Anorexia and nausea [6]

Anorexia is a very common accompaniment of terminal cancer, and there is, of course, no long-lasting remedy. There is, however, much that can be done to relieve the anxiety which the patient feels about the continued wasting [7]. Small meals should be offered, particularly the patient's favourite dishes, and a glass of wine or sherry may stimulate appetite. One of the great ironies of faddish 'alternative' diets is the denial of the simple pleasure of eating and drinking in the final weeks of a patient's life. Steroids may be extremely valuable and are underused in this situation. Steroid side-effects will not be a problem if the prognosis is a matter of weeks. Dexamethasone is probably the drug of choice (2 mg given three or four times a day), although lower doses may be adequate. Other helpful drugs are progestogens (especially megesterol), anabolic steroics and phenothiazines.

Treatment of nausea (and vomiting) may be difficult and depends on the cause (Fig. 7.3). Drug-induced nausea (due to morphine) may require treatment with metoclopramide, haloperidol or phenothiazines. Nausea due to intestinal obstruction or other causes of gut stress is often difficult to treat. Metoclopramide may help, as may domperidone. Rectal administration is often effective. 5-Hydroxytryptamine-3 ($5\text{-}HT_3$) antagonists can also be valuable in treatment of nausea in advanced cancer. If there is a mechanical cause, such as intestinal obstruction from an intra-abdominal mass, a fine-bore nasogastric tube may have to be passed for aspiration of stomach contents. In most cases symptomatic treatment with prochlorperazine, chlorpromazine or metoclopramide, given regularly before meals, may help. Rectal administration may occasionally be necessary.

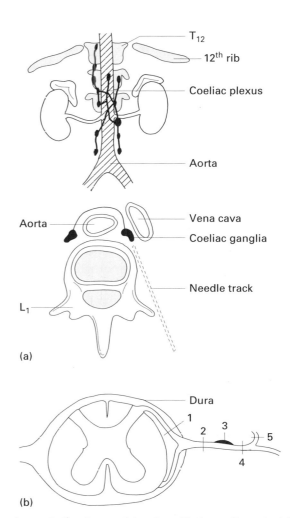

Fig. 7.3 Coeliac plexus and dorsal root blocks to relieve pain. (a) Anatomical relations of coeliac plexus. The plexus is comprised of a number of ganglia situated in front of T12 and L1. The injection is made in front of the anterior border of the body of L1. The needle is inserted below the 12th rib. (b) Dorsal root block and section. (1) Block of root inside dura. (2) Block of dorsal root outside dura. (3) Excision of dorsal root ganglion. (4) Coagulation of nerve trunk. (5) Coagulation of medial branch of primary ramus.

Oral mucositis

This distressing and under-recognized symptom frequently accompanies chronic ill-health or the administration of chemotherapy [8], paticularly with methotrexate, fluorouracil, beomycin or doxorubicin. Principles of management include both prevention (oral hygiene and use of a regular mouthwash), and treatment with ice chips during chemotherapy, to decrease oral mucosal bloodflow.

Constipation

There are many causes of constipation in patients with cancer. One of the most common is anorexia and low bulk intake. This can sometimes be helped by dietary fibre supplements if tolerated. Lack of fluid intake leads to hard stools and can be helped by increasing fluid intake and by a stool-softening agent such as docusate or a lubricant (liquid paraffin). Drugs (morphine, codeine and derivatives) are a very frequent cause of constipation and require a combined stimulant and stool softener such as a codanthramer or senna, as well as a review of analgesic dosage.

Intestinal obstruction [9]

This common complication of advanced intra-abdominal malignancy is often a cause of great distress and is difficult to treat. The tumour is usually diffusely scattered on the bowel surface, infiltrating the wall and the mesentery. A stiff, immobile bowel results in areas which are encircled and compressed. If a localized obstruction cannot be relieved by laparotomy, then pain control must be achieved by opioids and antispasmodics, antiemetics will be needed for nausea, and a stool-softening agent (without stimulating laxatives) for constipation. Octreotide may help control vomiting and a nasogastric tube may be needed if vomiting is intractable and cannot be relieved by other means. Most patients can be made more comfortable for a time, but this is often a miserable complication of cancer.

Depression and anxiety

Most patients will have episodes of depression and anxiety, and sympathetic conversation with family, friends, doctors and nurses will usually help the patient through bad days. Persistent, disturbing or suicidal depression (fortunately very uncommon) may require additional treatment with tri- or tetracyclic antidepressants, and occasionally skilled psychiatric help is needed. Some authorities find amphetamines are helpful in special circumstances. Benzodiazepines are useful for acute or persistent anxiety.

The care of the dying

In England and Wales alone, 135 000 people die each year from cancer, accounting for some 20% of all deaths. Of these about 60% die in district general hospitals, 30% at home and the remainder in hospices, nursing homes and private hospitals. About half of all cancer patients present with incurable conditions at the time of diagnosis, and in the more fortunate half with potentially curable cancers, the majority develop recurrent disease and require palliative symptomatic care. The World Health Organization has estimated that about 3.5 million people are suffering worldwide from cancer pains each day—a sad reflection on the quality of care available to the majority of cancer patients.

It has become increasingly apparent that patients dying from cancer have particular needs which are often poorly served by traditional means of support. Even the most well-meaning doctors frequently find themselves out of their depth either through inadequate training in the use of the appropriate drugs (particularly analgesics) or because of the difficulties of exploring patients' needs. It is against this background that interest and expertise in the management of terminally ill patients has developed and, as so often happens, it is the determined work of a few individuals which has identified the problem and developed principles which are now widely adopted.

First and foremost, it is always wrong for a doctor to say, or feel, that there is nothing more that he or she can do. The enthusiastic oncologist may feel that his or her work is over when the specific anticancer treatment is at an end. The patient will, in general, make a much less clear distinction between active and supportive treatment so that, from the patient's point of view, careful treatment with analgesics, concern about appetite, constipation, mobility and so on, may be equally important. Second, it is largely through the work of hospice staff that we are beginning to learn the critical importance of adequate symptom control. The symptoms most commonly causing distress are pain, anorexia, nausea and vomiting, constipation, weakness and lassitude.

Terminal care: home, hospice and support teams

Many patients like to remain at home for as long as they can and to die there if possible. Familiar surroundings and family life offer great comfort. The care of a dying patient is, however, extremely demanding and a great deal of support is always required if home care is to be achieved successfully. Women generally look after dying men much better than men care for dying women. There are many factors which determine the feasibility of home care. These include whether the patient lives alone; the continued presence of family or friends to provide support (the spouse or partner may have to go to work); whether there are young children at home to be cared for; the availability of adequate local support services such as nursing, laundry, home helps and meals on wheels; and the degree and nature of the patient's disability and symptoms. It may be necessary to provide specialized aids to nursing and mobility, such as handrails in the bathroom, commodes, a ripple or water bed, a hoist or a wheelchair.

A flexible approach is essential. Even if the intention is to care for the patient at home, the circumstances may change and the situation become more difficult, making hospital or hospice care necessary. This may lead to feelings of guilt or of defeat in the family; the doctor should realize this and explain that continuous care of the dying patient is a highly skilled task, that professional help is often needed and that the change in plan is not a sign of failure.

There has been a considerable expansion of palliative care teams and inpatient hospices such that palliative care has now emerged as a new medical specialty. Hospices for terminally ill cancer patients have taught us the importance of careful pain control, attention to patients' physical and spiritual needs, and the important ways in which medical, nursing and other staff can make enormous contributions by spending a little more time with patients, often just by listening or simply being there. Nevertheless, the hospice movement is itself aware of the disadvantages of hospice care. Hospices are expensive to set up and maintain, and demand a high staff to patient ratio. Some patients find the concept of moving to a 'terminal home' difficult to accept, even though the majority are content once they arrive. Psychologically, many patients find it difficult to accept that the doctor who has been treating them, in whom they have had trust and confidence, no longer has any treatment to offer. Doctors with a genuine interest in the management of terminally ill cancer patients often find it upsetting if they are made to feel that they have no further role, as sometimes happens when a hospice support team takes the view that it should be entirely responsible for a patient. For the general practitioner who will have to look after the family after the death of the patient with cancer, this sudden role change can create real difficulty.

The traditional alternative, and the place where many cancer patients die, has been the general hospital ward.

Undoubtedly there are advantages—in particular, the continuity of care afforded by familiar staff and surroundings. Some patients might gain comfort from the fact that many of the patients on the ward will be suffering from non-malignant conditions, and that the general atmosphere is likely to be brisk and active. However, most of us would agree that for patients in the final stages of their illness, the ideal environment would be more tranquil and the staff rather less busy, so that there is more time for reflective discussion. It is well known that on many general medical or surgical wards, the cancer patient is all too often hurriedly passed by, particularly by the medical staff, who perhaps feel pressured and unable to help, and embarrassed or discomfited by this inadequacy.

A solution is the setting up of community- or hospital-based supportive care teams, which consist of medical and nursing staff, usually with a social worker. Such teams exist to help both hospital specialists and local general practitioners, by providing expertise, assistance and time for terminally ill cancer patients, maintaining continuity of support whether the patient has been admitted to a hospital bed or is at home under the care of the local practitioner. From our own experience of working with such a team it is apparent that there are benefits both for the patient and for his or her family. Supportive care teams can assist by providing an expert service regarding, for example, choice of analgesic or antiemetic, as well as arranging for essential facilities such as commodes, home oxygen, rapid installation of telephone services and so on. Although all of these roles could be undertaken by general practitioners, district nurses or social workers, there is no doubt that the presence of a team entirely committed to the improvement of standards in terminal care enormously improves the efficiency of the service. Many teams also take on a bereavement counselling role and remain closely in touch with bereaved relatives, particularly if problems have been perceived before the death of the patient. Although there is no ideal time to refer patients to such a team, we feel that early referral is to be encouraged so that possible problems can be rapidly identified, and a close relationship quickly established.

Cancer quackery

Quackery: the pretensions or practice of a quack
Quack: shortened form of quacksalver—a charlatan
Quacksalver: one who quacks about his salves (derived from Dutch)
Patients with cancer may decide to abandon medical treatment and opt for false or unproven remedies such as

dietary manipulation, 'natural' or herbal medicines, homoeopathy, faith healing, visualization therapy, immunizations, multivitamin supplements and enemas. They may be urged to do so by relatives or other cancer patients, and they sometimes try these treatments in addition to conventional methods.

Patients who do this are usually frightened and anxious; some may see doctors as members of a conspiratorial establishment who have closed minds to any alternative approach. They may have strong ideas about the way their body works or what causes cancer, believing for example that the disease is the result of lifestyle, diet, psychological stress or pollution. However, even if dietary factors are important in aetiology it is illogical to expect that the cancer can therefore be cured by alterations in diet or emotional attitude, or by taking natural products such as herbal remedies. Sadly, giving up smoking does not cure lung cancer. Many august personages are prepared to lend their support to these notions, their names often being more impressive than their intellectual credentials.

There is also no shortage of doctors, naturopaths or homoeopaths to support the public in these beliefs, as well as some more tough-minded charlatans out to make money. There are many damaging aspects to their activities.

First, there is no evidence that any of these remedies work. No evidence for antitumour activity is presented, no evaluation of results and no independent or critical assessment of data. Instead, cases are quoted, anecdotes offered and spurious facts and figures are produced. In one of the few controlled studies of alternative cancer treatments, Laetrile (amygdalin), a 'harmless yet effective' remedy approved by most alternative cancer 'authorities', was found to be entirely without benefit and with significant side-effects when assessed in over 500 cancer patients [10]. High levels of oral vitamin A, sometimes offered as part of a dietary supplement, are known to be teratogenic [11]. Chinese herbs, increasingly used for cancer patients in the UK and USA, can be dangerously nephrotoxic [12–14]. Randomized trials of the 'holistic' approach against conventional treatment have not been undertaken partly due to reluctance by the practitioners of alternative medicine to put their beliefs to the test, and partly due to the ethical difficulties. Two case–control studies have been carried out in advanced cancer, neither of which has shown any benefit for survival in the 'alternative' approach, and one of which showed no improvement in quality of life either [15]. Vitamin C was shown in a randomized trial to be of no value in advanced cancer. Objective but uncontrolled studies of macrobiotic diets and immunoaugmentative

therapy have found no evidence of efficacy. Furthermore, even homeopathic remedies with high dilution may represent a potential hozard to the patient [16], although generally the risk is admittedly low.

Second, the proponents may say that they do not pretend to offer a cure-all, but some patients believe that they will be cured or the disease arrested. The process of mental adjustment to the diagnosis may be badly shaken by false optimism followed by despair at failure. The term *alternative medicine* is in itself a lie when it is used to imply that a proven method of treatment is being offered. Third, the patient may delay conventional treatment, occasionally with tragic consequences in the case of a potentially curable tumour. Fourth, the treatment is often expensive and patients may waste a lot of money. Finally, these 'remedies' may create a great deal of conflict within the family. Patients with advanced cancer can be cajoled or even bullied by their well-meaning relatives into taking an entirely 'natural' diet; then find it intolerable and lose what remaining interest they may have in nutrition. They may even feel that they have to continue in order not to let their children down.

It must be admitted, however, that one reason why patients seek these remedies is a dissatisfaction with conventional medicine or with their doctor, which may in part be well founded [17,18]. Patients will often say that they tried these treatments because they were given no hope or emotional support, because they found the prospect of radiotherapy or chemotherapy unnatural, because there was inadequate explanation and reassurance or because treatment was being unreasonably and thoughtlessly prolonged or aggressive without any hint of benefit. The first question a doctor should ask himself or herself when faced with a patient who has decided to undergo a quack treatment is whether he or she has given enough explanation and reassurance.

If a patient or relative decides to discontinue treatment it is, of course, essential to say what the consequences might be, but cruel to overstate the case in order to browbeat the patient into continuing [19]. Much cancer treatment is palliative and no great harm may be done by stopping it. It is kind to make it clear that, although the proposed alternative is bogus, the patient will be welcome to come back at a later date.

References

1 Levy MH. Pharmacologic treatment of cancer pain. *N Engl J Med* 1996; 335: 1124–32.

2 Saunders CM, Sykes N. *The Management of Terminal Malignant Disease.* London: Edward Arnold, 1993.

3 Hanks GW, Hoskin PJ. Opioid analgesics in the management of pain in patients with cancer. A review. *Palliative Med* 1987; 1: 1–25.

4 Twycross R. Guidelines for the management of nausea and vomiting. *Palliative Care Today* 1999; 32.

5 Baines M. Pain relief in active patients with cancer. analgesic drugs are the foundation of management. *Br Med J* 1989; 298: 36–8.

6 Bruera E, Higginson I, eds. *Cachexia-Anorexia in Cancer Patients.* Oxford: Oxford University Press, 1996.

7 Rimmer T. Treating the anorexia of cancer. *Eur J Palliative Care* 1998; 5: 179–81.

8 Mead GM. Management of oral mucositis associated with cancer chemotherapy. *Lancet* 2002; 359: 815–16.

9 Baines M. The pathophysiology and management of malignant intestinal obstruction. In: Doyle D, Hanks GW, McDonald N, eds. *Textbook of Palliative Medicine.* Oxford: Oxford University Press, 1998.

10 Moertel CG, Fleming TR, Rubin J *et al.* A clinical trial of amygdalin (Laetrile) in the treatment of human cancer. *N Engl J Med* 1991; 306: 201–6.

11 Rothman KJ, Moore LL, Singer MR *et al.* Teratogenicity of high vitamin A intake. *N Engl J Med* 1995; 333: 1369–73.

12 Lord GM, Cook T, Arit VM, Schmeiser HH, Wiliams G, Pusey CD. Urothelial malignant disease and Chinese herbal nephropathy. *Lancet* 2001; 368: 1515–16.

13 Lord GM, Tagore R, Cook T *et al.* Nephropathy caused by Chinese herbs in the UK. *Lancet* 1999; 354: 481–2.

14 Steuer-Vogt MK, Bonkowsky V, Ambrosch P *et al.* The effect of an adjuvant mistletoe treatment programme in resected head and neck cancer patients: a randomised controlled clinical trial. *Eur J Cancer* 2001; 37: 23–31.

15 Cassileth BR, Lusk EJ, Guerry P *et al.* Survival and quality of life among patients receiving unproven as compared with conventional cancer therapy. *N Engl J Med* 1991; 324: 1180–5.

16 Kirby BJ. Safety of homeopathic products. *JR Soc Med* 2002; 95: 221–2.

17 Cassileth B, Lush EJ, Strouse TB *et al.* Contemporary unorthodox treatment in cancer medicine: a study of patients, treatments and practitioners. *Ann Intern Med* 1984; 101: 105–12.

18 Downer SM, Cody MM, McCluskey P *et al.* Pursuit and practice of complementary therapies by cancer patients receiving conventional treatment. *Br Med J* 1994; 309: 86–9.

19 Fried TR, Bradley EH, Towle VR, Allore H. Understanding the treatment preferences of seriously ill patients. *N Engl J Med* 2002; 346: 1061–6.

8 Medical problems and radiotherapy emergencies

Acute and often life-threatening medical problems may arise as a result of the cancer and its treatment. Iatrogenic deaths are not infrequent because many treatments, particularly intensive chemotherapy, are inherently very dangerous. Nevertheless, the majority of deaths are avoidable, and many oncologists prefer to look after their patients in specialized cancer units with staff skilled in anticipating, avoiding and managing these problems.

Bone marrow failure and its consequences

Cytotoxic drugs damage the reproductive integrity of cells. Bone marrow haemopoietic cells are among the most rapidly dividing cells in the body and are extremely sensitive to the action of most antineoplastic agents. Some drugs—for example, vincristine and bleomycin—produce only slight bone marrow depression, while the majority impair haemopoiesis. With drugs such as doxorubicin, myelosuppression is one of the major toxicities. Cytotoxic agents affect different proliferative compartments within the marrow. This leads to non-uniform patterns of toxicity even within the same class of cytotoxic agent. For example, cyclophosphamide, administered as a single intravenous injection, causes predictable granulo-cytopenia 4–7 days later, with a less marked effect on platelet count. In contrast, melphalan and busulphan produce a slower marrow suppression with onset at 7–8 days and maximum depression of white count at about 2–3 weeks. Nitrosoureas such as *cis*-chloroethyl nitrosourea (CCNU) characteristically exert a delayed effect on the blood count at about 4–5 weeks.

The speed of onset and the severity with which the marrow is affected also depend on dose and timing of drug administration. Although the platelet count does not fall significantly with cyclophosphamide given in conventional doses, it will do so at much higher doses. Similarly, although neutropenia and thrombocytopenia usually occur at 4–5 weeks after CCNU administration in conventional doses, at very high doses such as those which have been used experimentally in the treatment of brain tumours, an earlier onset of neutropenia and thrombocytopenia may be seen, occasionally as early as 4–5 days after the drug has been given.

Although some agents (melphalan, busulphan, CCNU) may cause prolonged marrow suppression even when given on the first occasion, in a patient receiving intermittent cytotoxic chemotherapy for the first time the marrow depression is usually transient and the blood count normal in 2–3 weeks, when the next cycle can be given. With increasing duration of chemotherapy, however, the proliferative compartments in the marrow may become progressively more depleted and the nadir of the white count then becomes lower and recovery less rapid, so that chemotherapy cycles may have to be delayed or the dose reduced. In order to avoid life-threatening marrow suppression a familiarity with the cytotoxic regimen is essential, and the physician must be aware of the likelihood of increasing marrow depression with time.

However experienced the clinician, marrow depression does occur unexpectedly. With some treatment regimens — for example, during the induction of remission in acute myeloblastic leukaemia, or with the use of very high-dose chemotherapy in some solid tumours — pancytopenia is an inevitable consequence of treatment.

Granulocytopenia is symptomatic only when infection supervenes. There is usually fever, malaise, shaking and chills, sometimes accompanied by oral ulceration and perineal inflammation. If the platelet count is depressed the patient may develop epistaxis or purpura. It is unusual for symptoms of anaemia to occur acutely even if erythropoiesis ceases altogether as a result of cytotoxic agents, since the half-life of red cells (25 days) is such that the haemoglobin does not usually fall appreciably.

The management of marrow depression by blood component therapy

Blood transfusion [1]

Many patients undergoing combination intermittent chemotherapy for solid tumours develop moderate anaemia, with a haemoglobin of 10–12 g/dl. The blood count will recover when treatment is discontinued, and transfusion is not usually required unless the haemoglobin falls below 9 g/dl. In deciding whether to transfuse a patient, the symptoms of anaemia (fatigue, malaise and breathlessness) must be balanced against the risks of transfusion, in particular volume overload in elderly patients. There is some evidence that, in the presence of thrombocytopenia, a transfusion can precipitate episodes of bleeding — in particular, intracerebral haemorrhage. For this reason, many physicians prefer to use a platelet transfusion before giving blood or packed cells in severely thrombocytopenic patients.

Many patients with advanced malignant disease become anaemic due to an effect of the tumour itself or to marrow infiltration (for example, in myeloma, leukaemia or widespread bone secondaries). This occurs even when patients are not having treatment with chemotherapy or radiotherapy. Even if no active treatment for the tumour is planned, a patient may gain symptomatic relief from blood transfusion. Precise guidelines cannot be drawn, but in general transfusion should be considered only if the haemoglobin falls below 9 g/dl.

Platelet transfusion

The risk of bleeding is related to the platelet count and rises sharply below 20×10^9/l. Ecchymosis and purpura are characteristically found in pressure areas and on the shins. Major bleeding is life-threatening and intracerebral haemorrhage is often fatal.

Transfused platelets have a half-life of only a few days. Platelets have a variety of antigens on their surface, including human leucocyte antigens (HLAs). Repeated transfusion may be accompanied by immunization against these antigens, with the result that further platelet transfusions lead to rapid platelet destruction and a failure to elevate the platelet count. Nevertheless, platelet transfusion has been a major factor in decreasing the morbidity of intensive chemotherapy regimens and most patients can be protected during periods of hypoplasia without serious haemorrhage [2].

There is no single level of platelet count at which transfusion should be given. Platelet transfusion is rarely required at counts above 30×10^9/l. Indications for platelet transfusion are as follows.

1 A rapidly falling platelet count following the start of intensive chemotherapy in which it can be predicted that the circulating platelets will fall below 20×10^9/l within a 24-h period. This is particularly important when making arrangements for the care of patients at weekends. The trend of the platelet count will help in deciding if a further transfusion will soon be necessary.

2 If there is evidence of bleeding (such as widespread ecchymoses, epistaxis or gastrointestinal bleeding), platelet transfusion is essential, even at levels higher than 30×10^9/l.

3 Platelet transfusions are sometimes necessary at higher levels of platelet count (above 30×10^9/l), if there are other complicating factors such as anaemia, peptic ulceration or infection which predispose to bleeding.

Occasionally, patients will become refractory to platelet transfusions, with little or no rise in platelet count. Fever, infection and splenomegaly may all contribute to this, but the usual cause is immunization to platelet antigens. This can be avoided by using HLA-matched donors, generally obtained from the patient's family. In immunized patients a rise in platelet count can sometimes be produced by the use of corticosteroids.

Haemopoietic growth factors [3]

Short-term cultures of human bone marrow cells have allowed identification of progenitor cells which form colonies and whose growth is dependent on colony-stimulating factors (CSFs). The progenitor cells may form cells of several lineages but they are not the self-renewing stem cells (detected in the mouse spleen colony-forming assays). Cloning of the genes of these CSFs has led to the characterization of many of these molecules. Some of these are interleukins (see p. 95). CSFs are glycoproteins, active at extremely low concentrations (which usually interact between cells at short range) and which may stimulate a variety of functions in marrow precursor and mature cells. The chromosomal location and source of the factors are shown in Table 8.1.

The factors bind to specific, high-affinity receptors on the target cell. Granulocyte CSF (G-CSF) and macrophage CSF (M-CSF) stimulate the late stages of division and the differentiation of the granulocyte and macrophage lineage, respectively, and affect the function of mature cells. Other CSFs such as granulocyte/macrophage CSF (GM-CSF) stimulate several cell lineages earlier in differentiation. GM-CSF also increases neutrophil phagocytosis of bacteria and yeasts. Interleukin-1 (IL-1) and IL-6 act on early progenitor cells stimulating cell division and making cells more sensitive to GM-CSF, G-CSF and M-CSF by increasing the number of surface receptors. The earlier return of the white count may allow increased intensity of chemotherapy and possibly improve results of treatment. This has not yet been shown to occur in any chemo-curable cancer.

Clinical use of haemopoietic growth factors

Granulocyte colony-stimulating factor

GM-CSF has been shown to hasten the return of the neutrophil count with conventional myelosuppressive chemotherapy [4] and after autologous bone marrow transplantation (BMT). The platelet count is unaffected. G-CSF has become widely and rather uncritically used in cancer therapy. Before using G-CSF the physician should decide whether it is wise or necessary to use chemotherapy at a dose which will dangerously depress the white blood count. This is clearly not the case for palliative treatment. Using drugs intensively can only be justified if the cure rate is thereby increased. G-CSF may then have a role in improving treatment. There is no place for its routine use, the more so since it is very expensive and inconvenient. G-CSF is used when severe neutropenia has occurred, especially if accompanied by infection. It is used prophylactically when previous cycles have caused severe neutropenia.

Granulocyte/macrophage colony-stimulating factor

GM-CSF causes a rise in granulocyte and platelet count in patients not receiving chemotherapy. Immediately after injection it causes a fall in neutrophil count due to margination, especially in the lungs. It accelerates recovery following conventional chemotherapy and after autologous BMT. Fever and thrombophlebitis are side-effects. In spite of the more rapid recovery of the blood count, length of hospital stay and mortality do not appear to be reduced during autologous BMT. In patients undergoing combined radiotherapy and chemotherapy for small-cell lung cancer (SCLC) the use of GM-CSF was associated with more severe thrombocytopenia [5].

Erythropoietin

Anaemia due to malignant disease will improve recombinant human erythropoietin with amelioration of quality

Factor	Mol. wt	Chromosome	Source
G-CSF	18	17q11.2–21	Monocytes, endothelium
M-CSF	40–50	5q23–31	Monocytes, T cells, endothelium
GM-CSF	14–35	5q23–31	Monocytes, T cells
Endothelium			
EPO	36	7q11–22	Renal peritubular cells, macrophages
IL-3	14–28	5q23–31	T cells

Table 8.1 Haemopoietic growth factors: chromosomal location and cellular source.

of life. Erythropoietin has been shown to diminish the degree of anaemia and transfusion requirements in patients undergoing intensive chemotherapy for SCLC, and to decrease the period of transfusion dependence after allogeneic marrow transplantation [6]. A new form with more sialic acid side-chains has a much longer half-life allowing once weekly administration. Erythropoietin is extremely expensive and its routine use in mild anaemia is not justified.

Infections in the immune-compromised patient

Infections are a major cause of death in cancer. They not only occur frequently, but also are often more severe than in other patients, less responsive to therapy and sometimes produced by organisms which are not pathogens in healthy people. This susceptibility results from depression of host defence mechanisms produced by the tumour and its treatment.

The skin and mucosal surfaces are a barrier to infection. Tumour infiltration and local radiotherapy may lead to damage to lymphatic or venous drainage, with resulting susceptibility to local infection. The turnover of gastrointestinal epithelial cells is depressed by chemotherapy, leading to mucosal damage and ulceration, which allows gut organisms to escape into the portal system. The skin is breached by intravenous needles and cannulae, especially tunnelled subcutaneous lines. These are frequently sources of infection with skin organisms such as *Staphylococcus epidermidis*. Nasogastric tubes act as a focus for infection with *Candida albicans*.

Advanced cancer is sometimes associated with reduced function of both neutrophils and monocytes. Depression of chemotactic, phagocytic and bactericidal activity have all been described.

Impaired delayed hypersensitivity is common in advanced untreated Hodgkin's disease but less common in other malignancies. Lymphopenia is an invariable accompaniment of treatment with alkylating agents and extensive radiotherapy. Cell-mediated immunity is particularly important in host defence against fungi, viruses, tuberculosis and protozoa. Intensive cytotoxic chemotherapy leads to impaired production of antibody to bacterial and viral antigens.

Circulating bacteria are cleared by the phagocytic cells lining the sinuses of the reticuloendothelial system, especially in the liver and spleen. Antibody and complement are important for this clearance. Splenectomy increases

the risk of severe bacterial infection, especially pneumococcal septicaemia in young children and to a lesser extent in adults [7].

Bacteraemia and septicaemia [8]

Bloodstream infections are particularly frequent in granulocytopenic patients. Gram-negative bacteria (*Escherichia coli, Pseudomonas aeruginosa*), staphylococci and streptococci are frequent pathogens. Infections with Gram-positive bacteria have increased in frequency, especially *Staphylococcus epidermidis*. Patients with tunnelled subcutaneous lines are prone to infection with this organism. Fever in a neutropenic cancer patient is an indication for blood cultures, and cultures through the subcutaneous line. If there is an obvious source of the infection such as infected infusion sites, cultures should be taken and the cannula removed. Treatment should not be delayed in the neutropenic patient. Patients with febrile neutropenia at relatively low risk of developing serious complications are those who are being treated with short cycles of chemotherapy for solid tumours. These patients should be admitted to hospital. Recent trials have indicated that the oral amoxicillin–clavulanate combined with oral ciprofloxacin is as effective as intravenous chemotherapy in this group (70% of all patients). The high-risk patients (with uncontrolled cancer or inpatients on intensive therapy) are treated with intravenous antibiotics which include a β-lactam and an aminoglycoside, or ceftazidime.

Respiratory infection

Fever with pulmonary infiltration is a common occurrence in the severely immunocompromised patient. The major causes are given in Table 8.2. The difficulties in making a diagnosis can be considerable because sputum and blood cultures may be negative, and more invasive procedures such as transbronchial biopsy may be impossible because of thrombocytopenia or the general condition of the patient.

There are some clinical features which are helpful in diagnosis. Cavitation is more common with anaerobic bacteria, staphylococci and mycobacteria. *Pneumocystis* infection causes marked dyspnoea, and the chest X-ray shows bilateral infiltrates typically radiating from the hilum. The disease may, however, be indolent, and can cause lobar consolidation. Cytomegalovirus infection mainly occurs in severely immunodepressed patients, particularly during allogeneic BMT. The disease may also cause myocarditis, neuropathy and ophthalmitis. The

Table 8.2 Causes of fever and pulmonary infiltration in immune-compromised patients.

Bacteria	Streptococcus pneumoniae
Gram-negative organisms	Mycobacteria
	Legionella
Fungi	Aspergillus
	Candida
	Cryptococcus
Viruses	Cytomegalovirus
	Herpes simplex
	Measles
Protozoa	Pneumocystis
Treatment	Cytotoxic drugs
	Radiation pneumonitis

pulmonary infiltrate is usually bilateral. *Candida* infection can cause a wide variety of X-ray changes. There is often *Candida* infection elsewhere. Panophthalmitis may occur and the organism can sometimes be isolated from the blood. *Aspergillus* infection is usually rapidly progressive in these patients. Blood cultures are usually negative and the infiltrate can be in one or both lungs.

Faced with this diagnostic uncertainty the following scheme can be adopted.

In patients without neutropenia or thrombocytopenia, investigate with blood cultures, sputum culture, bronchoscopic washings and transbronchial biopsy, where possible. If blood and sputum cultures are negative, treat with broad-spectrum bactericidal antibiotics (usually with an aminoglycoside, penicillin and metronidazole or an equivalent combination). If *Pneumocystis* is a possible cause, high-dose cotrimoxazole should be given. If there is no response, consider aciclovir for herpes simplex infection and antifungal therapy with amphotericin or ketoconazole. Aciclovir is not effective against cytomegalovirus.

If blood or sputum cultures are positive treat as appropriate, but if there is no response consider a mixed infection.

In patients with neutropenia or thrombocytopenia, bronchoscopy can be carried out, but biopsy may not be possible and treatment may have to proceed along the lines indicated above without further diagnostic investigation. Before and after bronchoscopy, antibiotics and platelet transfusion may be necessary.

Urinary tract infections

Infection is common in patients with obstruction to out-

flow, particularly from the bladder. Obstruction may be by tumour or due to an atonic bladder in a patient with cord compression. Diagnosis is made by urine culture, and treatment is with antibiotics and relief of obstruction if possible.

Gastrointestinal infections

Oral thrush (infection with *Candida albicans*) is a frequent complication of chemotherapy. It is particularly likely to occur in immunosuppressed patients, in patients on steroids and in those treated with broad-spectrum antibiotics. The mouth and pharynx become very sore and white plaques of fungus are visible on an erythematous base. The infection may penetrate more deeply in some malnourished patients and extend down into the oesophagus, stomach and bowel. Oral nystatin, amphotericin or miconazole are usually effective.

Herpes simplex cold sores are often troublesome in leucopenic patients, and the lesions may become very widespread. Treatment is with aciclovir, given topically for minor infections in immunosuppressed patients and systemically for more serious infections.

Candida infection in the oesophagus requires treatment with oral nystatin suspension, but if this is ineffective treat with ketoconazole or a short course of amphotericin. *Candida* infections of the bowel should be treated with amphotericin.

Perianal infections are common in neutropenic patients. Preventive measures should always be employed, with scrupulous perineal hygiene and stool softeners to prevent constipation and anal fissures. Spreading perineal infection can be a life-threatening event, and urgent treatment with intravenous antibiotics active against Gram-negative and anaerobic bacilli is required.

Meningitis

Central nervous system (CNS) infections are rare, but patients with lymphoma or leukaemia occasionally develop meningitis due to *Cryptococcus neoformans*. The onset is insidious with headache. The organism can be detected by India ink staining of the CSF. Detection of *Cryptococcus* antigen in blood and CSF is possible in most patients. Many patients will improve with amphotericin and some will be cured.

Skin infections

Apart from infection introduced at infusion sites the most

common skin infection is shingles (varicella zoster). This infection, which is due to a reactivation of varicella zoster virus in dorsal root ganglia, is a dermatomal vesicular eruption which is particularly severe in immunocompromised hosts and which may disseminate as chickenpox and cause a fatal pneumonia. Patients should be treated with aciclovir as early as possible.

Prevention of infection in the leucopenic patient

When a patient is leucopenic reverse barrier nursing procedures are usually used. For most episodes of granulocytopenia, disposable aprons, face masks and careful washing of hands is probably satisfactory. For more persistent leucopenia (for example, with allogeneic BMT) a protected environment has much to commend it. Here the air is filtered free of bacteria and a laminar air flow is established from one end of the room to the other. The patients are 'decontaminated' before entry with oral antibiotics to kill intestinal bacteria, and cutaneous antiseptic cleansing. Protected environments can lower the infection rate but their contribution to overall reduction in mortality is small since the hazards of the disease and other effects of treatment are greater. The psychological stress and cost of isolation are other major disadvantages. Other important preventive measures are scrupulous hygiene in the placing of intravenous drugs, perineal hygiene and high standards of staff training.

Antibiotic prophylaxis has been studied extensively [9]. Several randomized trials have shown that ciprofloxacin is effective in preventing infection with Gram-negative organisms in neutropenic patients. The combination of ciprofloxacin and rifampacin with vancomycin has been shown to be effective prophylaxis in stem cell transplanta-

tion. Bacterial strains resistant to ciprofloxacin are, however, now beginning to occur in the community.

Prophylactic use of antibiotics has been shown to reduce the incidence of fungal infections in patients undergoing BMT. Fluconazole has been widely used; it reduces the frequency of *Candida* infection and is as effective as amphotericin in leukaemia induction treatment.

Aciclovir is effective in preventing varicella zoster in patients who are undergoing BMT and stem cell transplantation or who are in the recovery period. High-dose aciclovir and ganciclovir are also effective prophylactics for cytomegalovirus. In patients undergoing very intensive therapy trimethaprim/sulphamethoxazole prophylaxis helps prevent *Pneumocystis carinii* infection.

Cancer cachexia and the nutritional support of the cancer patient [10]

Weight loss is a common symptom of cancer, but profound and rapid weight loss usually indicates disseminated tumour. When cancer recurs and is widespread, loss of weight is an almost invariable accompaniment. This leads finally to the cachectic state in which the patient becomes wasted, weak and lethargic.

Pathogenesis of malnutrition in cancer

Anorexia is a major factor in reducing food intake (Table 8.3). The nausea and vomiting of chemotherapy are evident causes, as is depression anxiety. However, the mechanism of tumour-induced anorexia and cachexia is poorly understood. It frequently accompanies widespread disease, in particular the presence of hepatic metastases. Cy-

Table 8.3 Weight loss in cancer.

Reduced intake	Anorexia/cachexia syndrome
	Treatment induced effects: anorexia, nausea, oral ulceration
	Depression and anxiety
Nutrient malabsorption	Gut surgery
	Gut toxicity from radiation or drugs
	Bowel obstruction
	Malabsorption syndrome: obstructive jaundice, pancreatic carcinoma
Loss of protein and nutrients	Diarrhoea
	Ulceration of the gut mucosa by tumours
	Gut mucositis (drugs and X-rays)
Metabolic changes induced by tumour	Increased protein and fat metabolism
	Altered glucose metabolism induced by tumour
	Tumour consumption of carbohydrate and protein

tokines released by the tumour may contribute to the syndrome. These include tumour necrosis factor-α (TNF-α) and IL-6. Typically the patient loses all interest in food and has an altered perception of taste and smell such that the thought of eating can become repugnant.

Nutrient malabsorption may be due to mechanical causes such as surgical resection (partial gastrectomy or major gut resection), gut obstruction, or due to mucosal damage by drugs or radiation. Tumours ulcerating the gut and mucosal damage by treatment cause loss of blood and protein. Metabolic abnormalities have been found in advanced cancer but there is no uniform abnormality which is always present in cachectic individuals. The abnormalities which have been demonstrated are as follows.

1 An increased metabolic rate has been demonstrated in some patients. The mechanism is unknown. An overall increase in protein metabolism associated with a negative nitrogen balance has been demonstrated in some patients.

2 An abnormality of glucose metabolism in the tumour, a production of excess lactate, which is then reutilized to form glucose—a process wasteful of energy.

Maintaining nutrition

In considering nutritional support for an individual cancer patient, the objectives of treatment must be clear. If a potentially curative treatment is being considered either with surgery, chemotherapy or radiotherapy, there is evidence that effective nutritional support may improve the tolerance of treatment. Well-nourished cancer patients frequently lose weight as a result of cancer treatment, whether with surgery, chemotherapy or radiotherapy. If the effects of radical treatment are likely to persist over a week or more, and considerable weight loss can be anticipated, it is probable that nutritional supplements will decrease morbidity. If there is no prospect of cure, then nutritional support is a palliative procedure. Aggressive and uncomfortable means of maintaining nutrition are then completely inappropriate. There is no evidence at present that the progressive malnutrition and wasting which accompany advanced and incurable cancer can be reversed by any form of feeding. Every cancer patient should have an assessment of weight loss and appetite. If there has been loss of more than 10% body weight it is advisable to have a dietitian's advice in developing a plan for nutritional support.

Enteral nutrition

Attention to diet and to the foods available to the patient is of great importance. This involves discussions with the patient about favourite foods. Dietary advice from a dietitian and the support of the family in providing favourite foods are an essential part of the plan. Small but frequent meals are often helpful. Nutritional supplements can be added to the patient's diet, including high-calorie liquids such as Hycal and more complete protein and carbohydrate mixtures (for example, Complan or Clinifeed). Protein hydrolysates, providing small peptides and amino acid fragments, are also available (Vivonex). They provide calories in liquid form at a time when the patient finds it difficult to eat solid food. They can cause osmotic disturbances and for many patients they are quite unpalatable. Appetite stimulants such as medroxyprogesterone acetate and dexamethasone may be helpful in the short term.

Occasionally a patient may find it difficult to swallow or eat at all. Enteral support with liquid dietary supplements can be given by using a fine-bore flexible nasogastric feeding tube or by per-endoscopic gastrostomy feeding. The latter has been widely used in cancer of the head and neck, and of the oesophagus. The aim is to provide about 2000–3000 kcal/day. These supplements have a high osmolality. They can cause nausea and diarrhoea and provide a large solute load for renal excretion. Large amounts of fluid are required to excrete this solute load, even in the presence of normal renal function.

Total parenteral nutrition

It is now possible to provide adequate calories intravenously for patients who cannot take food by mouth or by nasogastric tube. Access is through a catheter placed in a deep vein, since parenteral nutritional solutions are irritant. The incidence of venous thrombosis when catheters are inserted into the subclavian vein is small. With all subcutaneous catheters there is a risk of infection which is particularly likely to occur in the immune-compromised individual. A variety of synthetic total parenteral nutrition solutions are available commercially, usually consisting of amino acid solutions with dextrose, vitamins, electrolytes and trace elements.

Several of the metabolic defects present in the malnourished patient can be reversed by total parenteral nutrition. Although it is difficult to demonstrate benefit, it is sometimes justifiable to support a patient with parenteral nutrition during intensive but potentially curative treatment. This includes patients undergoing major gastrointestinal surgery, or chemotherapy with marrow ablation. Total parenteral nutrition is complex, expensive and potentially hazardous. It is of no proven value as a routine measure in patients undergoing cancer therapies.

Acute metabolic disturbances

Hypercalcaemia

A raised plasma calcium is a frequent accompaniment of cancer. In a hospital population, carcinomas of the bronchus, breast and kidney are, together with multiple myeloma, the commonest malignant causes of hypercalcaemia. Life-threatening hypercalcaemia is usually due to cancer. Minor elevations of plasma calcium (up to 2.8 mmol/l) are not usually associated with any symptoms. As the plasma calcium rises, patients experience anorexia, nausea, abdominal pain, constipation and fatigue. There may be proximal muscle weakness, polyuria and polydypsia. With increasing hypercalcaemia, severe dehydration, confusion and finally coma may supervene.

Bone metastases are much the commonest cause of hypercalcaemia in cancer. Most patients with severe hypercalcaemia have demonstrable metastases on X-ray or on bone scanning. Bone marrow aspiration may show infiltration with tumour. Even if metastases are not detectable at presentation, they usually quickly become apparent. Metastases in bone stimulate osteoclast activity by the local release of parathyroid hormone-related protein (PTHrP). The bone resorption liberates factors such as transforming growth factor (TGF)-α, TGF-β, epidermal growth factor, and IL-1 (α and β forms) [11]. These factors may not only act locally to cause bone resorption but may also, in the case of breast cancer cause further release of PTHrP from tumour cells.

In addition to direct bone lysis by metastases, cancers may produce hypercalcaemia by remote, humoral mechanisms—the syndrome of humoral hypercalcaemia of malignancy (HHM). The syndrome is largely due to circulating PTHrP released from the tumour but other cytokines may also play a part, especially in lymphoma and myeloma. The protein has striking homology to PTH in the first 13 amino acids but differs in the remainder. It seems that alternatively spliced forms of messenger RNA may yield two or more different proteins. Most squamous carcinomas express the protein (whether the patient is hypercalcaemic or not). Its metabolic effect is similar to PTH, with increased bone reabsorption of calcium.

The treatment of hypercalcaemia in cancer may be a medical emergency, particularly in the elderly and in patients with myeloma. The raised plasma calcium may be accompanied by uraemia which is due to salt and water loss as a result of the effect of calcium on the distal tubule making it unresponsive to antidiuretic hormone. Hypokalaemia may also accompany hypercalcaemia, and may in part be due to a renal loss of potassium. Elderly patients, and those with impaired renal function, are unable to withstand the effects of the raised plasma calcium, and life-threatening renal failure may quickly develop. In myeloma it is particularly likely to occur since other causes of renal failure are present (see Chapter 27).

In severe hypercalcaemia, the first line of treatment is therefore with salt and water replacement using isotonic saline. In the first 24 h, 4–8 l may be required. This may be sufficient to lower the plasma calcium to normal. In the elderly, care must be taken not to overload the patient with fluids. If the plasma calcium does not begin to fall within 24 h, prednisolone given orally (30–60 mg/day) or hydrocortisone intravenously (50–100 mg 6-hourly) is often helpful in reducing the calcium, but not all patients will respond. Frusemide promotes calciuresis but care must be taken with volume replacement, to avoid further salt and water depletion.

Bisphosphonates reduce serum calcium by inhibiting bone resorption and are effective in hypercalcaemia due to metastases or PTHrP. Pamidronate is effective in 90% of patients. A dose of 60–90 mg given in a 2-h infusion is the usual procedure. It can be repeated every 2–3 weeks. Mild fever and skin irritation can occur, and it is preferable to use bisphosphonates after rehydration since temporary renal impairment can occur. Etidronate seems rather less effective—it is usually given as three infusions of 7.5 mg/kg. Clodronate in a dose of five daily infusions of 300 mg restores normocalcaemia in 90% of cases. Oral clodronate can be given (1600 mg/day) but causes gastrointestinal upset.

Mithramycin has been largely replaced by the bisphosphonates. The usual dose is 15–25 mg/kg, and a single injection usually causes a fall in plasma calcium after 24–48 h. Occasionally it may be necessary to use mithramycin on two or three successive days. This carries a risk of thrombocytopenia.

Intravenous or oral phosphate therapy is seldom necessary to control the plasma calcium, but phosphate infusions (usually with serum calcium of 4 mmol/l or more) may be helpful in patients who are gravely ill.

Calcitonin produces a more rapid fall in the plasma calcium but its effect is variable and its use is limited to patients with severe acute hypercalcaemia. The usual dose is 2–4 U/kg of salmon calcitonin subcutaneously 12-hourly, or 1–2 U/kg i.v. infusion every 6 h.

Although it is not usually difficult to diagnose the cause of malignant hypercalcaemia, diagnostic problems can occur when hyperparathyroidism is an alternative diagnosis in cancer patients who do not have evidence of disseminated disease. The steroid suppression test will not reduce the plasma calcium in hyperparathyroidism, but 75% of patients with cancer show a fall after 10 days of hydrocortisone administration. If serious doubt remains, elevation of plasma parathormone is found in 80% of patients with primary hyperparathyroidism, but not in patients with cancer.

Tumour lysis syndrome

An acute metabolic disturbance may occur as a result of the rapid dissolution of tumour following chemotherapy. This is particularly likely to occur in children with Burkitt's lymphoma or acute lymphoblastic leukaemia, and in non-Hodgkin's lymphomas in children, adolescents and young adults. The syndrome occurs when there is extreme sensitivity of the tumour to treatment, and is uncommon in adults with non-lymphoid neoplasms. When it occurs, tumour masses may disappear very rapidly, and as the cells are killed they release products of nitrogen metabolism, especially urea, urate and large amounts of phosphate.

The rapid reduction in tumour mass causes hyperuricaemia, hyperphosphataemia, hyperkalaemia and uraemia. Hyperuricaemia may result in acute urate deposition in the renal tubules (urate nephropathy), leading to acute renal failure or, less dramatically, to a reduction in glomerular filtration rate which exacerbates the hyperuricaemia. Occasionally, the syndrome can be sufficiently severe to cause an acute and prolonged uraemia. Hyperphosphataemia results in a reciprocal lowering of the plasma calcium and can result in tetany.

The syndrome is more likely to occur in children with Burkitt's lymphoma who have extensive disease, particularly if there are intra-abdominal masses, impaired renal function from tumour infiltration of the kidney or postrenal obstruction due to lymph node enlargement. The syndrome is rare in adults since the tumours are generally less sensitive to chemotherapy, and their dissolution less rapid. It may, however, occur if there is coincidental renal failure due to some other cause, ureteric obstruction or infiltration of the kidney with tumour.

Tumour lysis syndrome is usually preventable. Before beginning chemotherapy in a high-risk patient, allopurinol should be given (usually by mouth) in full dose (50–100 mg 8-hourly in children, twice this dose in adults)

for 24 h. This xanthine-oxidase inhibitor partly prevents the formation of uric acid. The precursors, xanthine and hypoxanthine, are therefore present in great excess but are much more soluble than uric acid and do not cause nephropathy. Allopurinol should be continued for the first few days of treatment and discontinued when the plasma urate is in the normal range. If 6-mercaptopurine is being given the dose should be reduced since allopurinol inhibits its metabolism. At the same time the patient should be given adequate fluids, usually in the form of intravenous saline, to establish a good diuresis. These measures should prevent both hyperuricaemia and hyperphosphataemia. In Burkitt's lymphoma, the induction chemotherapy is sometimes given at reduced dose until there has been considerable tumour shrinkage and then the full dose is administered. Allopurinol should be given to adults with high-grade lymphoma starting treatment with intensive chemotherapy; its use should be considered in other cases if there is any possibility of renal impairment.

If hyperuricaemia and acute renal failure develop these can usually be treated by cessation of chemotherapy, cautious administration of intravenous fluids with alkalinization of the urine to promote urate excretion, and allopurinol. If the blood urea and plasma urate continue to rise, peritoneal dialysis may be needed to tide the patient over the acute renal failure. If preventive measures are taken this should rarely be necessary.

Serous effusions

Many patients with cancer develop a pleural or pericardial effusion or ascites during the course of their illness. These can be difficult to treat and can be a major cause of discomfort and breathlessness. The effusions are exudates caused by the presence of tumour on the serosal surface. It is not clear how the increased permeability occurs. It is possible that it is due to factors produced by the tumour. The protein content is greater than 30 mg/l.

Pleural effusion

Pleural fluid must reach a volume of about 500 ml before it can be detected clinically, although lesser degrees can be radiologically apparent.

Typically the effusion is substantial in volume (1–4 l), accumulates rapidly, and may be blood-stained. It often causes dyspnoea with dry cough, sometimes with pleuritic chest pain. In addition to the fluid, there is usually a thick coating of malignant infiltrate on both pleural surfaces. The parietal layer can cause chest wall infiltration, pain and swelling. Although cytological demonstration of cells confirms the nature of the effusion, it is common for a malignant effusion to be repeatedly cytologically negative, in which case pleural biopsy will often be indicated if there is clinical doubt as to the diagnosis. However, pleural biopsy is only diagnostic in 50% of cases. Thoracoscopy increases the accuracy of biopsy—a diagnosis being made in 90% of cases of malignant disease. The frequency order of malignant disease causing pleural effusion is: lung cancer, breast cancer, genitourinary cancers, lymphoma and gastrointestinal cancer.

Occasionally, patients with cancer develop a pleural effusion from a non-malignant cause, and alternative explanations should always be considered if a patient with apparently controlled cancer unexpectedly develops a pleural effusion.

Management is rarely straightforward. Most patients require therapeutic aspiration (thoracocentesis) to improve symptoms of cough and dyspnoea, and large volumes (1–5 l) may have to be removed for worthwhile benefit. The fluid often forms sealed-off collections (loculations), especially when recurrent after aspiration. These loculated areas may make control of the effusion difficult. In patients with secondary pleural deposits, chemotherapy or endocrine therapy will be given as primary treatment (for example, in lymphoma or breast cancer). In these patients, this systemic treatment may prove effective in preventing reaccumulation of pleural fluid. In others, where effective systemic therapy is unavailable, the question of whether to instil an intrapleural sclerosant, to prevent or reduce fluid accumulation, will arise.

Pleurodesis with physical, antibiotic or bacterial sclerosants (talc, tetracycline, quinacrine or *Coryne bacterium parvum*) and cytotoxic drugs (such as bleomycin) are all commonly used. They depend on the production of an inflammatory reaction obliterating the pleural space. Each is effective only in a proportion of cases. Tetracycline can cause severe local pain, and bleomycin can cause fever and chills.

There are a few comparisons of one treatment with another. Talc instillation appears to provide the highest rate of control and is currently regarded as treatment of choice. It can be instilled under local or general anaesthetic after the effusion has been drained to dryness. It is a procedure requiring experience and care. Control rates of 90% are achieved. Simpler procedures, such as instillation of buomycin, tetracycline or *C. parvum* control 70% of effusions. They are indicated for patients whose condition is poor. Occasionally, pleurectomy will be required

for adequate control of an effusion due to pleural secondary deposits and should be considered if the patient's general condition warrants [12].

Pericardial effusion

This is an infrequent clinical problem and, in contrast to pleural effusion, pericardial effusions are less commonly due to malignancy than other causes such as infections, myxoedema, collagen disorders and rheumatoid arthritis. The diagnosis is often a radiological one, with 'globular' enlargement of the heart shadow. The clinical features are dyspnoea, orthopnoea, cough and central chest pain. The commonest signs are pulsus paradoxus, raised jugular venous pressure and hypotension. There may be a pleural rib, faint heart sounds and hepatomegaly. The diagnosis should be suspected in any patient with cancer who develops the rapid onset of unexplained breathlessness.

The commonest causes are carcinomas of breast and bronchus, and lymphoma including Hodgkin's disease. In patients with widespread metastases, it may occur concurrently with a malignant pleural effusion. The diagnosis can be simply confirmed by echocardiography, which also gives useful quantitative information regarding the volume of the effusion. Because pericardial aspiration is both more hazardous and technically more difficult than pleural aspiration, it should not be undertaken in asymptomatic patients where the diagnosis is certain.

Treatment is by means of the same chemicals that are used for pleural effusion including cytotoxic drugs and tetracycline. Talc is not used. There may in addition be a useful response to systemic chemotherapy or endocrine therapy. The formation of a surgical 'pericardial window' into the mediastinum is often beneficial if the effusion is persistent. The operation can be performed, if necessary, under local anaesthesia and high local control rates are achieved [13].

Ascites [14]

Ascites is a common clinical problem in cancer. The usual cause is widespread peritoneal seedlings which cause exudation of fluid and reabsorption block lymphatic drainage. Liver metastases are often present, and hypoalbuminaemia contributes to the accumulation of fluid by lowering plasma osmotic pressure. Common cancers causing ascites include carcinomas of ovary, breast, bronchus (especially small cell), large bowel, stomach and pancreas, and melanoma.

Patients usually present with abdominal distension,

bulging of the flanks and with peripheral oedema if there is associated hypoalbuminaemia and/or inferior vena caval obstruction. The umbilicus may be everted and some patients have a fluid thrill. It is important not to assume a malignant diagnosis, particularly when the tumour was previously thought to be localized or controlled by treatment. Important non-malignant causes include: portal hypertension (usually from cirrhosis or portal vein thrombosis), hepatic vein thrombosis (Budd–Chiari syndrome), raised systemic venous pressure as in long-standing cardiac failure and hypoalbuminaemia from other causes.

Diagnosis is by clinical examination, abdominal ultrasound and aspiration cytology. Ultrasound examination is a sensitive technique for demonstrating ascites and associated tumour masses. Malignant cells may be detected cytologically, though this examination is negative in 50% of cases of proven malignancy.

Treatment includes both therapeutic aspiration (paracentesis) and general measures designed to prevent recurrence. Some patients will have control of ascites, at least for a while, using spironolactone (50 mg 8-hourly) with or without frusemide. Slow drainage over several days, via a peritoneal dialysis catheter, may be necessary to give relief of symptoms. Instillation of cytotoxic agents is less frequently practised and less frequently successful than in malignant pleural effusion, but intraperitoneal bleomycin and quinicrine and TNF have all been used. Systemic chemotherapy (or endocrine therapy in breast cancer) may occasionally help to control ascites in appropriately sensitive cancers.

Surgical procedures such as peritoneovenous shunts (LeVeen and Denver shunts) can be helpful if the patient is likely to survive at least 3–6 months and suffering from repeated episodes of ascites. The initial success rate is about 70% but almost always occurs after a few months. The prognosis for patients with malignant ascites is poor, the majority dying within 6 months of diagnosis.

Carcinomatous meningitis [15]

This complication of cancer is increasingly recognized. Its frequency is not known with certainty, but some estimates suggest that as many as 5% of patients with solid tumours will be affected. It is commoner in lymphoma and leukaemia than in solid tumours. It is most frequently found in breast cancer (especially the lobular subtype) and SCLC but may occur in any tumour, including melanomas.

The tumour cells line the meninges in sheets and nodules, and penetrate into the substance of the brain, tracking down blood vessels. A dense fibrotic reaction may occur which may cause additional ischaemic neurological damage. The tumour cells reach the meninges either by direct extension from an underlying intracerebral metastasis, or possibly by direct haematogenous spread.

The presenting features are very varied and the diagnosis should be considered in any unexplained neurological disturbance in a patient with cancer. Central symptoms are altered consciousness, confusion, dysphasia, headache and meningism. Cranial nerve involvement is frequent (50% of cases), the oculomotor and facial nerves being the most frequently affected. Individual spinal nerve roots are very frequently involved, causing weakness and sensory disturbance. More generalized long tract signs occur due to cord involvement.

Investigation should include computed tomography (CT) or preferably magnetic resonance imaging (MRI) with gadolinium enhancement which is much more sensitive. The scans will also demonstrate hydrocephalus, which indicates that diagnostic lumbar puncture may be hazardous. MRI scans may show diffuse meningeal enhancement and focal deposits and nodules. In the spinal cord the investigation is less reliable, about 50% of cases showing a normal appearance.

Lumbar puncture will demonstrate tumour cells in most, but not all, cases. The sensitivity is increased by repeating the investigation if the first sample is abnormal but not diagnostic. The CSF protein is usually raised and the glucose level is reduced in 50% of cases.

Treatment is essentially palliative and there are no absolute guidelines. Certain drugs are useful. Methotrexate concentrations are much higher when the drug is administered directly into the CSF. The half-life is about 12 h and CSF drug concentrations have usually fallen to 0.1 μmol by 48 h, when it is safe to repeat the dose. The drug is usually given two to three times per week. There are difficulties with repeated administration, especially in the presence of malignant infiltration, and the distribution of the drug is less certain than when it is given prophylactically. Side-effects include arachnoiditis, transient paralysis, headache and vomiting. The use of intraventricular reservoirs does not appear to improve outcome, although they are reasonably well tolerated and convenient. Cytosine arabinoside can also be given intrathecally, with high concentrations being achieved in normal CSF. It is subject to the same limitations as methotrexate when given in carcinomatous meningitis. The half-life in the CSF is approximately 3.5 h, with a level of 1 μmol at 24 h below which the drug is not active. Thiotepa has been used in intrathecal treatment, but it is a prodrug whose intermediary metabolites are unknown. The usual regimens are twice weekly administration for 5 weeks and then weekly for 5 weeks.

Brain irradiation is often given, especially in those patients showing a response to intrathecal treatment. The usual regimen is 30 Gy in 10 fractions. Maintenance intrathecal treatment has not been shown to be of benefit, although, as with most aspects of treatment for this condition, there is a lack of data from randomized trials addressing this and other issues in management.

Patients treated with intrathecal treatment alone will often respond and survival may be improved. Dramatic responses may occur but are uncommon. The prognosis of carcinomatous meningitis remains very bad. The reported median survival is 6–12 weeks, but some patients survive much longer. Survival is worse in SCLC, in patients with widespread disease elsewhere, with poor previous performance status and with widespread neurological signs.

Progressive multifocal leucoencephalopathy

This rare syndrome is not always associated with cancer, but lymphoma is by far the commonest associated disorder. The clinical features are aphasia and dementia leading to coma, visual field loss which may progress to blindness, fits and focal paralyses. The differential diagnosis includes metastases, lymphomatous meningitis, herpes encephalitis and cerebrovascular disease. The CSF is usually normal.

The brain shows patchy demyelination throughout the white matter with abnormal oligodendroglia, the nuclei of which contain viral inclusions. Papova viruses (JC and SV40) have been isolated from these brains. Antibodies to these viruses may be present in blood or CSF and may help in diagnosis. The disease is usually fatal in 6–12 months, although some patients live for years. Responses to intrathecal and intravenous cytosine arabinoside have been reported.

Management of hepatic metastases

Many patients with cancer will develop hepatic metastases, and when these are widespread the expectation of life is only 2–3 months. In many cases there will be widespread dissemination and liver involvement will not be a separate medical problem. In some tumours such as

small-cell carcinoma of the bronchus, breast cancer or lymphoma there is a reasonable likelihood of a response to chemotherapy with symptomatic and biochemical improvement. There are, however, many occasions when the liver is involved with metastatic cancer for which chemotherapy is inappropriate due to primary or acquired drug resistance.

The usual symptoms are fatigue, weight loss, anorexia and right upper quadrant pain. There may be abdominal distension from ascites. Episodes of sudden severe pain may occur when there is haemorrhage into a metastasis. Later, jaundice develops with advancing cachexia. Survival is usually a few months, depending on the extent of involvement and rate of progression. Metastatic carcinoid tumours may be very slow growing, and in this disease hepatic metastases are compatible with survival of 3–5 years.

Almost all treatment of hepatic metastasis is palliative and the value of each approach depends on the circumstances of each patient. The main symptoms are anorexia, nausea, pain, fever and malaise. Jaundice is a late feature unless there is obstruction to the porta hepatis by a tumour or lymph node mass. Itching and steatorrhoea may then be major symptoms. The following approaches can be taken to relieve symptoms.

Pharmacological

Anorexia, fever and malaise may all be relieved for a time by corticosteroids. Prednisolone 20–30 mg/day is usually adequate, but the symptoms often recur after a few weeks and muscle wasting becomes profound if this dose is continued for long. Phenothiazines or metoclopramide before meals may help a little with the nausea, and aspirin or indomethacin may also relieve fever. Pain is treated with analgesics, as described in Chapter 7.

Radiotherapeutic

Although the liver does not tolerate large doses (above 35 Gy), radiotherapy has a useful role in palliation of pain and may also improve nausea and vomiting. With a dose of 20–35 Gy to the whole liver, over 70% of patients will experience some improvement, particularly relief of pain. In chemoresistant tumours the addition of chemotherapy or hypoxic cell sensitizers does not improve these results. Often a particularly painful metastasis can be treated with a local field using a few large fractions, producing quick relief of pain without adverse effects.

Chemotherapeutic

In the case of responsive tumours such as SCLC or breast cancer, chemotherapy may be very effective, with responses in 50–60% of patients. If the primary tumour is of a type not usually amenable to chemotherapy, it is unlikely that cytotoxic agents will be of much value. For metastatic adenocarcinoma of the bowel 5-fluorouracil (5-FU) has been most widely used, but the objective response rate is only 10–20%. Subjectively, particularly with respect to pain, the response rate is higher. Modern regimens use 5-FU in conjunction with folinic acid (p. 80), and prolonged infusion regimens may be preferable.

Surgical

Hepatic artery ligation or embolization can produce pain relief and shrinkage of metastases, but they recur rapidly with regeneration of the blood supply. Occasionally a slow-growing solitary metastasis is worth resecting in a fit patient with, for example, a carcinoid tumour. Surgical resection of isolated hepatic metastases has been increasingly performed in patients with colorectal cancer (see Chapter 16).

Radiotherapeutic emergencies

There are two common clinical situations which require urgent consideration by the radiotherapist. These are acute spinal cord compression and superior vena caval obstruction (SVCO).

Acute spinal cord or cauda equina compression [16,17]

This syndrome results from pressure on the cord, usually as a result of a tumour extending from a vertebral body to compress the cord from the epidural space (Fig. 8.1). Compression may also occur as a result of direct extension from a mediastinal tumour or the cauda equina from a retroperitoneal tumour. If the vertebra is weakened a crush fracture may precipitate cord compression. Very occasionally, intramedullary metastases will cause acute cord compression from within. Cord compression most commonly occurs in diseases where bony metastases (particularly vertebral metastases) are frequent. Myelomas and carcinomas of the prostate, breast and lung (particularly small-cell carcinomas) are the commonest causes. The thoracic vertebrae are the commonest site of com-

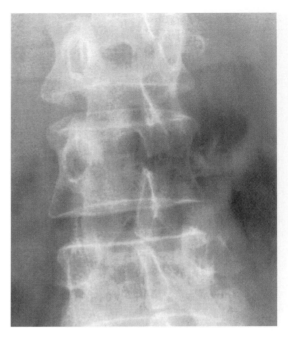

Fig. 8.1 X-ray of lumbar vertebrae showing destruction of the left pedicle L3.

pressive lesions (the cord ends at L1). Compression of the spinal venous drainage quickly leads to oedema and ischaemia of the cord.

The onset may be acute or gradual. Characteristically, the patient complains of back pain often with a root distribution, weakness of the legs, dribbling, hesitancy and incontinence of urine and sluggish bowel action. In most cases, only one or two of these symptoms will be present. Limb weakness and bladder dysfunction are later signs, but in many patients the symptoms will only have been present 48 h before paraplegia occurs. Higher cord lesions will also be accompanied by symptoms and signs in the upper limb (Table 8.4).

Cauda equina syndrome, where the compression occurs below the lower level of the spinal cord L1 or L2, is often difficult to diagnose. Features include leg weakness, sacral anaesthesia, retention of urine and erectile failure. Clinical diagnosis is particularly important since in this syndrome radiological studies, including myelography, often fail to demonstrate any definite abnormality. Careful neurological examination may reveal loss of sacral sensation (saddle anaesthesia) which will only be detected if perianal sensation is tested with a pin, and anal sphincter tone is assessed on rectal examination.

Table 8.4 Syndromes of spinal cord compression.

Complete compression
Sensory loss just below level of lesion
Loss of all modalities of sensation — variable in degree at first
Bilateral upper motor neurone weakness below lesion
Bladder and bowel dysfunction

Anterior compression
Partial loss of pain and temperature below lesion
Bilateral upper motor neurone weakness below lesion
Bladder and bowel dysfunction

Lateral compression (Brown–Séquard)
Contralateral loss of pain and temperature (touch much less
   affected)
Ipsilateral loss of proprioception and vibration
Ipsilateral upper motor neurone weakness

Posterior compression
Loss of vibration and position below lesion
Pain, temperature and touch relatively spared
Painful segmental paraesthesia at level of lesion

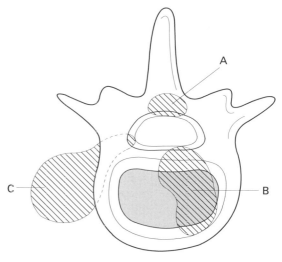

Fig. 8.2 Epidural compression of the cord may be caused by metastasis from the vertebral body (A and B) or from paravertebral metastasis penetrating through the intervertebral foramen (C). The vertebral body is the commonest site.

Spinal cord compression may occasionally occur at more than one site, giving rise to neurological signs (for example, a mixture of upper and lower motor neurone weakness) which would otherwise be difficult to explain on the basis of a single lesion.

Investigation should include plain X-ray of the spine, which may show evidence of multiple bone metastases, a paraspinal mass, a crush fracture at the site of pain, or less obvious changes such as erosion of a pedicle (Fig. 8.2). A normal X-ray is not uncommon; MRI is the most useful investigation. It demonstrates the site of blockage with great accuracy and usually gives a clear view of its extent (of the tumour inside and outside the spinal canal) and whether multiple lesions are present (Fig. 8.3). When MRI is not available, CT combined with myelography is a reliable alternative.

Cord compression is a medical emergency in which treatment must begin within hours, not days. Any patient with cancer who develops severe back pain with a root distribution is at very high risk and must be investigated at once.

Treatment of cord compression is by radiation therapy, surgery or a combination of both. For tumours that are radiosensitive (myeloma, lymphoma, SCLC, breast cancer) radiotherapy is usually the initial treatment. Dexamethasone is usually given before and during radiation. If there is evidence of neurological deterioration at any stage the need for surgery must be reassessed at once. For

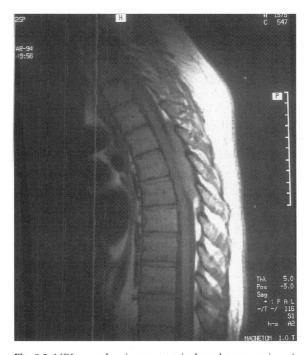

Fig. 8.3 MRI scan showing acute spinal cord compression. A large posterior mass, extending over three vertebrae, is compressing the spinal cord.

tumours insensitive to radiation, surgery may be the preferred initial treatment especially for solitary lesions. If the tumour is anterior, approaches to decompression are technically more difficult, but anterior approaches are now much more widely used. Posterior lesions are treated by decompressive laminectomy. Postoperative complications are not uncommon and instability of the spine occurs in 10% of cases.

The prognosis for patients with cord compression relates to the degree of neurological damage before treatment and to the underlying cancer. Delayed diagnosis results in a bad outcome. Speedy and efficient treatment are essential. If the patient has progressed to paraplegia before treatment, the chance that he or she will walk after treatment is less than 5%. Early diagnosis is essential since with less severe damage, 50% will be ambulatory. Widespread radioresistant tumour (for example, melanoma) has a bad prognosis. Chemotherapy plays no part in the initial management of cord compression.

Superior vena caval obstruction

This most commonly results from a right-sided carcinoma of the bronchus (particularly small-cell carcinoma). It also occurs in lymphoma (particularly Hodgkin's disease, in which mediastinal involvement occurs in about one-quarter of all patients), as well as carcinoma of the breast, kidney and other tumours which may metastasize to mediastinal nodes. Occasionally, it may be a presenting feature of a primary mediastinal tumour such as a thymoma, or a germ cell tumour. It is characterized by swelling of the face, neck and arms, with a typical plethoric cyanotic appearance. There is non-pulsatile engorgement of veins, and large collateral veins may be visible over the surface of the shoulders, scapulae and upper chest. Retinal veins may also be engorged, and there is often conjunctival oedema. The most constant physical sign is that of leashes of tiny bluish venules which occur over the chest wall, particularly in the precordial, subcostal and infrascapular regions. Patients are almost always dyspnoeic and hypoxic, and the chest X-ray usually shows a substantial right-sided mass (Fig. 8.4).

Urgent treatment with radiotherapy is the mainstay of management and is undoubtedly the treatment of choice for non-small-cell carcinomas of the bronchus and other tumours not amenable to chemotherapy, and where treatment must be started before the diagnosis is known. However, with the advent of effective chemotherapy for lymphoma and small-cell carcinoma of the bronchus, combination chemotherapy should be considered in

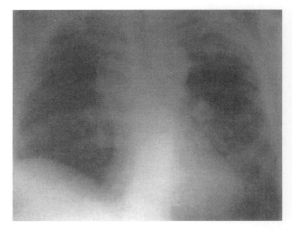

Fig. 8.4 Typical radiological findings in superior vena caval obstruction. The tumour is usually right-sided. In this case the diaphragm is raised because of involvement of the phrenic nerve.

SVCO due to these conditions and has a number of advantages. First, patients may be several kilometres from a radiotherapy centre; second, many of them will have extensive disease which would be left untreated by local irradiation; third, chemotherapy is given as a single intravenous injection, whereas radiotherapy has to be given daily for several days or weeks; and finally, the response to chemotherapy is often at least as quick as with radiotherapy, which can still be given if chemotherapy fails. Radiation dosage in treatment of SVCO should depend on the primary diagnosis. As with spinal cord compression, dexamethasone is a useful addition to treatment.

Other radiotherapy emergencies

Orbital or intraocular metastases most commonly occur in carcinoma of the breast and in malignant melanoma. They present with proptosis, oculomotor palsy or visual loss, which may be acute if there is bleeding into the eye from a choroidal deposit. These metastases may be bilateral. Early treatment with radiotherapy is important since permanent visual loss or ocular palsy may occur in a patient whose lifespan may be several years. Careful radiation planning is required in order to avoid treatment to the anterior half of the eyes and to the contralateral lens. A single lateral radiation field with a dose of 30 Gy in 10 daily fractions over 2 weeks of treatment is usually adequate. Chemotherapy plays no part in the management of these complications.

Primary or secondary cancers at other critical sites may

also lead to a necessity for urgent treatment. Impending collapse of a lung from severe bronchial narrowing may be the cause of an urgent referral from a chest physician who has been following an asymptomatic patient with known carcinoma of the bronchus for months or even years. The development of a unilateral monophonic wheeze, usually heard at its loudest over the main or lobar bronchus, is the most reliable physical sign. The sequence of chest X-rays often shows increasing shadowing and obstruction of part of the lung. Radiotherapy may well reverse this picture and relieve the patient's dyspnoea. The role of radiotherapy in carcinoma of the bronchus is more fully discussed in Chapter 12.

For the severe, localized and unremitting pain of bony metastases, radiotherapy is pre-eminently the treatment of choice. Palliative radiotherapy is often given as a matter of urgency in patients with severe bone pain who have not previously been treated maximally with radiotherapy to the painful site, especially if a single metastatic site is evident on clinical examination, X-ray or isotope bone scan. Analgesics (usually opiates) will need to be given during the course of treatment and often afterwards as well (see Chapter 7 for discussion of pain control). If an area of spinal cord is included in the field, the treatment is often fractionated over 2 weeks (30 Gy in 10 daily treatments), though shorter treatment periods are certainly acceptable for patients with a short lifespan and may be perfectly safe. Common regimens for the relief of bone pain include five fractions of 5 Gy calculated at depth, or four fractions of 6 Gy. Single-fraction treatments of 8–14 Gy are becoming more popular and are certainly more convenient [17]. It is becoming increasingly clear that such treatments are probably as effective as more conventional regimens [18].

Cancer during pregnancy [19]

Cancer is not uncommon in women during the childbearing years of life. Breast and cervical are the commonest tumours, but leukaemia, lymphoma, melanoma and colorectal cancers frequently affect this age group, especially as more women start families later. The approach to management will depend on the curability of the tumour, the stage of pregnancy and the wishes of the patient with respect to continuation of the pregnancy.

Treatment with cytotoxic drugs is especially hazardous during the first trimester. Pooled data suggest that the risk of fetal malformation if alkylating agents are used at this period is about 15%. For antimetabolites the figure is the same. Methotrexate is particularly likely to cause malfor-

mation. There are few data on other drugs. Large doses early in pregnancy will often cause abortion. The deformities are in skeletal and limb formation. There is no evidence of increased risk of malformation if treatment is in the second or third trimester, but it is not known if long-term consequences of drug treatment such as leukaemia will occur.

If the patient refuses termination and the cancer is curable with drug treatment then this must be given in full dosage (there is no evidence that drug combinations or full dosage carry a greater risk of fetal injury). Where possible, this treatment should be delayed to the second trimester. Local treatment, for example surgery for breast cancer, or involved field radiation for lymphoma can be given safely. Abdominal radiation must be avoided throughout pregnancy, and if given is very likely to lead to abortion. Radiation causes fetal growth retardation, CNS damage (microcephaly) and malformation of the eyes. The degree of microcephaly is related to radiation dose. The malformations can occur with irradiation at any stage in the pregnancy but are more severe earlier. Abdominal surgery for cancer can be performed but clearly presents major difficulties if the pregnancy is advanced. Safe delivery of the fetus can now usually be attained at 30 weeks gestation. This has made cancer management easier during the third trimester.

References

1 Petz LD. Red blood cell transfusion. *Clin Oncol* 1983; 2 (3): 505–27.

2 Kelton JB, Ali AM. Platelet transfusions—A critical appraisal. *Clin Oncol* 1983; 2 (3): 549–85.

3 Vose JM, Armitage JO. Clinical applications of haematopoietic growth factors. *J Clin Oncol* 1995; 13: 1023–35.

4 Gabrilove JL, Kubowski A, Scher H *et al.* Effect of granulocyte colony stimulating factor on neutropenia and associated morbidity due to chemotherapy for transitional cell carcinoma of the urothelium. *N Engl J Med* 1988; 318: 1414–22.

5 Bunn PA, Crowley J, Kelly K *et al.* Chemoradiotherapy with or without granulocyte-macrophage colony stimulating factor in the treatment of limited stage small cell lung cancer: a prospective phase III randomized study of the South West Oncology Group. *J Clin Oncol* 1995; 13: 1632–41.

6 Henry DH, Abels RI. Benefits of erythropoietin alfa in anemic cancer patients receiving chemotherapy. *J Clin Oncol* 1995; 13: 2473–4.

7 Weitzman S, Aisenberg AC. Fulminant sepsis after the successful treatment of Hodgkin's disease. *Am J Med* 1977; 62: 47–50.

8 Finberg RW, Talcott JA. Fever and neutropenia — how to use a new treatment strategy. *N Engl J Med* 1999; 341: 362–3.

9 Klastersky J. Prevention of infection in neutropenic cancer patients. *Curr Opin Oncol* 1996; 8: 270–7.

10 Bozetti F. Nutrition support in patients with cancer. In: Payne-James J, Grimble G, Silk D, eds. *Artificial Nutrition Support in Clinical Practice*. London: Edward Arnold, 1995: 511–33.

11 Mundy GR, Guise AT. Hypercalcaemia of malignancy. *Am J Med* 1997; 103: 134–45.

12 Fentiman IS. Diagnosis and treatment of malignant pleural effusions. *Cancer Treatment Rev* 1987; 14: 107–18.

13 Park JS, Rentschler R, Wilbury D. Surgical management of pericardial effusions in patients with malignancies. *Cancer* 1991; 67: 76–80.

14 Cheung DK, Raaf JH. Selection of patients with malignant ascites for a peritoneovenous shunt. *Cancer* 1982; 50: 1204–9.

15 Jayson GC, Howell A. Carcinomatous meningitis in solid tumours. *Ann Oncol* 1996; 7: 773–86.

16 Makvis A, Kunkler IH. Controversies in the management of spinal cord compression. *Clin Oncol* 1995; 7: 77–81.

17 Byrne NT. Spinal cord compression from epidural metastases. *N Engl J Med* 1992; 327: 614–19.

18 Hoskin P. Changing trends in palliative radiotherapy. In: Tobias JS, Thomas PRM, eds. *Current Radiation Oncology*, Vol. 1. London: Edward Arnold, 1994: 342–64.

19 Doll DC, ed. Cancer and pregnancy. *Seminars in Oncology*, 1989: 16 (5) (see reviews by Doll *et al.* (p. 337) for effects of cytotoxic drugs, and Brent (p. 347) for effects of radiation).

Paraneoplastic syndromes

Cancers are frequently associated with constitutional disturbances which are not due to the local effect of the tumour. For example, although cancer of the head of the pancreas will frequently cause obstructive jaundice leading to steatorrhoea and weight loss, these metabolic upsets are due to the physical presence of the tumour obstructing the common bile and pancreatic ducts. However, the tumour may occasionally give rise to a remote effect such as fever, thrombophlebitis or mood change. The mechanisms whereby these symptoms are caused are poorly understood. Such systemic metabolic effects of cancer are common and often add to the patient's symptoms. Sometimes these paraneoplastic syndromes may be the presenting feature of cancer and lead to other diagnoses being made in error, before a cancer is suspected. An awareness of these complications of cancer is therefore essential for correct management because the symptoms can often be controlled even when the primary tumour cannot be removed. Furthermore, the symptoms may be wrongly interpreted as being due to metastases and an opportunity for effective treatment of the primary tumour may be lost.

In recent years the pathogenesis of these syndromes has become clearer. The syndromes of ectopic hormone production have been further elucidated, antibody-mediated syndromes have been defined and syndromes due to secretion of colony-stimulating and growth factors have been described.

Table 9.1 illustrates some metabolic and paraneoplastic syndromes in non-endocrine neoplasms. The pathogenesis and management of weight loss, cachexia and hypercalcaemia are discussed in Chapter 8.

Fever due to malignant disease

Most patients with cancer who develop a fever do so because of infection. Fever is, however, a symptom of cancer itself and may be the presenting feature. Lymphomas, especially Hodgkin's disease, are often accompanied by fever and in these diseases the pyrexia usually indicates an aggressive and advanced tumour. The typical relapsing Pel–Ebstein fever is present only in a minority of patients with Hodgkin's disease. Non-specific intermittent or remittent fever is much more common. The pathogenesis is not well understood. Interleukin-1 (IL-1), IL-6 and tumour necrosis factor (TNF) are pyrogenic and are produced in cell culture of many tumours. They probably cause fever by inducing synthesis of prostaglandin E_2 in vascular endothelial cells in the hypothalamus which 're-sets' the temperature-regulating neurones.

Table 9.1 Metabolic paraneoplastic syndromes in nonendocrine neoplasms.

Syndrome	Tumour
Endocrine and metabolic	
Cushing's syndrome	Small-cell bronchogenic cancer, thymoma, bronchial carcinoid, neuroblastoma, phaeochromocytoma, medullary carcinoma of the thyroid
Inappropriate ADH secretion	Small-cell bronchogenic cancer, thymoma, lymphoma, duodenal carcinoma, pancreatic carcinoma
Gynaecomastia	Teratoma, large-cell lung cancer, adenocarcinomas (breast, pancreas and gut, tumours of liver and adrenal)
Hypoglycaemia	Retroperitoneal sarcoma and lymphoma, hepatoma
Hypercalcaemia (see Chapter 8)	All cancers with widespread bone metastases, squamous cancers, renal and ovarian carcinoma
Hyperpigmentation	Small-cell bronchogenic cancer
Cachexia, anorexia, altered taste	All tumours
Haematological	
Multiple thromboses	Pancreatic cancer, other adenocarcinomas
Erythrocytosis	Renal carcinoma, hepatoma, uterine cancer, cerebellar haemangioblastoma
Red cell aplasia	
Disseminated intravascular coagulation	Thymomas

Hypernephroma is conspicuous for its tendency to cause fever and leucocytosis and thus mimic a pyogenic infection. Other carcinomas may present similarly especially if they are metastatic to the liver and bone marrow. Sarcomas and primary liver cancer are also frequently associated with pyrexia.

When cancer is the cause of the presenting pyrexia it can usually be diagnosed fairly easily. When fever occurs on treatment the first priority is to exclude infection and then to investigate for tumour recurrence. If nothing can be done to treat the cancer itself, symptomatic relief can sometimes be obtained by aspirin, non-steroidal anti-inflammatory agents and steroids [1]. They probably act by blocking E_2 synthesis. The control of symptoms usually lasts a few weeks or months.

Ectopic hormone production in cancer [2]

Many cancers (perhaps the majority) produce hormone precursors and peptides, some of which have biological activity. In the formation of a hormone in an endocrine gland the precursor hormone (prohormone) is often the major storage form and is biologically inactive but is cleaved to the active hormone at the time of secretion. In the blood and tissues the hormone is degraded to the inactive carboxyl fragment and the amino fragment which may retain activity. Tumours may produce both inactive

prohormones and the active principle. They may also produce biologically active peptides such as human chorionic gonadotrophin (HCG) or variants of HCG which have a reduced carbohydrate content and which have lost activity. Similarly, a biologically active glycopeptide hormone may have two chains, both of which are necessary for biological activity.

If only one chain is made by the tumour it will be inactive.

The mechanism of ectopic synthesis is not clear, but may be due to abnormal gene activation as a result of malignant transformation. In this section, 'ectopic' hormone is taken to mean production of a hormone by a non-endocrine tumour. Clearly cancers of the adrenal, pancreas or endocrine cells in the gut may cause hormonal disturbances. These are discussed in the appropriate chapters.

Syndrome of inappropriate antidiuretic hormone (ADH) secretion

This occurs as a result of two separate mechanisms: (a) formation and release of ADH from the tumour, and (b) release of normal ADH from the pituitary as a stress response in ill patients.

Ectopic production of arginine vasopressin by the tumour—usually small-cell lung cancer (SCLC)—may cause profound hyponatraemia. An elevated level of ADH and impaired water handling are present in 30% of SCLC patients. The syndrome is characterized biochemically by a plasma sodium below 130 mmol/l with a low plasma and high urine osmolality. Clinically it usually becomes apparent only when the plasma sodium reaches 120 mmol/l or below, when the patient becomes tired, then drowsy and confused. The commonest underlying tumour is SCLC, which is usually apparent on chest X-ray. A computed tomography (CT) scan of the brain may be necessary to exclude cerebral metastases as a cause of the neurological picture, since they are common in SCLC.

Cyclophosphamide, vincristine and morphine can also cause hyponatraemia due to either pituitary ADH release or a direct effect on the renal tubule. Although 30% of patients have impaired water handling, only 10–20% have a plasma sodium below 130 mmol/l [3]. The ADH is identical with that produced by the neurohypophysis.

A low plasma sodium may be found in very ill patients regardless of cause. This is probably due to inappropriate ADH release from the posterior pituitary. This syndrome is occasionally difficult to distinguish from ectopic ADH production. In SCLC, marked hyponatraemia (assumed to be a reflection of ectopic ADH) is associated with a worse prognosis.

Treatment of the tumour with drugs and radiotherapy may improve the metabolic abnormality. While this is being done, demeclocycline (300 mg by mouth 6–8-hourly at first then 8–12-hourly) is effective in correcting the plasma sodium. It does this by rendering the distal tubule unresponsive to the ectopic ADH. This drug can impair renal function, and the blood urea should be measured regularly. In severe cases water restriction may be temporarily required, but this is difficult to sustain and is sometimes ineffective. In an acutely ill patient with life-threatening hyponatraemia, a 3% saline infusion combined with intravenous frusemide (to increase free water clearance) is an effective emergency treatment.

Ectopic adrenocorticotrophic hormone (ACTH) production

Excess production of ACTH is an uncommon metabolic complication of cancers which are normally neuroectodermal in origin. The commonest tumour to produce the syndrome is small-cell carcinoma of the bronchus. Small carcinoid tumours in the lung, thymus and pancreas may also cause the syndrome. Raised ACTH levels have been found in half of all patients with SCLC, and immunoreactive ACTH can be extracted from the majority of these tumours. Normal ACTH is derived from pro-ACTH which is, in turn, derived from pro-opiomelanocortin. In SCLC most of the immunoreactive ACTH is derived from these precursor molecules with little ACTH itself. Nevertheless, pro-ACTH can produce Cushing's syndrome.

In SCLC clinical manifestations of ectopic ACTH production are very unusual, and when they occur the clinical picture is usually different from classical Cushing's syndrome. There is usually hypokalaemia, glucose intolerance, hypertension, pigmentation and muscle weakness, but without the long-term weight gain of typical Cushing's syndrome. These patients usually have extensive disease with a poor prognosis. Estimates of the frequency of this syndrome in SCLC vary depending on the criteria used to define it.

In indolent or benign tumours such as bronchial or thymic carcinoid, typical Cushing's syndrome occurs. The syndrome also occurs rarely in squamous lung cancer, adenocarcinomas of the lung, gut or kidney and medullary carcinoma of the thyroid. It also occurs in thymoma and ganglioneuroblastoma in childhood. Some of these tumours contain molecules of a prohormone with a higher molecular weight than normal ACTH which may not be biologically active. Rarely, tumours can produce a corticotrophin-releasing factor which acts on the pituitary to produce Cushing's syndrome by ACTH release.

Clinically, the syndrome caused by SCLC is rarely confused with other forms of Cushing's syndrome. The diagnosis is more difficult when the tumour is a bronchial carcinoid. The urinary free cortisol is increased and plasma cortisol is greatly raised. In SCLC with ectopic ACTH, high-dose dexamethasone does not suppress the plasma cortisol level, in contrast to pituitary-dependent Cushing's syndrome. Some patients with ACTH from carcinoid tumours will show suppression with dexamethasone. The plasma ACTH will be very low with an autonomous adrenal adenoma or carcinoma. In the latter, the plasma cortisol may also fail to suppress with dexamethasone.

Treatment is to the primary tumour. If this is ineffective then aminoglutethimide and ketoconazole will block steroid synthesis. If total blockade is produced a replacement dose of hydrocortisone must be given. Metyrapone will also block 11-hydroxylation of corticosteroids, causing a fall in plasma cortisol. This drug can be useful in seriously ill patients before definitive treatment of the tumour begins, but neither drug will produce lasting benefit in the absence of treatment of the disease.

Hypoglycaemia

Hypoglycaemia is a very uncommon complication of some cancers. It occurs with large thoracic and abdominal sarcomas, especially those situated retroperitoneally, and with hepatomas, mesotheliomas, adrenal carcinomas and lymphomas [4]. It does not seem to be produced by insulin, which cannot be found in plasma or tumour extracts. Elevated plasma levels of somatomedin-like (insulin-like growth factor II) peptides have been found. These are peptides which are normally made in the liver as a result of growth hormone (GH) and which have an action like insulin. The insulin-like growth factor II peptides inhibit pituitary secretion of GH, thereby impairing the compensatory response to hypoglycaemia.

Hypoglycaemic attacks may be spontaneous or associated with fasting, and can be very severe. Emergency treatment requires glucose infusion. Clinically, the episodes are indistinguishable from those produced by islet cell tumours, but the plasma insulin is not raised. If the tumour cannot be completely removed the hypoglycaemia may be partially controlled by frequent feeding, diazoxide, glucagon or corticosteroids.

Gynaecomastia and gonadotrophin production

Gynaecomastia is an increase in the glandular and stromal tissue of the male breast. In most instances when it complicates a non-endocrine malignancy, it is probably caused by tumour-related HCG production. In women oligomenorrhoea may occur. In children precocious puberty may occur with hepatoblastoma or hepatoma. Teratoma and seminoma may both be associated with HCG production and so may carcinoma of the bronchus of all histological types. Other HCG-producing tumours include those of the pancreas (both exocrine and islet cell tumours), liver, adrenal and breast. In most cases of non-germ cell neoplasms, HCG is produced in amounts too small to be clinically significant, although it may occasionally be useful as a tumour marker. In other cases the hormone may not be glycosylated by the tumour, and this results in its rapid removal from the blood. Some tumours secrete free subunits which are not associated with biological activity. The increased oestrogen production which is the cause of the gynaecomastia is probably due to the action of the ectopic HCG on the testis or within the tumour itself. The correct treatment is removal of the tumour, but if this is not possible, or is incomplete, the HCG inhibitor danazol may be useful if the gynaecomastia is painful. Painful gynaecomastia can also sometimes be relieved by mammoplasty or local irradiation of the breasts. Further details on HCG are given in Chapters 4 and 19.

Other ectopic hormones

Bronchial carcinoids and pancreatic islet cell tumours may, rarely, produce GH-releasing substances over sufficient length of time to cause acromegaly. Galactorrhoea has been reported with cancer, due to hyperprolactinaemia. Hyperthyroidism may occur in trophoblastic tumours producing HCG. This does not appear to be due to thyroid-stimulating hormone (TSH) production, but the HCG may have TSH-like activity. Hypercalcaemia is discussed in Chapter 8.

Haematological syndromes

Anaemia

Anaemia is an almost universal accompaniment of advanced cancer. Many factors contribute, including gastrointestinal bleeding leading to iron deficiency, and poor appetite with resulting iron and folate deficiency. Even if there are no secondary deficiency states, anaemia can still develop and can be regarded as a 'paraneoplastic' syndrome. Characteristically it is similar to the anaemia of other chronic diseases. It takes a few months to develop and the haemoglobin does not usually fall below 8–9 g. The anaemia is normocytic and normochromic or slightly hypochromic. The serum iron is low but so is the total iron binding capacity (TIBC), in contrast to the anaemia of iron deficiency where the TIBC is high. The marrow shows stainable iron in macrophages. The red cell survival is often shortened without an increase in erythropoiesis sufficient to compensate for this. There also appears to be a block in release of iron from macrophages into the plasma. Serum erythropoietin (EPO) levels are low.

Treatment of the anaemia depends on the successful treatment of the cancer. If this is impossible, and there are no secondary deficiencies of iron or folate, the anaemia can be corrected, albeit temporarily, by blood transfusion. Response to EPO occurs but is temporary (see p. 114).

An autoimmune haemolytic anaemia (AIHA) which usually responds to treatment with steroids may complicate B-cell neoplasms and Hodgkin's disease. It is much less common to find AIHA associated with non-lymphoid neoplasms, but it has been reported as an association with cancers of many types.

Erythrocytosis

The commonest cancer to produce this syndrome is renal

carcinoma. Rarer causes include cerebellar haemangio-blastoma, hepatoma, uterine leiomyosarcoma and fibroids [5]. The explanation is the production of EPO. Only 2–5% of cases of renal cancer are associated with polycythaemia, though excess production of EPO occurs in over half of all patients. It is not clear if the hormone itself is inactive or if there is a block to its action.

If the investigation of a high haematocrit confirms a true polycythaemia a renal carcinoma should be excluded unless the patient is hypoxic.

Erythrocytosis usually responds to removal of the primary tumour whether or not it is due to EPO production by the tumour.

Thrombotic disorders [6]

Recurrent venous thromboembolism may occur with mucin-secreting adenocarcinomas usually of the gut. Rarely these may be multiple arterial occlusions. Substances produced by the tumour react with factor VII and provoke coagulation through the extrinsic pathway. Heparin is the most effective treatment but the rare syndrome of arterial occlusion is often unresponsive.

Carcinoma of the pancreas, especially of the body or tail, is occasionally associated with multiple thromboses, often in superficial veins and migratory in nature [7]. Other adenocarcinomas may give rise to the same syndrome of *migratory thrombophlebitis*. The tumours tend to be inoperable. The venous thromboses are sometimes in an unusual site such as the arm, and this may arouse suspicion of the underlying diagnosis. Pulmonary embolism seldom occurs.

Disseminated intravascular coagulation (DIC) [7]

This is a complication of malignancy which has been described in many different types of cancer, of which the commonest are adenocarcinomas (prostate, breast, pancreas, ovary) and other tumours such as metastatic carcinoid, neuroblastoma and rhabdomyosarcoma. It is probably due to the liberation of thromboplastin-like material from cancer cells, but some cancers secrete thrombin-like enzymes. Many patients with cancer have increased levels of fibrin degradation products in the blood, but the degree of intravascular coagulation is usually mild. Problems with haemorrhage are very unusual except in acute promyelocytic leukaemia, where DIC can be severe when treatment has been started. In solid tumours, where the DIC is chronic and low grade, treatment

is by removal of the cancer where possible. Occasionally the DIC can be associated with red cell fragmentation (microangiopathic haemolytic anaemia) especially in stomach cancer [8]. This syndrome may also be accompanied by acute renal failure (the haemolytic–uraemic syndrome).

Red cell aplasia

Acquired suppression of erythropoiesis has been described in adults as an accompaniment of tumours, particularly thymomas, although in many of these cases the thymoma is benign. It occurs rarely in association with a variety of other cancers such as carcinoma of the bronchus. The anaemia, which is often severe, is normocytic and erythropoiesis is selectively absent from the marrow. An immune suppression of erythropoiesis provoked by the tumour is the postulated cause. Fifty per cent of cases respond to thymectomy.

Neurological syndromes [9]

Cancers can be associated with neurological syndromes unrelated to direct compression or infiltration. Minor, or subclinical, manifestations are frequent in some cancers such as lung cancer. However, for the oncologist clinically significant non-metastatic neurological complications of malignancy are infrequently encountered. Most neurological complications of cancer are due to metastases or compression and it is a grave error to fail to treat a cancer causing, for example, seizures or spinal cord compression, because of a mistaken diagnosis of a non-metastatic manifestation of the tumour. The mechanism of damage is immunological, but ill-understood. Both humoral and T-cell mediated cytotoxicity appear to be involved. The major clinical syndromes are discussed briefly below.

Encephalomyelitis

This is a general term embracing a wide variety of paraneoplastic neurological syndromes affecting the brain and spinal cord. The commonest associated cancer is SCLC. Here the mechanism is immunological with polyclonal anti-Hu antibodies often present in the blood. The central lesions are sometimes associated with severe sensory neuropathy due to dorsal root ganglia involvement. Treatment is often ineffective even when the primary tumour is removed.

Limbic encephalitis is a rare variant. An underlying small-cell carcinoma is likely to be responsible. It is characterized by the fairly rapid onset of confusion, memory disturbance and agitation. There is temporal lobe degeneration with some perivascular infiltrate. Anti-Hu antibodies are usually present. As with cerebellar degeneration, the main differential diagnosis is from intracranial metastasis.

Cerebellar degeneration [10,11]

These rare syndromes are most commonly associated with carcinoma of the bronchus, ovary and uterus, and Hodgkin's disease. They differ from the chronic idiopathic cerebellar degenerations of adult life by being more rapid in evolution, sometimes progressing to severe disability in a few months, even before the primary tumour is apparent. Unsteadiness of gait, truncal ataxia, vertigo and diplopia (sometimes with oscillopsia and opsoclonus) occur. Long tract signs due to spinal cord degeneration may develop. Pathologically there are two variants. One is part of the encephalomyelitis spectrum with perivascular inflammatory infiltrate. In other cases there is Purkinje cell loss without inflammation. Anti-Yo antibodies are polyclonal anti-Purkinje cell antibodies typically present when the cause is breast or ovarian cancer. Anti-Hu antibodies are present when SCLC is the cause. Anti-Hu antibodies are associated with inflammation but anti-Yo is not. Treatment of the primary tumour, although necessary, does not usually help. A CT scan is essential to exclude a cerebellar metastasis as far as possible. The response to treatment of the tumour is very disappointing, most cases showing at best stabilization of the neurological process even when the disease is cured or is in remission.

Carcinomatous myelopathy

This exceedingly rare syndrome can present as a flaccid paraplegia of acute onset with loss of sphincter control. The primary tumour is usually lung cancer. There is necrosis of the cord with little inflammation. The mechanism is unknown and the damage irreversible. A less acute myelopathy can also occur, associated with loss of anterior horn cells and a slowly progressive lower motor neurone weakness. It is usually associated with lymphoma and lung cancer.

The diagnosis of carcinomatous myelopathy is difficult to make. Cord compression must be excluded and the CSF examined for malignant cells. Other diseases such as amyotrophic lateral sclerosis may cause a similar picture. The association with carcinoma may become apparent only late in the evolution of the disease.

Peripheral neuropathy

The commonest variety of neuropathy seen in association with cancer is a *sensory neuropathy*. Pathologically there is segmental demyelination of nerves, usually distally, and axonal degeneration. SCLC is the commonest association and anti-Hu antibodies are usually present. The neuropathy varies in its severity. There is a severe form occurring earlier, sometimes before the tumour is manifest and occasionally following an intermittent course. The cerebrospinal fluid (CSF) shows a modest increase in protein (1–2 g/l), without excess cells.

There is also a slowly progressive *sensory neuropathy*, associated with pains and paraesthesiae in the limbs, which may spread to the trunk and face. There is degeneration of dorsal root ganglia sometimes associated with a mononuclear cell infiltrate. Later, there is loss of the posterior columns leading to ataxia. The patient may become chair- or bed-bound before the primary tumour has declared itself. Cancer of the lung (especially SCLC) is the commonest tumour but lymphoma and many other cancers can be associated. Removal of the tumour usually does not produce improvement and the neuropathy is progressive. Steroids may sometimes help.

A pure motor neuropathy may occur in association with Hodgkin's disease but is rare.

An *acute ascending paralysis* of the Guillain–Barré type may also occur, and has been noted in Hodgkin's disease especially.

The diagnosis of carcinomatous neuropathy is often very difficult. Infiltration of the meninges with carcinoma and lymphoma may occasionally cause peripheral sensory and motor damage. The CSF should therefore always be examined for malignant cells. In young patients with lymphoma, where the risk of central nervous system (CNS) involvement is high, it is usually best to treat the patient for CNS relapse if there is doubt about the diagnosis. The presence of anti-Hu antibodies is strongly suggestive of the diagnosis.

Paraneoplastic retinopathy

In this disorder patients with SCLC develop a rapid loss of visual acuity, impaired colour vision, night blindness and restricted visual fields. An antibody to a protein in retinal photo-receptive cells is present and there is loss of rods and cones with immunoglobulin in the ganglion layer of the retina.

Lambert–Eaton myasthenic syndrome [12]

In this rare syndrome, which is found almost exclusively with SCLC, the patient complains of weakness, aching and fatigue in the shoulder and pelvic girdle muscles, and sometimes impotence. It resembles myasthenia except that the relationship of fatigue to repeated muscular activity is less clear-cut and the electromyogram shows an increase in muscle action potentials at higher rates of nerve stimulation. The ocular and bulbar muscles are usually spared. The syndrome may appear before the tumour. Unfortunately there is little response to oral anticholinesterases. The syndrome is produced by immunoglobulin G (IgG) antibodies to voltage-gated calcium channels which impair calcium influx and acetylcholine release. Treatment of the tumour may help. Plasma exchange and intravenous immunoglobulin may produce improvement as may 3,4-diaminopyridine, which prolongs calcium channel activation.

Muscle and joint syndromes

Many patients with cancer complain of fatigue and sometimes of aching in the muscles which is occasionally out of proportion to the amount of weight loss. It has often been postulated that some of these patients have a more specific muscle disturbance. Conversely, unequivocal myopathic syndromes are unusual. Arthritic complications of cancer are also uncommon.

Polymyositis and dermatomyositis

A syndrome which is typical of polymyositis, and which may be associated with skin changes indistinguishable from dermatomyositis can, rarely, accompany cancer. All types of tumours have been reported in association. The likelihood of an occult, localized and remediable tumour being discovered is, however, small, only 10–15% of cases being associated with a neoplasm. One therefore has to judge the extent to which investigation should be undertaken in each patient. A cancer is much more likely to be present in men over the age of 50 and when the syndrome is dermatomyositis. In this group, bronchial carcinoma is by far the commonest associated malignancy. A reasonable policy is to carry out a minimum of investigations in middle-aged patients presenting with dermatomyositis.

These would include chest X-ray, acid phosphatase and abdominal ultrasound in a man and pelvic ultrasound and mammograms additionally in a woman. Clinical indications such as rectal or vaginal bleeding or persistent cough should, of course, be further investigated.

The syndromes are characterized by symmetrical proximal muscle weakness which is slowly progressive. The skin changes consist of facial erythema and oedema, especially over the nose and around the eyes. The chronic contractures and calcification typical of the childhood disease do not usually have time to occur. Steroids produce temporary improvement, and azathioprine may also be of benefit. Where possible, the underlying cancer should be treated.

Hypertrophic pulmonary osteoarthropathy [13]

Nowadays, bronchogenic carcinoma is almost exclusively the cause of this uncommon syndrome although it can occur with lung metastases. The periosteum at the ends of the long bones (tibia, fibula, radius and ulna especially) is raised, thickened and inflamed, and periosteal new bone formation is shown by a typical layer of calcification parallel to, and 2–3 mm above, the periosteal surface of the bone. The bone is tender and the neighbouring joints may be hot and swollen, and clubbing is usually present. The pathogenesis of the syndrome is unknown, but it may regress on treatment or removal of the cancer. A rare form of the syndrome may be associated with features of acromegaly, with raised GH levels in the plasma.

Polyarthritis

An asymmetrical polyarthritis is a rare complication of cancer, particularly lymphoma and lung cancer. The differential diagnosis is from rheumatoid arthritis, but tests for rheumatoid factor are negative and the arthritis is less erosive. The syndrome may subside with removal of the tumour.

Dermatological syndromes

The skin manifestations of malignancy are extremely varied. First, the skin may be infiltrated by primary or secondary cancer. Second, it may be indirectly affected by general metabolic consequences of cancer at other sites (for example, due to obstructive jaundice or steatorrhoea). Third, some inherited disorders are associated with skin manifestations and an increased likelihood of developing cancer (Table 9.2). Finally, some skin eruptions are non-specific manifestations of internal malignancy. Some of these (such as dermatomyositis and thrombophlebitis) have previously been described in this chapter. The following is a brief account of some dermatological syndromes not discussed elsewhere.

Acanthosis nigricans

This is a brown/black eruption in the armpits, groins and on the trunk which has a velvety surface and multiple papillary outgrowths. A familial form occurs which is not associated with cancer, and the syndrome can develop without any underlying malignancy in middle age. However, when it occurs in adult life, a cancer is often present, usually an adenocarcinoma and often a gastric neoplasm. Lymphomas are also associated. The skin lesion may antedate the cancer and, when it recurs after treatment, may herald a recurrence.

Hypertrichosis (lanuginosa acquisita)

Very rarely an adenocarcinoma of the lung, breast or gut, or a bladder carcinoma, may be associated with lanugo, which is fine downy hair on the face, trunk or limbs. The syndrome may be associated with acanthosis nigricans or ichthyosis. The hair growth does not usually regress after treatment of the primary tumour.

Erythroderma

A generalized, red, maculopapular rash may complicate cancer and the underlying disease is nearly always a lymphoma. The condition may progress to exfoliative dermatitis. Control of the underlying lymphoma is essential in treatment. As the rash fades it becomes slightly scaly and bran-coloured. Relapses of the lymphoma may result in further skin rash.

Sweet's syndrome is a febrile disorder with erythema of the face and trunk associated with leukaemia and lymphoma.

Vasculitis

Many variants of vasculitis (polyarteritis, leucocytoclastic vasculitis) may be associated with underlying cancer. Hairy cell leukaemia is the tumour with the closest association and the skin disorder may precede the clinical appearance of the malignancy.

Tumour	Marker
Disorders of pigmentation	
Hyperpigmentation	MSH-producing carcinoma (usually bronchial)
Vitiligo	Melanoma
Hodgkin's disease	
Acanthosis nigricans	Adenocarcinomas, lymphomas
Erythema and inflammation	
Dermatomyositis	Most cancers
Thrombophlebitis	Adenocarcinomas
Thrombophlebitis migrans	Adenocarcinomas, especially pancreas and ovary
Erythroderma	Lymphomas
Pyoderma gangrenosum	Myeloproliferative syndromes, leukaemia, myeloma, lymphoma
Erythema	Carcinoid, glucagonoma
Fat necrosis	Pancreatic carcinoma
Bullous eruptions	Lymphoma
Vasculitis	Hairy cell leukaemia, other lymphomas, many solid tumours
Generalized pruritus	Lymphoma, leukaemia, polycythaemia
Acquired ichthyosis and hypertrichosis	
	Hodgkin's disease
	Lung cancer
	Breast cancer

Table 9.2a Non-metastatic dermatological manifestations of malignancy.

Table 9.2b Inherited disease (associated with cancer and with non-malignant skin lesions).

Gardner's syndrome: epidermal cysts and dermoids with multiple colonic polyps leading to carcinoma

Neurofibromatosis: neurofibromas, café-au-lait patches and other skin lesions, with sarcomatous change, medullary carcinoma of thyroid and phaeochromocytoma

Tylosis palmaris: hyperkeratosis of palms and soles with oesophageal cancer

Peutz–Jeghers syndrome: buccal, oral and digital pigmentation with multiple intestinal polyps leading uncommonly to gut carcinomas, ovarian tumours

Ataxia-telangiectasia: telangiectases on neck, face, behind elbows and knees with cerebellar ataxia, IgA deficiency and increased incidence of lymphoma and leukaemia

Chediak–Higashi syndrome: defective skin and hair colour, recurrent infections, high incidence of lymphoma and leukaemia

Wiskott–Aldrich syndrome: eczema, purpura, pyoderma, thrombocytopenia, low IgM, leukaemia and lymphoma

Tuberose sclerosis: adenoma sebaceum on cheeks, mental retardation and epilepsy. Hamartomas and astrocytoma

Bloom's syndrome: photosensitive light eruptions, facial erythema, dwarfism, leukaemia, squamous cell carcinoma of the skin

Adult progeria (Werner's syndrome): thickened tight skin, soft tissue calcification, growth retardation; soft-tissue sarcomas

Fanconi's anaemia: patchy hyperpigmentation, skeletal abnormalities, anaemia leading to acute myelomonocytic leukaemia

Pyoderma gangrenosum

This is an infrequent complication of malignancy and can occur with other diseases such as ulcerative colitis. The lesions start as red nodules and then expand rapidly, breaking down in the centre to form necrotic, painful, infected ulcers with a rolled, erythematous edge. Although the condition responds to steroids, the dose needed is usually very high. An underlying lymphoma or myeloproliferative syndrome is the most commonly associated malignancy, and the skin lesion may regress with successful treatment of the tumour.

Bullous eruptions

Very uncommonly, typical bullous pemphigoid and dermatitis herpetiformis are associated with underlying cancers, usually lymphomas.

Ichthyosis

Hodgkin's disease, other lymphomas and occasionally cancer of the lung, are occasionally associated with thickened and flaking skin, usually affecting the face and trunk. The skin changes appear after the clinical appearance of the disease. Histologically there may be epidermal atrophy or hyperkeratosis.

Tylosis palmaris is an inherited hyperkeratosis of the palms associated with oesophageal cancer.

Alopecia

Patchy alopecia occasionally accompanies lymphoma (usually Hodgkin's disease). There may be follicular mucinosis. The disorder may be self-limiting.

Generalized pruritus

Occasionally patients present with a generalized itching without any rash. Although cancer is not a frequent cause of this problem, it is an important one and the itching may precede the clinical appearance of the tumour, sometimes by a few years.

Hodgkin's disease is one of the commonest cancers to be associated and the itching can, in this disease, become intolerable. Pruritus is usually worse at night, and in the case of polycythaemia, worse after a hot bath. Lung, colon, breast, stomach and prostate are other primary tumours. Effective treatment of the cancer will often alleviate the condition and will certainly do so in Hodgkin's disease.

Nephrotic syndrome

The kidney may be involved by cancer in many ways but clinically evident non-metastatic manifestations are unusual, apart from amyloidosis complicating myeloma (see Chapter 27). Massive proteinuria leading to nephrotic syndrome may occur as a direct result of glomerular damage [14]. In membranous lesions it is thought that complexes of tumour products and antibody are deposited in the glomeruli. In the elderly especially, a small proportion of patients with membranous glomerulonephritis have an underlying cancer, removal of which results in remission of the renal lesion. The cancer is usually an adenocarcinoma (breast, colon, stomach). Hodgkin's disease is also associated, although here there is usually minimal-change glomerulonephritis.

References

1 Tsavaris N, Zinellis A, Karablis A *et al.* A randomized trial of the effect of three non-steroidal anti-inflammatory agents in ameliorating cancer-induced fever. *J Intern Med* 1990; 228: 451–5.

2 Pierce ST. Paraendocrine syndromes. *Curr Opin Oncol* 1993; 5: 639–45.

3 List AF, Hainsworth JD, Davis BW, Hande KR, Greco FA, Johnson DH. The syndrome of inappropriate secretion of antidiuretic hormone (SIADH) in small cell lung cancer. *J Clin Oncol* 1986; 4: 1191–8.

4 Ron D, Powers AC, Pandian MR, Godine JE, Axelrod L. Increased insulin-like growth factor II production and consequent suppression of growth hormone secretion: a dual mechanism for tumour-induced hypoglycaemia. *J Clin Endocrinol Metabolism* 1989; 68: 701–6.

5 Laski ME, Vugrin D. Paraneoplastic syndromes in hypernephroma. *Semin Oncol* 1987; 7: 123–30.

6 Lesher JL. Thrombophlebitis and thromboembolic problems in malignancy. *Clin Dermatol* 1993; 11: 159–63.

7 Naschitz JE, Yeshurun D, Eldar S, Lev LM. Diagnosis of cancer-associated disorders. *Cancer* 1996; 77: 1759–67.

8 Antman KH, Skarin AT, Mayer RJ *et al.* Microangiopathic haemolytic anaemia and cancer. A review. *Medicine* 1979; 58: 377–84.

9 Posner JB. *Neurologic Complications of Cancer.* Philadelphia: FA Davis, 1995.

10 Peterson K, Rosenblum MK, Kotanioes H, Posner JB. Paraneoplastic cerebellar degeneration. I. A clinical analysis of 55 anti-Yo-antibody-positive patients. *Neurology* 1992; 42: 1931–7.

11 Hammack J, Kotanioes H, Rosenblum MK, Posner JB. Paraneoplastic cerebellar degeneration. II. Clinical and immunologic findings in 21 patients with Hodgkin's disease. *Neurology* 1992; 42: 193–83.

12 Lang B, Newsom-Davis J. Immunopathology of the Lambert–Eaton myasthenic syndrome. *Semin Immunopathol* 1995; 17: 3–15.

13 Burstein HJ, Janicek MJ, Skarin AT. Hypertrophic osteoarthropathy. *J Clin Oncol* 1997; 15: 2759–60.

14 Boulton-Jones JM. Renal complications of malignant disease. *Bailliere's Clin Oncol* 1988; 2 (2): 347–73.

10 Cancer of the head and neck

Introduction, aetiology and epidemiology

Carcinomas of the upper air and food passages are a varied and important group of tumours with particular epidemiological features [1]. Worldwide, head and neck cancer is the sixth commonest type of malignancy, and its incidence is rising [2]. These tumours pose exceptionally difficult management problems, and account for approximately 4% of all carcinomas in the UK. Figure 10.1 shows age-specific incidence rates for the UK.

Important aetiological factors include excessive intake of tobacco either by smoking or chewing (a common practice in many parts of Asia and India where, as a result, oral cancer is among the commonest of all tumours). Alcohol, particularly spirit, ingestion is also an important contributing agent [3] and these two factors are clearly synergistic (Fig. 10.2). Syphilitic leucoplakia was previously an important predisposing factor in carcinoma of the tongue. Dental and mechanical trauma have also been incriminated, but with improvements in oral and dental hygiene these factors are less important now [2]. The Paterson–Kelly (Plummer–Vinson) syndrome of chronic anaemia, glossitis and oesophageal web is known to predispose to postcricoid carcinoma, particularly in women. More recently, adenocarcinoma of the nasal cavity has been described in hardwood workers in the furniture industry. Several clusters have now been reported.

Important racial differences have also emerged, particularly in relation to carcinoma of the nasopharynx, commonly seen in the Chinese, particularly those of the Mongolian race. It is especially common in Hong Kong and south China, and in male Taiwanese is by far the commonest cause of death, three times the rate of any other neoplasm. It is also common in the Philippines, Malaysia, Greenland, Malta, North Africa and Saudi Arabia. Curiously, it often develops at a far younger age than other head and neck cancers, with a bimodal age distribution. Of all cases 20% (in high-prevalence areas) are diagnosed in patients (usually male) under the age of 30 years.

Alterations of the tumour suppressor gene *p53* and its protein product have been noted in head and neck cancers. Genetic mutations are also present both in normal oral mucosa and tumour tissues with evidence of a tumour-associated *p53* mutation [4]. Aetiologically, environmental agents have been implicated, including dietary factors such as salted fish and vegetables popular among many Chinese, Inuit (Eskimo) and North Africans. Case–control studies in Chinese patients have suggested a link between salted fish consumption and incidence of nasopharyngeal carcinoma [5].

Apart from possible dietary causes of nasopharyngeal

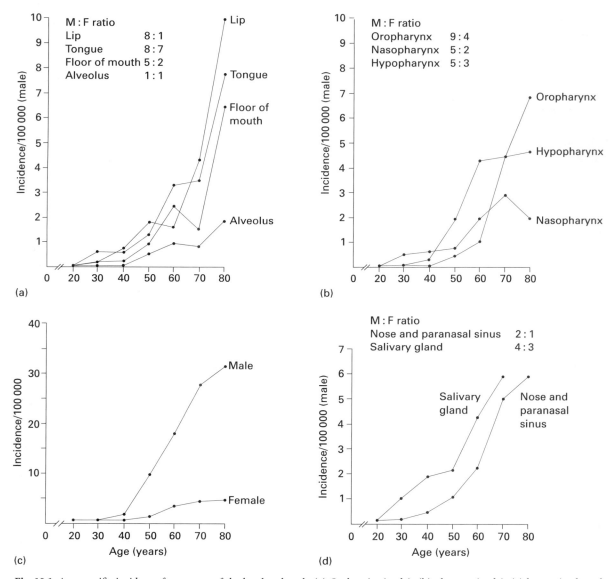

Fig. 10.1 Age-specific incidence for cancers of the head and neck. (a) Oral cavity (male); (b) pharynx (male); (c) larynx (male and female); and (d) nose and paranasal sinuses and salivary gland (male).

carcinoma, it is also known that patients with this condition generally have evidence of Epstein–Barr virus (EBV) genome in the epithelial tumour cells [6] and a characteristic EBV antibody pattern with a rise in immunoglobulin A (IgA) and IgG antiviral capsid antigen and EBV-associated nuclear antigens.

In head and neck cancers there is a male predisposition (except possibly for postcricoid carcinomas), with a male : female ratio of approximately 3 : 1. For some sites, notably

carcinoma of the larynx, the male : female ratio has been reportedly as high as 10 : 1.

Improvements in dental and oral hygiene led for a period (1960–80) to a falling incidence of cancers of the head and neck, though the incidence now appears to be rising again. American data provide age-adjusted incidence rates of 17.3 per 100 000 (white males) and 5.6 (white females). Approximately 40% of these tumours prove fatal. In the UK, Scandinavia, Germany, Japan and

Israel the figure is somewhat lower, but elsewhere in north-west Europe (France, Switzerland, Italy and Scotland) the death rate is slightly higher. These survival figures probably correlate with alcohol intake.

Pathology

The overwhelming majority of these tumours are squamous cell carcinomas, though frequency of other histological types and degree of differentiation vary with site. Nasopharyngeal carcinoma is clearly an exception, and differs from other head and neck cancers in a number of ways. For example, in one large series the commonest tumours from this primary site were anaplastic and

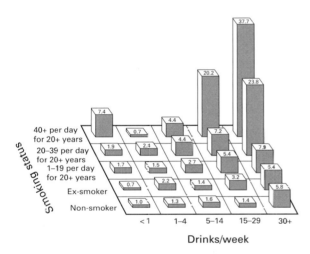

Fig. 10.2 Relative risk of oral/pharyngeal cancer in males by alcohol and tobacco consumption. From Cancer Research Campaign Factsheet (1993) on oral cancer, with permission.

squamous cell carcinomas, though lymphoepithelioma (undifferentiated squamous cell carcinoma), malignant lymphoma, adenoid cystic carcinoma (cylindroma) and plasmacytoma also occurred, as well as rarer tumours such as melanoma or undifferentiated sarcoma. Together, these constituted a significant group of carcinomas of non-squamous origin amounting to almost 30% of all cases. By contrast, in a series of over 2000 cases of carcinoma of the larynx, 95% were squamous, showing varying degrees of differentiation and including 97 patients with carcinoma *in situ*. Of patients with head and neck carcinomas 20% or more develop multiple primary lesions, most notably within the oral cavity.

Malignant lymphoma can arise anywhere within the head and neck but particularly from Waldeyer's ring. In such cases special care should be taken to establish the correct histological diagnosis since prognosis and management of lymphoma is very different from epithelial carcinoma.

Clinical staging

Careful staging is essential, both as a reminder to carry out full clinical and radiological assessment in each case, and also in order to develop logical treatment strategies and to document for case comparison [7]. In Europe, the proposals of the Union Internationale Contre le Cancer for standard tumour node metastasis (TNM) staging have gained wide acceptance [8]. This has been facilitated by the adoption of the same staging notation for lymph node status regardless of the primary head and neck site (Table 10.1). Unfortunately this uniformity of notation has not been possible for T staging, where some primary sites are still staged according to their spread (see Tables 10.2 and 10.3 for examples).

Table 10.1 Staging of nodes and metastases in head and neck cancers [7].

The definitions of the N categories for all head and neck sites except thyroid gland are:

N *Regional lymph nodes*

N_x Regional lymph nodes cannot be assessed

N_0 No regional lymph node metastasis

N_1 Metastasis in a single ipsilateral lymph node, 3 cm or less in greatest dimension

N_2 Metastasis in a single ipsilateral lymph node, more than 3 cm but not more than 6 cm in greatest dimension, or in multiple ipsilateral lymph nodes, none more than 6 cm in greatest dimension, or in bilateral or contralateral lymph nodes, none more than 6 cm in greatest dimension

     N_{2a} Metastasis in a single ipsilateral lymph node, more than 3 cm but not more than 6 cm in greatest dimension

     N_{2b} Metastasis in multiple ipsilateral lymph nodes, not more than 6 cm in greatest dimension

     N_{2c} Metastasis in bilateral or contralateral lymph nodes, none more than 6 cm in greatest dimension

     N_3 Metastasis in a lymph node more than 6 cm in greatest dimension

T stage	N stage
T_x not assessed	N_x not assessed
T_0 no primary found in nasopharynx	N_0 no palpable lymph nodes
T_1 tumour confined to nasopharynx	N_1 N < 3 cm ipsilateral
T_2 tumour extends to soft tissue of oropharynx	N_2 N 3–6 cm ipsi- or bilateral and/or nasal fossa
T_{2a} without parapharyngeal extension	N_3 N > 6 cm
T_{2b} with parapharyngeal extension	M stage
T_3 tumour invades bony structures and/or paranasal sinuses	M_x not assessed
T_4 tumour with intracranial extension and/or involvement of cranial nerves, infratemporal fossa, hypopharynx or orbit	M_0 no distant metastases

Table 10.2 Current UICC staging system in nasopharyngeal carcinoma (1997).

M_1 distant metastases present.

Table 10.3 TNM staging for oropharyngeal and oral cavity carcinoma.

T—Primary tumour
T_{is} Pre-invasive carcinoma (carcinoma *in situ*)
T_0 No evidence of primary tumour
T_1 Tumour 2 cm or less in its greatest dimension
T_2 Tumour more than 2 cm but not more than 4 cm in its greatest dimension
T_3 Tumour more than 4 cm in its greatest dimension
T_4 Tumour with extension to bone, muscle, skin, antrum, neck, etc.
T_X The minimum requirements to assess the primary tumour cannot be met

N—Regional lymph nodes
See Table 10.1 for N staging notation

M—Distant metastasis
M_0 No evidence of distant metastasis
M_1 Evidence of distant metastasis
M_x The minimum requirements to assess the presence of distant metastasis cannot be met

Stage grouping

Stage I	T_1	N_0	M_0
Stage II	T_2	N_0	M_0
Stage III	T_3	N_0	M_0
	T_1, T_2, T_3	N_1	M_0
Stage IV	T_4	$N_0 N_1$	M_0
	Any T	$N_2 N_3$	M_0
Any T	Any N	M_1	

Distant metastasis

The definitions of the M categories for all head and neck sites are:
M   Distant metastasis
M_x Presence of distant metastasis cannot be assessed
M_0 No distant metastasis
M_1 Distant metastasis.

Routine assessment and staging should always include careful inspection of the primary site, with measurement of its dimensions and examination for direct extension into adjacent tissues and local lymph node areas. Although a reasonable attempt at clinical examination and staging can be made with indirect laryngoscopy and nasopharyngoscopy with mirror techniques, most patients require an examination under anaesthetic, with direct endoscopic evaluation, before firm conclusions can be drawn. This is particularly true of nasopharyngeal carcinoma, since mirror examination of the postnasal space can be demanding for the patient, and unreliable even in the hands of an expert. Outpatient fibreoptic nasendoscopy has become standard practice since the mid-1980s. Histological confirmation must ideally be obtained in every case.

Investigation

Plain radiography, computed tomography (CT) and MRI scanning are of great value. In carcinomas of the larynx and hypopharynx, for example, the soft-tissue lateral

X-ray of the neck often gives a useful indication of the anatomical extent of the lesion, of particular value in subglottic tumours of the larynx, where extension or origin of the lesion may be difficult to assess. CT and magnetic resonance (MRI) scanning have made a dramatic impact on the accuracy with which deep-seated lesions can now be visualized, particularly those of the nasopharynx, parotid gland, retro-orbital area and paranasal sinuses, and where there is involvement of the skull base or other evidence of bone erosion (Fig. 10.3).

Haematogenous spread is uncommon at presentation, but when it does occur the lungs are the most common site of spread. The risk is highest with advanced tumours and in cases of nasopharyngeal carcinoma. A chest X-ray is essential and will also disclose the occasional simultaneous carcinoma of the bronchus. A routine blood count and liver function tests should also be performed.

These tumours are best managed jointly by a surgeon and a radiotherapist with particular interest in this area, since they present technical problems of management unequalled by those at any other site. Because of the extreme variation in presentation, natural history and response to treatment, this chapter only gives a brief outline of general principles of management; for those with a particular interest, specialist texts can be recommended [9].

Carcinoma of the larynx

In the Western world, carcinomas of the larynx form the largest numerical group. Historically, the first laryngectomy for carcinoma is generally credited to Billroth in 1873.

The human larynx is an unusually complex organ (Fig. 10.4) combining the role of a protective sphincter for keeping the lower respiratory tract free from foreign bodies, with the highly sophisticated function of speech production. This demands extraordinary precision in the tone of the laryngeal musculature and in the approximation of the vocal cords themselves.

Laryngeal cancer accounts for about 2–3% of all malignant disease, but the distress it causes is disproportionately high because of the severe social consequences of loss of speech. Indeed, the quality of voice and speech production is an important factor in choice of treatment. The larynx is sufficiently accessible to be viewed directly with ease, using mirror techniques (indirect laryngoscopy), nasendoscopy or by direct vision under anaesthesia. It contains epithelial and mesodermal tissue components which lend themselves well to the study of radiation effects on both normal and abnormal tissues. For these reasons, the larynx has always been of particular interest to the radiotherapist.

Cigarette smoking is undoubtedly the most important aetiological factor, accounting for the male predominance. There is a known correlation between premalignant laryngeal mucosal changes and the number of cigarettes smoked. The rise in incidence of laryngeal carcinoma has been shown to parallel the rising incidence of carcinoma of the bronchus, and in patients cured of early

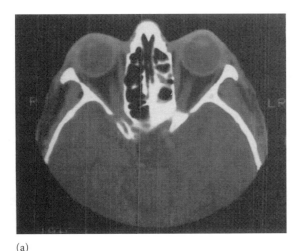

(a)

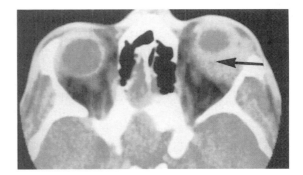

(b)

Fig. 10.3 CT scanning in head and neck tumours. (a) CT scan through nose and paranasal sinuses showing a large tumour of left maxilla with extensive local invasion and bone destruction

(see also Fig. 4.5, p. 42); (b) CT scan through orbits showing large left-sided tumour (arrowed) displacing the globe forwards and downwards.

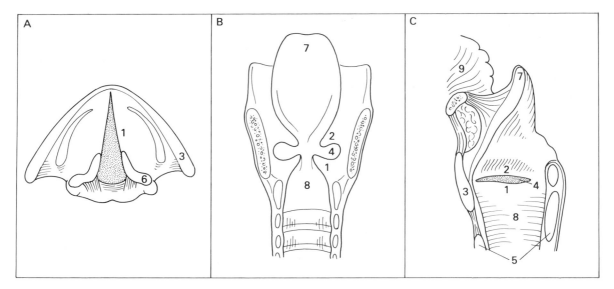

Fig. 10.4 Anatomy of the larynx. (A) From above; (B) coronal plane; (C) median sagittal plane. (1) True vocal cord; (2) false vocal cord; (3) thyroid cartilage; (4) laryngeal ventricle; (5) cricoid cartilage; (6) arytenoid; (7) epiglottis; (8) subglottic area; (9) base of tongue.

laryngeal carcinoma but continuing to smoke, bronchial carcinoma has become the commonest cause of death.

Hoarseness is the principal and often the only symptom, and any patient with hoarseness of more than 3 weeks duration should be referred for immediate laryngoscopy since early (T_{1-2} N_0) carcinomas can almost always be cured by radiotherapy (see below). Dysphagia is much less common, though important in patients with supraglottic carcinoma, particularly when there is extension to the oropharynx. Dyspnoea, sometimes with stridor, is a feature of subglottic carcinoma where early obstruction is the rule and immediate tracheostomy frequently required before definitive management can be undertaken.

Carcinomas can arise from any of the three anatomical regions of the larynx, though not with equal frequency (Fig. 10.5). Lesions of the glottis are much the commonest, followed by supraglottic and finally subglottic cancers. Though early supraglottic cancer is uncommon in the UK, these tumours are commoner than cancer of the glottis in some parts of Europe including Spain, Italy and Finland. In glottic lesions, the commonest site is the anterior third of the cord, often with extension to anterior or (more rarely) the posterior commissure. The whole cord can, however, be involved. Direct spread can take place upwards via the laryngeal ventricle to the false cord and then to the remainder of the supraglottic region, or downwards

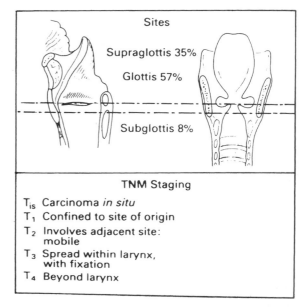

Fig. 10.5 Relative frequency and TNM staging system in laryngeal cancer.

directly to the subglottic area. Lymph node metastases are uncommon in early glottic carcinoma since the lymphatic drainage of the true cord is so sparse, but prognosis is highly dependent on the T stage. Most patients with T_1

and T_2 tumours are curable, whereas the majority of T_3 and T_4 lesions are not. Tumours of the epiglottis are usually advanced at presentation because there is little anatomical hindrance to direct tumour extension, particularly into the pre-epiglottic space. They do not cause hoarseness initially, and may elude diagnosis at laryngoscopy, particularly if the tumour arises on the inferior surface.

Management and prognosis

Carcinoma of the glottis

Radiotherapy to a *minimum* radical dose of 66 Gy (daily fractions over $6\frac{1}{2}$ weeks, or equivalent) will cure the majority of patients where the vocal cord remains mobile (T_1 well over 90% and T_2 70%). Many centres now increasingly employ routinely higher doses, around 70 Gy. Where failure occurs with radiotherapy treatment, salvage surgery is curative in over half of all cases. Total laryngectomy is usually necessary but some cases can be treated successfully by partial laryngectomy with preservation of the voice, particularly if the initial tumour was well localized. Although conservative surgery (usually by partial vertical laryngectomy) can deal effectively with most early glottic carcinomas, the resulting voice is inferior to what can be achieved with radiotherapy. There are few drawbacks to radiotherapy, for early cases, since the field of treatment is small (often only 5×5 cm) with no need—at least in T_1 tumours—to irradiate local lymph node areas.

Treatment of the *advanced* case is more difficult, requiring full discussion between surgeon and radiotherapist. There is an increasing emphasis on laryngeal preservation, which seems fully justified by recent data [10]. Surgery is occasionally required as an emergency procedure, particularly with subglottic extension. Many centres still employ a policy of planned radiotherapy and surgery in combination for the majority of these advanced lesions, especially if there is evidence of cartilage invasion, perichondritis, extralaryngeal spread or nodal metastases where the ultimate prospect for cure is so poor. However, radiotherapy in combination with multiagent chemotherapy has gradually replaced this approach whenever possible (see below), reserving 'salvage' surgery for cases in which non-surgical treatment had been unsuccessful. This has become more widely practised in recent years, and has led to a higher proportion of patients cured of the carcinoma yet with retention of the larynx and satisfactory speech production [10]. Adverse prognostic factors such as fixation of the primary tumour, early local inva-

sion, extrinsic spread and lymph node metastasis are interrelated and often occur together. The potential role of chemotherapy is discussed below (p. 154). For the majority of these patients, even the most intensive combinations of surgery, radiotherapy and chemotherapy will fail to cure, and the ultimate 5-year survival rate for T_3 lesions is about 25%.

Carcinoma of the supraglottis

These tumours are more difficult to treat. They often present late because early symptoms are few. Dysphagia may not develop until ulceration and local extension take place. Both local invasion and lymph node involvement are more common than with glottic carcinomas, and almost a quarter of supraglottic lesions extend down to the glottis. By locally invading in other directions, these tumours frequently involve the oropharynx (particularly the posterior third of the tongue) and the hypopharynx (particularly the pyriform fossa). For early lesions, a policy of radical irradiation with salvage surgery (total laryngectomy) where required (as for glottic tumours) is usually recommended, though surgery may be preferable for accessible lesions, such as those at the tip of the epiglottis. Conservative surgery is not normally possible. An important difference in radiotherapy technique between treatment of this region and the true glottis is that the radiation fields should routinely include the local lymph node areas, since clinical and occult lymph node metastases are common. For more advanced supraglottic lesions, the combination of total laryngectomy with preoperative radiotherapy has traditionally been employed, and a 5-year survival rate of around 60% has been achieved. However, histological examination of the specimen may show that the preoperative radiation had already produced a probable cure. For this reason it may be preferable to withhold surgery until there is evidence of recurrence or residual disease after radiation.

Carcinoma of the subglottis

The outlook is much less satisfactory with these difficult tumours. Often there is vocal cord fixation at diagnosis, and invasion of the cricoid cartilage is common. Involvement of the thyroid gland or paratracheal lymph nodes occurs in about half of all cases, and surgical excision, if undertaken, must be radical. Such operations are performed less often nowadays, in favour of a planned combination of radiotherapy and chemotherapy, with surgery reserved for residual or recurrent disease.

Conservative surgery in laryngeal cancer

Although long-term survival in patients with laryngeal cancer has remained almost unchanged for the past 20 years, the quality of life of survivors has improved considerably. Where surgery proves necessary in radiotherapy failures, it is sometimes possible to offer conservative surgery [11], offering the patient some chance of reasonable speech production. With *horizontal* supraglottic laryngectomy (Fig. 10.6), the upper part of the larynx is removed but the cords preserved. In *vertical* partial laryngectomy, the surgeon removes one vocal cord, the false cord and the vocal process of the arytenoid with part of the adjacent thyroid cartilage, and if necessary up to one-third of the contralateral vocal cord. Success in these procedures lies in accurate evaluation of tumour extent even though preoperative assessment can never be completely reliable.

Rehabilitation

Following laryngectomy, social and vocal rehabilitation is of great importance (see Chapter 7, p. 101). With the appropriate training of oesophageal voice technique and stoma care, most patients can look forward to a full life, usually with an adequate voice. Although this is difficult to

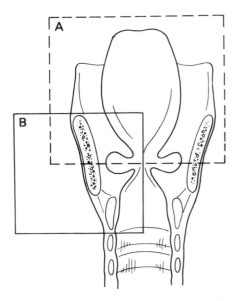

Fig. 10.6 Conservative laryngectomy operations in laryngeal cancer. (A) Horizontal supraglottic laryngectomy; (B) vertical partial laryngectomy.

define, the ability to speak on the telephone is often used as an important criterion.

Permanent vocal prostheses are often now used in patients who find it difficult to develop adequate oesophageal speech [12]. These devices contain valves which sometimes offer a striking improvement in voice quality. An example is the Blom–Singer valve, which requires a permanent pharyngeal puncture with placement of a small tube which is brought forward to the skin of the anterior neck. By occluding the opening with a finger, many patients can produce adequate speech, although care of the valve can be difficult and a high standard of hygiene is essential.

Carcinoma of the pharynx

Anatomy and patterns of metastasis

The pharynx is best considered as a passage with two distal sphincters serving the function of channelling both food and air in the right directions—the digestive and respiratory passages. During deglutition the respiratory tract is effectively closed off by laryngeal constriction, protecting the trachea and bronchi from inhalation of food or foreign bodies. The pharynx has three concentric coats: an internal mucous membrane, a supporting fibrous tunica and a muscular coat with a series of deficiencies for entry of vessels and nerves. These defects are important because they are the principal sites through which malignant tumours of the pharynx spread to adjacent tissues, particularly lymph nodes, in the neck.

Anatomically, the pharynx is usually described in three contiguous parts (Fig. 10.7). The *nasopharynx* is situated behind the nasal cavity and extends from the base of the skull above to the superior aspect of the soft palate below. It is bounded posteriorly by prevertebral fascia, extending anteriorly to the junction of the hard and soft palate. The *oropharynx* is situated behind the oral cavity, extends inferiorly to the floor of the vallecula sulcus and includes the posterior third of tongue, vallecula, soft palate, uvula, faucial pillars and tonsils. The *laryngopharynx* (or *hypopharynx*) is situated behind the larynx, extending from the floor of the vallecular sulcus above to the level of the lower border of the cricoid cartilage below, where it joins the oesophagus. It includes the pyriform fossae, posterior pharyngeal wall and postcricoid area. The whole pharynx has a rich lymphatic drainage and early nodal involvement is common, with a predictable clinical pattern (Fig. 10.8). The important but inaccessible node of Rouvière is

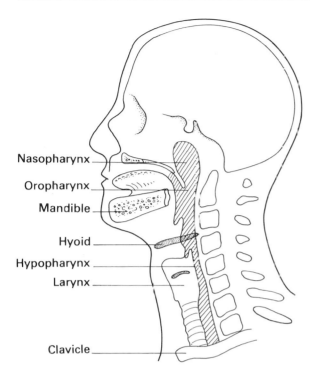

Fig. 10.7 Anatomical divisions of the pharynx.

Nasopharynx

Oropharynx

Mandible

Hyoid

Hypopharynx

Larynx

Clavicle

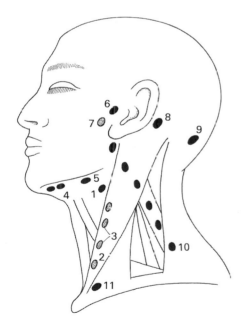

Fig. 10.8 Lymphatic drainage of the head and neck. (1) Jugulodigastric; (2) jugulo-omohyoid; (3) deep cervical; (4) submental; (5) submandibular; (6) preauricular; (7) parotid; (8) postauricular; (9) occipital; (10) posterior triangle; (11) supraclavicular.

situated in the lateral retropharyngeal area, closely related to the jugular foramen and situated over the lateral masses of the atlas. Its importance lies in its critical position, making it an early site of invasion, particularly by nasopharyngeal tumours.

Most pharyngeal carcinomas are squamous in origin (oropharynx 60%, hypopharynx 75%) although primary cancers arising from the nasopharynx are typically poorly differentiated or undifferentiated, or even anaplastic. Three-quarters of all nasopharyngeal lesions present with obvious lymphadenopathy, whereas in hypopharyngeal cancer almost half of all cases are clinically free of nodes [13]. Lymphomas are also relatively common in the oropharynx (particularly the tonsil) and nasopharynx.

Carcinoma of the nasopharynx

Although relatively uncommon in the Western world, these tumours are the commonest of all malignant tumours in many parts of China, accounting in some areas for half or more of all cancers (see pp. 6,8). Clinical staging is more difficult than in any other head or neck site because of the inaccessibility of the lesion and its drainage routes. The TNM staging system is now widely used.

Cancers of the nasopharynx often have an insidious onset and present late, often with nodal disease in the neck. Nasal obstruction, usually unilateral, and secretory otitis media are also common. Bone erosion or destruction is common because of the close proximity of the nasopharynx to the base of the skull, many patients presenting with cranial nerve involvement, particularly nerves III–VI, which pass through the cavernous sinus. The IX–XII nerves may also be involved by direct tumour extension where they pass through the parapharyngeal space in proximity to the lateral nasopharyngeal wall. Other extrapharyngeal sites of extension include the paranasal sinuses, nasal cavity, orbit and middle ear. Involvement of these regions causes pain, nasal stuffiness or discharge, unilateral deafness and ophthalmoplegia.

Treatment is by radical radiotherapy, with or without chemotherapy (see below). The irradiation volume must be large in order to encompass likely sites of local extension and nodal involvement. This must be achieved without any concession in total dosage, which should be at least 60 Gy delivered within 6–6.5 weeks. Higher doses may be delivered to the primary site but the many challenging technical difficulties include avoidance of the upper part of the spinal cord and temporal lobe of the brain (both of which have limited radiation tolerance yet are unavoidably included in the treatment portals), as well as the minimization of mucosal reaction as far as possible. The classical approach of Lederman (Fig. 10.9) is still widely employed and aims at non-uniform high-dose irradiation to the primary and bilateral cervical nodes. Lateral and anterior fields are employed, with appropriate shielding and field changes to avoid dangerous overtreatment of the upper cervical spinal cord without compromising the dosage to the lymph nodes. Even with this technique, a small portion (usually about 4 cm) of the spinal cord may inevitably receive a dose of 50 Gy, and treatment complications will be inevitable in some cases. Other complications of treatment such as perichondritis or radionecrosis are uncommon with careful fractionation and avoidance of overdosage. It is important to avoid removal of teeth during or shortly after treatment. Surgery has no place other than biopsy of the primary lesion, and occasionally in removal of residual lymph node disease by block dissection if the primary appears controlled.

Results of treatment are closely related to stage (Table 10.2); median disease-free 5-year survival, even in patients with early disease, is less than 50%. The largest single group ($T_2 N_{0-1}$), with an intermediate prognosis, have a 5-year disease-free survival of about 30%. A significant number of patients alive at 5 years will ultimately die of recurrence, and prolonged control followed by late relapse is common in this tumour. With $T_{3-4} N_{2-3}$ disease very few patients survive 5 years. Overall 5-year survival is better in younger people and in women. Recent attempts to improve results have included the use of intracavitary caesium implants to increase the dose to the primary site. The role of chemotherapy is discussed below (p. 154), but is now regarded by many authorities as a standard part of treatment for nasopharyngeal carcinoma.

Carcinoma of the oropharynx

These tumours are somewhat more accessible, and in many ways simpler to treat. The important sites include the soft palate, faucial pillars, tonsil, posterior third of tongue and pharyngeal wall. The relative incidence and TNM staging are shown in Fig. 10.10 (Table 10.4). Presenting symptoms include dysphagia with pain as well as aspiration of liquids. There may also be dysarthria with large tumours of the posterior tongue. The tumour is usually visible providing the anterior portion of the tongue is carefully retracted, but cancers arising from the posterior third tongue can be notoriously difficult to

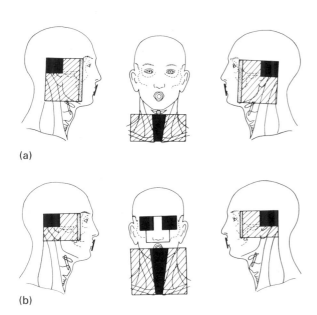

(a)

(b)

Fig. 10.9 Typical radiation for radical treatment of carcinoma of the nasopharynx. (a) First phase of treatment (40 Gy in 4 weeks); (b) second phase of treatment (to 60 Gy total dose in 6 weeks). From [14] with permission.

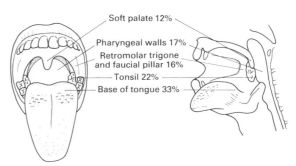

Soft palate 12%
Pharyngeal walls 17%
Retromolar trigone and faucial pillar 16%
Tonsil 22%
Base of tongue 33%

Fig. 10.10 Carcinoma of the oropharynx: relative frequency at different sites.

Table 10.4 Tumours of the orbit (excluding globe).

Benign	Malignant
Haemangioma	Lymphoma
Lachrymal gland tumours	Rhabdomyosarcoma
Meningioma	Optic nerve glioma
Lymphangioma	Metastases
Neurofibroma	Angiosarcoma and other sarcomas
Dermoid cysts (pseudotumour)	Myeloma

visualize, cervical lymph nodes may be enlarged [15] and sometimes precede definition of the primary site by more than a year. Radiological assessment can be very useful, using plain lateral views of the neck, tomography, barium contrast studies and CT scanning. There are differences in the presenting stage of tumours at different sites within the oropharynx; lesions of the tonsillar fossa are more often locally advanced (T_3 and T_4) at presentation than tumours of the retromolar trigone or anterior faucial pillar.

Combinations of surgery and radiotherapy are routinely used in managing these lesions, though increasingly the emphasis has been on radical radiotherapy (sometimes in combination with chemotherapy), with surgery reserved for radiotherapy failures. The radiotherapeutic technique is much simpler than with carcinoma of the nasopharynx since direct extension of tumour can usually be dealt with simply by extension of the field in the appropriate direction. A recent randomized study from Europe [16] has suggested a real advantage in tumour control following hyperfractionated radiotherapy using two fractions of treatment per day (see also Chapter 5). Difficult problems arise when there is extension into the hard palate, mandible, tongue or larynx, and these are usually best dealt with by high-dose radiation (with or without chemotherapy), or by surgery if treatment by irradiation and chemotherapy is unable to control the primary tumour. This is also true of lymphatic metastases. *En bloc* radical neck dissection may be required and can even be performed bilaterally if necessary.

Surgery and radiation are probably equally effective in controlling both the primary and the node metastases though with a far better functional result in patients treated by radiotherapy. Combined surgery and radiation may be valuable in more advanced tumours, particularly those arising in the anterior faucial pillar. For tonsillar tumours, excision biopsy of the whole tonsil is usually advisable for reliable histology, and may be sufficient if the resection margins are unequivocally clear.

For patients with local recurrence surgical removal offers the only prospect of cure. These operations are complex and require careful consideration, demanding close co-operation between the head and neck surgeon who will undertake the radical excision and the plastic surgeon responsible for the reconstruction. Modern techniques, for example using jejunal replacement of the pharynx, have improved the functional results, but rehabilitation of oropharyngeal function, especially deglutition, can be exceptionally difficult. Patients may need many months of skilled support and may suffer long-term problems with

oral lubrication since the radiation fields frequently cover the parotid glands.

Lymphoma of the pharynx

A significant proportion of nasopharyngeal and tonsillar tumours will prove histologically to be lymphomas rather than epithelial tumours. Invariably these are non-Hodgkin's lymphomas, usually lymphocytic B-cell neoplasms. It is wise to undertake full investigation as for non-Hodgkin's lymphomas at other sites, because distant spread occurs. The stomach is involved in 20% of cases at some stage but spread to the marrow and other extranodal sites is unusual at presentation. Nasopharyngeal lymphomas also have a tendency to spread directly to the paranasal sinuses and nasal fossae. Routine treatment of these contiguous areas is often recommended whenever a primary nasopharyngeal lymphoma is encountered. Although this represents an unusually large treatment volume, local control can usually be achieved with a more modest dose than for epithelial tumours. Generally 40 Gy in 4 weeks is adequate.

Carcinoma of the laryngopharynx (hypopharynx)

These are at least as common as those of the oropharynx, and as with other sites, excessive cigarette and spirit consumption are the chief aetiological factors. Common symptoms include dyspnoea, dysphagia, anorexia, inanition and sometimes stridor. Most are well-differentiated squamous carcinomas and are locally advanced at presentation. Palpable lymph nodes are present in about half—a quarter of these are bilateral.

Although the prognosis in general is poor, some sites are prognostically more favourable than others. Carcinomas of the upper part of the laryngopharynx, including the aryepiglottic fold and exophytic lesions of the pharyngolaryngeal fold, have a better prognosis than those of the more infiltrating or ulcerative variety, arising from the pyriform fossa, cervical oesophagus and posterior pharyngeal wall. They have a poor prognosis despite intensive treatment with radiotherapy, surgery and chemotherapy (in patients whose general condition warrants it). Five-year survival rates remain no better than 10–15% overall, regardless of the specific hypopharyngeal subsite or method of treatment. A small subgroup has a better prognosis, including a remarkable 5-year survival rate of 50% for early ($T_1 N_0$) lesions of the pyriform fossa. Although good results with radiotherapy alone have occasionally been claimed for individual patients with advanced disease, it is clear that the chief use of radiotherapy lies in palliation, and the avoidance of mutilating surgery which would in all probability fail to cure. Radical surgery is, however, occasionally indicated in patients with operable lesions and in good general health; these individual decisions are best made by a surgeon and radiotherapist working jointly in a combined clinic. Most patients ultimately die of local or regional recurrence (rarely because of lymph node disease alone) although an increasing proportion have evidence of more widespread dissemination.

Radiation technique is complicated by the large volume frequently required. Delineation of the lower extent of spread in laryngopharyngeal tumours is often very difficult. The technique usually consists of lateral opposed field treatment with either open (direct) or wedged fields (see Chapter 5). A major technical problem arises when the tumour has extended below the thoracic inlet since easy access by lateral fields is limited by the shoulders. These tumours pose some of the greatest technical challenges in clinical radiotherapy, particularly with postcricoid primary tumours. For treatment to be curative, a minimum radical dose of 60 Gy in 6 weeks, or equivalent, is always necessary. As with laryngeal cancers, an increasing number of centres routinely advocate a higher dose.

Tumours of the oral cavity

Tumours of the oral cavity include those arising from the lip, the mobile portion of the tongue (anterior to the circumvallate papillae), buccal mucosa, alveolae (gingiva), floor of mouth, hard palate and retromolar trigone. They are among the commonest tumours seen in many combined head and neck oncology clinics (Fig. 10.1), and are often surprisingly advanced at presentation. The incidence is rising, particularly among younger men [17], and there is evidence that use of retinoids in high-risk populations may prevent the development of dysplastic premalignant intraoral lesions into frankly invasive tumours [18].

The commonest symptom is of a non-healing ulcer on the lip, tongue, cheek or floor of mouth. Cancers of the lip can arise on the upper or lower vermillion border, or an adjacent area such as the philtrum, with direct involvement of the lip itself. The primary lesion can be raised, ulcerated, excavated, pigmented, well or poorly demarcated, painful or painless. Many oral cavity lesions are first diagnosed by a dentist and are sometimes hidden by dentures. Leucoplakia is a predisposing cause. On exami-

nation the usual findings are of a raised erythematous ulcerated lesion, often with an area of necrosis. Large tumours of the tongue may reduce mobility and interfere with speech.

Clinical examination should include careful bimanual palpation and the lesion should always be measured. Examination of the neck may reveal enlarged lymph nodes.

Investigation should include chest X-ray, full blood count and liver function tests. In patients with tumours of the floor of mouth or lower alveolus, investigation should always include radiological examination (orthopantomogram) of the lower jaw since asymptomatic involvement can occur, even when the lesion is not tender. Fine-needle aspiration cytology of neck nodes is easily performed.

The clinical behaviour and probability of metastases varies with the site [15]. Carcinomas at the tip of the tongue are far easier to control than tumours of its lateral margins: cancers of the dorsum are most difficult of all (Fig. 10.11). In general, tumours of the floor of the mouth, buccal mucosa, hard palate and alveolus show similar and relatively low metastatic rates, whereas tumours of the oral tongue have a higher propensity for nodal spread.

Metastases are more frequent with poorly differentiated tumours. Larger tumours (above 4 cm in diameter) are more difficult to control and likely to be accompanied by cervical node metastases. Bilateral node involvement is common with lesions of the floor of the mouth and faucial arch. The anatomical position of the abnormal nodes varies with the primary site. For carcinomas of the oral

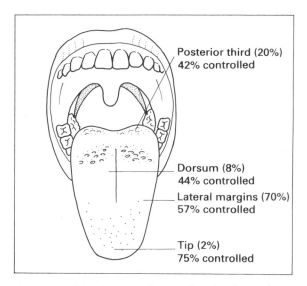

Fig. 10.11 Relative frequency (in parentheses) and control rates in carcinoma of the tongue.

tongue and floor of mouth, the commonest sites are the jugulodigastric and submaxillary nodes, whereas palatine and retromolar trigone lesions are more frequently accompanied by lymphadenopathy at the angle of the jaw. Second primary cancers are relatively common within the oral cavity [4].

Management

Optimum management is best achieved in joint consultative clinics staffed by a surgeon, radiotherapist and medical oncologist [19]. Principles of management are similar for the major sites within the oral cavity and will be considered together, except for carcinomas of the lip (see p. 152).

Small accessible tumours (T_1) of the oral cavity

These have an excellent cure rate with radical radiotherapy, with very good preservation of function. Interstitial implantation techniques are often ideal for intraoral tumours (that is, excluding those of the lip), since the treatment volume can be kept small and a high dose to be given safely. Implants of radium, caesium, gold, tantalum and iridium are all satisfactory. Intraoral sites often treated by interstitial irradiation include tongue, buccal mucosa, floor of mouth, palate and lower alveolus. Very small lesions (less than 1 cm) can be treated with an interstitial implant alone, without external beam irradiation, though most radiotherapists use a combination of interstitial and external irradiation in larger tumours which are still small enough to implant (T_1 and small T_2 cancers). With an interstitial implant, a tumour dose of 60 Gy is usually given over 4–7 days. Where interstitial and external radiation are used together, many authorities recommend that the volume implant is taken to 50 Gy in 5–7 days, followed by external beam irradiation to 30 Gy in 3 weeks. In some clinics, excisional surgery is preferred for small tumours of the anterior tip of the tongue, sometimes using the laser-excision technique.

Larger tumours of the oral cavity (T_2–T_4)

In these tumours, external beam irradiation has traditionally been the mainstay of treatment, though a dual modality approach using combined radiation and chemotherapy is increasingly being employed (see below). With external irradiation, doses of 60 Gy over 6 weeks are usually considered essential; tolerance is related to the volume irradiated. Radiation technique involves treatment by lateral open (direct) or wedged fields, to include both the primary tumour and the initial drainage node group. For cancers of the tongue, floor of mouth and lower jaw, the palate can safely be excluded from treatment by means of a mouth gag which depresses the tongue.

The proper management of metastases in neck nodes remains contentious. Many clinics recommend routine radical neck dissection in patients with mobile nodes, and prophylactic node dissection in clinically node-negative patients has revealed a significant incidence of micrometastatic tumour. In patients without evidence of neck node involvement (N_0), most radiotherapists give prophylactic treatment to the neck, to a slightly lower dose (50 Gy in 5 weeks or equivalent) than radical dosage, on the grounds that occult nodal spread is common and that nodal recurrence is reduced by such treatment. Most centres employ external beam irradiation, sometimes in combination with surgery, to control metastatic neck nodes, though ultimate survival rates in patients with N_2 and N_3 nodes are poor whatever the approach.

Patterns of recurrence and overall survival are clearly dependent on the size and stage of the tumour. In one large study the cumulative 3-year survival in mobile tongue and floor of mouth lesions without lymphadenopathy was 57%, whereas for patients with palpable lymphadenopathy the survival rate fell to 42% [20]. Where lymph node involvement is obvious at presentation, failure at the primary site is common despite intensive radiotherapy.

Occasionally it is possible to control a limited relapse (usually the primary site) with an interstitial radioactive implant, though radical surgery is usually required later since durable control is rarely achieved.

In the UK, surgery is usually undertaken if local relapse occurs after primary radiation therapy, though increasingly some centres recommend primary surgical excision instead of radical irradiation because of the long-term problems of radiation damage within the oral cavity. A wide resection is invariably required, with immediate reconstruction.

The advent of free flap grafting with microvascular anastomosis has dramatically improved the cosmetic results. However, complete surgical extirpation of the initial area at risk has to be undertaken, often resulting in substantial local damage with loss of function. A typical operation for a recurrent lesion of the floor of the mouth might include a hemiglossectomy, excision of the floor of the mouth, hemimandibulectomy, and neck dissection (commando procedure) with pedicle and/or microvascular free flap grafting in order to achieve adequate healing—

a major undertaking in patients who are often debilitated enough to require hyperalimentation before surgery. Intensive rehabilitation and speech therapy are also critically important. Chapter 7 (pp. 100–2) provides a fuller discussion of patient rehabilitation. For persistent radiation-induced dry mouth (xerostomia) the use of oral pilocarpine has been shown to increase salivary production, generally with fairly minor side-effects such as sweating and urinary frequency [21].

Chemotherapy may also be valuable in the primary or secondary management of these tumours and is further discussed in the final section of this chapter.

Carcinoma of the lip

These are almost always squamous cell carcinomas, often well differentiated and presenting relatively early since the tumour is usually visible. The incidence has fallen rapidly during the past 25 years, and less than 300 new cases are now seen annually in the UK. Cancers of the lower lip are much commoner than those of the upper lip (20:1) but upper lip cancers are relatively commoner in women.

Metastasis is relatively uncommon, and is to local lymph nodes. About 7% of patients have involvement of local nodes at diagnosis, and the same proportion will develop metastases in local lymph node groups after primary treatment. Nodal invasion is usually directly to the submaxillary or submental nodes and metastases rarely occur elsewhere.

Treatment

Treatment is by surgery or radiotherapy. Most carcinomas of the lip are curable by radiation therapy, particularly where the tumour is small (T_1). External beam therapy with photons or electrons, and brachytherapy with radium moulds or interstitial iridium implants, have all been used, all with high cure rates. Surgery also offers excellent local control, though the cosmetic result may be slightly less satisfactory, particularly where excision of a substantial portion of the lip needs to be undertaken. In larger tumours (T_2), radiotherapy is generally accepted as a better method of treatment both cosmetically and functionally, since surgical excision often leads to poor closure of the mouth and may interfere with phonation. With large destructive cancers of the lip (T_3, T_4—now relatively uncommon), it is difficult to achieve an adequate cosmetic and functional result by either method of treatment, and the incidence of local recurrence is higher. Healing

may be excellent even following large doses of radiation therapy, but surgical reconstruction is often necessary.

External beam irradiation is most commonly employed, using either electron beam therapy or moderate-energy photons, though the lip is also one of the classic sites for brachytherapy. As with treatment of skin cancer, an individually designed lead cut-out can be used to allow for external beam treatment of any size and shape of field. Treatment schedules are varied, though the best cosmetic schedules include 40 Gy applied dose in 10 fractions daily over 2 weeks, 50 Gy applied dose in 20 fractions over 4 weeks, 45 Gy in 10 fractions (given on alternate weekdays over 3.5 weeks) or, in centres preferring lengthy radical dosage, 60 Gy in 30 consecutive daily fractions over 6 weeks. This latter regimen is probably the most suitable for large volumes.

In the rare patient with nodal metastases, radical neck dissection is the treatment of choice, though radiotherapy can also be effective. With radical radiation therapy, surgery or a combination of both techniques, the results in carcinoma of the lip are excellent, and virtually all patients without lymph node involvement should be considered curable. Even with lymph node metastases, the overall survival is 60–70% at 5 years.

Nasal cavity and paranasal sinuses

These uncommon tumours, where presentation is often late and accompanied by early invasion of critical structures, are among the most difficult of all tumours of the head and neck region. The exposed nature of these facial cancers demands great skill both in eradicating the tumour, and providing acceptable reconstruction. They tend to be slow-growing, well-differentiated squamous carcinomas, in which local recurrence is the major problem. Melanoma of the nasal cavity accounts for almost 10% of nasal cavity cancer. Tumours of the nasal cavity/paranasal sinuses spread locally and to the nasopharynx (Fig. 10.12). Although late presentation is the rule, those originating from within the nasal cavity tend to present earlier, usually with nasal obstruction, stuffiness or offensive discharge.

Anatomically, the commonest tumours are those of the maxillary antrum, followed by nasal cavity and echinoid sinus.

Localized tumours of the maxillary antrum are usually asymptomatic; symptoms such as swelling and erythema of the cheek should raise a suspicion of extension beyond the confines of the primary site. Erosion of the floor of the

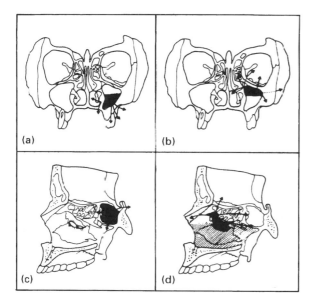

Fig. 10.12 Pathways of local spread of tumours of the nasal cavity and paranasal sinuses. (a) and (b) lower and upper maxillary tumours spreading to orbit, nasal fossa, palate, upper alveolus and soft tissues; (c) sphenoid sinus tumours (lateral view) into nasopharynx, base of brain, ethmoid and nasal cavity; (d) nasal fossa tumours (lateral view) into orbit, base of skull, sphenoid and posterior choana. From [21] with permission.

orbit and displacement of the globe may occur, leading to diplopia and ophthalmoplegia. Spread downwards (into the oral cavity) or posteriorly (into the pterygoid region) are also common, and other adjacent sites such as nasal cavity, ethmoid and sphenoidal sinuses are often involved (Fig. 10.12).

Little is known of the predisposing factors, though excessive alcohol intake, cigarette smoking and oral hygiene are held to be important. Adenocarcinoma of the nasal cavity is an occupational hazard in hardwood furniture makers, presumably due to inhalation of an occupational carcinogen. Staging by TNM or other conventional criteria has been disappointing but CT and MRI scanning give far more practical information (Fig. 10.3).

The concept of combined modality treatment is well established. In 1933, Ohngren advocated treatment by a combination of surgery and irradiation on the grounds that this gave better results than either treatment alone. In general, this approach has been validated and remains the standard policy in many large centres, particularly for treatment of the maxillary antrum. Surgical healing, even after radical doses of radiotherapy, is not usually a problem at this site, since the head and neck region is so well

vascularized. Conversely, there seems little prospect of reducing the extent of surgery for tumours which have usually spread beyond their primary confines at the time of diagnosis. No worthwhile comparative trials have been reported, but several series have demonstrated a 5-year survival of up to 40% with combined treatment. In patients too frail to undergo an operation, a 5-year survival of 20% has been achieved with the use of radiotherapy alone. Modern prosthetics have allowed many of these patients to face the world with a reasonably normal appearance despite substantial anatomical deficiencies.

Tumours of the middle ear

Cancer of the middle ear is extremely unusual, chiefly occurring in middle-aged men with a history of chronic otitis media, often making diagnosis difficult since the symptoms may be little more than an accentuation of the chronic discharge, with the addition of bleeding and pain. Direct local spread to mastoid air cells or external auditory canal is the rule, sometimes producing severe pain particularly if bone erosion has occurred. The tumours are usually squamous carcinomas, arising as a result of squamous metaplasia of the columnar epithelial cells normally present. Adenocarcinoma is very rare. Complete surgical removal is often impossible, and local control difficult to achieve. Extension beyond the temporal bone makes the prognosis very poor. Local extension to the brain may occur. Since survival rates are similar (about 25% at 5 years) whichever local method of treatment is employed, radical irradiation is usually preferred. Other rare tumours include soft-tissue sarcomas and primary tumours of bone. In these cases, radical surgery is seldom possible and the mainstay of treatment is radiotherapy.

Glomus jugulare tumours arise from neuroendocrine chemoreceptors of the jugular bulb, and should be considered with similar tumours (chemodectoma, paraganglioma) arising at other sites such as the bifurcation of the carotid artery (carotid body tumour) or posterior mediastinum. They are three times commoner in women, and may sometimes be bilateral. Although histologically benign, these tumours invade locally. Surgery is hazardous, since they are highly vascular and usually involve the middle ear and petrous temporal bone. Presentation is with a classical cluster of symptoms including deafness, cranial nerve palsies, local pain and tinnitus. Radiotherapy is often the treatment of choice and modest doses (40–50 Gy in 4–5 weeks) are adequate though regression may be slow.

Carcinoma of the pinna and external auditory canal

Tumours of the external auditory canal are usually squamous cell carcinomas, but on the pinna (much the commoner site) the commonest cell type in the UK is the basal cell carcinoma, though squamous carcinomas are commoner in the USA. Malignant melanoma is occasionally encountered. Usually there is a visible lesion of the pinna or, in the case of tumours of the external canal, crusting, discharge or unilateral deafness occur. Pain is unusual. Local extension may occur to preauricular structures, tympanic membrane, middle ear or mastoid.

Although radical surgery can be curative, it is widely accepted that treatment by radical radiotherapy is equally effective and offers a better functional result, even though mucosal oedema, sterile fluid collections in the middle ear and perforation of the eardrum may occur with high-dose radiation.

Chemotherapy in squamous carcinomas of the head and neck [23]

Although both surgery and radiotherapy can be curative for localized squamous cancers of the head and neck (and even in some cases with lymph node involvement), the prognosis of patients with recurrent or disseminated disease is very poor [24]. The first attempts at using cytotoxic chemotherapy in these patients were made at least 30 years ago, often using intra-arterial perfusion. More recently, interest has shifted from the use of single agents to combination chemotherapy, and from treatment of recurrent disease to the use of adjuvant chemotherapy in the initial management. Both of these approaches remain controversial [25].

Active drugs include methotrexate, cisplatin, bleomycin, 5-fluorouracil (5-FU) and mitomycin C. All of these show some degree of activity and in the past few years there has been a tendency towards combination chemotherapy for recurrent disease, increasingly employing cisplatin 5-FU or methotrexate–bleomycin combinations, although the duration of response tends to be short. There is no definite evidence that multidrug regimens are superior in survival to single agent therapy [26]. Other newer agents with activity include paclitaxel, docetaxel (see Chapter 6, p. 84 for a fuller discussion), vinorelbine, gemcitabine and topoisomerase inhibitors such as topotecan.

A major area of controversy surrounds the use of adjuvant combination chemotherapy immediately following (or in some cases preceding) local treatment with surgery or radiotherapy [24,27]. Both American and European groups have reported better local control and survival by comparison with historical controls. Indeed, randomized studies have been reported, using chemoradiotherapy compared with conventional radical irradiation [28,29] and increasingly suggesting a possible benefit for the combined modality group, especially in terms of freedom from local recurrence. In a large study from the Christie Hospital, Manchester, the addition of two pulses of single-agent methotrexate proved clearly beneficial in a series of over 300 patients with advanced disease. A large prospective meta-analysis [24] has confirmed the following.

1 Over 11 000 patients were included in analysis, from 76 trials.

2 34% were classified as UICC/TNM stage III; 56% stage 4.

3 There was a small, but significant improvement in overall and event-free survival in favour of chemotherapy (blank percentage vs. overall survival).

4 The benefit appeared dependent on timing of chemotherapy—synchronous chemoradiation clearly produced better results.

5 There is no evidence of benefit with neoadjuvant or subsequent chemotherapy.

6 No obvious advantage for platinum-containing programmes compared with other regimens.

Several uncontrolled series have investigated cisplatin–5-FU combinations and found them both active and feasible in combination with radical irradiation. Other active agents include carboplatin and ifosfamide. Despite encouraging data from a number of studies and meta-analyses it remains difficult to evaluate the role of chemotherapy in primary treatment until larger-scale randomized trials have been completed. This study suggested an overall 6.5% increase in survival overall (all trials taken together) but almost double this figure (12.1%) with synchronous chemoradiation therapy. Chemotherapy for advanced disease should probably not be used outside controlled clinical trials [25].

Patients with nasopharyngeal carcinoma undoubtedly have a higher response rate to chemotherapy. Attention has naturally turned to the use of chemotherapy as an adjuvant to primary treatment by radical irradiation. Although at least one large study has proven positive [30], the most recent information from the large Asian–Oceanic Oncology Group reported on a prospectively randomized trial of 330 patients, and were unable to demonstrate an improvement either in relapse-free survival or overall survival between two treatment arms [31]; however, in the subgroup of 49 patients with very bulky neck lymph nodes (greater than 6 cm) the results of multimodal treatment were superior, the chemotherapy apparently doubling the survival rate from 37 to 73%. However, a recent overview of all of the published randomized studies concluded that 'chemotherapy might improve survival and that this improvement is more apparent for single-agent chemotherapy given synchronously with radiotherapy' [32]. This study suggested an overall 6.5% increase in survival overall (all trials taken together) with synchronous chemoradiation therapy. It is now widely accepted that synchronous schedules are superior, that radical chemoradiation programmes are well tolerated by the majority of patients and that disease-free survival is improved. Choice of agents remains controversial; the Pignon meta-analysis does not favour platinum-containing regimens over the chemotherapy.

Tumours of salivary glands

Although uncommon, accounting for about 2% of all neoplasms, salivary tumours are of great interest since they are of such varied histology and present technical problems in management. The most common primary site is the parotid (almost 80% of all cases), though the other major (submandibular and sublingual) and minor salivary glands can be affected. Occasionally, tumours of minor salivary glands can grow to a large size, mimicking cancers of the nasopharynx or palate.

The parotid gland is an accessible organ, overlying the styloid process, situated between mastoid and mandible, and mostly lying anterior to the pinna. Its deep boundary is close to the parapharyngeal space and lateral pharyngeal wall. Superiorly, it rarely extends beyond the zygomatic arch. The gland is divided by the facial nerve and it branches into a superficial and deep lobe; excision is often limited for fear of surgical damage to this nerve. The submandibular gland lies beneath the horizontal portion of the mandible, and the sublingual gland (the smallest of the three major salivary glands) lies in the floor of the mouth, in contact with the inner surface of the mandible, often extending to the midline where it meets the contralateral gland.

Pathologically, the wide variety of histological types of salivary tumour encompasses both benign and malignant disorders (Table 10.5). Three-quarters are benign, mostly pleomorphic adenomas or 'mixed salivary tumours',

which is much the commonest tumour in the parotid gland and less frequently found in other sites (only 40% of tumours in minor salivary glands). About 65% occur in women, mostly in the 50–65 age group, though pleomorphic adenomas of the parotid have been reported even in children. The tumours are histologically varied, often with several populations of cells. However, the overall pattern, though bizarre, pleomorphic and disorganized, is not one of malignancy.

Twenty-five per cent of parotid tumours are malignant. *Malignant mixed tumours*, or pleomorphic adenocarcinomas, often resemble pleomorphic adenomas histologically though foci of malignant change are typically scattered throughout the specimen. These patients usually give a history of slow-growing and painless parotid swelling, often for several years, followed by a sudden change, with increased swelling and pain. This well-recognized development represents one of the best examples of malignant change within an area of benign neoplasia—a most unusual phenomenon at other sites. *Adenoid cystic carcinomas* or cylindromas are rather more common (about 15% of malignant salivary tumours) and arise in major salivary glands but also quite typically in the minor glands, for example in the palate. Characteristically, these tumours spread by direct extension along perineural spaces, a feature which may lead to unusual clinical presentations. *Mucoepidermoid carcinomas* are well recognized, and consist histologically of two distinct populations of cells, with both mucus secretion together with typical epidermoid morphology. These often tend to be less malignant tumours and the lowest grade ones are clinically benign, though at the other end of the spectrum is the high-grade mucoepidermoid carcinoma which can be difficult to control and may be rapidly fatal. *Acinic cell tumours* are rare, more common in females, with a slow clinical

Table 10.5 Histological types and prognosis in salivary gland tumours.

	Frequency (%)	5-year survival
Pleomorphic adenoma	75	96
Adenocarcinoma	8	50
Mucoepidermoid		
low grade	3	90
high grade	3	20
Adenoid cystic	4	60
Malignant mixed	2	55
Acinic cell	1	80
Squamous	3	25

evolution and an unusual histological picture suggesting an origin in acinic epithelial cells. Squamous cell and *anaplastic carcinomas* of the salivary glands must be diagnosed with caution, since there is a problem in distinguishing these from secondary deposits arising from a head and neck tumour site of more typical squamous origin. Histologically, the squamous or anaplastic element may be one component of a mixed malignant or other type of salivary tumour. True anaplastic or squamous tumours of the salivary gland are among the most malignant of tumours, with a very poor prognosis. *Lymphoma* of the parotid is occasionally seen, but it is difficult to be sure if its site of origin is the parotid itself or an adjacent lymph node. *Adenolymphoma* (Warthin's tumour) is an unusual lesion, sometimes misdiagnosed as an abscess, and of doubtful origin. It is never malignant, may even be degenerative, and is characterized by large pink-staining cells surrounded by a lymphoid 'follicle', often with a centrally cystic area.

Clinical features and management

Benign salivary tumours usually present with a slowly-growing painless mass. The onset of pain or a facial palsy is a sinister development suggestive of malignancy. The most rapidly growing tumours are anaplastic and squamous carcinomas, other malignant salivary tumours typically presenting with a more insidious onset. With adenoid cystic carcinomas, pain is a common feature due to the perineural spread. Lymph node involvement is unusual in salivary tumours though reportedly more common in high-grade mucoepidermoid carcinoma. Haematogenous spread is, however, well recognized, particularly with anaplastic, mixed malignant tumours and cylindromas.

Surgical excision is undoubtedly the most important approach for both benign and malignant salivary tumours. For benign parotid tumours (occurring most commonly in the superficial portion of the gland), superficial parotidectomy with preservation of the facial nerve is the operation of choice, giving excellent results if complete excision is achieved. When excision is incomplete, postoperative radiotherapy will reduce recurrence rates and is mandatory in this situation. Although some surgeons recommend follow-up observation after incomplete excision, this policy carries the disadvantage that a second operation may then be required, with the consequent risk of damage to the facial nerve. It is far safer to offer routine postoperative radiotherapy to patients with incompletely excised parotid tumours. At other sites such

as the submandibular and sublingual glands, wider excision may be possible since there is no risk of facial nerve trunk damage.

The indications for routine radiotherapy in malignant tumours are: inadequate surgical excision margins; tumours of high grade (particularly squamous, anaplastic and mixed malignant lesions); when surgery has been performed for recurrent disease; and for malignant lymphoma of the parotid, where surgery plays no part in the management, other than for biopsy. There is justification for the suggestion that postoperative radiotherapy should be offered in all cases of malignant salivary tumours. Lymphomas and adenocarcinomas are generally the most radiosensitive types of salivary tumour. Occasionally, surgery is contraindicated, for example in unfit or elderly patients, or in those with malignant tumours of the minor salivary glands in the nasopharynx or palate. In these circumstances, long-term control can sometimes be achieved with radiotherapy alone.

The radiotherapy technique may be technically demanding since large volumes of tissue need to be uniformly irradiated and care is required to avoid overtreatment to sensitive structures — the brainstem, eye and mucous membranes. The usual arrangement is a wedged pair of fields. Particular care must be taken to avoid irradiation of the contralateral eye from the exit beam. A dose of 50–55 Gy in 5–5.5 weeks is adequate treatment for residual benign tumours. Malignant parotid tumours need higher doses. If there is residual disease postoperatively 60–70 Gy in 6–8 weeks is recommended. Because of the initially large volume, a shrinking field technique may be necessary (see Chapter 5). The whole parotid bed should be treated up to the zygomatic arch and inferiorly to the level of the hyoid, to include both the jugulodigastric and upper cervical nodes. For submandibular and sublingual tumours, large treatment volumes are also required since the whole gland will need to be irradiated. Adenoid cystic lesions must be irradiated generously in view of the perineural invasion; with parotid cylindromas, the mastoid should always be treated.

Should the whole of the cervical node chain be irradiated in patients with malignant parotid tumours? Since the frequency of lymph node involvement varies with the histology, routine cervical node irradiation is only necessary in patients with squamous or anaplastic tumours, adenocarcinomas or mucoepidermoid and malignant mixed tumours of high grade. In some clinics, particularly in the USA, these patients are treated by elective lymph node dissection.

Prognosis

The outcome depends on the histological type [32] as well as operability. Routine use of postoperative radiotherapy increases local control in all of the major types, but squamous, anaplastic and high-grade mucoepidermoid carcinomas carry a poor prognosis because of both local recurrence and metastatic spread. Better results are seen with low-grade mucoepidermoid tumours and acinic cell tumours, with adenoid cystic and malignant mixed tumours carrying an intermediate prognosis. Overall, women have a better prognosis than men (10-year survival: 75% and 60%, respectively).

Further surgical excision is sometimes possible for localized recurrent disease while for distant metastases, palliative radiotherapy may be useful, particularly with less aggressive slow-growing tumours. Pulmonary and other distant metastases are encountered, particularly with adenoid cystic carcinoma. Treatment with chemotherapy has no established role.

Tumours of the orbit and eye [33]

Orbit

Both primary and secondary neoplasms occur in the orbit (Table 10.4). Lymphoma and rhabdomyosarcoma are the commonest primary tumours. Soft-tissue sarcoma, nerve and nerve sheath tumours (including optic nerve gliomas) and meningiomas are all seen occasionally. Orbital secondary deposits are likely to be due to carcinomas of the breast, bronchus or thyroid.

Clinical features

Because of the orbit's rigid structure, forward displacement of the globe (proptosis) is the cardinal physical sign. Ophthalmoplegia may also occur because of interference with the external ocular muscles or, less commonly, because of a third cranial nerve palsy, particularly with posteriorly placed tumours. Proptosis can be extreme and disfiguring, particularly in children. Chemosis and infection are common and may lead to a misdiagnosis of cellulitis. Panophthalmitis can lead to perforation of the globe and unilateral blindness is common with advanced tumours. The rapid onset of chemosis and lid oedema suggest that the tumour is malignant. Marked proptosis with normal ocular movement usually indicates a slow-growing benign tumour. Tumours within the muscle cone produce less disturbance of ocular movement but more proptosis and greater visual loss; those outside the cone produce eccentric proptosis and affect vision later.

INVESTIGATION

Plain X-rays and tomography can be extremely helpful and give good views of the orbital margins and optic canals. Greater detail is obtained with CT scanning, which gives information on the site, size and degree of intra- and extraorbital spread as well as a clear indication of bony erosion and soft-tissue tumour invasion (Fig. 10.3). Ultrasound examination may be helpful in providing rapid demonstration that a tumour is present. Biopsy confirmation of the diagnosis should be obtained where possible, but there may be formidable difficulties, with a risk of tumour spillage, haemorrhage and blindness. If the tumour is encapsulated it is usually best to excise it entirely.

Lymphoma

Malignant lymphomas of the orbit are almost always of the non-Hodgkin variety and may be isolated or encountered as part of a more generalized lymphoma (see Chapter 26). Full investigation is required as for any other lymphoma, since evidence of systemic disease will sometimes be found. Biopsy is usually straightforward since they tend to be anteriorly placed, and treatment with radiotherapy is usually successful. Even where systemic lymphoma is discovered, radiotherapy is used as an addition to systemic treatment in order to prevent local recurrence, and modest doses of the order of 30 Gy over 3 weeks are usually adequate.

Orbital pseudotumour

This condition usually presents as a painful ophthalmoplegia often accompanied by swelling of the eyelids. Computed tomography scanning shows a retro-orbital mass, often ill defined and surrounding the optic nerve. Histologically there is a pleomorphic inflammatory infiltrate but occasionally monotypic B cells can be demonstrated, indicating a low-grade lymphoma.

The disease responds rapidly to steroids which may prevent visual loss. Relapses occur and the 'tumour' may spread back through the orbital fissure to the base of the brain. Radiotherapy may help but, in rare cases, the disease can be relentlessly progressive.

Rhabdomyosarcoma

This is usually embryonal in type, occurring chiefly in infants, young children and adolescents, slightly more commonly in males. Local spread involves the maxilla, paranasal sinuses, frontal bone or even the brain, via the anterior or middle cranial fossae. Haematological spread is primarily to lung or bone but is less common than with rhabdomyosarcomas from other sites. Lymph node involvement, present in 25% of cases, usually involves upper deep cervical or preauricular nodes. These tumours often advance rapidly, leading to particularly severe proptosis with chemosis and lid oedema. Wherever possible, full pretreatment staging, including bone marrow aspiration, should be performed. Surgery was formerly used for control of the primary lesion, but radiotherapy has become increasingly preferred and has a low local recurrence rate. High doses of the order of 50 Gy over 5–6 weeks are required and a high proportion of these patients preserve useful vision provided that the lachrymal apparatus is shielded to ensure against xerophthalmia (see below).

Adjuvant chemotherapy is now an established part of treatment, with combinations of cyclophosphamide, vincristine and actinomycin D or doxorubicin. At least one course of combination chemotherapy is given before the orbital radiation, because of the high probability of extraocular spread and also because rapid resolution occurs which will make the child more comfortable and the radiotherapy technically easier. The chemotherapy should normally be continued for about 1 year. Local irradiation is important as a means of ensuring local control even when metastases are present. Routine use of chemotherapy has improved 5-year survival from 40% using surgery and radiotherapy alone to about 75%, with a particular improvement in tumours of younger children, which were previously notorious for their high probability of dissemination (see Chapter 24).

Lachrymal gland tumours

These are usually considered with orbital tumours, though they are extremely rare. Commonest in young adults, their histological spectrum is reminiscent of that of salivary gland tumours, with pleomorphic adenomas and adenoid cystic carcinomas the most frequently encountered types. There is usually a long history (longer than a year) of a slowly expanding, hard, painless mass. With more rapidly growing lesions, a biopsy is imperative and complete surgical removal of the tumour should be carried out if possible. Where total removal of the lachrymal

gland cannot be performed (for a patient with either a pleomorphic adenoma or any of the malignant tumours) radiotherapy should also be given. Local recurrence is very common even after a high dose, so every effort should be made to remove these tumours. True carcinomas of the lachrymal gland are rare, and extraorbital spread tends to occur early. Malignant lachrymal gland tumours are a miscellaneous group, difficult to treat and with a poor overall prognosis and a 5-year survival rate in the order of 20%. Mucosa-associated lymphoid tissue (MALT) lymphoma also occurs at this site, often accompanied clinically by Sjøgren-like syndrome (see Chapter 26). This prognosis is usually excellent as this variety of non-Hodgkin lymphoma is characteristically indolent.

Optic nerve glioma

This is discussed on p. 163.

Radiation techniques for tumours of the orbit

Although lead shielding of the cornea, lens and lachrymal sac is routinely recommended, it is impossible to arrange for homogeneous irradiation of the whole of the orbital content as well as adequate shielding of sensitive structures. A wedged pair of fields (see Chapter 5) is the usual arrangement. Great care must be taken to avoid irradiation of the contralateral eye, even though useful vision is often retained in the treated one. It is useful to ask the patient to look directly into the beam during treatment both to fix the gaze and to avoid the inevitable build-up effect of the closed lid. With supervoltage beams, the maximal energy deposition is deep to the cornea and may even partly spare the lens. Partial or complete corneal shielding can usually be achieved with a simple cylindrical shield, and conjunctival damage is uncommon particularly as low doses of radiation are well tolerated by this part of the eye. Where shielding is impossible, painful keratitis, sometimes with iridocyclitis or even corneal ulceration, may occur. Failure to shield the lachrymal gland will usually pose a greater threat to the integrity of the eye since the lachrymal apparatus has a lower tolerance, and doses of greater than 30 Gy over 3 weeks will cause significant reduction of tear production with consequent dryness of the eye, requiring regular instillation of lubricant drops.

The most radiosensitive structure in the eye is the lens itself (see Chapter 5, p. 61) and cataracts can develop after doses of a few Grays though clinically important lens opacity is rarely seen with doses below 15 Gy. With doses above 25 Gy, progressive cataract is almost invariable;

fortunately, these cataracts can be removed and an intra-ocular lens implanted. Other parts of the eye such as the retina and the sclera have a much higher radiation toler-ance closely similar to that of the central nervous system, and clinically important changes are uncommon where doses of less than 60 Gy are given by carefully fractionated external beam therapy.

Tumours of the eyelid and conjunctiva

Tumours of the eyelid are not uncommon and include basal cell and squamous cell carcinomas mostly occurring in elderly patients. The lower lid and inner canthus of the eye are the commonest sites (see Chapter 22). In the con-junctiva both melanoma and squamous cell carcinoma are occasionally encountered, and are important to diag-nose early since small lesions can be effectively treated by radiation, with conservation of the eye and preservation of vision. In general, local surgical excision is advisable, followed by radiotherapy using an applicator carrying a radioactive source, often ^{90}Sr. It is important to dis-tinguish true melanomas from precancerous ocular melanosis (a diffuse flat pigmented lesion) which can be clinically diagnosed with confidence, and should be observed without biopsy since malignant change may take years to develop. Overall prognosis of conjunctival melanoma is good (5-year survival about 75%), though patients with bulky lesions have a high risk of early fatal dissemination. Squamous carcinomas have an even better prognosis provided that adequate surgery and/or radio-therapy are expertly given.

Tumours of the globe

The two most common tumours are retinoblastoma and uveal (choroidal) melanoma. Retinoblastoma is discussed in Chapter 24.

Malignant melanoma of the uveal tract is the common-est intraocular tumour of adults (6 per million per year). Blood-borne metastases are common, but may not be-come clinically apparent for many years. Only 15% arise in the ciliary body and iris, but these present earlier and are more easily visible. Choroidal melanoma (85% of the total) may cause no symptoms at first unless arising from the macula. At other sites a peripheral field defect may go unnoticed. Retinal detachment may occur.

The diagnosis is normally made on inspection. Primary choroidal melanoma must be distinguished from secondary deposits since the choroid is a known site of metastasis of cutaneous melanoma.

In the past, immediate enucleation has been preferred to biopsy in the belief that biopsy was dangerous. A more conservative approach is now adopted, especially in the elderly. Small melanomas can probably be watched and surgery only considered when the tumour enlarges. Treat-ment is then by photocoagulation, cryotherapy, local ir-radiation to a high dose or surgery. In small lesions and tumours of the iris, enucleation can sometimes be avoided though it may be necessary for large lesions or where there is macular or optic nerve involvement or retinal detach-ment. Pain, local extension and secondary glaucoma are also indications for enucleation.

References

1 Fovastiere A, Koch W, Trotti A, Sideransky D. Medical progress. head and neck cancer. *N Engl J Med* 2001; 345: 1890–900.
2 Shah JP, Lydiatt W. Treatment of cancer of the head and neck. CA. *Cancer J Clin* 1995; 45: 352–68.
3 Grønbaek M, Becker U, Johansen D *et al.* Population based cohort study of the association between alcohol intake and cancer of the upper digestive tract. *Br Med J* 1998; 317: 844–8.
4 Brennan JA, Mao L, Hruban R *et al.* Molecular assessment of histopathological staging in squamous cell carcinoma of the head and neck. *N Engl J Med* 1995; 332: 429–35.
5 YuMC, Ho JHC, Lai S *et al.* Cantonese-style salted fish as a cause of nasopharyngeal carcinoma: a case control study in Hong Kong. *Cancer Res* 1986; 46: 956–61.
6 Vokes EE, Liebowitz DN, Weichselbaum R. Naso-pharyngeal carcinoma. *Lancet* 1997; 350: 1087–91.
7 Janot F, Klinjanienko J, Russo A *et al.* Prognostic value of clinico-pathological parameters in head-and-neck squamous cell carcinoma: a prospective analysis. *Br J Cancer* 1996; 73: 531–8.
8 Union Internationale Contre le Cancer. Sobin LH, Wittekind Ch, eds. *TNM Classification of Malignant Tumours*, 5th edn. New York: Wiley-Liss, 1997.
9 Shah JP. *Head and Neck Surgery*, 2nd edn. St Louis: Mosby, 1996.
10 Lefebvre J-L, Bonneterre J. Current status of larynx preserva-tion trials. *Curr Opin Oncol* 1996; 8: 209–14.
11 Chevalier D, Piquet JJ. Subtotal laryngectomy with cricohy-oidopexy for supraglottic carcinoma. review of 61 cases. *Am J Surg* 1994; 168: 472–3.
12 Jassar P, England RJA, Stafford ND. Restoration of voice after laryngectomy. *J Royal Soc Med* 1999; 92: 299–302.
13 Don DM, Anzai Y, Lufkin RB *et al.* Evaluation of cervical lymph node metastases in squamous cell carcinoma of the head and neck. *Laryngoscope* 1995; 105: 669–74.
14 Lederman M, Mould RE. Radiation treatment of cancer of

the pharynx: with special reference to telecobalt therapy. *Br J Radiol* 1968; 41: 251–74.

15 Martinez-Gimeno C, Rodriguez EM, Vila CN, Varela CL. Squamous cell carcinoma of the oral cavity: a clinicopathologic scoring system for evaluation risk of lymph node metastasis. *Laryngoscope* 1995; 105: 728–33.

16 Horiot JC, Le Fur R, N'Guyen T *et al.* Hyperfractionation vs. conventional fractionation in oropharyngeal carcinoma: final analysis of a randomized trial of the EORTC cooperative group of radiotherapy. *Radiother Oncol* 1992; 25: 229–32.

17 MacFarlane GJ, Boyle P, Scully C. Rising mortality from cancer of the tongue in young Scottish males. *Lancet* 1987; 2 (8564): 912.

18 Lippman SM, Batsakis JG, Toth BB *et al.* Comparison of low-dose isotretinoin with beta-carotene to prevent oral carcinogenesis. *N Engl J Med* 1993; 328: 15–20.

19 Hutchison I. Complications of radiotherapy in the head and neck: an orofacial surgeon's view. In: Tobias, JS, Thomas, PRM, eds. *Current Radiation Oncology*, Vol. 2. London: Edward Arnold, 1996: 144–77.

20 Montana FS, Hellman S, von Essen CF, Kligerman MM. Carcinoma of the tongue and floor of the mouth: Results of radical radiotherapy. *Cancer* 1969; 23: 1284–9.

21 Johnson JT, Ferretti GA, Netuery WJ *et al.* Oral pilocarpine for post-irradiation xerostomia in patients with head and neck cancer. *N Engl J Med* 1993; 329: 390–5.

22 Robin PE, Powell DJ, Stansbie JM. Carcinoma of the nasal cavity and paranasal sinuses: incidence and presentation of different histological types. *Clin Otolaryngol* 1979; 4: 431–56.

23 Lamont EB, Vokes EE. Chemotherapy in the management of squamous-cell carcinoma of head and neck. *Lancet Oncol* 2001; 2: 261–9.

24 Pignon JP, Bourhis J, Domengue C, Designe L. Chemo-therapy added to locoregional treatment for head and neck squamous cell carcinoma: three meta-analyses of updated individual data. *Lancet* 2000; 355: 949–55.

25 Vokes EE, Weichselbaum RR, Lippman SM *et al.* Medical progress: head and neck. *N Engl J Med* 1993; 328: 184–94.

26 Tobias JS. Current issues in cancer. Cancer of the head and neck. *Br Med J* 1994; 308: 961–6.

27 Munro AJ. An overview of randomized controlled trials of adjuvant chemotherapy in head and neck cancer. *Br J Cancer* 1995; 71: 83–91.

28 Gupta NL, Swindell R. Concomitant methotrexate and radiotherapy in advanced head and neck cancer: 15 year follow-up of a recognized clinical trial. *Clin Oncol* 2001; 13: 339–44.

29 Merlano M, Vitale V, Rosso R *et al.* Treatment of advanced squamous-cell carcinoma of the head and neck with alternating chemotherapy and radiotherapy. *N Engl J Med* 1992; 327: 1115–21.

30 Chua DTT, Sham JST, Choy D *et al.* Preliminary report of the Asian-Oceanian Clinical Oncology Association randomised trial comparing cisplatin and epirubicin followed by radiotherapy vs. radiotherapy alone in the treatment of patients with loco-regionally advanced nasopharyngeal carcinoma. *Cancer* 1998; 83: 2270–83.

31 Al-Sarraf M, LeBlanc M, Shanker Giri PG *et al.* Chemoradiotherapy vs. radiotherapy in patients with advanced nasopharyngeal cancer: phase III randomised intergroup study 0099. *J Clin Oncol* 1998; 16: 1310–17.

32 Hickman R, Cawson RA, Duffy SW. The prognosis of specific types of salivary gland tumours. *Cancer* 1984; 54: 1620–4.

33 Hernandez JG, Brady LW, Shields JA *et al.* Radiotherapy of ocular tumours. In: Tobias, JS, Thomas, PRM, eds. *Current Radiation in Oncology*, Vol. 1. London: Edward Arnold, 1994: 101–25.

11 Brain and spinal cord

Brain tumours

Brain tumours are among the most devastating of all malignant diseases, frequently producing profound and progressive disability leading to death. In addition, they are often difficult to diagnose and are invariably challenging to treat. The incidence appears to be rising steadily, at least in the USA; peak incidence is in the first decade of life and at age 50–60 years. Brain tumours are one of the most important groups of childhood tumours, second only to the leukaemias and lymphomas in frequency. In the UK the incidence is approximately six per 100 000, with 2200 deaths each year.

Very little is known of the aetiology. An increase in both benign and malignant brain tumours has been noted following radiation of the scalp for benign conditions in childhood. Cranial radiation (together with antimetabolite therapy) has also been implicated as a cause of brain tumour development in children given central nervous system (CNS) prophylaxis for acute leukaemia [1]. Significant differences exist in the frequency of brain tumours throughout life, suggesting the possibility of different aetiological factors in their causation [2]. Clearly, childhood and adult CNS tumours have different biological behaviour; only haemangioblastoma has an equal incidence in both childhood and adult life. Hormonal influences in pituitary adenoma and meningioma may explain the earlier peak age incidence of these tumours in females, and to some extent account for the apparent sex ratio differences.

Primary cerebral lymphoma has become far more frequently diagnosed with the advent of the acquired immune deficiency syndrome (AIDS) pandemic over the past decade. The other important recent aetiological factor in cerebral lymphoma is the increase over the past 20 years in successful organ transplantation.

Over the past 25 years, neurosurgical and radiotherapeutic techniques have improved with, in some instances, a positive impact on prognosis or a reduction in treatment morbidity. More recently, a possible role for cytotoxic agents has begun to emerge, although their contribution is not yet fully established.

Cellular biology of brain tumours

The growth kinetics of malignant brain tumours have been widely studied in recent years, mostly using incorporation of radiolabelled DNA precursors such as ^{3}H-thymidine or bromodeoxyuridine (BUdR) and quantifying the result by immunological techniques with a specific anti-BUdR-DNA monoclonal antibody. Higher-grade tumours have much higher labelling indices [3], and are more likely on flow cytometry studies to exhibit aneuploidy.

Oncogene analysis has also proven valuable, in over 50% of glioblastoma multiforme, for example, amplification of N-myc, C-myc, N-ras or other oncogenes is present, often with simultaneous overexpression of more than one. In addition, the epidermal growth factor receptor (EGFR; see Chapter 3) is usually highly expressed, and encoded for by the erb-B oncogene [4].

At least six specific and frequently occurring molecular genetic alterations have been identified in the pathogenesis of gliomas. In the amplification of EGFR, a specific gene appears responsible. In high-grade tumours, hemi- and homozygous deletion of interferon loci at chromosome 9p has been demonstrated. Major karyotypic alterations also occur: in primitive neuroectodermal tumours including medulloblastoma, deletion of the short arm of chromosome 17 is common. Loss of heterozygosity on chromosome 10 is also frequent, with a specific association with glioblastoma [5]. Tumour suppressor gene(s) are present on the distal portion of this chromosome's long arm.

Other specific aberrations are beginning to emerge, particularly involving chromosomes 1, 3, 7 and 22 [6]. One particularly well-studied tumour is the meningioma, which frequently displays monosomy 22.

Pathological classification of brain tumours

The majority of brain tumours are gliomas, thought to arise from malignant change of mature glial elements, usually with differentiation towards one particular type of glial cell [7]. Although it now seems clear that tumour progression can occur, for example from astrocytoma to glioblastoma, no predisposing premalignant states have been recognized in human glioma—unlike many other human solid tumours.

Taken together, astrocytomas, ependymomas, oligodendrogliomas and medulloblastomas comprise over 90% of all primary brain and spinal cord tumours. In cases where the tumour is well differentiated, there is usually no difficulty in recognizing the type of cell from which the tumour has arisen.

These tumours are classified according to the cell of origin and a widely accepted working classification is given in Table 11.1. Other more detailed classifications have been proposed by the World Health Organization, but the simpler system outlined in Table 11.1 is used in this chapter.

Gliomas

ASTROCYTOMAS

These are much the commonest variety and arise from astrocytes which are the supporting cells of the brain. They are divided into four grades (according to Kernohan) on the basis of cytomorphological characteristics. Grade I is the least malignant. Grades II–IV show progressively more malignant characteristics, with the degree of malignancy assessed according to histological features such as invasion, tumour necrosis, cellularity, pleomorphism and mitotic activity. Low-grade gliomas (Fig. 11.1a) chiefly occur in the frontal, parietal and temporal lobes and in the brainstem and cerebellum of children. Local destruction is unusual, in contrast to high-grade gliomas, in which degeneration, necrosis, haemorrhage, infarction and local destruction are characteristic.

Biopsy specimens are not always representative of the whole tumour: mixed varieties are common. Descriptive terms are sometimes used where a particular morpholog-

Table 11.1 Simplified classification of brain tumours.

Primary tumours		Secondary tumours
Gliomas	*Pineal tumours*	*Common sites of origin*
Astrocytoma	Pinealoblastoma	Lung
Glioblastoma multiforme	Pinealocytoma	Breast
Ependymoma	Germinoma	Melanoma
Oligodendroglioma	Teratoma	
Primitive neuroectodermal		*Less common sites of origin*
tumours (including	*Intracranial lymphoma*	Ovary
medulloblastoma)	'Histiocytic' lymphoma	Testis
Pituitary tumours	Microglioma	Gut
Pituitary adenoma		Bladder
Craniopharyngioma	*Acoustic*	Kidney
Pituitary carcinoma		Pancreas
	Chordoma	Liver
Meningioma		Leukaemia and lymphoma
Benign	*Neuronal tumours*	
Malignant	Ganglioneuroma	*Miscellaneous*
(meningiosarcoma)	Ganglioglioma	Langerhans' cell
	Colloid cyst	histiocytosis (LCH)

ical feature predominates—the terms *fibrillary, protoplasmic, gemistocytic* or *pilocytic* are used to describe relatively well-differentiated types of astrocytoma. These subdivisions may have considerable prognostic significance (see below). In highly malignant gliomas it may be impossible to recognize the initial cell of origin—they are among the most bizarre and undifferentiated of all tumours, often termed *glioblastoma multiforme* (Fig. 11.1b). Growing rapidly by direct extension they are always much larger than suggested by imaging studies such as computed tomography (CT) or magnetic resonance imaging (MRI). They are rarely operable, do not as a rule respond impressively to irradiation and are usually fatal within a year. By contrast, low-grade gliomas enlarge much more slowly and can often be excised completely, though local recurrence does sometimes occur. They comprise over 30% of all childhood brain tumours [8].

True grade I gliomas are, however, extremely unusual—most low-grade gliomas are grade II. Gliomas at different sites may behave quite differently despite a similar histological appearance. For this reason, localized gliomas of the optic nerves are often left untreated and may regress spontaneously while gliomas of the pons or brainstem are much more aggressive and demand urgent attention with wide-field irradiation.

EPENDYMAL TUMOURS

These comprise about 5% of all primary brain tumours and are derived from the ciliated lining cells of the CNS cavities. The tumour cells form characteristic rosettes (Fig. 11.1c). This most commonly occurs in childhood and early adult life, just over half arising from infratentorial sites. Tumour spread occurs by direct invasion and also by seeding throughout the CNS, particularly with high-grade ependymoma and where the primary tumour is infratentorial. Although tumour grading is perhaps less important than with astrocytomas, low-grade ependymomas have a far better prognosis than the higher grades. Most aggressive of all is the ependymoblastoma.

OLIGODENDROGLIOMAS

These are derived from other supporting cells and are usually very indolent in their growth pattern, with a long history, often calcifying. The cells have a typical appearance (Fig. 11.1d) with a clear zone around the nucleus, the cells appearing 'boxed in'. Typical sites are the frontal, parietal and temporal lobes. The commonest age range is 40–60 years. The clinical history is often lengthier than with astrocytomas, and these tumours can be surprisingly radiosensitive.

MEDULLOBLASTOMA

The term *primitive neuroectodermal tumour* is now increasingly preferred to describe these, and certain other, embryonal tumours. Cytogenetically there is a characteristic loss of genetic information often from chromosome 17. They comprise 3% of all brain tumours and are predominantly diagnosed in childhood and young adult life, with few cases occurring after the age of 25 years. There is a peak age incidence of 4–10 years, and the tumour chiefly arises in the posterior fossa, from the vermis, cerebellar hemispheres or the fourth ventricle. Patients usually present with raised intracranial pressure (see below). Because of close proximity to the cerebrospinal fluid (CSF) the tumour metastasizes via the CSF either to the spinal cord or elsewhere in the brain. Occasionally, distant metastases are seen outside the CNS, and bone metastases (mostly osteosclerotic) and marrow involvement are occasionally encountered. Other sites include lung and lymph nodes.

Pituitary tumours

Comprising about 10% of primary intracranial neoplasms, these usually arise from the glandular epithelial cells, producing tumours which are histologically classified according to the staining characteristics of the cytoplasmic granules. Granular staining is mostly absent (chromophobe tumours, Fig. 11.1f) but in a minority there is characteristic acidophilic or basophilic staining. Increasingly, however, these tumours are pathologically classified using functional and immunological criteria. Non-epithelial pituitary tumours arise from cell rests from Rathke's pouch, producing tumours known as *craniopharyngiomas*. This part of the brain is also a common site of secondary cancer, chiefly from breast cancer and small-cell lung cancer (SCLC).

Chromophobe adenomas comprise about three-quarters of all pituitary tumours, and are more common in adult life. They tend to be non-functional (endocrine-inactive), though adrenocorticotrophic hormone (ACTH), growth hormone (GH), prolactin and other hormones are sometimes produced. They frequently attain a large size, particularly if non-functioning, and may extend upwards out of the sella, to involve the optic chiasm leading to the characteristic visual disturbance of bitemporal hemianopia (Fig. 11.2). Of the chromophil tumours, the acidophil adenomas are chiefly associated with excessive production of GH, leading either to acromegaly if the tumour arises in adult life, or very rarely to gigantism when the tumour occurs in childhood. Basophilic tumours tend to be smaller, usually secreting ACTH and/or melanocyte-

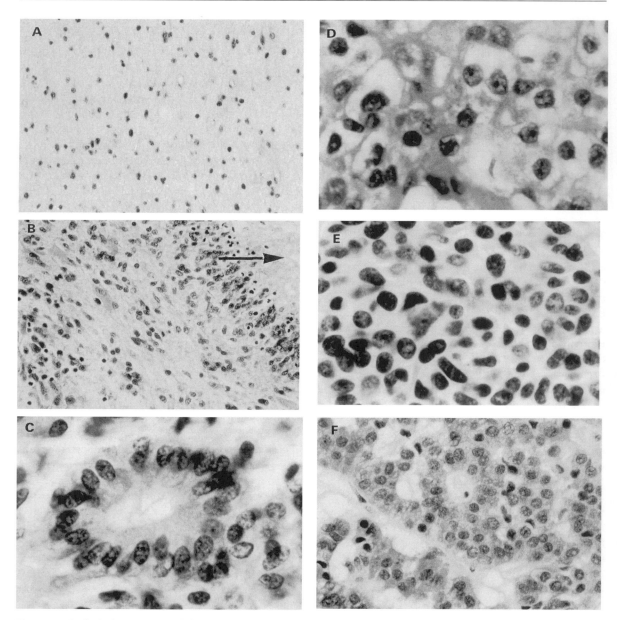

Fig. 11.1 Histological appearance of the commoner brain tumours. (A) Low-grade glioma showing sparse cellularity with no vascular proliferation (original magnification × 200). (B) High-grade glioma showing cellular pleomorphism and necrosis (arrowed) (× 200). (C) Ependymoma: tumour forms typical rosettes (× 400). (D) Oligodendroglioma showing typical 'boxed-in' cell appearance (× 400). (E) Medulloblastoma showing small, darkly staining, closely packed cells (× 400). (F) Pituitary adenoma: appearance is characteristic of endocrine tumours (× 250).

stimulating hormone, leading to Cushing's syndrome sometimes with hyperpigmentation. These tumours are usually small and rarely involve the suprasellar area, so visual signs are unusual.

Meningioma

These comprise about 10% of all brain tumours and arise from the meninges. There is a predilection for certain

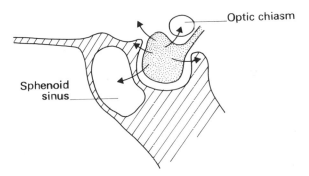

Fig. 11.2 Local effects of pituitary tumours. Extension commonly produces pressure on the optic chiasm, base of brain and anterior and posterior clinoid processes. Extension occurs inferiorly and laterally, to sphenoid and cavernous sinuses.

sites, particularly the parasagittal region and sphenoid ridge. They often cause cerebral compression but frank invasion is very uncommon except for the rare malignant meningioma, sometimes referred to as meningiosarcoma. Pressure outwards may cause erosion of the inner table of the skull, while inward displacement of the brain may lead to epilepsy as an early feature. Meningiomas may be chiefly fibrous in nature (fibroblastic meningioma) or very vascular (angioblastic meningioma), the latter having a more rapid evolution and more frequent malignant transformation. A specific genetic abnormality, monosomy 22, is present in up to 70% of cases.

Others

TUMOURS OF THE PINEAL AND THIRD VENTRICLE
This is a highly diverse group of tumours arising either from the pineal itself, the third ventricle, or less commonly from ectopic sites of pineal tissue, particularly in the hypothalamus. Common types include the *pinealoblastoma*, which histologically resembles medulloblastoma; the *pinealocytoma*, which is a tumour of mature pineal cells; and *germ cell tumours*, which can be either pure seminoma (pineal germinoma) or teratoma, often contain highly differentiated mesenchymal structures. These latter tumours may produce α-fetoprotein (AFP) and human chorionic gonadotrophin (HCG) which can be measured in CSF or blood often critical for diagnosis and management (see Chapter 4). At the anterior end of the third ventricle, the histological types are even more varied and include *pituitary tumours, germinomas, meningiomas, optic nerve glioma*, LCH and *non-malignant granulomas* which can occasionally cause diagnostic difficulty, such

as tuberculosis and sarcoidosis. In proven pineal and suprasellar germinomas there is a high risk of spinal seeding (20–30%), possibly aggravated by attempts at surgical excision.

INTRACEREBRAL LYMPHOMAS (see also Chapter 26)
These are unusual, but now far more common as one of the recognized AIDS-related malignancies. The two main types are the 'histiocytic' lymphoma, which can occur at any site in the brain and appears more frequently in immune-suppressed patients such as renal transplant recipients; and the microglioma, a rare intracranial lymphoma not seen outside the CNS.

THALAMIC AND BRAINSTEM TUMOURS
These are usually gliomas, though surgical biopsy is generally regarded as inadvisable. Thalamic gliomas are seen both in children (usually well-differentiated tumours) and adults (usually glioblastoma multiforme). Brainstem tumours are also chiefly encountered in children and are usually astrocytomas of variable differentiation.

TUMOURS OF CRANIAL NERVES AND NERVE SHEATHS
Acoustic neuroma is a tumour of adult life, rather more common in females, and arising from the VIII cranial nerve, usually in its vestibular part. These tend to be slow-growing tumours which present with unilateral deafness, vertigo, tinnitus, and involvement of other cranial nerves. Although strictly benign, they exert a local space-occupying mass effect. Other less common neuronal tumours include the ganglioneuroma and ganglioglioma which are also typically benign though dangerous because of local pressure effects.

CHORDOMAS
These uncommon malignant tumours originate from the remnants of the embryonic notochord. Although occasionally encountered in children and young adults, the peak age of incidence is 50–60 years and the characteristic sites are in the extremes of the spinal cord: a spheno-occipitocervical group (40% of all cases) and a sacrococcygeal group (equally frequent). The tumour consists of very characteristic solid cords of polygonal or mucin-containing 'physaliperous' cells, sometimes with a lobulated pattern. Local pressure symptoms are common, including bulbar, occipital or neck symptoms from tumours at the upper end of the spine, or constipation and low back pain from sacrococcygeal tumours. Extensive bone destruction may occur.

Clinical features

Brain tumours can be difficult to diagnose. The onset of symptoms may be late, particularly in tumours situated in less critical areas of the brain, where they often grow to a substantial size before diagnosis, only producing subtle changes in personality, muscular power or co-ordination. In more critically sited tumours, obvious symptoms such as convulsions, ataxia or sensorimotor loss lead to much earlier diagnosis.

Symptoms can be divided into four main groups.

1 The tumour can exert a *mass effect* and lead to raised intracranial pressure, with headache, drowsiness, nausea and vomiting as the cardinal symptoms. The headache is often worse in the morning, typically clearing by lunchtime. Vomiting may be sudden, unexpected and not preceded by nausea. Tumours situated around the fourth ventricle, in the cerebellum and around the pons are particularly likely to lead to raised intracranial pressure (Fig. 11.3) often with ventricular enlargement.

2 There is a large group of *focal symptoms* caused by damage to local structures. These are determined by the site and size of the tumour. In a relatively small space, occupying lesions can cause devastating symptoms if sited in the motor cortex, Broca's area or the base of the brain. Accurate siting of tumours is often possible as a result of these specific symptoms: myoclonic seizures, development of late-onset grand mal epilepsy and hemiparesis all point to lesions in the motor cortex, whereas lip-smacking, hallucinations and other psychotic disturbances are typical of a temporal lobe lesion. For tumours situated more deeply, visual disturbances occur due to interruption of the visual pathways. At the base of the brain, the classical features are those of cranial nerve lesions, often multiple. Tumours near the jugular foramen cause a specific pattern of cranial nerve palsies since many of the lower cranial nerves exit at or near this point. Ataxia, nystagmus and diplopia are typical of cerebellar lesions, often coupled with nausea and headache due to raised intracranial pressure.

3 The third group of symptoms results from *remote endocrine effects*, occurring with tumours of the pituitary and hypothalamus. Damage to local structures is of great importance in pituitary tumours which can extend upwards to the suprasellar area and optic chiasm, inferiorly into the sphenoid sinus or laterally to the cavernous sinus or beyond, sometimes into the middle or posterior fossa (Fig. 11.2). Damage to the III, IV and VI cranial nerves may occur. Bleeding into a pituitary tumour (pituitary apoplexy) results in sudden deterioration of vision, severe headache and hypopituitarism. Lesser degrees of panhypopituitarism are common in pituitary tumours, though different end organs may be variably affected. The florid syndrome includes hypothyroidism from reduction in thyroid-stimulating hormone (TSH) production, hypocorticism with hypotension from reduction in ACTH and hypogonadism with loss of secondary sexual characteristics, libido and amenorrhoea with infertility. Sophisticated endocrinological investigations are often required to determine the full extent of the pituitary syndrome, but simple measurements of tri-iodothyronine (T3), thyroxine (T4), TSH, cortisol and gonadotrophins (and GH in children) are usually sufficient for demonstration of the basic defects.

4 Tumours of the CNS occasionally *metastasize*. This usually occurs late in the disease: although very unusual in adults, metastases are well recognized in children with

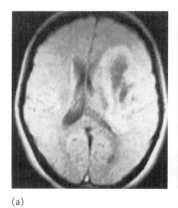
(a)

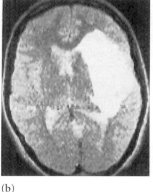
(b)

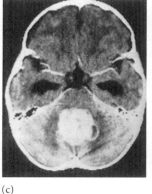
(c)

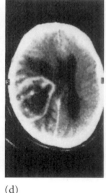
(d)

Fig. 11.3 (a) CT scan showing a large mass (glioma) in the left hemisphere. (b) MRI scan from same case as (a). (c) CT brain scan showing large midline tumour of the posterior fossa. This was a medulloblastoma. (d) CT brain scan showing large parieto-occipital glioma. Note the obvious rim of contrast with oedema and ventricular dilatation.

medulloblastomas and poorly differentiated ependymomas. Secondary spread from these tumours is almost always via the CSF, usually presenting as spinal or meningeal deposits. Bone metastasis is also a well-recognized complication of medulloblastoma.

The accurate diagnosis of brain tumours has been revolutionized by the advent of contrast-enhanced CT and MRI scanning (Fig. 11.3). Both carry the advantages of high definition and easy repeatability, CT brain scanning does, however, have its limitations, particularly in tumours of the posterior fossa and brainstem. In these sites, MRI is clearly superior. Pituitary tumours require high resolution since they are often small and close to bony structures. Most CT scanning machines can reliably detect lesions greater than $1\,cm^3$ but low-grade gliomas are sometimes poorly visualized. Angiography is still indicated to exclude arteriovenous malformations and occasionally to visualize posterior fossa, deep-seated and thalamic lesions and other sites poorly visualized by CT or MRI scanning. In addition, preoperative angiography may be helpful in defining the tumour's vascular supply. Digital subtraction techniques provide excellent images in these situations.

Management of brain tumours

Surgical removal or biopsy is desirable both for histological diagnosis and sometimes for definitive treatment. Radical excision can, however, be extremely hazardous and Stereotactic CT-guided biopsy is used for histological confirmation in inoperable cases. Where hydrocephalus is present surgical decompression by ventriculoperitoneal drainage results in dramatic improvement. For deep-seated (for example, thalamic, pineal and brainstem) tumours even a biopsy may be out of the question. Urgent reversal of acute cerebral oedema may be necessary, which may include the use of intravenous urea, mannitol, or high doses of dexamethasone (see p. 173 for management details). Radiotherapy is frequently employed as an adjunct to surgery and sometimes as the definitive treatment both in adults [9] and children [8]. The role of chemotherapy is still debatable, though cytotoxic drugs are increasingly used.

Gliomas

LOW-GRADE (KERNOHAN GRADES I AND II)
Complete surgical excision is often attempted since these lesions tend to be well localized and can often be removed from adjacent structures without causing too much damage. In many cases surgery is the sole method of treatment.

However, late local recurrences may occur, sometimes at a higher tumour grade. Routine irradiation is now established as an important mode of treatment in incompletely resected tumours, at least in adults. One recent study (from the Mayo Clinic) of 167 low-grade astrocytomas showed that in the pilocytic group (41 cases) there was a good prognosis regardless of postoperative treatment. In the remainder, radiotherapy clearly prolonged survival especially if the tumour dose exceeded 53 Gy, in which case the 5-year survival rate was 68% compared with 21% when radiotherapy was not given [10]. Interestingly, complete surgical excision did not appear critically important so radiotherapy may become the dominant therapeutic modality in low-grade gliomas. In childhood brain tumours the same general principles seem to apply (see also Chapter 24).

Although postoperative irradiation is now increasingly recommended in all cases, a recent large-scale European multicentre study has failed to demonstrate a clear-cut radiation dose–response for low-grade cerebral glioma [11]. Three hundred and seventy-nine patients were randomly assigned to treatment either with low (45 Gy over 5 weeks) or high-dose (59.4 Gy over 6.6 weeks) radiotherapy, with a median follow-up of 74 months; overall survival (58%) and progression-free survival (48%) were similar in both groups.

HIGH-GRADE (KERNOHAN GRADES III AND IV)
For these tumours radiotherapy is almost always employed as an adjunct to surgery (Fig. 11.4) — first, because complete surgical removal is rarely possible; and second, because the results of surgery alone are so poor. Recent studies of postoperative irradiation for glioblastoma multiforme have demonstrated that, although at 1 year

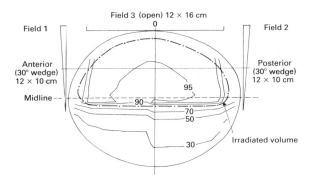

Fig. 11.4 External beam radiation for cortical glioma. Typical three-field plan treating whole hemisphere. The irradiated volume is shown by the broken line (– • –).

there are no survivors with surgery alone, almost one-fifth of patients receiving postoperative radiation are still alive. Large radiation volumes are required, sometimes including the whole of the brain. Doses of 40–50 Gy in 4.5–6 weeks are often used (Fig. 11.4), or higher doses if the target volume can be sufficiently focused [12]. However, the ultimate prognosis remains very poor, less than 6% of patients with grade IV disease surviving for 5 years. For patients with grade III tumours, the survival is better, and over half of the surviving patients achieve an independent life (Fig. 11.5).

Attempts to improve these dismal figures have led to the use of wide-field irradiation or treatment to higher dosage, since local recurrence at the initial tumour site is almost always the cause of death. If a safe means of increasing the dose could be found, better local control might be possible and there is increasing interest in at least three novel radiation techniques: interstitial brachytherapy, stereotactic external beam irradiation and hyperfractionated radiotherapy.

1 Interstitial brachytherapy, often using ^{125}Ir or ^{60}Co sources, permits the delivery of high doses of radiotherapy to the volume without unnecessary treatment of large areas of normal brain, and can be used in conjunction with stereotactic surgery. A large series from San Francisco suggested that this technique might be valuable both for primary treatment and also recurrent disease [13], particularly in grade III lesions, though the excellent results from this group probably reflect careful selection of tumours which are limited by size and the performance status of the subject. Indeed, these features, together with age and clinical history, are known to be important prognostic factors [12]. Unfortunately, however, the use of

high-dose brachytherapy has failed to prevent a familiar pattern of locoregional failure [14].

2 External beam stereotactic radiosurgery has been widely tested in recent years [15,16]. Compared with interstitial irradiation, it has the advantage of non-invasiveness and can also be employed together with more conventional wide-field external beam therapy—even including whole-brain irradiation. Only a limited number of patients are suitable for treatment by radiosurgery but the technique seems promising with small tumours which, due to their precise location, are unsuitable for surgical resection (for example, brainstem, thalamus, optic tract). The precision of stereotactic radiosurgery offers the hope of a higher-dose treatment to a more restricted volume than would be possible by other external beam approaches.

Cytotoxic agents are sometimes used as an adjuvant to surgery and radiotherapy for high-grade gliomas. The nitrosoureas *bis*-chloroethyl nitrosourea (BCNU) and *cis*-chloroethyl nitrosourea (CCNU) have received most attention, since they are known to be lipid-soluble and cross the hypothetical blood–brain barrier (see Chapter 6). Assessment of response of brain tumours to chemotherapy is difficult, but there is no doubt that some patients with recurrent disease benefit, though most of these responses are short-lived. In a large prospective multicentre trial, Walker and coworkers showed that routine use of BCNU as an addition to surgery and radiotherapy prolonged the median survival only by a few weeks [17]. Treatment by surgery and chemotherapy (but no irradiation) was much less successful. There is a possible slight superiority for CCNU over BCNU.

Temozolomide is a recently introduced, cytotoxic, new drug active against gliomas. It is an alkylating agent and is a derivative of mutozolomide but less toxic, with myelosuppression as the main side-effect. It is more active in recurrent glioblastoma than procarbazine [17]. Its role in newly diagnosed glioblastoma multiforme (GBM) is being evaluated.

In spite of many small randomized trials over 30 years the role of chemotherapy in high-grade malignant glioma is still uncertain. A meta-analysis using updated individual patient data has now been performed and shows a 6% increase in 2-year survival if chemotherapy is given [18]. This result will undoubtedly stimulate further study of chemotherapy in these tumours. Intra-arterial drug treatment has proved to be unacceptably toxic.

Other agents with known activity are temozolamide, vincristine and procarbazine. These drugs have the added advantage of being relatively non-toxic. Cisplatin and

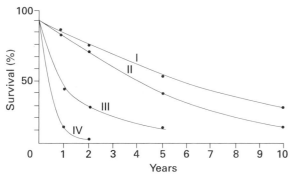

Fig. 11.5 Survival related to grade in malignant glioma. Note the small proportion of 10-year survivors even with low-grade tumours.

vepesid (VM26) have recently been shown to have some activity.

One commonly used combination is procarbazine, CCNU and vincristine (PCV), a well-tolerated regimen often used as adjuvant therapy and given on a 6-weekly outpatient basis.

EPENDYMOMA

This is far less common than astrocytoma and behaves differently. It arises from cells lining the ventricles and central canal of the spinal cord, and has a tendency to seed throughout the subarachnoid space, giving rise to symptomatic spinal deposits in about 10% of patients, particularly in patients with high-grade lesions, especially if arising from the fourth ventricle. For this reason, routine craniospinal irradiation is usually recommended in all patients with high-grade ependymomas and for ependymomas of the posterior fossa regardless of grade (see p. 170 for details of technique and toxicity). The primary site should receive a high dose (50 Gy or greater in 5–7 weeks) with full craniospinal treatment in patients with high-grade tumours. Spinal cord primaries tend to be of lower grade than intracerebral tumours, with a better survival rate.

The overall survival is better than with astrocytomas, over 50% of patients surviving 5 years. In a report by Phillips and coworkers [19] the 5-year survival of patients given *intensive* radiotherapy was almost 90%, twice the overall survival rate of 40% (which included those who died postoperatively without treatment as well as patients who received inadequate irradiation dosage). The exceptionally rare choroid plexus carcinoma is also best treated by surgery with routine postoperative radiotherapy [20].

OLIGODENDROGLIOMA

These uncommon tumours are often relatively well differentiated, slow growing and amenable to complete surgical removal. Postoperative irradiation is advisable where there has been incomplete surgical excision or where there are histologically aggressive features (sometimes termed *oligodendroblastoma*). In a group of over 30 patients, reported by Sheline and coworkers, the 5-year survival with surgery alone was 31%, compared with an 85% survival rate in patients receiving postoperative irradiation [20]. From these and other data, the 10-year survival rate is of the order of 35%.

For recurrent oligodendroglioma there is increasing evidence of chemoresponsiveness, using either PCV or cisplatin [21].

DEEP-SEATED GLIOMAS

Gliomas situated deep to the cerebral cortex present particular problems of diagnosis and management. Important sites include the thalamus and hypothalamus, pons, brainstem, pineal region and optic nerves. Histological confirmation is often impossible because surgical intervention could be so hazardous, though gliomas of the pineal area are increasingly considered suitable, particularly since histology at the site is so critical to management.

Their clinical behaviour varies greatly. Optic nerve gliomas, which usually present with proptosis or blindness, are often thought to be benign and unresponsive to radiotherapy. However, in some cases the tumours are bilateral, involve the optic chiasm or extend backwards to the ventricles, sometimes with hydrocephalus. These should be treated with radiotherapy. Although uncomplicated lesions may be self-limiting, radiotherapy may produce complete relief of distressing proptosis, and objective response verified on CT or MRI scanning. Pierce *et al.* [22] reported a series of 24 children with optic nerve glioma with lengthy follow-up (median 6 years) and an overall 6-year survival rate of 100%. Over 90% of patients had improvement or 'stabilization' of vision.

For thalamic tumours, radiotherapy is almost invariably indicated since surgical excision or even histological confirmation is so dangerous at this site. The prognosis appears to vary with age, though, as expected, histological grade (usually obtained only at autopsy) is also important. The 5-year survival rate in young patients with grade III lesions is about 25%.

Tumours of the pons and brainstem carry a particularly poor prognosis, often presenting with florid symptoms including cranial nerve palsies, ataxia or involvement of the long tracts. These are usually high-grade astrocytomas and infiltrate widely, often attaining a large volume before diagnosis. They are a challenge to the radiotherapist since they are surgically untreatable, but often present with urgent problems in management. The majority show a symptomatic response to radiotherapy, but the ultimate survival rate (approximately 15%) is poor. A large review of patients with brainstem tumours showed an average survival of 4 years for irradiated patients, compared with only 15 months if untreated. With a documented response to treatment, average survival was over 5 years. Large lateral opposed fields are required since the tumour has usually spread throughout the whole of the pons, brainstem and medulla and often to the upper cervical spine. Doses of 40–55 Gy in 4–5 weeks daily treatment are usually recommended although some centres employ fewer fractions, for example a total dose of 45–48 Gy in 15 daily fractions.

MEDULLOBLASTOMA (AND OTHER PRIMITIVE NEUROECTODERMAL TUMOURS)

Surgical treatment alone is unsuccessful, and postoperative radiotherapy has been routinely employed since the 1920s, when the marked radiosensitivity of this tumour was first noted. With increasingly accurate treatment planning, the use of supervoltage equipment and prophylactic irradiation of the whole brain and spinal cord, the 10-year survival rate has improved and is close to 50% [23].

An attempt at surgical removal is bound to increase the complication rate. However, although these tumours are radiosensitive, they do recur at the primary site, and removal of tumour bulk appears to reduce the rate of local recurrence. Most neurosurgeons excise as much tumour as is safely possible and it is now routine practice to offer postoperative irradiation. The whole of the craniospinal axis should be treated as soon after surgery as possible. Treatment planning must be meticulous, taking particular care to treat the base of the brain, retro-orbital area and brainstem (Fig. 11.6). These sites can be undertreated if adult surface anatomical boundaries are used without regard to the anatomy of the developing brain. The technique which we employ is carried out as follows.

1 Irradiation of the whole brain with large lateral opposing fields, including the midbrain and upper cervical vertebrae as far as the lower limit of C2, to a midline dose of 30 Gy in 3 weeks.

2 Boosting of the posterior fossa and midbrain as far anteriorly as the anterior clinoid process, to 45 Gy at the same rate.

3 At the same time as the posterior fossa boost is commenced, spinal irradiation is begun, from the lower border of the cerebral fields to the lower border of vertebra S2 so that the entire spinal cord, including the conus medullaris and cauda equina, is treated. A dose of not less than 30 Gy is given to the spine over 4–5 weeks.

4 For the final part of treatment, the posterior fossa is boosted to a still higher dose. The final brain doses are as follows: posterior fossa, 50–55 Gy in 6–7 weeks; midbrain, 45 Gy in 5–6 weeks; cerebral hemispheres and anterior part of brain, 35 Gy in 4 weeks; and spinal cord, 30 Gy minimum dose in 4–5 weeks.

5 Further boosting of limited areas of the spine if shown to be positive for tumour seeding, using myelographic or MRI.

It is important to monitor the blood count during treatment of the spine, but with this technique and dose rate

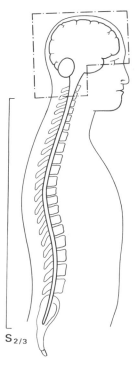

$S_{2/3}$

Fig 11.6 Craniospinal irradiation. Schematic representation of the field arrangement for craniospinal irradiation in medulloblastoma and other tumours which seed through the CSF.

the treatment rarely has to be discontinued, although the white blood count frequently falls to about 2×10^9/l by the end of treatment.

Irradiation of the whole neuraxis carries a number of drawbacks. Fortunately, skull growth is usually almost complete by the time of treatment, so permanent reduction in skull volume is very rare. Nevertheless, some degree of shortness of stature (particularly sitting height) must be expected from irradiation of the whole spine coupled with pituitary irradiation (see Chapter 5). In addition, midline organs such as the thyroid, larynx, oesophagus, thymus and heart are directly in the path of the exit beam, and the kidneys and female gonads are also likely to receive significant scattered irradiation despite the most careful planning. The need for whole-spine irradiation has therefore been questioned, especially as only 10% of children will develop spinal cord metastases.

Despite these hazards and the possible added problem of cognitive/learning defects, over 75% of surviving children lead independent and active lives and at least one study has shown that intellectual achievement in these children is not impaired. In the context of curative treatment by whole CNS irradiation there is little doubt that possible hazards of treatment have to be accepted [24].

Chemotherapy has mainly been used for treatment of recurrent disease and as initial treatment in very young children (under 2 years) in whom CNS irradiation carries particular toxicity. Lipid-soluble agents have been used both singly and in combination. Responses are usually short-lived, and combination chemotherapy may be difficult if relapse follows soon after craniospinal irradiation because of the volume of irradiated bone marrow. Methotrexate, which may be of some value, may be hazardous within 6 months of irradiation as it can cause leucoencephalopathy.

Combination chemotherapy is increasingly preferred to single-agent treatment, and response rates up to 75% have been reported. It has recently been established that both cisplatin and carboplatin are active agents. Chemotherapy is also increasingly used for recurrent childhood malignant glioma, and a few studies have produced encouraging results using CCNU, vincristine and prednisone [25].

Cytotoxic chemotherapy has also been used as an adjuvant to surgery and radiotherapy. The International Society for Paediatric Oncology has undertaken a large trial to assess the role of adjuvant chemotherapy with vincristine and CCNU [26]. From a series of over 330 cases, the main beneficiaries appear to be those where the tumour was incompletely removed, with brainstem spread and below 3 years of age.

It is often possible to obtain symptomatic improvement in patients with recurrence by further radiotherapy, particularly if the initial treatment was given at least 3 years beforehand.

Pituitary tumours [27]

For small tumours without suprasellar extension, many surgeons now favour resection via the trans-sphenoidal route, which avoids the complications of craniotomy, although infection and CSF rhinorrhoea are occasionally encountered. Over 90% of patients with visual field defects have satisfactory postoperative reversal of the visual symptoms with only a few requiring craniotomy after trans-sphenoidal resection, even with relatively large non-active macroadenomas with suprasellar extension. For larger tumours and those with extension outside the pituitary fossa, craniotomy still may be necessary. In children with craniopharyngioma, surgery can be particularly difficult (see p. 163).

Postoperative irradiation for patients with pituitary tumours decreases the likelihood of local recurrence. Chromophobe adenomas are more radiosensitive than chromophil tumours. In patients with acromegaly (almost always due to a chromophil tumour), arrest or reversal of the syndrome can be achieved with surgery and postoperative irradiation in 75% of cases. Pituitary irradiation is clearly the treatment of choice after unsuccessful surgery for patients with Cushing's disease [28]. Craniopharyngioma requires a high local dose for eradication (50–60 Gy in 5–7 weeks).

Multifield planning and attention to localization detail are essential for successful radiation treatment. A three-field plan is normally employed, with particular care to avoid overtreatment of the eyes and optic chiasm. For most tumours the field size can be limited, although chromophobe pituitary adenomas can reach a very large size. In some centres a rotational plan is used. The radiation technique is the same regardless of whether the patient is treated postoperatively as an adjuvant to surgery, or later for recurrence—though in the latter instance, the treatment volume may have to be larger. Complications of radiotherapy are relatively unusual but include visible impairment, hypopituitarism and radiation carcinogenesis [29].

Alternatives to the use of conventional external beam irradiation include interstitial yttrium-seed irradiation, gamma-knife radiosurgery [16] and heavy-particle (proton or α-particle) irradiation.

The use of bromocriptine has been advocated in recent years as an alternative to surgery and/or radiotherapy. This agent is particularly useful for small tumours producing prolactin only (prolactinomas). Although widely used, patients on bromocriptine do sometimes develop frank recurrence; it is also uncertain how long the drug needs to be continued. If bromocriptine fails, prolactinomas may have to be removed surgically.

Meningioma

Meningiomas should be surgically excised. If inaccessible and difficult to remove, postoperative irradiation should be given, and reduce the rate of local recurrence. As these tumours are not very sensitive to radiation, high doses are usually required (50–60 Gy over 5–7 weeks). For patients with 'malignant' meningioma, radiotherapy is always required, though the overall prognosis in these cases is very poor. Occasionally they metastasize to distant sites. Recent reports have suggested a possible benefit from chemotherapy with oral hydroxyurea [30].

Pineal tumours

These present particular problems of management since they are often not biopsied by the surgeon for fear of causing irreparable damage. Many pineal tumours are curable by radiotherapy (particularly the 'pure' non-teratomatous pineal germinomas), and in patients without histological verification of the type of pineal tumour a brief trial of radiotherapy is often justified unless there is strong evidence of a teratomatous tumour such as raised markers (α-fetoprotein (AFP) or β-HCG, see below) or clear-cut radiological heterogeneity within the primary tumour. Germinoma and pinealoblastoma are the most radiosensitive of pineal tumours, and repeat CT or MRI scanning after as little as 2 weeks' treatment often shows dramatic reduction in size. In which case, it can reasonably be assumed that the diagnosis is either germinoma or pinealoblastoma since other pineal tumours (generally glioma or pineal teratoma, pinealocytoma) are far less radiosensitive. Radiotherapy technique varies with the type of tumour and in verification germinoma there is an increasing tendency to treat with platinum-containing chemotherapy in the first instance [31] (for chemotherapy details see Chapter 19). With the radiosensitive group, there is a tendency for involvement by tumour seeding throughout the CNS, and full craniospinal irradiation should be employed. This is not required with other pineal tumours, though if radiotherapy is selected as the treatment of choice, they do require a high local dose to the primary itself. Biopsy or even total removal of pineal tumours, may be possible providing accurate histological diagnosis. For the less radiosensitive group, total surgical removal offers the best result. Pineal teratomas, like teratomas at other sites, can produce AFP and HCG both in CSF and in the blood.

Overall survival of pineal tumours (including unbiopsied cases) is close to 80% in patients under the age of 30, reflecting the high incidence of radio- or chemo-curable germinomas in this group. For older patients the prognosis is much worse, of the order of 25%, due no doubt to the higher incidence of gliomas and other less radiosensitive tumours.

Intracranial lymphoma

Microgliomas and histiocytic lymphomas are also radiosensitive. The surgical approach depends on the site of the lesion and surgery is sometimes complete. Nevertheless, radiotherapy should be offered in all high-grade cases and a remarkable degree of radiosensitivity is sometimes encountered, although durability of response is often disappointing (see Chapter 26). In general, the best results have been obtained with high dosage, and full craniospinal irradiation is often advocated since these tumours can spread throughout the nervous system.

Chordoma

Surgical removal is essential though often difficult because of the anatomy of the tumour. These tumours often have a 'dumb-bell' appearance with an intraspinal component, making total removal impossible. Postoperative radiotherapy is therefore usually necessary, although these lesions are rather insensitive. High radiation dose is particularly difficult to achieve in the cervical spine, though sacral chordomas can be treated to a higher dose since there is no danger of damage to the spinal cord. Despite the marginal radiosensitivity of chordomas, long survival has occasionally been documented in patients treated by subtotal surgical removal and radical postoperative radiotherapy.

Other tumours

Acoustic neuromas, and other neuronal tumours, are best treated surgically or by fractionated sterotactic 'radiosurgery' [32]. Conventional postoperative radiotherapy should certainly be considered where surgery has been incomplete. The surgical approach depends both on the site of the tumour and also on the degree of hearing loss. The prospect for preservation of functional hearing is much better with tumours under 2 cm and where auditory brainstem responses and other audiological assessments are only minimally abnormal. With elderly patients or poor operative risk candidates, sequential MRI may allow for a conservative non-intervention policy without significant danger. Recently, a large study of radiosurgery (162 patients) from the USA has claimed a 98% control rate with low toxicity [32].

Treatment on relapse

For recurrent brain tumours, the question of retreatment radiotherapy often arises. When the disease-free interval has been short, as with high-grade gliomas, there is little value in retreatment since only a modest radiation dose can be safely achieved—of doubtful benefit where more intensive radiotherapy has already failed. However, in patients with low-grade glioma of any type, or those with medulloblastoma, late recurrences are common. Feasibility of retreatment increases with time from initial treatment, and if a sufficient time has passed (10 years or more), a complete retreatment dose can be contemplated. Chemotherapy is increasingly used as the first type of relapse treatment, and sometimes has the virtue of delaying for as long as possible a second course of radiotherapy. With medulloblastoma particularly, widespread late primary, cerebral and spinal metastases can develop, with continued responsiveness to repeated courses of radiotherapy. Dexamethasone often provides valuable symptomatic relief. Chemotherapy may produce transient responses and is discussed above.

Prognosis of brain tumours

For malignant gliomas, the prognosis is heavily dependent on tumour grade and on other well-established prognostic factors (see Fig. 11.5). Patients with malignant glioma fall chiefly into two prognostic groups since those with grade I and II tumours have a relatively good prognosis and 5- and 10-year survival rates of approximately 65 and 35%, whereas those with grade III and IV tumours have a 5-year survival rate of under 10% (Fig. 11.5), with a much worse prognosis in the grade IV category. In all grades incomplete removal is associated with a worse prognosis.

In medulloblastoma, a variety of factors contribute to prognosis. Age at diagnosis and completeness of excision are both important; children over 15 years of age have a better prognosis. Children with spinal metastases at presentation are not usually cured. The adequacy of the irradiation, both in technique and dose, is crucial and 5-year survival rates of over 40% should now be achieved with modern techniques.

In ependymoma, prognosis depends on tumour grade. The median survival following surgery in low-grade ependymoma is approximately 10 years. Recurrences are frequently of a higher histological grade, and median overall survival in high-grade ependymoma is no better than 2–3 years.

Both pituitary tumours and meningiomas have an excellent prognosis following surgical removal and, where appropriate, postoperative radiotherapy. Few large series of pineal tumours have been reported. Survival is very variable (see above). In chordoma, the prognosis is poor since these tumours are not usually entirely resectable or fully radiosensitive. In children with high grade glioma a recent study has suggested that overexpression of p53 protein is strongly associated with an adverse outcome, independently of clinical or pathological features [33].

Secondary deposits in the brain

Cerebral metastases are common and account for about one-third of all brain tumours. Common primary sites include carcinoma of the breast and bronchus, and melanoma. In each of these tumours, autopsy series confirm that the probability of dissemination to the brain is very much greater than the frequency of premortem diagnosis. About 60% of all patients with SCLC have demonstrable brain metastases at autopsy, and in melanoma about three-quarters of patients who die from disseminated disease have brain metastases. Many other tumours can metastasize to the brain, though at a much lower frequency (Table 11.1).

Metastases may be either single or multiple and diagnostically (particularly when solitary) may be difficult to distinguish from primary brain tumours, or when, as occasionally occurs, there is no known primary.

Cortical, cerebellar, thalamic and pituitary deposits are all encountered. As with primary brain tumours, the characteristic symptoms are those of raised intracranial pressure, focal neurological damage and convulsions. The diagnosis is usually suggested by contrast-enhanced MRI or CT scanning. Although local oedema is often present, this is usually less than that seen with high-grade primary brain tumours. In patients with known cancer, particularly lung, breast or melanoma, further investigation is not usually indicated, especially where the primary diagnosis has been made within the previous 5 years, although alternative diagnoses should always be considered. With apparently solid metastases, the most important differential is from a benign brain tumour, particularly meningioma (especially, of course, if the tumour is anatomically located at a common meningioma site). In cases of multiple metastases, the presumed diagnosis is almost always correct, though occasional confusion with intracerebral abscesses may occur.

Treatment

REVERSAL OF OEDEMA

Treatment with dexamethasone, often at high oral dosage (6 mg every 6 h, or if necessary by intramuscular or intravenous administration) can provide rapid, even dramatic relief from symptoms of raised intracranial pressure. Response to this powerful agent is a useful indicator that an intracerebral tumour is present, and a helpful pointer to the likelihood of response to radiotherapy. Its effect is rapid, and can often be reduced in dosage within a week or two. It is a great mistake to allow patients to remain on dexamethasone for too long because of the inevitability of steroid complications, particularly proximal myopathy and facial swelling. In general, we usually recommend gradual discontinuation of dexamethasone over 3–6 weeks, though this policy occasionally results in patients redeveloping symptoms and signs of raised intracranial pressure because of too rapid reduction—in which case, the dose can easily be increased again. There is considerable variation in the rapidity with which patients can be weaned off dexamethasone. In those where dexamethasone is ill advised or dangerous (for example, where there is a history of bleeding peptic ulcer, severe hypertension or diabetes) it is sometimes possible to achieve the desired reduction in cerebral oedema by the use of intravenous urea (1 g/kg, in dextrose solution), mannitol (2 g/kg as a 20% solution) or oral glycerine which can be made palatable by making it up in a 50% mixture with lemonade. Most patients dislike this latter treatment because it rapidly induces diarrhoea, but it can be highly effective in improving symptoms of raised intracranial pressure. Occasionally, the dexamethasone dose may need to be elevated still further—with benefit—over a very short period, up to a dose of 24 mg/day.

RADIOTHERAPY

Radiotherapy is indicated in a high proportion of patients with secondary brain deposits, though the decision to treat requires careful thought. Patients likely to benefit include those with known radiosensitive tumours (particularly SCLC of the bronchus and to a lesser extent carcinoma of the breast); those in whom there has been a good response to dexamethasone; those whose general condition is good (particularly if there is no other evidence of distant metastases); and those with multiple intracerebral deposits in whom there can be no question of surgery.

The choice of fractionation and dosage remains contentious. Recent large multicentre studies have shown no advantage for prolonged fractionation, and a total dose of 12 Gy in two consecutive daily fractions is as effective as much more prolonged regimens, is more convenient for patients, requires less transportation as these patients are often too unwell to attend independently, and frees up valuable resources. Patients with less radiosensitive tumours (adenocarcinomas, melanoma and others) may require higher doses particularly in the case of surgically unsuitable single metastatic deposits where the relatively limited volume can be treated to a higher dose.

SURGERY

Neurosurgical removal of metastases is occasionally performed in the mistaken supposition that the surgeon is dealing with a primary brain tumour. In these cases, where there has been complete macroscopic removal, treatment with postoperative radiotherapy is usually given as well, in case of unrecognized deposits elsewhere in the brain. Surgical removal of metastases is valuable in a small proportion of patients. Relative indications include: young fit patients with a solitary brain metastasis without evidence of disease elsewhere; where there has been a long treatment-free interval (often the case in patients with breast cancer); and where the single metastasis is unlikely to be radiosensitive (as, for example, in adenocarcinoma of the bronchus or thyroid). In this selected group, surgical removal is probably the treatment of choice [34].

CHEMOTHERAPY

In chemosensitive tumours such as small-cell carcinoma of the bronchus or testicular germ cell tumours, intravenous chemotherapy is effective in producing tumour response [35]. The role of chemotherapy requires further definition. The long-held concept of a blood–brain barrier may be erroneous, because the changes in vasculature following establishment of a secondary deposit result in a breach of the physiological boundary. Intrathecal chemotherapy is of no value for intracerebral metastases.

Overall survival is poor, particularly where the primary diagnosis is SCLC or melanoma. In other cases, such as breast cancer and adenocarcinoma from other sites, survival may be more prolonged, particularly where neurosurgical removal of a solitary metastasis is possible, and in patients where the cranial involvement represents a late solitary site of recurrence.

Lymphomatous or carcinomatous meningitis is discussed in Chapter 8.

Tumours of the spinal cord

Primary tumours of the spinal cord are very uncommon, though secondary deposits involving the cord are frequently encountered. Table 11.2 shows the main types of spinal cord tumour. Ependymoma is the commonest, astrocytoma much less frequently seen. Schwannomas, vascular tumours and meningiomas are the other relatively common types. Secondary deposits may be intramedullary but are more often extramedullary (usually extradural), frequently resulting from direct spread from an adjacent involved vertebral body. Management of acute cord compression is also dealt with in Chapter 8.

Table 11.2 Classification of tumours of spinal cord (with percentage frequency).

Intradural (55%)	Extradural (45%)
Extramedullary	Metastases (25%)
Meningioma (15%)	Myeloma (6%)
Neurofibroma (10%)	Lymphoma (5%)
Congenital and others (7%)	Sarcomas (5%)
	Others (5%)
Intramedullary	
Ependymoma (5%)	
Astrocytoma (5%)	
Angiomas (6%)	
Others (7%)	

Symptoms

Pain and tenderness may be presenting symptoms (especially with metastasis) and is generally felt directly over the cord lesion, though the site of pain can be misleading. More laterally situated tumours (often involving the nerve roots as well) may cause more specific and focally sited pain than centrally placed tumours, for example fusiform intramedullary lesions which can extend in a clinically silent way throughout several segments. Sensorimotor loss is frequently present, with defects of both power and sensation at and below the level of involvement. There may be obvious sensory loss (especially evident in lesions of the dorsal and lumbar spine involving loss of sensation over the trunk). Muscular weakness in the upper limbs is a feature of lesions of the cervical spine. Below the affected area of an incomplete cord compression there may be partial preservation of function with less obvious neurological abnormalities and only patchy sensory loss but complete cord compression or major interruption of the vascular supply leads to paraplegia or severe paraparesis. Loss of sphincter function is a late sign with a poor prognosis (see Chapter 8), but lesser degrees occur earlier and their significance is often missed.

Tumours situated below the lower end of the spinal cord (vertebral level L1 or L2) may produce a typical *cauda equina syndrome* with sacral anaesthesia, sciatic pain (often bilateral), gluteal weakness, wasting, impotence and bladder dysfunction with retention and overflow incontinence. Most cases are less symptomatically clear-cut and in practice the diagnosis is often very difficult, although MRI scanning has made such cases easier. A myelogram is likely to be normal and cannot reliably exclude the diagnosis. Ependymomas constitute the largest single group of primary tumours at the lower end of the cord

(conus medullaris and filum terminale). Lateral compression of the spinal cord may cause a complete or partial Brown–Séquard syndrome with ipsilateral spastic weakness, reduced vibration sense and proprioception, together with contralateral insensitivity to pain and temperature change. Tumour progression causes an increasingly florid clinical picture with weakness, sensory loss, hyperreflexia and autonomic dysfunction (see Table 8.4). Acute spinal cord compression is discussed in Chapter 8.

Destructive secondary deposits, which more often involve the vertebral column than the spinal cord, produce more local pain and tenderness than some of the less common primary cord lesions. Common primary sites of vertebral or cord metastases include carcinoma of the bronchus (particularly small-cell), carcinoma of the breast and myeloma. Less common primary sites include thyroid, large bowel malignancies, kidney and cutaneous melanoma.

Differential diagnosis

Although the clinical syndrome of spinal cord compression usually implies a malignant aetiology, a few non-malignant lesions can produce a similar clinical picture. These include inflammatory cord lesions (particularly transverse myelitis, infectious polyneuropathy or Guillain–Barré syndrome), anterior spinal arterial occlusion, abscess of the cord, syringomyelia and haemorrhage into the cord (haematomyelia). Very occasionally an acutely prolapsed intervertebral disc may produce symptoms of cord compression.

Investigation

Radiological investigation is essential. Plain X-rays of the spine may show an obvious lytic deposit in the vertebrae) at the level of compression, but X-ray changes may be very subtle, with loss of the pedicle of the spine but no other significant features. Myelography used to be widely used, gives good anatomical demonstration of the spinal cord lesion and will show whether the block is partial or complete (Fig. 11.7) but has now been almost completely replaced by MRI scanning (see Fig. 8.3). With a complete block, it is difficult to be certain of the upper extent of the abnormality, and very occasionally a cisternal myelogram will need to be performed if full anatomical definition is considered important for therapy. Metrizamide gives good definition of root pathology but, being water-soluble, is rapidly cleared so that re-examinations require a further lumbar puncture. In tumours with doubtful or

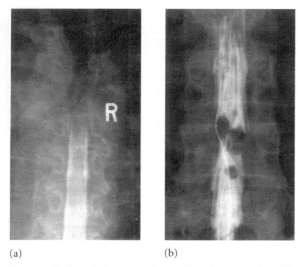

(a)   (b)

Fig 11.7 Radiological changes in spinal cord compression: (a) complete cord compression; (b) partial cord compression due to multiple deposits from an ependymoma.

difficult physical signs, CT scanning can be invaluable. This investigation can be even more informative when combined with metrizamide myelography. In general, however, MRI scanning has rapidly become the imaging modality of choice with spinal tumours. Myelography is now largely outmoded.

Management

For primary tumours of the spinal cord, surgical removal is the treatment of choice if it can be safely attempted without permanent neurological deficit. However, major technical difficulties are often encountered, and in-tramedullary tumours are almost always unresectable. Surgical decompression is invaluable even where the tumour cannot be removed, and this is generally achieved by laminectomy, often encompassing several segments. Biopsy will be diagnostically valuable even if little more can be surgically achieved. Spinal neoplasms often extend over a considerable length of the cord. These are typically low-grade gliomas and can sometimes be fully excised. Many benign or extramedullary and intradural tumours of borderline malignancy can be removed without need for further treatment. This group includes meningiomas, low-grade gliomas, neurofibromas and tumours of the coverings of the cord (angiomas, fibromas and lipomas).

For more malignant tumours and in patients with secondary deposits involving the spinal cord, surgical decompression followed by postoperative radiotherapy is usually the treatment of choice. If rapid transfer to a neurosurgical centre is difficult or if the patient is unfit or unsuitable for surgery (perhaps because of widespread malignant disease), intensive radiotherapy can often provide excellent palliation, particularly if the cord lesion is a secondary deposit of a radiosensitive tumour. In malignant primary cord tumours such as high-grade glioma, total surgical removal is usually impossible and postoperative radiotherapy is mandatory. A high radiation dose will be required since these tumours are not usually very radiosensitive, generally to the tolerance dose (see below). Very careful judgement of anatomical details, field length, fractionation and total dose is always required.

High doses of dexamethasone are invaluable in reducing cord oedema, making intensive radiotherapy safer. The role of chemotherapy is not established and it has no routine place in the management of spinal cord tumours.

Tumours of the peripheral nerves

These are rare tumours, more often benign than malignant. Multiple neurofibromatosis (von Recklinghausen's disease), the commonest peripheral nerve tumour, is most frequently encountered. In 5–10% of cases, sarcomatous change takes places (neurofibrosarcoma). Tumours of the nerve sheath (Schwannomas) can occur in both cranial and peripheral nerves, particularly the acoustic nerve, spinal nerve roots, peripheral nerves and occasionally the V, IX or X cranial nerves. These may occasionally undergo malignant change. *Neuroepithelioma* is an exceedingly rare malignant tumour of peripheral nerve, sometimes occurring in conjunction with von Recklinghausen's disease. The histological appearance suggests a neural crest origin, and metastases are frequent.

Treatment of peripheral nerve tumours is by surgical excision if the tumour is producing troublesome pressure symptoms or where there is any suspicion of malignant change. Routine surgical excision of neurofibromas in patients with von Recklinghausen's disease should be discouraged unless there is a sudden increase in size of one of the peripheral lesions. Management of sarcomatous tumours is discussed in Chapter 23.

Radiation damage in the brain and spinal cord

With radical radiotherapy, particularly of midline tumours, the treatment volume may include the spinal cord.

For example, in lung cancer a portion of the cord is usually irradiated. Radiation tolerance of the brain and spinal cord are of great clinical importance since this frequently sets the dose limit [36,37]. Both acute and late damage may occur, the latter being of much greater importance. In the brain, early effects include headache, nausea, vomiting and lassitude from raised intracranial pressure, both as a result of the tumour itself and also from acute cerebral oedema produced by the radiotherapy. Drowsiness and irritability have been described as side-effects of whole-brain irradiation in children (somnolence syndrome) but are transient and self-limiting. An early syndrome of demyelination may develop but is extremely rare. Late changes include haemorrhage, gliosis, demyelination and necrosis of the brain. The clinical features are those of progressive focal or generalized neurological damage, occurring months or even years after radiation. Damage to the optic chiasm is well recognized in patients treated for pituitary tumours and is clearly dose-related, with minimal risk when daily fraction size is kept between 1.8 and 2.0 Gy.

Early radiation damage to the spinal cord is more frequently encountered and usually transient. The commonest feature is Lhermitte's syndrome, characterized by 'electric shock' sensations in the extremities (usually the feet), particularly marked on flexion of the neck. It usually occurs a few weeks after the treatment, and is usually self-limiting and without long-term effects.

With late radiation damage, myelopathy can cause progressive motor and sensory changes at the irradiated site, leading to paraparesis, anaesthesia and, in exceptionally severe cases, a paraplegia with physiological transection of the cord. If less than the total width of the cord has been irradiated, a Brown–Séquard syndrome may result. These changes are due to direct damage to neurological tissue with loss of anterior horn cells, other neurones and oligodendroglia as well as direct vascular damage leading to infarction of the cord. Progressive and chronic radiation myelopathy is usually irreversible and leads to spastic paraplegia with sphincter disturbance. This is fatal in over 50% of cases, particularly where the lesion is in the cervical or upper dorsal cord.

Radiation tolerance of the cord is inversely related to the length of cord irradiated. It is generally accepted that for a 10-cm length of cord, a dose of 40 Gy in daily fractions over 4 weeks is safe, though this dose may have to be exceeded in patients with relatively insensitive lesions which cannot be completely excised, for example a chordoma. Fraction size is clearly important since treatment to 50 Gy in daily fractions over 5 weeks is usually safe, where-as many cases of cord damage have been documented following treatment to a dose of 40 Gy in daily fractions over 3 weeks [40].

References

1 McKeran RO, Williams ES, Thornton-Jones H. The epidemiology of brain tumours. In: Thomas DGT, ed. *Neurooncology*. London: Edward Arnold, 1990: 135–40.
2 Relling MV, Rubnitz JE, Rivera GK et al. High incidence of secondary brain tumours after radiotherapy and antimetabolites. *Lancet* 1999; 354: 34–9.
3 Hoshino T, Nagashima T, Cho KG et al. Variability in the proliferative potential of human gliomas. *J Neuro-Oncol* 1989; 7: 137–43.
4 Nishikawa R, Ji XD, Harmon RC et al. A mutant epidermal growth factor receptor common in human glioma confers enhanced tumorigenicity. *Proc Natl Acad Sci USA* 1994; 91: 7727–31.
5 James CD, Olson JJ. Molecular genetics and molecular biology advances in brain tumours. *Curr Opin Oncol* 1996; 8: 188–95.
6 Bigner SH, Mark J, Burger PC et al. Specific chromosomal abnormalities in malignant gliomas. *Cancer Res* 1988; 48: 405–11.
7 Russell DS, Rubenstein LJ. *Pathology of Tumors of the Nervous System*, 4th edn. Baltimore: Williams & Wilkins, 1982.
8 Freeman CR, Farmer JP, Montes J. Low-grade astrocytoma in children: evolving management strategies. *Int J Radiation, Oncol Biol Physics* 1998; 41: 979–87.
9 Black PM. Medical progress: brain tumors. *N Engl J Med* 1991; 324 (1471–6): 1555–64.
10 Shaw EG, Daumas-Duport C, Scheithauer BW et al. Radiation therapy in the management of low-grade supratentorial astrocytomas. *J Neurosurgery* 1989; 70: 853–61.
11 Karim ABMF, Maat B, Hatlevoll MD et al. A randomised trial on dose–response in radiation therapy of low-grade cerebral glioma: EORTC study 22844. *Int J Radiation Oncol Biol Physics* 1996; 36: 549–56.
12 Bleehen NM, Stenning SP (MRC Brain Tumour Working Party). A Medical Research Council trial of two radiotherapy doses in the treatment of grades 3 and 4 astrocytoma. *Br J Cancer* 1991; 64: 769–74.
13 Larson D, Gutin P, Leibel S et al. Stereotaxic irradiation of brain tumors. *Cancer* 1990; 65: 792–9.
14 Schupak K, Malkin M, Anderson L et al. The relationship between the technical accuracy of stereotactic interstitial implantations for high-grade gliomas and the pattern of tumor recurrence. *Int J Radiation Oncol Biol Physics* 1995; 32: 1167–76.
15 Brada M, Graham JD. Stereotactic external beam radiotherapy in the treatment of glioma and other intracranial lesions. In: Tobias, JS, Thomas, PRM, eds. *Current Radia-*

tion Oncology, Vol. 1. London: Edward Arnold, 1994: 85–100.

16 Plowman PN, Doughty D. Stereotactic radiosurgery X. Clinical isodosimetry of gamma knife versus linear accelerator X-knife for pituitary and acoustic tumours. *Clin Oncol* 1999; 11: 321–9.

17 Walker MD, Green SB, Byar DP *et al.* Randomized comparisons of radiotherapy and nitrosoureas for the treatment of malignant glioma after surgery. *N Engl J Med* 1980; 303: 1323.

18 Glioma Meta-Analysis Trialists Group. A systematic review and meta-analysis of individual patient data from 12 randomised trials. *Lancet* 2002; 359: 1011–18.

19 Phillips TL, Sheline GE, Boldrey E. Therapeutic considerations in tumours affecting the central nervous system: ependymomas. *Radiology* 1964; 83: 98–105.

20 Sheline GE, Boldrey EB, Karlsberg P, Phillips TL. Therapeutic considerations in tumours affecting the central nervous system: oligodendrogliomas. *Radiology* 1964; 82: 84–9.

21 Bouffet E, Jouvet A, Thiesse P *et al.* Chemotherapy for aggressive or anaplastic high grade oligodendrogliomas and oligoastrocytomas: better than a salvage treatment? *Br J Neurosurg* 1998; 12: 217–22.

22 Pierce SM, Barnes PD, Loeffler JS *et al.* Definitive radiation therapy in the management of symptomatic patients with optic glioma. *Cancer* 1990; 65: 45–52.

23 Thomas PRM. Medulloblastoma—progress and pitfalls. In: Tobias JS, Thomas PRM, eds. *Current Radiation Oncology*, Vol. 2. London: Edward Arnold, 1996: 202–17.

24 Livesey EA, Hindmarsh PC, Brook CGD *et al.* Endocrine disorders following treatment of childhood brain tumours. *Br J Cancer* 1990; 61: 622–5.

25 Sposto R, Ertel IJ, Jenkin RDT *et al.* The effectiveness of chemotherapy for treatment of high-grade astrocytoma in children: results of a randomised trial. *J Neurooncol* 1989; 7: 165–77.

26 Tait D, Thornton-Jones H, Bloom HJG *et al.* Adjuvant chemotherapy for medulloblastoma: the first multicentre controlled trial of the International Society for Paediatric Oncology. *Eur J Cancer* 1990; 26: 464–9.

27 Powell MF, Lightman SL, eds. *Management of Pituitary Tumours: a Handbook*. Edinburgh: Churchill Livingstone, 1995.

28 Estrada J, Boronat M, Mielgo M *et al.* The long-term outcome of pituitary irradiation after unsuccessful trans-sphenoidal surgery in Cushing's disease. *N Engl J Med* 1997; 336: 172–7.

29 O'Halloran DJ, Shalet SM. Radiotherapy for pituitary adenomas: an endocrinologist's perspective. *Clin Oncol* 1996; 8: 79–84.

30 Schrell UMH, Rittig MG, Anders M, Koch UH, Marschalek R, Riesewetter F, Fahlbusch R. Hydroxyurea for treatment of unresectable and recurrent meningiomas. II. Decrease in the size of meningiomas in patients treated with hydroxyurea. *J Neurosurg* 1997; 86: 840–4.

31 Balmaceda C, Heller G, Rosenblum M *et al.* Chemotherapy without irradiation—a novel approach for newly diagnosed CNS germ cell tumors: results of an international cooperative trial. *J Clin Oncol* 1996; 14: 2908–15.

32 Kondziolka D, Lunsford LD, McLaughlin MR *et al.* Long-term outcomes after radiosurgery for acoustic neuromas. *N Engl J Med* 1998; 339: 1426–33.

33 Pollack IF, Finkelstein SD, Woods J *et al.* Expression of p53 and prognosis in children with malignant gliomas. *New Engl J Med* 2002; 346: 420–7.

34 Bindal AK, Bindal RK, Hess KR *et al.* Surgery vs. radiosurgery in the treatment of brain metastasis. *J Neurosurg* 1996; 84: 748–54.

35 Twelves CJ, Souhami RL, Harper PG *et al.* The response of cerebral metastases in small cell lung cancer to systemic chemotherapy. *Br J Cancer* 1990; 61: 147–50.

36 Wara WM, Phillips TL, Sheline GE *et al.* Radiation tolerance of the spinal cord. *Cancer* 1975; 35: 1558–62.

37 Constine LS, Woolf PD, Cann D *et al.* Hypothalamic-pituitary dysfunction after radiation for brain tumors. *N Engl J Med* 1993; 328: 87–94.

12 Tumours of the lung and mediastinum

Carcinoma of the bronchus

Introduction

Carcinoma of the bronchus is by far the commonest cancer in the Western world, having increased steadily in incidence since the 1930s. It had an overall incidence in the UK of 102 per 100 000 males and 46 per 100 000 females in 1990. The incidence is strongly related to age (Fig. 12.1). As a result of the increasing prevalence of cigarette smoking since the First World War, carcinoma of the bronchus has become the leading cause of cancer death in males over the past 50 years. In recent years, more women have become cigarette smokers, with the result that lung cancer has become increasingly common in women, and mortality continues to rise [1]. In 1952, the male:female ratio for lung cancer incidence was 13:1; in 1990 the figure stood at 2:1.

Although several aetiological factors have been implicated, including exposure to radioactivity and possible environmental hazards, these are insignificant compared with the highly carcinogenic effect of prolonged exposure to cigarette smoke. Recent studies have shown that non-smokers married to lifelong smokers are at double the expected risk for developing lung cancer. Case–control studies have also suggested an increased incidence in lung cancer in non-smokers who lived in a household of heavy smokers during childhood and adolescence.

A great deal of political debate has followed the demonstration of an incontrovertible link between cigarette smoking and lung cancer, in which health education, cost of treatment, possible loss of tax revenue, reduction in productivity resulting from ill health and freedom of choice have been the principal points for discussion. At an international level, there have been a wide variety of approaches towards the restriction of smoking, stemming from the differing philosophies of different countries. In many Scandinavian countries, for example, it is now almost socially unacceptable to smoke in public places, and cigarettes have become extremely expensive, with the result that smoking-related illnesses are beginning to decline. There is a clear inverse relationship between the cost of cigarettes and the amount smoked (Fig. 12.2). In the UK, restriction of smoking in public areas has been a protracted and uphill battle. There is now a clear inverse relationship both in the UK and the USA between socioeconomic status and incidence of lung cancer. The death rate from this disease is disproportionately high in comparison to incidence because of the low cure rates currently achieved (less than 10% at 5 years overall). So far, attempts at screening, even in high-risk groups, have met with very little success. In developing countries, cigarette consumption is rapidly rising and high-tar brands which are no longer popular in this country are widely advertised. Despite overwhelming evidence of the dangers of cigarette smoking, major tobacco companies are urging farmers in developing countries to change from production of staple arable crops to growing tobacco.

Fortunately, the carcinogenic effects of cigarette smoke are to some extent reversible. In their classic study of the smoking habits of British doctors, Doll and Hill [1] were able to demonstrate a gradual reduction in mortality of British doctors who gave up smoking. Lung cancer declines in incidence when smokers give up the habit. After

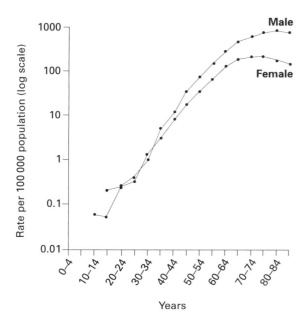

Fig. 12.1 Cancer of the lung: age-specific incidence rates for men and women.

12 years of total abstinence from cigarette smoking, the risk of developing lung cancer is almost as low as in non-smokers, except for heavy smokers (more than 20 per day), in whom the risk never falls to that of the non-smoker. In the lower age groups (30–45 years), there is at least some evidence for a slight fall in death rate over the past 15 years (Fig. 12.2). Since there has been little decrease in the number of cigarettes smoked in the UK, this reduction may possibly be due to the wider use of low-tar brands. Nevertheless, insufficient time has elapsed since the introduction of these brands for us to be confident that the risk is indeed lower. Attempts to prevent the development of lung cancer by the administration of retinoids to high-risk individuals have been unsuccessful; indeed, lung cancer deaths were increased [4].

Other aetiological factors, thought or known to have a role, include asbestos exposure, industrial pollution, ionizing radiation, occupational hazards and others (see also Chapter 2). Of these, asbestos exposure is probably the most critical, both for lung cancer and also mesothelioma (see p. 195). This is particularly important when combined with cigarette smoking: in smokers with occupational exposure to asbestos, the risk of lung cancer is 45 times above that of the normal population.

The molecular pathology of lung cancer

The carcinogens in cigarette smoke cause mutations in genes, some of which result in further genomic instability. By the time the cancer is clinically apparent numerous mutations in dominant or recessive growth-regulatory genes are apparent. Many types of abnormality occur, including deletions, rearrangements, point mutations, splicing errors and amplification. Figure 12.3 shows diagrammatically some of the abnormalities which are consistently observed at the various stages of tumour growth during the progression from hyperplasia/dysplasia to invasive cancer in non-small-cell lung cancer (NSCLC). The genes deleted at chromosomes 3p and 9p21 are not yet defined, but will clearly prove to be of great interest in understanding lung cancer growth.

Pathology of lung cancer

Histological types

Lung cancer is only rarely a tumour of the true lung parenchyma, arising far more frequently in large and medium-sized bronchi. There are many histological types of lung cancer. It is, however, convenient to consider the commonest varieties in four major groups, although there is substantial histological variation within each of these (Table 12.1). There has been considerable debate as to whether the cell of origin is different in the different histological types. There is, however, a great deal of circumstantial evidence to suggest that the cancers arise from a common precursor cell which has the capacity to differentiate into a variety of histological types.

SQUAMOUS CELL CARCINOMA
This is the commonest histological type and is characterized by the presence of keratinization and/or intercellular bridging, and is often subdivided on the basis of differentiation. Most of these tumours arise proximally in large bronchi (though they may also arise peripherally), and tend to be polypoid or infiltrating, often with distinct borders. Since the bronchi at this level are not normally lined by squamous epithelium, it is likely that neoplastic change at this site is preceded by squamous metaplasia, though studies of carcinoma *in situ* have suggested that this may not always occur. Mutations and loss of heterozygosity of the *p53* gene have been found in many tumours.

SMALL-CELL LUNG CANCER (SCLC)
Small-cell lung cancer is characterized by a diffuse growth of small cells with fine granular nuclei, inconspicuous nu-

Mortality trends 1941–1990 males, England and Wales

Mortality trends 1941–1990 females, England and Wales

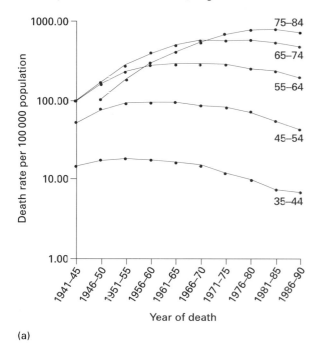

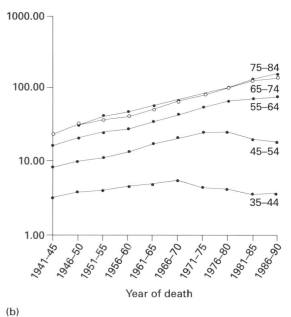

(a)

(b)

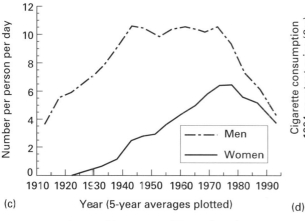

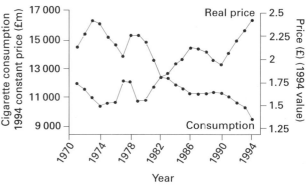

(c)

(d)

Fig. 12.2 Smoking and lung cancer. (a) Trends in lung cancer mortality for men and women of different ages (England and Wales). From [2] with permission. (b) Age-adjusted lung cancer mortality rates (United States). (c) Smoking prevalence and lung cancer mortality in men and women (England and Wales). From [3]. (Copyright ©1975 by Scientific American, Inc. All rights reserved.) (d) Relative risk of lung cancer according to daily cigarette consumption.

cleoli, and scanty cytoplasm. The cells tend to be tightly packed or moulded, with little evidence of supportive tissue. Occasionally, combinations of small-cell and squamous cell carcinomas are seen, though many pathologists

think that such tumours should be classified as poorly differentiated squamous cell carcinoma. Neurosecretory granules are often present on electron microscopy (Fig. 12.4). These may be the site of origin of the hormones

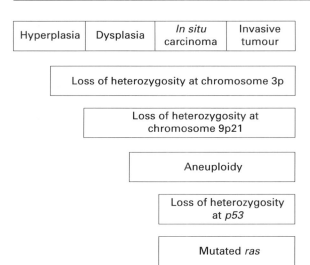

Hyperplasia	Dysplasia	*In situ* carcinoma	Invasive tumour

Loss of heterozygosity at chromosome 3p

Loss of heterozygosity at chromosome 9p21

Aneuploidy

Loss of heterozygosity at *p53*

Mutated *ras*

Fig. 12.3 Genetic changes which accompany progression to invasive lung cancer.

Table 12.1 Histological classification of lung cancer*.

	Frequency (%)
Squamous carcinoma	35–45
Small-cell carcinoma	20
Adenocarcinoma (bronchogenic, acinar bronchioloalveolar)	15–50†
Large-cell carcinoma (with or without mucin, giant and clear cell variants)	10
Mixed forms	10–20
Other tumours (carcinoid, cylindroma, sarcoma and mixed histological types)	2

*Adapted from World Health Organization classification.
†Geographical variation.

such as adrenocorticotrophic hormone (ACTH), antidiuretic hormone (ADH) and calcitonin which are sometimes produced and give rise to ectopic hormone syndromes which may be clinically significant (see Chapter 9). Small-cell carcinomas express other markers of neural differentiation. Chief among these is the presence on the cell surface of the neural-cell adhesion molecule (NCAM). The cells secrete autocrine growth factors such as gastrin-releasing peptide (the mammalian homologue of bombesin) which, after secretion, binds to receptors on

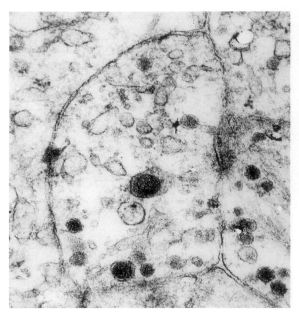

Fig. 12.4 Electron microscopy appearances in small-cell carcinoma. Dense neurosecretory granules are shown in cell processes (×52 250).

the tumour cell surface and causes a mitotic stimulus. Numerous other peptide hormones also bind to receptors on the SCLC cell surface and there has been considerable recent interest in the possible therapeutic effects of blocking such autocrine growth mechanisms. The tumours also show overexpression or amplification of one or more *myc* family oncogenes. Karyotypically, there is an almost universal deletion of part of the short arm of chromosome 3 (bands 14–23), and loss of heterozygosity at the site of the *p53* gene (17p). As in NSCLC, *p53* mutations occur frequently. Small-cell carcinomas typically develop in proximal large bronchi and are characterized by extensive local invasion associated with early blood-borne and lymphatic metastases, making them almost invariably unsuitable for surgery as a definitive treatment. Many tumours are diagnosed by biopsy of supraclavicular or cervical lymph nodes.

ADENOCARCINOMAS

These show the typical features of neoplastic cells derived from glandular epithelium, with formation of acini, papillae and mucus. Many adenocarcinomas are peripheral in site of origin, frequently invading the pleura. These cancers sometimes arise in scar tissue, and may occur in fibrotic lung disease. Adenocarcinoma is less clearly related to cigarette smoking than either squamous cell or small-cell carcinoma, and was the predominant cell type before the advent of cigarette smoking. Unlike other forms of lung cancer, it is slightly commoner in females. There is some evidence that it is increasing in frequency. In some large series from the USA adenocarcinoma now accounts for 50% of all NSCLC. The uncommon bronchioalveolar carcinoma sometimes presents as a multicentric tumour with alveoli lined by neoplastic columnar cells.

LARGE-CELL CARCINOMA

Large-cell carcinoma refers to undifferentiated tumours with a variety of appearances. The cells are large, often with featureless cytoplasm and show little tendency towards keratinization or acinar formation. In a proportion of these tumours there is evidence of mucus production, and there may also be other ultrastructural characteristics which are reminiscent of adenocarcinoma. The tumour borders are generally well defined, and the tumour itself may arise from a subsegmental or more distal bronchus.

MIXED HISTOLOGIES

Approximately 20% of tumours show a mixed histological appearance (small/large-cell, adeno/squamous, squamous/small-cell). Of interest is the finding that 10–20% of typical adenocarcinomas have some cellular features of neuroendocrine cells such as expression of chromogranin (found in dense core granules), NCAM and neurone-specific enolase. There have been some studies which purport to show that these tumours may, like SCLC, show sensitivity to chemotherapy, but the issue is not settled.

Pathological diagnosis

In over 80% of patients with lung cancer, malignant cells are found in the sputum, using standard exfoliative cytology techniques. The likelihood of a positive sputum diagnosis increases from 58% with a single specimen, to 78% when four specimens are obtained. This proportion is also increased when specimens are obtained at bronchoscopy either from trap, brush or lavage specimens. The four major categories can be distinguished with an accuracy of 80% by either cytological or histological methods. Occasionally a mixture of cell types is seen, for example mixed small-cell and large-cell carcinoma or adenosquamous tumours. About one-quarter of autopsy cases show mixed histologies, although this high proportion may be related to a treatment-induced change in the histology [5]. Cases with mixed histology are one line of evidence suggesting

that these carcinomas do not arise from different cells, but that the cancer-inducing event results in cells which can differentiate along more than one pathway.

The clinical distinction between primary adenocarcinoma of the bronchus and secondary pulmonary deposits from primary adenocarcinomas at other sites may be a difficult one, especially if no endobronchial lesion is seen at bronchoscopy. Similarly, the clear-cell carcinoma variant of large-cell carcinoma can be mistaken for metastatic hypernephroma. One important clinical feature of squamous cell carcinomas is that they may cavitate and can therefore be confused with a lung abscess.

Patterns of local invasion and metastasis

Carcinoma of the bronchus spreads by local invasion and by lymphatic and haematogenous routes (Fig. 12.5). Locally, the tumour may spread into the mediastinum or through the bronchial wall, lung parenchyma and to the pleural space and chest wall. There may be erosion of overlying ribs. Apical tumours typically spread from the apex of the lung to involve the brachial plexus, with erosion of upper thoracic ribs and local nerves such as the thoracocervical sympathetic chain (Pancoast syndrome). At the hilum of the lung the tumour may damage the phrenic or left recurrent laryngeal nerve. It may also erode posteriorly into the oesophagus or vertebrae.

Lymphatic spread within the chest is chiefly to hilar and mediastinal, subcarinal, tracheobronchial and paratra-

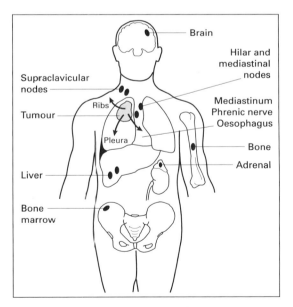

Fig. 12.5 Local and metastatic spread in lung cancer.

cheal nodes. Beyond the chest, involvement of supraclavicular, cervical and axillary nodes may occur. Lymphatic involvement below the diaphragm is frequent in small-cell carcinoma, especially to upper para-aortic nodes.

Blood-borne spread is especially frequent in small-cell carcinoma and typically occurs earlier than with other lung cancers. The skeleton is frequently involved, particularly vertebrae, ribs and pelvis, and widespread infiltration into bone marrow occurs, especially in small-cell carcinoma where estimates of frequency vary from 5 to 30%, depending on the number of marrow aspirations, the extent of the tumour and the sensitivity of the methods used to detect the infiltrating cells. Other common sites include the brain (65% of autopsies in small-cell carcinoma), liver and adrenals, but secondary deposits can be found in any organ. Early and rapid dissemination is particularly characteristic of small-cell carcinoma, which also has the most rapid volume doubling time.

Clinical features

Most patients with lung cancer present with symptoms directly related to the tumour such as haemoptysis, cough, dyspnoea or chest pain. Since many are smokers, some of these symptoms (particularly a cough) will already be present as a result of chronic bronchitis and emphysema. This may delay them in seeking advice, though a substantial number are sufficiently aware of the increased intensity of their symptoms to give up smoking, often after a lifetime of being unable to do so. The cough is often persistent, nocturnal and may be productive. Sputum may be blood-streaked or persistently discoloured as a result of infection which cannot resolve due to atelectasis beyond an obstructing endobronchial tumour. Haemoptyses, though intermittent, usually become increasingly severe. Pain, usually aching, is present in over 50% of patients. It seems to be commoner in patients with mediastinal involvement or atelectasis, and is much commoner than the typical, sharper, pain of bone metastases.

More peripheral tumours often present rather late, when already of significant size. They may cause pain in the chest wall by direct extension to the pleura or periosteum of the ribs, often trapping or invading intercostal nerves. Direct tumour invasion of the left recurrent laryngeal nerve may result in hoarseness of the voice, which is a frequent presenting symptom. Pleural effusion, phrenic nerve palsy, and lobar or total lung collapse may all contribute to increasing dyspnoea. Pneumonias that fail to resolve completely after antibiotics raise the suspicion of underlying cancer. Dysphagia may result from enlarged mediastinal lymph nodes which compress the oesophagus, usually at its mid or lower third, or by direct invasion. Wheeze and stridor are important signs of obstruction of large airways, generally due to proximal tumours.

Tumours at specific sites may produce typical syndromes. A Pancoast tumour, situated at the apex of the lung, causes severe pain in the shoulder, chest wall and arm as a result of relentless local invasion which destroys ribs and infiltrates the brachial plexus. Weakness of the small muscles of the hand may occur, with paraesthesiae on the inner aspect of the arm, due to $C_{5/6}$, T_1 motor loss. Tumours of the right main or right upper lobe bronchus (often with associated right paratracheal node enlargement) may compress the great veins leading to superior vena caval obstruction (SVCO), producing a typical clinical syndrome consisting of swelling of the face, neck and upper arms, plethora or cyanosis and rapid development of a visible collateral circulation over the scapula and upper chest wall. In severe cases, conjunctival oedema (chemosis) occurs. The majority of cases of SVCO are caused by small-cell carcinomas and prompt treatment may produce a gratifying resolution of these symptoms (see Chapter 8).

Some patients notice a 'mass' in the neck due to lymph node enlargement. In other patients the presenting symptoms are caused by secondary deposits, especially in small-cell cancer. Pain in the back may be due to vertebral collapse, and is particularly important since cord compression with paraplegia may develop with great rapidity unless the diagnosis is made and treatment started promptly. Other typical metastatic presentations include neurological symptoms and signs (focal lesions, raised intracranial pressure, cerebellar syndromes) and weight loss and nausea from hepatic involvement.

Constitutional symptoms are also common and most patients with lung cancer complain of anorexia, weight loss, weakness and fatigue. Although many patients do not notice clubbing of the fingers, this is a common manifestation particularly associated with squamous cell carcinoma and rare in small-cell carcinoma. Pain in the limbs may result from the much less common hypertrophic pulmonary osteoarthropathy which can be severe.

A wide variety of paraneoplastic non-metastatic syndromes have been described in association with lung cancer. These are discussed in Chapter 9. Many of these syndromes are uncommon. Hypercalcaemia (without obvious bone metastases) is most frequently found in squamous cell cancer, and the syndromes of inappropriate ADH secretion and ectopic ACTH production are both commoner in small-cell carcinoma. The symptoms and management of hypercalcaemia are discussed in Chapter 8 and of ectopic hormone production in Chapter 9.

Staging notation

Although complex, the tumour node metastasis (TNM) staging system and stage grouping is widely used in NSCLC (Table 12.2) and has been shown to be useful prognostically. It has little value in small-cell carcinomas, in which local and distant dissemination is so common, and the role of surgery so limited that staging systems have little relevance.

Investigation and staging

Non-small-cell lung cancer

Most patients with suspected lung cancer are first seen by

Table 12.2 TNM staging system for NSCLC.

T—primary tumour

T_0	Primary tumour not demonstrable
T_x	Positive cytology but tumour not demonstrable
T_{is}	Carcinoma *in situ*
T_1	Tumour less than 3 cm in diameter, no proximal invasion
T_2	Tumour more than 3 cm in diameter, or invading pleura or with atelectasis, more than 2 cm from carina
T_3	Tumour of any size with extension into the chest wall, diaphragm, mediastinal pleura or within 2 cm of carina
T_4	Tumour of any size with invasion of mediastinal organs or vertebral body

N—regional lymph nodes

N_0	Nodes negative
N_1	Ipsilateral hilar nodes
N_2	Ipsilateral mediastinal and subcarinal nodes
N_3	Contralateral mediastinal or hilar nodes, scalene or supraclavicular nodes

Stage grouping				*5-year survival**
Stage IA	T_1	N_0	M_0	61
Stage IB	T_2	N_0	M_0	38
Stage IIA	T_1	N_1	M_0	34
Stage IIB	T_2	N_1	M_0	24
	T_3	N_0	M_0	
Stage IIIA	T_{1-3}	N_2	M_0	13
Stage IIIB	T4	Any N	M_0	5
	Any T	N_3	M_0	
Stage IV	Any T	Any N	M_1	1

*Figures from [6].

a chest physician and the diagnosis made by fibreoptic bronchoscope. This instrument has the advantage of permitting good access to lobar and segmental bronchi and is especially helpful in evaluating upper lobe tumours out of biopsy range of the rigid bronchoscope. The rigid instrument is, however, sometimes useful since it may give a better view of proximal bronchi and allows a larger biopsy in doubtful cases.

Staging of NSCLC is important since a crucial distinction between operable and inoperable tumours has to be made. To the surgeon, the most important criteria are the tumour site, absence of metastases and the general fitness of the patient. Before any consideration of surgery, the maximum amount of information must therefore be obtained. Chest X-ray may indicate that the tumour is inoperable. Findings indicating inoperability include large central primary tumours particularly extending across the midline; widening of the superior mediastinum due to enlargement of paratracheal nodes; intrapulmonary, rib or other bony metastases; pleural effusion; and bilateral tumours. Further assessment is often needed; bronchoscopic evaluation is usually required to make the diagnosis and is essential to assess operability.

At bronchoscopy, some tumours can be shown to be inoperable. Features indicating inoperability are: endobronchial tumour within 2 cm of the main carina; extrinsic compression and widening of the angle of the main carina indicating mediastinal spread; and paralysis of the left vocal cord resulting from recurrent laryngeal nerve palsy.

With very few exceptions, mediastinal involvement is a strong contraindication to surgery. Assessment of the mediastinum is therefore essential in any patient being considered for operation. Clinical evidence of involvement includes a hoarse voice with a typical 'bovine' cough, resulting from recurrent laryngeal palsy, Horner's syndrome from involvement of the cervical sympathetic chain, pain in the shoulder, SVCO, cardiac dysrhythmia and dysphagia. Further assessment can be made by tomographic views of the mediastinum, and by barium swallow which may show enlarged mediastinal nodes causing extrinsic oesophageal compression. Computed tomography (CT) scanning is a useful aid in the preoperative assessment of tumour extent, sometimes demonstrating unexpected lymph node involvement or direct invasion of other structures (Fig. 12.6). Chest wall involvement, for example, usually indicates inoperability. It is, however, important not to rule out surgery on the basis of an equivocal CT scan since not all lymph node enlargement will prove to be neoplastic at thoracotomy.

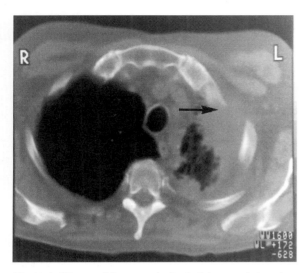

Fig. 12.6 CT scan of thorax, at the level of the manubrium, in a patient with squamous carcinoma of the lung. The tumour is shown extending through the pleural space into the chest wall, eroding the ribs (arrowed).

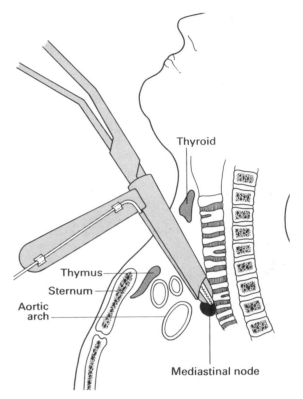

Fig. 12.7 The technique of mediastinoscopy.

Table 12.3 Chemotherapy in NSCLC.

Agent	Response rate (%)
Single agents	
Ifosfamide	15
Mitomycin	15
Vinorelbine	20
Cisplatin	12–15
Gemcitabine	20
Paclitaxel	20
Doxorubicin	12
Etoposide	10–12
Combination therapy in advanced disease	
Mitomycin, ifosfamide and cisplatin	45
Mitomycin, vinblastine and cisplatin	40
Cisplatin, vindesine or vinorelbine	25–35

The mediastinum can be directly visualized by mediastinoscopy (Fig. 12.7). In this procedure the surgeon makes a small incision in the suprasternal notch and the mediastinum is inspected through a mediastinoscope. Biopsies of the nodes are taken where possible. For left-sided tumours an additional mediastinotomy may be necessary, and it is generally performed through the bed of the second intercostal cartilage. In patients whose mediastinoscopy is negative the resectability rate is at least 85% and in over 50% of cases the nodes will not be involved at thoracotomy. In a further 30% the stage will be N_1 only (Table 12.3). Clearly, if the diagnosis has been made from supraclavicular node biopsy or biopsy of metastatic lesions, these patients are unsuitable for surgery. Other signs of obvious distant spread, such as abnormal liver function tests combined with an abnormal liver scan or hepatic ultrasound, are also obvious contraindications to operation. If the liver function tests are normal and there are no neurological symptoms or signs, ultrasound scan of the liver or CT brain scan will seldom be positive and are therefore not routinely indicated. A bone scan may, however, show unsuspected metastases.

Finally, the surgeon needs to know whether his or her patient is likely to withstand a surgical operation. Routine exercise testing, spirometry and other lung function tests such as ventilation/perfusion scanning can all be valuable. Patients with poor pulmonary reserve may have to be excluded from surgery even though their tumours are operable by other criteria. As a rough guide, patients with forced expiratory volume less than 1.2 l/s do not withstand pneumonectomy, though this also depends on age, sex, size and especially height. Patients over 70 years of age also tolerate pneumonectomy poorly (particularly right-sided).

Small-cell lung cancer

For patients with SCLC, the rationale for staging is altogether different. The characteristic early and widespread dissemination of this tumour makes surgical intervention inappropriate in the large majority of cases, although the occasional instance of 'surgically resectable' SCLC is encountered.

In some patients, determination of the degree of spread in SCLC is both logical and necessary. For example, although radiotherapy alone is no longer considered to be the best treatment for this disease (see below), it is sometimes used in patients considered unsuitable for chemotherapy. More commonly, in patients undergoing treatment with chemotherapy, radiotherapy is often given to those with 'limited' disease in whom no metastases can be demonstrated and disease is confined to one hemithorax. If the proposed treatment is only with cytotoxic drugs, irrespective of extent of disease, then routine staging is unnecessary, although investigation of specific symptoms is sometimes indicated on clinical grounds.

If staging in SCLC is to be undertaken, the most useful investigations include liver function tests (including measurement of serum albumin), plasma electrolytes and calcium determination, full blood count, isotope bone scanning and ultrasound liver scanning in patients with abnormal liver function tests. CT scanning of the brain in asymptomatic patients is seldom abnormal and not performed as routine. Bone marrow examination is positive (using conventional stains) in only 5% of patients with limited disease and normal blood counts. The proportion rises if staining with monoclonal antibodies is used. Marrow examination is therefore not always used in staging, and contributes nothing if the disease is already known to be disseminated.

Treatment

The principles of treatment of NSCLC and SCLC are very different. SCLC is seldom surgically resectable, usually widespread at presentation and is both more chemosensitive and more radiosensitive. For these reasons their management is considered separately.

Non-small-cell lung cancer

SURGERY

For NSCLC, surgical resection offers the best hope of cure. The percentage of operable cases varies with the philosophy of the surgeon, but the criteria for operability are not usually met in more than about 30% of cases. Approximately 50% of tumours are obviously unresectable by chest X-ray or bronchoscopic criteria. Physiological evaluation, biochemical testing and mediastinoscopy raises the unresectability rate still further (see above).

For patients in whom surgery is possible, the choice of operation depends on the location of the tumour and the patient's respiratory capacity. If the tumour is peripheral with no evidence of local extension, a wedge or segmental resection may occasionally be sufficient, particularly in patients whose pulmonary reserve is poor. In patients with more centrally located tumours contained within a single lobe, lobectomy is the usual procedure, provided the hilar nodes are clear. An adequate margin of normal-looking lung should be removed where possible. Pneumonectomy is necessary for tumours originating within the main stem bronchus, where the primary tumour involves more than one lobe, or where the hilum is involved. Clearly, these patients should undergo careful measurement of respiratory function before such an operation can be contemplated.

Although patients with evidence of local spread are usually considered to have inoperable lesions, many surgeons are prepared to undertake an operation in Pancoast tumour since cancers at this site (superior sulcus) may be biologically more favourable. Despite local invasion of pleura and ribs, they can sometimes be removed surgically, and regional lymphatic metastases appear to be unusual.

The mortality (5%) and morbidity associated with pneumonectomy are greater than with a lesser operation such as a lobectomy (2% mortality); many surgeons do not operate in patients over the age of 70 years, since mortality rises steeply with advancing age.

There is considerable controversy over the role of surgery when mediastinal nodes are involved (N_2). Many surgeons are now prepared to operate on some of these patients, especially after previous (neoadjuvant) chemotherapy (discussed below). The results of randomized trials comparing this approach with radical radiotherapy are awaited.

RESULTS OF SURGICAL TREATMENT

The results of surgical treatment depend largely on the

degree of patient selection; surgeons using the most strin-gent criteria for operability will have the best results. Histological type and stage of the tumour were important prognostic criteria [6]. Patients with squamous cell carci-noma have the best survival, 37% of all patients surviving 5 years. Patients with adenocarcinoma or large-cell carci-noma do less well, the overall 5-year survival being 27%. The importance of tumour stage is shown in Table 12.2. For patients with stage I disease, the 5-year survival rate is over 60% for all histologies (but approaching 80% for T_1 squamous carcinomas), suggesting that in NSCLC tu-mour stage is more important than histology in determin-ing survival. In patients with squamous cell carcinoma, the presence of local nodal involvement does not always imply early death from metastases. In these patients, radical surgery may be possible if the mediastinal node involvement was limited. Early mediastinal nodal involve-ment should not be regarded as an absolute contraindica-tion to surgery. Nevertheless, despite modern operative techniques and more careful case selection, the data in 1997 are only slightly better than those obtained in the 1950s.

RADIOTHERAPY

Although patients with NSCLC have always formed a large part of the radiotherapist's work there is continued debate regarding the indications for the use of this treatment. In judging which patients are suitable for treatment, the radiotherapist has to decide whether the intention is radi-cal or palliative. In the majority of cases, palliation is the only realistic expectation, though long-term survival is occasionally seen in patients irradiated only with palliative intent.

Palliative radiotherapy The majority of patients with NSCLC have inoperable disease. Palliative radiotherapy is often recommended for locoregional disease considered unsuitable for surgery but without evidence of distant metastases. Such patients include those with tumours of the main stem bronchus within 1 cm of the carina, those with invasion of important mediastinal structures such as the recurrent laryngeal or phrenic nerves, and those with troublesome symptoms including haemoptysis, obstruc-tion of a major bronchus, severe cough and pain. Finally, in patients in whom obstruction to a bronchus is immi-nent or where SVCO is present, radiotherapy is indicated, whether the patient is symptomatic or not.

Relative contraindications to radiotherapy include metastases beyond the locoregional nodes, multiple le-sions, bronchial fistula, supraclavicular node involvement

or a large tumour mass. Even under these adverse circum-stances, palliative treatment may still offer benefit, if the patient's symptoms demand it. If the patient is sympto-matic, treatment should be given as soon as possible.

When should treatment be used in asymptomatic pa-tients with inoperable disease? In an early study, treatment with radiotherapy, chemotherapy or both was compared to no initial treatment. Survival was the same in all groups (approximately 8.5 months), with no advantage for active treatment unless specific symptoms were present. Delay-ing radiotherapy until the onset of a specific symptom frequently allowed a patient 4–5 months before treatment proved necessary, and this group had the best palliation of all. Some radiotherapists in the UK therefore delay pallia-tive treatment, but this is not the practice in many large centres especially in North America and other European countries. Increasingly, palliative radiotherapy schedules have become shortened and simplified without apparent loss of benefit.

Radical radiotherapy Occasionally, patients with operable lung cancer are referred for radiotherapy either because they decline the offer of surgery, or because of coexistent medical conditions which would make surgery hazardous. In these operable cases and other inoperable localized tumours where the tumour can be encompassed by the radiation fields, radical irradiation may be justifiable, though even in these selected patients the 5-year survival following radiotherapy alone is only about 10%.

It seems likely therefore that radiotherapy can occa-sionally cure patients with carcinoma of the bronchus, particularly those with small, technically operable tu-mours. In these patients, a radical approach should be employed, requiring treatment to a higher dose than generally employed for palliation of symptoms, in the region of 50–60 Gy over 5–6 weeks in daily fractions or equivalent (see Chapter 5, Fig. 5.8). Such treatments may be accompanied by side-effects including dysphagia, peri-carditis and skin reactions. In addition, irradiation of a portion of spinal cord is unavoidable even with the most sophisticated planning techniques. With careful tumour imaging and the use of multifield techniques this problem can be minimized. Radiation damage to the spinal cord is discussed on pp. 176–7.

There have been several new approaches to radical radiation treatment. A recent trial of continuous hyper-fractionated accelerated radiotherapy (CHART) has re-cently reported improved survival for this technique compared with conventional radiotherapy [7]. In another approach a European trial used cisplatin as a radiation sensitizer during radiotherapy and, in a randomized trial [8], provided some evidence of improved survival. Neither technique is yet standard practice, but both results emphasize that effective local treatment may have an impact on survival.

Outside controlled clinical trials there is no place for routine preoperative radiotherapy in operable lung cancer. Occasionally a patient with stage III disease, with mediastinal involvement, may achieve a useful clinical regression with radiotherapy. However, even in such cases, it is exceptional for surgery to become a practical proposition. Combined treatment with surgery and preoperative radiotherapy is often recommended for Pancoast tumour (see above), but overall the results do not appear better than those of surgery alone.

CHEMOTHERAPY

Several drugs have been shown to have some activity in NSCLC (Table 12.3). The response rates are relatively low and no survival advantage has been shown for any of these drugs used as a single agent. Attempts have therefore been made to try and improve response rates by using drugs in combination. Typical combinations are shown in Table 12.3.

Of the various combination regimens that of mitomycin, ifosfamide and cisplatin appears to be among the most active, but is associated with considerable toxicity. Most of the active regimens include cisplatin, with its concomitant nausea and vomiting. Newer active regimens include carboplatin and gemcitabine, and carboplatin with etoposide or paclitaxel.

In advanced metastatic disease, the value of chemotherapy is questionable. The survival benefit is small, compared with best supportive care, but this oversimplifies the issue. The toxicity of chemotherapy (which is reduced in the more recent regimens) is balanced against improvement in symptoms which accompanies response. Responses are more frequent, long lasting and complete in patients who are fit, and many patients have a strong wish for active treatment. A meta-analysis has indicated that there may be a benefit in median and 1-year survival for the use of chemotherapy [9].

There has been considerable interest in the combination of chemotherapy before surgery in localized, initially inoperable, tumours and of chemotherapy before radical radiotherapy for localized tumours. There is no doubt that preoperative chemotherapy is associated with a higher response rate (up to 60%) than in metastatic disease, that some tumours are rendered operable and there may even be no viable tumour at resection. The impact on survival is not yet known. Large-scale trials will be necessary to determine this. A few small trials have suggested benefit, but others have not. Chemotherapy before or after radical radiation has been assessed in several randomized trials, but these were too small for a convincing survival difference to be shown (see, for example [10]). The meta-analysis [9] of all data from these trials indicates a potential benefit of 2–7%. It seems that a similar benefit of chemotherapy is present in all stages of localized NSCLC treated with surgery or radiotherapy. Such small differences are nevertheless very important in such a common disease. The value of concomitant radiotherapy and chemotherapy is still undecided and awaits large-scale randomized trials.

Small-cell lung cancer

The majority (two-thirds) of patients present with extensive disease—that is, thoracic disease involving more than one hemithorax or with metastatic spread. In these patients radiotherapy has a palliative role only and even with modern chemotherapy the prognosis is very poor. In patients with limited disease (confined to one hemithorax) chemotherapy is the mainstay of treatment.

CHEMOTHERAPY

It has long been apparent that SCLC is a rapidly dividing tumour, usually metastatic at the time of presentation. For this reason a systemic approach to treatment is essential. SCLC is relatively sensitive to cytotoxic agents and chemotherapy has become the mainstay of treatment. An early randomized prospective study comparing radiation alone with radiation and combination chemotherapy showed a clear short-term survival advantage for the patients treated with both chemotherapy and radiation compared with radiation alone.

Numerous single agents have since been shown to have activity. Cyclophosphamide and ifosfamide are the most useful alkylating agents. Many other drugs such as etoposide, taxanes, irinotecan, vinca alkaloids, cisplatin, and anthracyclines also have activity (Table 12.4).

Single-agent chemotherapy has largely been discarded except under special circumstances (discussed below). Numerous trials of combination chemotherapy, using a wide variety of regimens and schedules have shown a high rate of complete (25–50%) and partial (30–50%) responses (Table 12.5).

The duration of conventional chemotherapy has been assessed in three large studies. The balance of evidence suggests six cycles of conventional chemotherapy to be

Table 12.4 Single-agent chemotherapy in SCLC (the response data are approximate and depend on case selection).

Agent	Response rate (%)
Carboplatin	60
Etoposide	40–70
Irinotecan	45
Paclitaxel	35
Cyclophosphamide	35
Ifosfamide	35
Cisplatin	35
Doxorubicin	30
Docetaxel	25
Gemcitabine	20
Methotrexate	20
Vincristine	15
CCNU	10

Table 12.5 Combination chemotherapy in SCLC.

Regimen	Approximate response rate (%)
Cisplatin and etoposide	80
Ifosfamide, cisplatin and etoposide	75
Vincristine, doxorubicin and cyclophosphamide	70
Cisplatin, doxorubicin and etoposide	85
Doxorubicin, cylophosphamide and etoposide	80

Table 12.6 Adverse prognostic factors in SCLC.

Poor performance status
Extensive disease
Low plasma albumin and sodium
Raised alkaline phosphatase or lactate dehydrogenase
Brain metastases
Marrow infiltration or anaemia

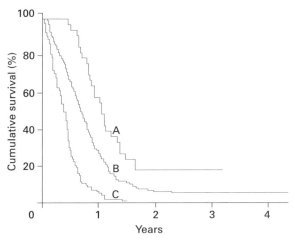

Fig. 12.8 Prognostic factors in SCLC. In A all patients had good performance status and normal biochemistry (see Table 12.6). In C patients had poor performance status and more than two biochemical abnormalities. Group B is by exclusion. From [12] with permission.

adequate. Neutropenia is a major dose-limiting toxicity which can be partially overcome by the use of haemopoietic growth factors. Recently completed randomized trials have assessed survival is improved by increasing dose intensity. This has been approached either by acceleration of cycles or by dose increase with the use of haemopoietic growth factors. Some of these trials have shown a survival benefit but the issue is not yet decided.

Attempts to increase the intensity of chemotherapy by giving drugs weekly have not improved survival. Similarly the use of very high-dose chemotherapy with peripheral blood stem cells as initial treatment is of unproven value, although the overall response rates with these approaches are high.

The toxicity of chemotherapy is considerable and the gains in survival are as yet modest. With limited disease it is now possible to achieve survival of 2 years in 15–20% of patients. A survey of survival in SCLC [11] has shown that 8% of limited disease (LD) patients and 2.2% of extensive

disease (ED) patients will be alive at 2 years. Relapse of SCLC occurs for 6 years, at which point only 2.6% of all patients are alive. Even though there is a chance of long survival and possibly cure with chemotherapy, the morbidity of treatment is sufficient to justify more palliative approaches, especially in elderly or ill patients. Such approaches must be judged critically since the symptoms of the disease are a major component of poor quality of life. Oral etoposide, for example, was widely promoted as a simple palliative treatment, yet two randomized trials showed it produced worse response and survival, worse toxicity and worse quality of life. Treatment should not be reduced without evidence of equivalent benefit.

There are certain factors which are known to be associated with a poor prognosis in SCLC, and these are listed in Table 12.6. Of these, the most important are ED, poor performance status, low plasma albumin and sodium and abnormal liver function tests (Fig. 12.8). In elderly patients, in whom these poor prognostic factors are often present, it is unwise to persist with chemotherapy beyond the first two or three cycles unless there is a clear improvement in the tumour and in the patient's well-being. For younger patients with LD and in whom there are no adverse prognostic features, intensive combination chemotherapy offers the best chance of long-term survival. There will be many patients who fall between these two extremes, and here the physician must decide on a case-by-case basis what appears to be the best policy.

RADIOTHERAPY

Small-cell lung cancer is radiosensitive, with complete radiological response of the primary tumour in over 80% of cases. Even large primary lesions associated with massive hilar and mediastinal lymphadenopathy may regress completely, following moderate doses of radiotherapy (40–50 Gy over 4–5 weeks). There has been interest in the use of twice-daily (hyperfractionated) radiotherapy but without proof of benefit in randomized studies.

Although the initial response to radiotherapy is usually gratifying, recurrence in the irradiated area is frequent and long-term local control of the disease is not always achieved. As might be expected, there is evidence that more durable local control may be obtained by higher radiation dosage although at the cost of greater toxicity, particularly if chemotherapy is also used.

The combination of chemotherapy and radiotherapy for the primary tumour has been investigated in several randomized trials in which patients treated with chemotherapy were assigned either to receive thoracic irradiation or not. The studies were too small to detect a moderate difference reliably, but an overview [13] in which individual data have been reanalysed has shown a 5% benefit in survival at 3 years (from 7 to 12%) — a 60% relative improvement. The morbidity of thoracic irradiation may be considerable in combination with chemotherapy. Nevertheless, thoracic irradiation now has an established role in patients with limited disease who are fit enough to receive it and who are responding to chemotherapy. Concomitant radiotherapy and chemotherapy, but no substantial improvement in survival, has been shown in the first randomized trial. The optimum timing of irradiation is also unclear. Although a recent Canadian study [14] has suggested a benefit for early treatment, other studies have not and the meta-analysis [13] showed no difference in survival with respect to time.

In summary, thoracic irradiation should be considered under the following circumstances.

1 In patients with LD, where there is an incomplete response to chemotherapy but no evidence of distant disease.

2 In patients with LD who are responding to chemotherapy.

3 For local recurrence.

4 For SVCO unresponsive to chemotherapy.

Radiotherapy is of great palliative value in SCLC, and is the treatment of choice for painful bone metastases and for brain metastases. Clinical evidence of brain metastases occurs in 25% of patients with SCLC and is demonstrable in about two-thirds of patients at autopsy. Treatment with radiotherapy to the whole brain to a total dose of 20 Gy in five fractions in a week is often effective and well tolerated; there seems to be no advantage for more prolonged regimens. Similar fractionation is usually satisfactory for painful bony deposits.

Symptomatic brain metastases are frequent in SCLC This has led to the assessment of prophylactic cranial irradiation (PCI). Two large-scale randomized trials have shown that routine use of PCI has decreased the clinical frequency of brain metastases from 40% to less than 10% with a small benefit for survival [15]. Prophylactic cranial irradiation therefore reduces the undoubted morbidity of brain metastasis. Conversely, PCI is itself associated with short-term toxicity (confusion, unsteadiness, memory loss) and a possible long-term neurological morbidity, although this seems very uncommon. The usual policy is to offer PCI to patients who have had a good response to chemotherapy, thereby avoiding unnecessary cerebral irradiation in non-responding patients whose survival time will be short.

SURGERY

Very uncommonly SCLC presents as a small peripheral tumour without mediastinal node involvement. Such tumours can be resected and it is usual to give postoperative chemotherapy. Clinical trials have shown that there is no benefit in surgery after chemotherapy as a 'debulking' procedure. The role of surgical intervention is therefore small in SCLC generally.

Tumours of the mediastinum [16]

The mediastinum lies at the centre of the chest and is bordered by the thoracic inlet superiorly, the diaphragm inferiorly, the vertebral column posteriorly, the sternum anteriorly and the pleural reflections laterally (Fig. 12.9). A great variety of tumours can arise in the mediastinum and tend to occur at different sites within it.

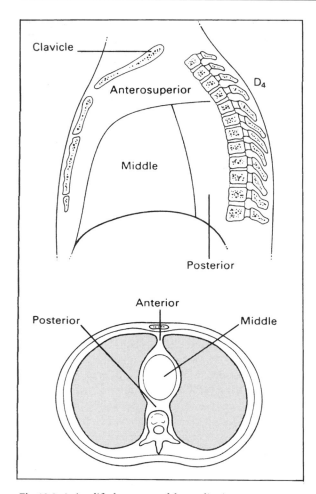

Fig. 12.9 A simplified anatomy of the mediastinum.

Table 12.7 Tumours of the mediastinum.

Anterosuperior
Thymoma
Teratoma
Thyroid and parathyroid tumours
Sarcoma (haemangiosarcoma, haemangiopericytoma)
Mesothelioma
Lipoma

Middle
Malignant lymphoma
Tumours of the heart
Secondary lymph node involvement
Pericardial tumours

Posterior
Neurofibroma, neurilemmoma, Schwannoma
Neuroblastoma
Neurofibrosarcoma
Phaeochromocytoma
Chordoma
Paraganglioma

The *anterosuperior compartment* of the mediastinum is bounded inferiorly by the diaphragm, anteriorly by the sternum and posteriorly by the vertebral column down to the fourth thoracic vertebra, and then by the anterior pericardium. It contains the upper trachea and oesophagus, the aortic arch and the thymus and may also include a retrosternal portion of a normal thyroid gland, with parathyroid structures and embryonic cell rests. The *middle compartment* of the mediastinum is bounded anteriorly by the anterior pericardium and posteriorly by the oesophagus, and extends downwards to the diaphragm. It contains the heart, ascending aorta, main bronchi, hila and carina, and the subcarinal and other closely related tracheobronchial lymph nodes. The *posterior mediastinum* lies between the vertebral column and posterior pericardium and contains the oesophagus, the descending thoracic aorta and the sympathetic nerve chains. The pattern of tumours arising in the mediastinum reflects these anatomical divisions (Table 12.7).

Anterosuperior mediastinum [17]

The commonest malignant tumours are thymomas and germ cell tumours, including teratomas of various types and seminomas. In addition, thyroid and parathyroid adenomas occur at this site and can cause diagnostic difficulties, and carcinomas of the thyroid may occasionally arise from the retrosternal portion of the gland. Symptoms from superior mediastinal tumours are usually caused by pressure on local structures such as the oesophagus, trachea and laryngeal or phrenic nerves. Dysphagia, dyspnoea, stridor, cough and SVCO are relatively common, and vocal cord palsy and/or diaphragmatic paralysis are sometimes seen. These symptoms occur less frequently with slow-growing tumours (such as retrosternal goitre and some thymomas).

Thymoma

Thymic tumours form a mixed histological picture often including more than one population of cells. Lymphocytes, epithelial cells and spindle cells tend to predominate, and 'typical' thymomas may contain lymphocytic and epithelial components as apparently distinct populations. Unfortunately, thymic tumour histology is a poor predictor of the behaviour of the tumour, though the macroscopic appearance is more valuable. Some thymic tumours grow very slowly over many years. Others grow more rapidly with local invasion and pleural spread.

The criteria for malignancy are difficult to define in thymomas, and the tumours are usually described as invasive or non-invasive. Distant metastases are unusual. Occasionally, Hodgkin's disease can arise from thymic tissue, without the evidence of lymphadenopathy elsewhere. In these cases surgical excision is less important than with other types of thymic tumour. Thymic *carcinomas* are rare tumours which show clear histological features of malignancy. Many variants have been described (squamous, clear cell, spindle cell, small, mucoepidermoid, adenocystic).

A variety of clinical syndromes are associated with thymomas. The commonest is *myasthenia gravis*, which occurs in 44% of patients. Myasthenia may be the presenting feature of the tumour which is benign or malignant. Myasthenia gravis is associated with antibodies to acetylcholine receptors, but its relationship to the tumour is not well understood. Removal of the thymoma results in remission of the myasthenia in approximately 30% of cases. *Red cell aplasia* occurs in 4% and may be associated with leucopenia and/or thrombocytopenia. A spindle cell thymic tumour is the commonest pathology. Occasionally the aplasia recovers after removal of the tumour. Other syndromes include hypogammaglobulinaemia, connective tissue diseases, pernicious anaemia and autoimmune thyroiditis. Together, associated diseases occur in 80–90% of thymomas, with myasthenia gravis and cytopenias being the commonest.

Diagnosis may be difficult since a core biopsy is usually necessary. Investigation includes chest X-ray (Fig. 12.10) and CT scan of the chest, which may show pleural metastases. Treatment is by surgical removal whenever possible. Complete removal is usually achieved if the tumour is encapsulated and in such cases local recurrence is unusual. Capsular invasion, direct extension to the pleura or pericardium and incomplete resection are all indications for postoperative radiotherapy, which reduces the local recurrence rate. Doses of 40–50 Gy in 3–5 weeks in 25 fractions are often used. More distant spread of recurrence after radiotherapy is sometimes treated by chemotherapy, although experience is limited and the results are often poor. The most active agents appear to be ifosfamide, cisplatin and etoposide. Cisplatin-containing regimens have been used and responses occur in 70% of cases, 40% being complete. Responses usually last from 2 to 3 years [18].

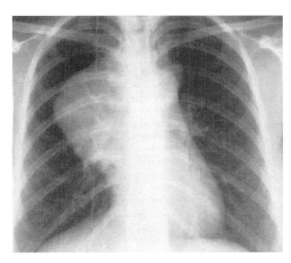

Fig. 12.10 Typical posteroanterior chest X-ray appearance in a patient with a thymic tumour. There is a well-demarcated tumour mass and the lung fields are clear.

Encapsulated thymomas have an excellent prognosis and 60% of patients are alive 20 years later. Invasive thymomas have a much worse prognosis, and only 50% of patients are alive after 5 years.

Carcinoid of the thymus

This tumour is uncommon and probably develops from neuroendocrine cells within the thymus (see Chapter 15). These rare tumours may give rise to Cushing's syndrome by producing ACTH and causing adrenal hyperplasia. They are occasionally malignant and are much more common in men. Although they may be completely resected, they often recur locally and metastasize. They do not cause carcinoid syndrome. The prognosis is not good, with 5-year survival as low as 15% in some series.

Germ cell tumours

Primary germ cell tumours of the mediastinum are uncommon but are potentially curable. Although teratomas and mixed tumours are the commonest, pure seminoma is also described. The tumours may produce β-human chorionic gonadotrophin (β-HCG) and α-fetoprotein (AFP) as do testicular tumours (see Chapter 19). As with thymomas, the usual clinical presentation is with local pressure symptoms, chiefly dyspnoea, cough and dysphagia. Occasionally, gynaecomastia is the presenting feature. Haematogenous metastasis is unusual, lung and brain being the commonest sites. Local lymphatic invasion may occur. Any young male with an unexplained superior mediastinal tumour of uncertain origin should have plasma tumour markers (AFP and β-HCG) measured since histological interpretation can be difficult even in experienced hands and these tumours can be misdiagnosed as adenocarcinoma. There is an association between Klinefelter's syndrome (XXY) and mediastinal germ cell tumours.

Plain chest X-ray and CT scanning are essential to delineate the tumour and for following progress after treatment. CT lung scanning will occasionally reveal unsuspected metastases. The principles of management are essentially as for testicular germ cell tumours (see Chapter 19). Primary treatment is with combination chemotherapy (currently using combinations including cisplatin, bleomycin, vinblastine and etoposide). Seminomas are in some cases curable by local radiotherapy; 40 Gy in 20 daily fractions over 4 weeks is the usual dose, although chemotherapy is now considered an essential component of treatment.

In mediastinal teratomas, the role of radiation for residual disease is uncertain. Surgical removal of suspicious residual masses should always be considered, ideally when tumour markers have returned to normal. Previous treatment with large doses of bleomycin may lead to pulmonary toxicity with stiff lungs and poor lung compliance, which may make the post-thoracotomy period particularly hazardous. Recent reports of combined chemotherapy and surgical treatment have been encouraging, with several long-term survivors (probable cures), in contrast to earlier reports in which cure was rare.

Middle mediastinum

In the middle compartment of the mediastinum, lymphomas are the commonest malignant tumours, and both Hodgkin's disease and non-Hodgkin's lymphomas occur. The differential diagnosis includes an important group of non-malignant conditions—pericardial and bronchogenic cysts, mediastinal lipoma, tuberculosis, sarcoidosis and infectious or malignant causes of hilar and/or mediastinal lymphadenopathy. In the absence of palpable lymphadenopathy in an accessible site, the diagnosis is usually made by mediastinoscopy or limited thoracotomy. Tissue diagnosis is essential and examination of fresh (unfixed) tissue is valuable for the histopathologist since the use of immunocytochemical stains can help distinguish difficult lymphomas from each other and from anaplastic carcinomas (see Chapter 3).

Staging and management of mediastinal lymphomas follow similar principles to those at other sites (see Chapter 26). Surgical excision has no place in the routine management of these tumours, which are sensitive both to chemotherapy and radiotherapy. Occasionally, mediastinal lymphoma causes severe SVCO which requires emergency treatment (see Chapter 8).

Two particular characteristic non-Hodgkin's mediastinal lymphomas occur. The first is T-cell convoluted, lymphoblastic, diffuse lymphoma, seen predominantly in adolescent males. The second is a sclerosing B-cell lymphoma, occurring most frequently in young women (Chapter 26). Hodgkin's disease of the mediastinum, usually in association with obvious lymphadenopathy in the neck and/or axilla, occurs in about 30% of all supradiaphragmatic cases, but the mediastinum may occasionally be the sole site of involvement.

Posterior mediastinum

Tumours of the posterior mediastinum are chiefly neurogenic in origin, and usually arise from the thoracic sympathetic chain or intercostal nerves (Table 12.7). They are frequently asymptomatic but may cause back pain, dysphagia or ptosis due to Horner's syndrome. Neurofibromas are the commonest, and can usually be removed surgically. They can arise sporadically or in patients with von Recklinghausen's disease. Other neurogenic tumours include schwannomas (both benign and malignant) and neurofibrosarcoma. These neurogenic tumours may extend through the intervertebral foramina (dumb-bell tumours) and cause cord compression. This is suggested by vertebral erosion on lateral chest X-ray. Ganglioneuromas are probably the commonest of the sympathetic nerve tumours and are generally well differentiated, encapsulated and surgically resectable. In some cases, urinary vanillyl mandelic acid may be raised and can be useful for monitoring progress. A less well-differentiated form (ganglioneuroblastoma) is also encountered, and has a worse prognosis because of local recurrence and metastases. Phaeochromocytoma, another hormonally active tumour, frequently presents with symptoms of catecholamine excess rather than with pressure symptoms, such as paroxysmal hypertension, headache, palpitation, chest pain and excessive sweating. It should be surgically excised where possible. In children, neuroblastoma is a common cause of posterior mediastinal tumour, accounting for about one-fifth of all childhood neuroblastomas. The management of neuroblastoma is discussed in Chapter 24.

Of the rare tumours, chordoma occasionally presents as

a posterior mediastinal tumour, and its management is discussed in Chapter 11. Paraganglioma (chemodectoma) is rare and may be locally invasive, usually involving the great vessels.

Diagnosis of posterior mediastinal tumours requires careful radiological assessment (sometimes with contrast studies such as aortography or contrast CT scanning) as well as precise tissue diagnosis, which usually requires thoracotomy. Management is by surgical removal of the tumour wherever possible. For incompletely excised malignant tumours, postoperative radiotherapy is usually recommended.

Mesothelioma

This relentlessly progressive malignant tumour arises from the surface of the pleura, occasionally remaining well localized at the primary site but more often spreading diffusely and involving a substantial area of the pleura including the inner surface of the visceral pleura, thereby encroaching on to the pericardium. Pleural effusion is common, and the disease is occasionally bilateral. Primary peritoneal mesothelioma, without pleural involvement, may also occur, and peritoneal disease occasionally develops in patients in whom the pleura is the main or primary site of disease. Most patients with mesothelioma give a history of asbestos exposure, though there is characteristically a delay of 20 years or so before the disease becomes apparent. The incidence of mesothelioma is rising, presumably because of the widespread use of asbestos products. Although the past 10 years have seen increasingly stringent constraints on the use of asbestos, the full impact of this substance has not yet been felt [19]. Crocidolite is thought to be the most carcinogenic fibre. A staging system is shown in Table 12.8.

Pathology

Pathologically the tumours may appear sarcomatous, often with both fibrous and epithelial elements which may be so anaplastic as to be almost indistinguishable from a poorly differentiated carcinoma. The degree of anaplastic change correlates poorly with clinical behaviour. In other cases the distinction from adenocarcinoma may be very difficult. Direct extension is characteristic, and mesotheliomas typically invade ribs and chest wall. Early and widespread involvement of intercostal bundles probably accounts for the severe pain so typical of this tumour. In addition, extension through the diaphragm, invasion of

local lymph nodes and distant blood-borne metastases are all commonly found.

Clinical features

Patients typically complain of increasing chest pain, which can be very severe, coupled with shortness of breath on exertion. The dyspnoea tends to be progressive and unremitting, often leading to severe incapacity even at rest. On examination there are signs of diminished chest movement and pleural effusion. Radiologically, the most typical feature of asbestos exposure is the pleural plaque, often multiple, and usually associated with pleural effusion (Fig. 12.11). In mesothelioma there is extensive pleural infiltration extending into the mediastinum and causing 'crowding' of the ribs on the affected side because of contracture caused by the tumour.

Diagnosis

The diagnosis can usually be confirmed by pleural biopsy. In cases with such widespread involvement that surgical resection is impossible, diagnostic thoracotomy should be avoided, particularly since tumour seeding of thoracotomy scars is common and can produce additional severe pain. Computed tomography scanning is of great importance for definition of the tumour anatomy, particularly with respect to the juxtapericardial reflection of the pleura and the adjacent pericardium, which are often poorly visualized by plain X-ray of the chest.

Table 12.8 Staging for mesothelioma. From [20].

T_1	Ipsilateral parietal pleura
T_2	Parietal and visceral pleura (including mediastinal and diaphragmatic pleura)
T_3	Locally advanced but potentially resectable tumour. Both pleural surfaces, extends into mediastinal fat
T_4	More extensive unresectable tumour
N_0	No regional nodes
N_1	Ipsilateral bronchopulmonary nodes
N_2	Mediastinal nodes (ipsilateral)
N_3	Contralateral nodes

Stage grouping

Stage I	T_1	N_0	M_0
Stage II	T_2	N_0	M_0
Stage III	Any T_3		M_0
	Any N_{1-2}		M_0
Stage IV	Any T_4, N_3 or M_1		

Radiotherapy is of very little value, though pain relief and apparent reduction in the rate of tumour growth occasionally occur. Adequate irradiation of the whole pleural surface is technically difficult because of the proximity of the lung, but new methods of tangential arc irradiation may allow this technique to be explored further. A wide variety of chemotherapeutic agents have been used in mesothelioma but with no long-term success, although responses to doxorubicin, cisplatin and other agents occasionally occur [21]. Responses to α-interferon are also reported. Combinations of cisplatin and interferon produce responses in about 20% of patients, and some responses last for many months. Intrapleural chemotherapy is occasionally attempted for control of the malignant pleural effusion, but the results are discouraging. Overall median survival is fractionated over 1 year [22]; negative prognostic factors include sarcomatous histology, male gender, poor performance status and a raised white cell count at diagnosis.

The very poor results of treatment argue strongly for rigid control of the use of asbestos products, and patients with mesothelioma and a clear history of industrial asbestos exposure are usually considered by independent tribunals to be strong candidates for compensation.

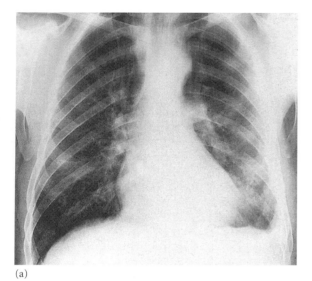

(a)

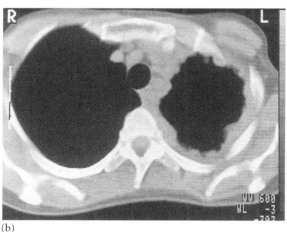

(b)

Fig. 12.11 Mesothelioma. (a) Typical X-ray findings, including pleural shadowing with nodulation behind the heart, in the costophrenic angle and along the lateral chest wall, together with partial destruction of ribs. Courtesy of Prof M.E. Hodson. (b) Typical CT scan appearance, with involvement of the whole of the pleura of the left lung and complete sparing on the right.

Treatment

Treatment of mesothelioma is highly unsatisfactory. Surgery is possible only in a very small minority of cases with localized involvement, though surgical cures can be obtained. Local recurrence is common, and most surgeons favour wide excision where possible, including sacrifice of part of the chest wall, diaphragm, pericardium and adjacent lobe of lung where necessary.

References

1 Doll R, Hill AB. Mortality in relation to smoking. ten years' observation on British doctors. *Br Med J* 1964; 1: 1399–410.

2 Doll R. *Harveian Oration.* London: Royal College of Physicians, 1982.

3 Cairns J. *Smoking Prevalence and Lung Cancer.* Scientific American.

4 Omenn GS, Goodman GE, Thornquist MD *et al.* Effects of a combination of beta carotene and vitamin A on lung cancer and cardiovascular disease. *N Engl J Med* 1996; 334: 1150–5.

5 Thatcher N, Girling DJ, Hopwood P *et al.* Improving survival without reducing quality of life in small-cell lung cancer patients by increasing the dose-intensity of chemotherapy with granulocyte colony-stimulating factor support: results of a British Medicine Research Council Multicenter randomized trial. *J Clin Oncol* 2000; 18: 395–404.

6 Mountain CF. Revisions in the International Staging System for Lung Cancer. *Chest* 1997; 111: 1710–17.

7 Saunders M, Dische S, Barrett A *et al.* Continuous hyperfractionated accelerated radiotherapy (CHART) versus conventional radiotherapy in non-small-cell lung cancer: a randomised multicentre trial. *Lancet* 1997; 350: 161–5.

8 Schaake-Koning C, van den Bogaert W, Dalesio O *et al.* Effects of concomitant cisplatin and radiotherapy on inoperable non-small-cell lung cancer. *N Engl J Med* 1992; 326: 524–30.

9 Non Small Cell Lung Cancer Collaborative Group. Chemotherapy in non-small cell lung cancer. a meta-analysis using updated data on individual patients from 52 randomised trials. *Br Med J* 1995; 311: 899–909.

10 Dillman RO, Seagreen SL, Propert KJ *et al.* A randomized trial of induction chemotherapy plus high-dose radiation vs. radiation alone in stage III non-small-cell lung cancer. *N Engl J Med* 1990; 322: 940–5.

11 Souhami RL, Law K. Longevity in small cell lung cancer. *Br J Cancer* 1990; 61: 584–9.

12 Souhami RL, Bradbury I, Geddes DM, Spiro SG, Harper PG, Tobias JS. Prognostic significance of laboratory parameters measured at diagnosis in small cell carcinoma of the lung. *Cancer Res* 1985; 45: 2878–82.

13 Pignon J-P, Arriagada R, Ihde DC *et al.* A meta-analysis of thoracic radiotherapy for small-cell lung cancer. *N Engl J Med* 1992; 327: 1618–24.

14 Murray N, Coy P, Pater JL *et al.* Importance of timing for thoracic irradiation in the combined modality treatment of limited-stage small cell lung cancer. *J Clin Oncol* 1993; 11: 3363.

15 Auperin A, Arriagada R, Pignon JP *et al.* Prophylactic cranial irradiation for patients with small-cell lung cancer in complete remission. *N Engl J Med* 1999; 341: 476–84.

16 Harper PG, Addis B. *Unusual Tumours of the Mediastinum.* In: Williams CJ, Krickorian JC, Green MR, Raghavan D, eds. *Textbook of Uncommon Cancer.* Chichester: Wiley, 1988: 411–49.

17 Mullen B, Richardson JD. Primary anterior mediastinal tumours in children and adults. *Ann Thoracic Surg* 1986; 42: 338–45.

18 Tomiak EM, Evans WK. The role of chemotherapy in invasive thymoma: a review of the literature and consideration for future trials. *Crit Rev Oncol Haematol* 1993; 15: 113–24.

19 Peto J, Hodgson JT, Matthews FE, Jones JR. Continuing increase in mesothelioma mortality in Britain. *Lancet* 1995; 345: 535–9.

20 Rusch VW. Prosposed new international TNM staging system for malignant pleural mesothelioma. *Lung Cancer* 1996; 14: 1–12.

21 Kraruf Hansen A, Hansen HH. Chemotherapy in malignant mesothelioma: a review. *Cancer Chemotherapy Pharmacol* 1991; 28: 319–30.

22 Curran D, Sahmoud T, Therasse P *et al.* Prognostic factors in patients with pleural mesothelioma: the European Organisation for Research and Treatment of Cancer experience. *J Clin Oncol* 1998; 16: 145–52.

13 Breast cancer

Incidence, aetiology and epidemiology

Breast cancer is the commonest of all malignant diseases in women, with an annual incidence of 21 000 new cases in England and Wales and 143 000 new cases in the USA. The incidence has risen steadily over the past 50 years with a striking geographical variation across the world. Incidence figures in the developed Western world are much higher than in poorer, developing countries (Fig. 13.1). The age-related incidence is shown in Fig. 13.2. One woman in 10 will develop breast cancer during her lifetime, making it the leading cause of death from malignant disease in Western women. In the UK the prevalence of breast cancer is so high that approximately one-half of all live female cancer patients are suffering from this single disease.

There are a number of known aetiological factors [1–3]. Women with a first-degree relative with breast cancer have a three-fold increase in risk. In particular, a history of breast cancer diagnosed premenopausally confers on the patient's daughters an additional risk of 3–11 times the normal rate. Women bearing their first child over the age of 30 are three times more likely to develop breast cancer than those who do so when under 20 years, and there is an increased risk in patients who have a history of benign breast disease, particularly epitheliosis and benign cellular atypia. Early menarche and late menopause predispose to a higher incidence, whereas oophorectomy, carried out early in life, offers some degree of protection. It is also

clear that prophylactic oophorectomy in women with a *BRCA1* or *BRCA2* mutation considerably reduces the risk of their developing breast cancer [3]. Although the evidence relating to use of oral contraceptives has been contentious, it seems likely that breast cancer is not more common in patients who have used these [4]. A large-scale recent study from the USA (Women's Health Initiative, WHI) confirmed an additional risk of 26% after 5.2 years of use of a combination of oestrogen/progestin medication, as well as additional risks of stroke and heart disease [4]. Follow-up of victims of Hiroshima has shown a late increase in incidence of breast cancer. Demographic differences are probably due more to dietary, cultural or geographical variability than to racial characteristics since Japanese and Hawaiian women who settle in the USA have daughters and granddaughters whose breast cancer prevalence follows the American pattern after as little as two generations. A high-fat diet as a causal agent in breast cancer has been strongly questioned by a negative cohort analysis from an international group of epidemiologists [5]. Conversely, a link has emerged between breast cancer incidence and alcohol intake. Recent cohort studies have suggested a reduced risk of breast cancer in women who are physically active, exercising regularly, but an increased risk in women taking hormone replacement therapy (HRT) either with oestrogens alone or in combination with progestins [6]. The small additional risk may be offset, at least in part, by other clinical advantages, including a clear reduction in the risk of osteoporosis, and has virtu-

Location

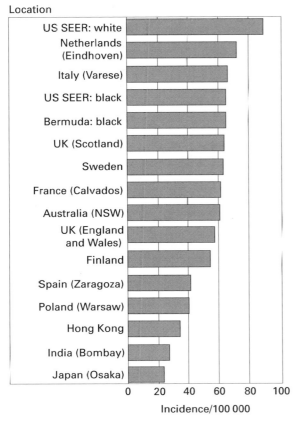

Fig. 13.1 Incidence of breast cancer. Directly standardized rates per 100 000 world population.

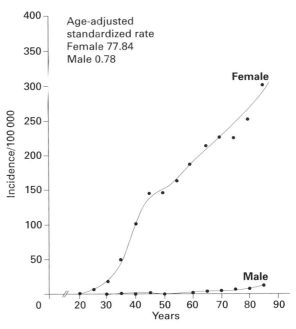

Fig. 13.2 Age-specific incidence of breast cancer.

ally disappeared after 5-year cessation of HRT. A recent large study has clarified the important protective role of breastfeeding [7]. There was a clear relationship between the duration of breastfeeding and the subsequent risk of breast cancer, with a relative reduction decreasing 4.3% for every 12 months of breastfeeding, and a decrease of 12% for each birth. This was true for women in both developed and developing countries, with no variation by age, menopausal status, ethnic origin, age at first live birth, or the total number of births. The authors estimated that the cumulative incidence of breast cancer in developed countries could be reduced by more than half, from 6.3 to 2.7 per 100 women by age 70, if women had the average number of births and lifetime duration of breastfeeding that had been prevalent in developing countries until recently. In the author's view, breastfeeding could account for almost two-thirds of this estimated reduction in breast cancer incidence.

Overall, there is strong evidence of a recent fall in breast cancer mortality, probably from earlier diagnosis and better treatment, and predating the application of the UK national screening programme [8].

Identification and cloning of *BRCA1* and *BRCA2* has led to a rapid increase in understanding of the molecular events in hereditary breast cancer [9]. Possession of *BRCA1* or *BRCA2* implies a 50–85% probability of the disease developing at some point during a patient's life, usually during the postmenopausal period (and also an ovarian cancer risk of 15–45%). The overwhelming majority of sporadic breast cancer cases are not, however, related to *BRCA1* or *BRCA2* and there are other genes such as *p53* which also confer a predisposition to the disease. Heterozygotes for mutations in the ataxia-telangiectasia gene may also be at increased risk. The *BRCA1* gene itself is a large gene, encoded by 5592 nucleotides distributed over a genomic region of approximately 100 kb.

Pathology and mode of spread

Almost all breast cancers arise from the glandular epithelium lining the lactiferous ducts and ductules, and are therefore typical adenocarcinomas. True intraduct carcinomas (or ductus carcinoma *in situ*, DCIS) do occur, particularly in screen-detected cases (see below), but most primary breast cancers have invaded into the stroma of the breast by the time of diagnosis (invasive carcinoma). The great majority of these present as breast lumps, although a very small number have eroded through the skin of the breast by the time they are first seen, presenting as fungating tumours. Lesser degrees of skin involvement lead to skin dimpling or tethering and *peau d'orange* in which skin infiltration leads to local lymphatic obstruction. The wide variability in histological appearance has led to classifications of these tumours according to microscopic characteristics (recently with the help of histochemical stains). Tumour grade, essentially the degree of differentiation, is of great prognostic importance [10].

Intraduct carcinomas of the breast (DCIS and lobular carcinoma *in situ*), without evidence of true invasiveness, are undoubtedly premalignant in a proportion of cases often with widespread abnormalities within the breast [11]. With the advent of mass screening, DCIS is now encountered far more frequently, indeed, pure intraduct carcinoma is rightly regarded as a 'new disease'. There is still considerable uncertainty about its natural history, but both radiotherapy and tamoxifen appear to reduce the risk of development towards invasive disease [12,13].

Modes of spread in breast cancer (Fig. 13.3) have been the subject of great controversy. The main focus of dispute previously was whether or not breast cancer always spread 'centrifugally' or by direct lymphatic dissemination, before more widespread involvement in the bloodstream; or whether the latter route was possible even in the absence of local nodal involvement. It is now clear that blood-borne metastases do occur independently, though axillary node involvement is highly predictive of probability of haematogenous spread. Local dissemination may occur to the underlying chest wall and related structures (ribs, pleura and brachial plexus), or to overlying skin. Lymphatic spread is to axillary lymph nodes and the supraclavicular, internal mammary or contralateral groups. Blood-borne metastasis occurs particularly to bone (especially the axial skeleton), liver, lung, skin and central nervous system (both brain and spinal cord). Intra-abdominal and pelvic metastases, including ovarian and adrenal deposits, are common. Many patients manifest particular patterns of spread, for example widespread bone involvement without evidence of soft-tissue disease. Some patients develop relentless local recurrence of disease, cancer *en cuirasse*, without distant metastasis but with a deep fungating ulcer affecting much of the chest wall. The reasons behind these patterns are unclear and apparently unrelated to histological characteristics or pathological grade.

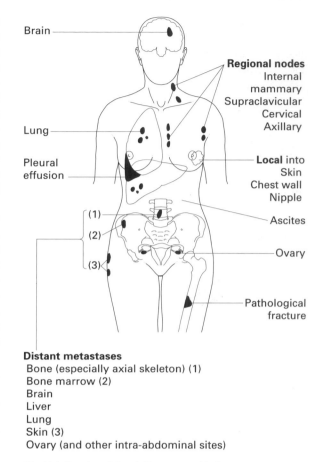

Distant metastases
Bone (especially axial skeleton) (1)
Bone marrow (2)
Brain
Liver
Lung
Skin (3)
Ovary (and other intra-abdominal sites)

Fig. 13.3 Local, nodal and distant spread in breast cancer.

Haematogenous spread is of crucial importance, since patients die from distant metastases rather than from uncontrolled local disease. The likelihood of axillary lymph node metastases correlates closely with the size of the primary tumour. There is a quantitative relationship between the number of metastatic lymph nodes and survival; see also Figs 4.2 and 13.7. Internal mammary node involvement is an important early site of spread of medially placed tumours, which have a reputation for higher risk of relapse and death than tumours located elsewhere in the breast [14]. The finding of supraclavicular lymphadenopathy at diagnosis is a particularly adverse clinical sign. Recent evidence suggests that detection of tumour cells in the bone marrow carries considerable prognostic weight [14]. Such cells presumably disseminate via the haematogenous route. Observations relating to the natural history of breast cancer using evidence from screening programmes have suggested that breast cancer does indeed behave as a progressive disease, that time of diagnosis is important in determining outcome; and that local treatment can sometimes be totally effective for small tumours [15]. Assessment of individual risk has also become increasingly precise [15].

Clinical features

Most women with breast cancer present to their family doctor with a lump in the breast, although screen-detected cases are increasingly frequent since the widespread adoption of mass population screening (see below). Most breast lumps are benign and the commonest causes are cysts, fibroadenomas or areas of fibroadenosis. Although a skilled surgeon often gives the correct clinical diagnosis, all breast lumps should be regarded as potentially malignant and firm histological diagnosis is nearly always necessary. Not all women with breast cancer present with a lump; pain in the breast, discharge or bleeding from the nipple, and pain or swelling in the axilla are also occasionally encountered.

Signs suggesting malignancy include: an asymptomatic impalpable but radiologically typical lesion, with microcalcification and an opacity with radiating fibrous strands; a change within the breast noticed by the patient herself; or signs of locally advanced disease. These include a large mass, tethering to skin and/or chest wall, axillary or supraclavicular lymph node enlargement, *peau d'orange*, nipple inversion and skin infiltration. Although cancers are typically firm or indurated, this may also be true of a simple cyst. Although women now present more often with relatively early disease, the lump is sometimes deliberately ignored, and can even be present for years before it becomes a fungating mass, though this now fortunately has become less common. Patients may present with symptoms from a secondary deposit, for example in the spine or brain. These may include pain in the back, due to vertebral metastasis leading to vertebral collapse and/or spinal cord compression (see pp. 124–6). General symptoms such as lassitude and anorexia may reflect advanced and widespread disease, particularly liver involvement.

Confirming the diagnosis

There are several methods of confirming the diagnosis. Aspiration of cysts is easy and frequently performed. The finding of a cyst with typical greenish fluid and disappear-ance of the lump after aspiration makes the diagnosis of cancer extremely unlikely. Aspiration cytology from solid lesions is fully established as a reliable diagnostic technique and it is even possible to provide prognostically useful cytological grading. If there is real diagnostic uncertainty, a much larger piece of tissue can be obtained by core biopsy with a 'Tru-cut' or other percutaneous biopsy needle, which usually yields an adequate core of tissue for histology. If the diagnosis cannot be obtained in this way, excision biopsy will be necessary. It is unjustifiable to proceed to mastectomy without giving the patient an opportunity to consider both the implications of the diagnosis and the alternative approaches for primary control of the tumour.

Mammography is widely used. On the whole, carcinomas have a characteristic mammographic appearance, with fine calcification and areas of obvious radiological irregularity; fixation of deep lesions either to chest wall or skin can sometimes be seen. The permissible radiation dose for a mammogram has now been reduced to a mean glandular dose of 3 mGy (maximum) (the equivalent of 10 standard chest X-rays). There is no longer any need to compromise exposure time for fear of radiation exposure. Moreover, radiation exposure is generally lower still; in our own hospital, for example, the average dose using state-of-the-art equipment is only 0.8 mGy. Mammography is particularly valuable to exclude synchronous primary cancers within the breast, a finding which would have considerable bearing on the choice of operation.

Preoperative investigation

A good deal of controversy has surrounded the question of preoperative investigations which are helpful in influencing management. In some centres patients are extensively investigated with isotope bone, liver and brain scans, together with skeletal X-rays, tumour marker analyses and estimations of urinary hydroxyproline. However, the general view at present is that the most valuable tests are a chest X-ray, full blood count, simple assessment of liver function and abdominal (hepatic) ultrasonography. In short, staging is only important if it defines 'early' breast cancer, distinguishing it clearly from more advanced cases unlikely to be surgically curable. Increased scepticism regarding the role of routine (and expensive) staging investigations has led to a reduction in their use.

Staging notation

There have been several attempts to devise a simple stag-

Table 13.1 Staging systems in breast cancer.

Stage	Description
TNM staging notation for breast cancer	
T_1*	Tumour less than 2 cm in diameter
T_2*	Tumour 2–5 cm in diameter
T_3*	Tumour more than 5 cm
T_4	Tumour of any size with direct extension to chest wall or skin
N_0	No palpable node involvement
N_1	Mobile ipsilateral nodes
N_2	Fixed ipsilateral nodes
N_3	Supraclavicular or infraclavicular nodes or oedema of arm
M_0	No distant metastases
M_1	Distant metastases

*T_1, T_2 and T_3 tumours further divide into (a) no fixation, and (b) with fixation to underlying pectoral fascia or muscle.

ing system, most of the classifications depending on the tumour size, the presence or absence of axillary node metastases, and the confirmation of distant metastases. The tumour node metastasis (TNM) staging system proposed by the Union Internationale Contre le Cancer has become widely accepted (Table 13.1). Future modifications are likely to take account of more detailed information regarding the pathological grade of the tumour, and its endocrine receptor status.

Hormone receptors in breast cancer

A proportion of breast cancers carry cellular receptors for oestrogen and other steroid hormones (including progestogen) both in their cell nuclei and also the cytoplasm. These receptors are present in 65% of cancers in postmenopausal women but only 30% of those premenopausal *BRCA1*-associated tumours are generally negative for both oestrogen and progesterone receptors (PR) whereas *BRCA2* tumours are characteristically positive [9]. Hormone dependence of some breast cancers can be demonstrated clinically by alteration of the hormonal environment (see p. 208). It is now established that the presence of an oestrogen receptor (ER) in a breast cancer cell correlates with the probability of hormone dependence in an individual tumour, making it possible to predict response to hormonal treatments. This has considerable clinical implications. Oophorectomy, for example, can be avoided in patients who are known to have an ER-negative tumour. It is not entirely clear whether ER status is the reflection of a genuine and fundamental difference between 'negative' and 'positive' breast cancers

or whether there is a continuum from ER-rich tumours to those with no detectable ERs whatever. The evidence at present favours the latter view, and ER 'positivity' is normally used to describe tumours in which the level of ER is greater than a certain defined figure, usually 5 fmol/mg cytoplasmic protein, or 25 fmol/mg nuclear DNA (see Chapter 6).

Oestrogen receptor positivity is associated with well-differentiated tumours (particularly tubular, lobular or papillary types) and with microscopic elastosis in the tumour. Clinically, it is apparent that slow-growing tumours tend to be ER-positive. Both primary tumours and metastases show similar ER content, though ER-negative metastases are sometimes encountered from an ER-positive primary tumour. The reverse is rarely true.

How successful have ER measurements been in the prediction of hormone responsiveness? At most, only 5–7% of ER-negative tumours respond to hormone manipulation. Conversely, 55% of ER-positive tumours will respond, so ER positivity, although useful, is not entirely reliable. There is, however, a detectable semiquantitative response; tumours very rich in ERs are clinically hormone-dependent in 90% of cases. Tumours rich in PRs are usually clinically hormone-responsive (more than 80% of cases).

Screening for breast cancer

The general principles of cancer screening have been discussed in Chapter 2. At first sight, breast cancer would appear to be an ideal tumour for a screening programme: relatively common (1–2 cases per 1000 women per year); and relatively accessible to clinical examination by doctors, nurses, paramedical staff and by the patient herself. In addition, mammography often demonstrates a breast cancer before it is clinically evident. Furthermore, there are known groups of patients at relatively high risk: those with a strong family history of breast cancer, those with late first pregnancies and those with a history of benign breast disease.

However, unselected mass clinical and mammographic screening has not yet been unequivocally justified by the results [16]. Apart from the considerable cost, it is not clear if the cure rate would be appreciably higher as a result of the earlier detection, although several studies have suggested a reduction in mortality in patients over 50 years, presumably from detection of the cancer at an earlier stage. Screening of selected high-risk patients may, however, be more worthwhile. In the UK, the Forrest Report recommended regular screening of all women between the ages of 50 and 64 years (the highest-risk age group), in line with the results published in the 1980s. Taking all age groups together, the overall results so far are not entirely encouraging. The value of screening appears particularly dubious in young women who, in more than one report, have had an overall worse survival than the unscreened group—perhaps due to a more rapid cancer growth rate in the younger patient, coupled with a sense of false security between routine scanning appointments. Breast self-examination, though widely practised, cheap and easily repeated, does not appear beneficial. Regrettably, international evidence remains substantially inconsistent [17].

Several studies have now confirmed an increased rate of mammographic detection of early cancers with a probable survival advantage over unscreened cases, though the false positive rate is considerable, the cost high and the anxiety produced distressing [18]. When a screening programme begins, about 20 (prevalent) cases are detected per 1000 women. When these 'screened' women are followed up, the new (incident) cases are about two per 1000 per year; the cost of incident screen-detected cases is therefore between £10000 and £25000, and the cost of each life saved as a result of screening is perhaps 2–5 times this figure. Breast screening is clearly not a panacea, although it may prove justifiable for certain defined groups [19]. The effectiveness of screening depends heavily on the population uptake, and is more clear-cut in a compliant, well-motivated group than, for instance, an inner-city population who might be harder to reach because of their greater social or demographic mobility.

An important recent surgical advance is the recognition that the sentinel node—those nodes (sometimes a single one) first receiving drainage from a tumour—can be removed by very limited surgery [20]. These findings correlated closely with more formal axillary dissection, allowing the possibility of avoiding axillary dissection altogether, though the technique is not yet fully established. Important questions relating to screening techniques, interval and management of intraduct non-invasive lesions have yet to be answered. The 3-yearly interval recommended in the UK is probably too long, since a large number of 'interval' cancers still develop [21].

Management of the primary tumour in 'early' breast cancer

Surgical operations for breast cancer

A good deal of controversy has previously surrounded the choice of operation in patients with 'early' breast cancer—

as it does, to some extent, even now. It is worth remembering that the principle of surgery in breast cancer is 'adequate control of locoregional disease' and there is no doubt that very good results, in terms of freedom from local recurrence, are achieved by mastectomy. In patients with axillary node involvement the additional use of postoperative radiotherapy will reduce the local recurrence rate still further but at the cost of an increased risk of arm swelling (lymphoedema).

With increased understanding that patients with breast cancer die not from uncontrolled local disease but from distant blood-borne metastases, there is now a much greater readiness to offer less mutilating procedures than mastectomy, wherever possible. In the USA and western Europe, conservative breast-preserving procedures are routinely employed, and regarded as the treatment of choice (see below) though simple mastectomy with axillary dissection is still required in about 20% of cases—a dramatic difference even from 10 years ago. Patients requiring mastectomy include those with large or retroareolar tumours (especially in a small breast), widespread intraduct carcinoma, and patients with multiple lesions within the same breast. Surgical reconstruction of the breast has advanced considerably over the past 10 years and there are a variety of techniques now available. The most commonly used are silicone prostheses and myocutaneous flap reconstruction. The improved contour is valuable and helps both confidence and self-image. However, the cosmetic result can be mediocre by comparison with the best results from radiotherapy, and reconstruction of the nipple is not generally performed, which is a further drawback. Myocutaneous flap reconstruction is cosmetically the most successful surgical method, but it is a far lengthier procedure than simple insertion of a silicone prosthesis.

Combinations of surgery and radiotherapy
(Table 13.2) [22]

Following treatment by surgery alone, local recurrence of disease in the chest wall, ipsilateral lymph nodes or residual breast occurs with a frequency of 7–30%. It is more common with large tumours (above 5 cm) and with axillary node involvement. Postoperative radiotherapy greatly reduces the frequency of local recurrence, particularly in patients with axillary node-positive disease [23]. However, most studies have shown no *survival* benefit from the routine use of radiotherapy in axillary node-positive cases, although an extremely important randomized study of postoperative radiotherapy in high-risk premenopausal women suggested a genuine survival ad-

Table 13.2 Five-year survival rates in operable breast cancer.

Operation	5-year survival rate (%)
Extended mastectomy (Urban)	67
Radical mastectomy (Halsted)	69
Total mastectomy (Patey)	67
Simple mastectomy and radiotherapy (McWhirter)	66
Radical radiotherapy with local excision of tumour (Calle)	74

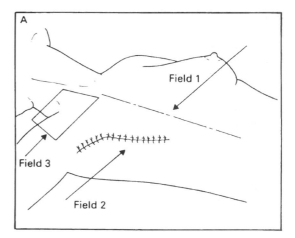

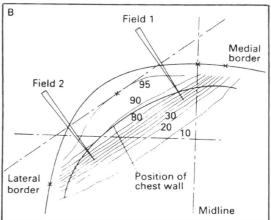

Fig. 13.4 Postoperative irradiation following mastectomy. (a) Use of two wedged fields tangentially applied to irradiate chest wall, axilla and internal mammary nodes. Field 3 irradiates the supraclavicular and lower cervical nodes using a directly applied radiation beam. Many other field arrangements are in common use; (b) transverse view showing isodose distribution from the two tangential fields (1 and 2) in relation to the breast and the chest wall.

vantage [24]. All patients (a total of 1708) received adjuvant chemotherapy following mastectomy with axillary dissection. At 10 years postmastectomy, local recurrence (9 vs. 32%), overall survival (54 vs. 45%) and disease-free survival (48 vs. 34%) were significantly better in the irradiated group. This and similar studies will stimulate a fresh look at our current understanding of the biology of breast cancer since localized treatments are not generally held to contribute greatly to freedom from distant recurrence and overall survival. From the point of view of local recurrence, it is clear that local irradiation plays a crucially important role, an observation well documented by the large Cancer Research Campaign (CRC) King's/Cambridge study which compared simple mastectomy with simple mastectomy plus local irradiation in a prospectively randomized study [25]. The clear result is that local recurrence is indeed reduced by radiotherapy (from 30 to 11% at 10 years) but that survival is unchanged, at least up to 10 years from initial treatment.

Techniques of postoperative irradiation vary widely. For example, some authorities omit regional node irradiation entirely (unless there is histological evidence of axillary disease), treating only the chest wall in patients who have undergone mastectomy [26]. Axillary irradiation should usually be avoided in patients who have undergone axillary node dissection—unless there is major involvement or extranodal disease. An example of a field arrangement with dose distribution is shown in Fig. 13.4.

The initial impetus towards minimal surgical excision with breast preservation came from Keynes in London and later, Baclesse in Paris and Crile in the USA. Subsequently, large series from Calle (Institut Curie, Paris) and others have lent strong support to the safety and effectiveness of these approaches. In Calle's series [27] of over 1000 cases the results at 5 and 10 years are certainly within the range achieved by more traditional surgical approaches, and only the minority of patients in this series later required surgical resection for local recurrence. About half

requiring 'salvage' mastectomy subsequently proved to be long survivors, suggesting that local recurrence following 'adequate' initial treatment may not necessarily be accompanied by widespread metastases.

An important American study on the role of breast-conserving primary treatment was initially reported in 1985, and later updated [23]. These data give strong support for the concept of breast preservation. Over 1800 patients were randomized to undergo treatment either with simple mastectomy alone, or local excision ('lumpectomy') with or without postoperative radiotherapy. After full axillary node dissection, patients with node-positive disease were given adjuvant chemotherapy. Five-year disease-free survival after local excision plus radiotherapy was better than with simple mastectomy alone. Furthermore, overall survival with local excision was, if anything, also slightly better. Ninety-eight per cent of node-positive patients treated by local excision, axillary dissection, radiotherapy and adjuvant chemotherapy remained free of local recurrence, compared with 64% without radiotherapy.

The conventional approach for early breast cancer has sharply altered over the past decade, in favour of these more conservative treatments. In general the cosmetic result of radical irradiation is highly satisfactory in the majority of cases, unlikely to be equalled by surgical reconstruction techniques. The psychological and sexual implications of mastectomy are beginning to be understood, and it is likely that the demand for radiotherapy as an alternative to mastectomy will increase. The question of local excision vs. mastectomy has largely been answered both by the changing preferences of surgeons and also by the patients themselves. Long-term follow-up is essential, especially since features have already emerged which might, in the individual case, argue against local excision with breast preservation rather than mastectomy. These include large primary size, inadequate excision with positive margins, high *in situ* component and high tumour grade.

Adjuvant hormone and cytotoxic therapy are discussed on pp. 206–7.

Management of the primary tumour in advanced breast cancer

For patients with locally advanced disease (T_3, T_4 and the majority of patients with N_{1B} or N_2 disease) the results of mastectomy have been disappointing. Surgery is contraindicated apart from debulking operations (often referred to as 'toilet' mastectomy) which can be extremely valuable together with radiotherapy, chemotherapy and hormone treatment to give the best possible chance of local control. Such surgical procedures are particularly helpful with fungating bulky exophytic cancers.

Radiotherapy is generally preferred; given cautiously, a high dose can often be achieved, with a local control rate as high as 90% at 5 years, although the overall survival in such patients is only 20–25%. The probability of local control is inversely related to the size of the primary

tumour [27], and features such as fixation to the chest wall, fixed axillary lymphadenopathy or involvement of supraclavicular lymph nodes contribute both to inoperability and also a higher probability of local recurrence. A high local dose is essential. In one recent retrospective series, treatment to a dose of 60 Gy or more resulted in a local control rate of 78% whereas a lower dose achieved local control in under 40%, the addition of chemotherapy reducing the local recurrence rate still further.

In many cases, particularly with elderly patients, radiotherapy can initially be withheld and the patient treated with tamoxifen. This agent can produce remarkable responses even in patients with advanced fungating local disease, and it is usually clear by 6 weeks after starting treatment whether or not she is responding. In younger women, treatment with chemotherapy may give a more rapid response and is usually regarded as a treatment of choice (see below); even elderly patients should be considered for chemotherapy since tolerance in this age group can be surprisingly good, with appropriate antiemetics and other supportive measures.

Complications of local treatment

Lymphoedema

This is due to lymphatic and venous obstruction and is a frequent (about 10%) and troublesome sequel to treatment for breast cancer, particularly when both radical surgery and radiotherapy have been used. Other factors contributing to its development include infection and recurrent or persistent disease. If lymphoedema appears years after primary treatment, axillary recurrence of tumour is the likely explanation. Apart from the disfigurement, the swelling can be very uncomfortable, and can also be a focus for spreading subcutaneous infection (cellulitis).

Management of the swollen arm is difficult and often unsuccessful. The patient should be instructed in isometric exercises with the arm elevated, in an attempt to improve the muscle pump. Avoidance of infection is essential; the patient must take care not to damage the skin of the affected arm, and wear gloves for tasks such as gardening. Cellulitis must be treated promptly with antibiotics. If local recurrence of tumour is confirmed it is usually better treated with systemic treatment rather than further radiotherapy, in order to avoid additional radiation damage. Compression sleeves are sometimes helpful in massaging fluid out of the limb but they often need to be used for several hours to be effective. Nocturnal elevation of the arm (for example, by a roller towel arrangement or by resting on pillows) is often recommended if the patient can tolerate it. Nurse-led lymphoedema clinics skilled in management of this complication are an important part of the oncology department — an effective but labour-intensive aspect of care.

Stiff or frozen shoulder

Patients undergoing mastectomy should be given a programme of graded exercises postoperatively, to increase shoulder mobility, prevent stiffness and help prevent lymphoedema. The aim is to develop normal elevation and rotation in the shoulder joint. Abduction and elevation of the arm are most important. If a frozen shoulder has developed, physiotherapy and short-wave diathermy are helpful.

Restoring a normal breast contour

Most women adapt well to an external prosthesis. For those who do not, breast reconstruction or an internal implant should be considered. It is often helpful to reassure patients who are about to undergo mastectomy that early breast reconstruction is feasible, and regarded by the surgeon as part of the primary treatment, if the patient so wishes. Of the various alternative techniques, simple silicone or saline implant (with a tissue expander if necessary) is the most straightforward but more complex surgery including the latissimus dorsi or transverse rectus abdominis muscle (TRAM) flap, though more demanding for the patient, do provide a better final result. Nipple reconstruction is best achieved by use of pigmented skin transfer (from upper thigh) but remains a difficult surgical challenge.

Psychological disturbance

Any form of mastectomy is mutilating, especially radical mastectomy. The incidence of depression and psychosexual disorders is about 25% during the first year and are more severe in women who place particular emphasis on their body image. Pre- and postoperative counselling is certainly helpful and the role of patient support and counselling groups is discussed in Chapter 7. Although patients undergoing treatment without losing the breast clearly suffer a range of psychological disturbances, these seem to be different from those encountered in patients who have required mastectomy. The most difficult period is generally the initial 6 months after primary treatment.

Adjuvant hormone therapy and chemotherapy

Since patients with breast cancer often develop disseminated disease from undetectable micrometastases present at the diagnosis, initial increasing attention has been paid to the concept of adjuvant systemic therapy following primary local treatment. The aim is to eradicate these deposits before they become clinically apparent, an approach supported by animal data suggesting that small metastases are more chemosensitive. Although most of the initial trials were far too small to detect the difference with certainty, more recent studies have clarified the degree of benefit and long-term outcome from adjuvant systemic treatment [28,29].

Adjuvant hormone therapy

Following the demonstration that oophorectomy caused regression of advanced breast cancer, several studies of the effect of ovarian ablation as an adjuvant to mastectomy have been performed. Its effect in randomized comparisons of patients with ER-positive disease has now been convincingly demonstrated. The large 1998 overview of all prospectively randomized studies of tamoxifen (and adjuvant chemotherapy as well) has now shown unequivocally that there is a real long-term survival benefit in patients given tamoxifen for at least 2 years after initial treatment (Fig. 13.5) [29]. This applies to both node-negative and node-positive patients and clearly persists for up to 15 years following therapy. Unexpectedly, the benefit appears to be even greater at 10 than at 5 years, and it now seems clear that at least 5 years of tamoxifen is required for maximum effect. The benefit is limited to patients with hormone-receptor positive disease (over 75% of all cases). There may also be additional benefits from the cholesterol-lowering effect of tamoxifen (with reduction in frequency of death from myocardial infarction) and from the significant protection it appears to produce against postmenopausal bone loss. Recent fears regarding the carcinogenic potential of tamoxifen on the uterine endometrium should not be exaggerated; the complication is extremely rare. However, a recent large-scale study using anastrozole (1 mg orally per day) has shown that it is both more effective and less toxic than tamoxifen, though the data are still preliminary. Thirteen patients developed endometrial carcinoma in the group of 3125 patients treated with tamoxifen, compared with only three in the similar-sized anastrozole group [30].

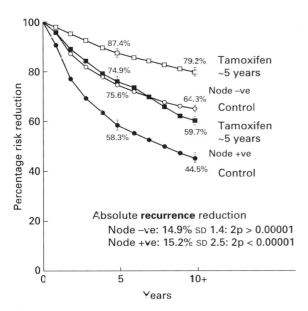

Fig. 13.5 Absolute reduction in risk of recurrence of breast cancer following tamoxifen. Open symbols: node −ve cases. Closed symbols: node +ve cases. From [28].

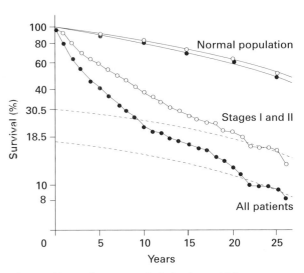

Fig. 13.6 Twenty-five year survival of patients with breast cancer. Dashed lines are an extrapolation parallel to the indicated proportion 'cure' at 25 years. From [28] with permission.

Adjuvant chemotherapy

The earliest study, that of Nissen-Meyer and coworkers at the Oslo Cancer Institute [31], suggested that cyclophosphamide given immediately after surgery could improve survival at 10 years.

The unpredictable nature of breast cancer and the need for lengthy follow-up make interpretation of more recent studies extremely difficult, but it is clear (again from worldwide data generated by the Early Breast Cancer Trialists Collaborative Group) that adjuvant chemotherapy had a substantial impact on both disease-free and overall survival (Fig. 2.12) in node-positive premenopausal patients, particularly in women aged 30–40 years (Fig. 13.6). As Peto has pointed out, small improvements in survival may be translated into thousands of lives saved in a condition such as breast cancer where the incidence is so high. Subgroups of node-negative patients with adverse features such as large or high-grade primary tumour also benefit from adjuvant chemotherapy. Adverse prognostic features include tumour size greater than 3 cm, poorly differentiated tumours, nuclear pleomorphism, hormone receptor negativity, high proliferation rate and expression of *erb*-B2 protein. Young patients, diagnosed under the age of 35 years, should also be treated with adjuvant chemotherapy regardless of node status or other features,

since they have much to gain from chemotherapy. More recently, 'neoadjuvant' therapy has been tested for breast cancer in a number of randomized control trials. In this approach, the chemotherapy is given as primary treatment, prior to surgery or radiotherapy. Although an interesting concept in breast cancer, it is too early to know whether such preoperative treatment will prove in the long run more effective than the conventional sequence of treatment. In patients with smaller, operable tumours, however, it now seems clear that administering adjuvant chemotherapy should take precedence over postoperative radiation therapy [32]. This means that for a large proportion of premenopausal women (including virtually all node-positive cases) the current sequence of therapy should be: local surgical excision plus axillary dissection; combination chemotherapy; and, finally, radiation therapy—a dramatic change even from 10 years ago. Patients should also receive tamoxifen if they are ER-positive.

The difficulty in assessment of early results of adjuvant therapy is discussed more fully in Chapter 2. These problems are particularly acute in breast cancer, in view of the lengthy follow-up required. It is not a simple matter to give an unqualified answer to the question whether adjuvant chemotherapy is of benefit to *all* patients with early breast cancer. The advantage is probably confined to subgroups of patients, and may not be substantially greater than with adjuvant hormone therapy, generally a far less toxic form of treatment. The toxicity of combination chemotherapy can be considerable (although many patients have little difficulty), so this is clearly an area where a possible benefit must be weighed against the quality of the patient's life (see Chapter 7). Using hormone therapy in ER-positive premenopausal patients clearly has a major role, possibly as great as chemotherapy [33, 34].

Only 10 years ago, current practice in the UK did not generally favour the routine use of adjuvant chemotherapy, but the situation has altered sharply. Adjuvant chemotherapy, generally with six courses of CMF (cyclophosphamide, methotrexate and 5-fluorouracil), is now widely employed in node-positive premenopausal patients; in patients with additional risk factors, particularly more than four axillary nodes positive, more intensive doxorubicin-based regimens are customary. Tamoxifen is now recommended for virtually all postmenopausal patients regardless of node status (certainly all those known to be ER-positive), with the possible exception of those with small (T_1) low-grade tumours. Five years of treatment has become the standard recommendation.

Treatment of metastatic disease

In most patients with apparently localized breast cancer it is probable that the disease is in fact systemic or generalized at presentation and that metastatic disease will later develop. This view is supported both by the common occurrence of widespread metastases, often many years after mastectomy has been undertaken, and by long-term follow-up studies of patient cohorts (Fig. 13.6). In the classic study by Brinkley and Haybittle, the overall survival was only 20% after 25 years [35]. Even in women deemed suitable for mastectomy (the 'early' operable group), the survival was only 30%. The appearance of metastases usually prove fatal within 3 years, though many women who respond to treatment do live longer. The likelihood of dissemination is strongly linked to the presence or absence of histologically positive axillary lymph nodes at the time of operation, and a quantitative relationship between the number of positive axillary lymph nodes and the probability of metastatic disease has been established.

Options for hormonal manipulation
(see Chapter 6)

Since the first therapeutic oophorectomy by Beatson in 1896, it has become clear that at least one-third of patients with advanced disease gain symptomatic benefit from hormonal manipulation. A wide variety of procedures have been used, including oophorectomy, ovarian irradiation (sometimes referred to as 'artificial menopause'), treatment with oestrogens, antioestrogens, luteinizing hormone-releasing hormone (LHRH) antagonists (for example, goserelin), anabolic steroids, glucocorticoids and progesterones, surgical treatment by adrenalectomy or hypophysectomy and treatment with aromatase inhibitors such as anastrozole or letrozole.

The conventional approach is largely based on the menstrual status of the patient. In most premenopausal and perimenopausal patients, surgical or radiation-induced ovarian ablation was traditionally employed for metastatic disease, but the advent of LHRH antagonists has led to these approaches being far less frequently employed nowadays since these agents provide adequate reduction of circulating oestrogen and render patients hormonally postmenopausal within 2 months of first administration. Goserelin is given monthly by intramuscular injection. Conversely, the use of laparoscopy oophorectomy—a safe and simple procedure requiring only a single night in hospital—has repopularized the surgical approach as a serious alternative. This is all the more true as patients are now much more carefully selected on the basis of ER-positivity, filtering out those who could not benefit from oophorectomy. In postmenopausal patients, tamoxifen (which probably acts as an antioestrogen, but perhaps has directly cytotoxic activity as well) is the most widely used agent because of the relative lack of side-effects [36]. For almost 20 years it has been used as a standard adjuvant therapy (see below).

Given by mouth at a standard dose of 20 mg daily, the drug is slowly cumulative. Side-effects, although uncommon, include flushing, nausea, hypercalcaemia, a disease 'flare', thrombocytopenia, fluid retention and menstrual disturbances. Most patients gain a pound or two in weight while taking tamoxifen, and some notice changes in the quality of their skin, hair or nails.

Patients with ER-positive tumours are very much more likely to demonstrate a significant response to hormonal manipulation; patients with ER-negative tumours rarely respond. Patients who are ER-positive have a different natural history from the ER-negative group, with a longer disease-free interval and overall survival. Simultaneous measurements of ER and PR give an even better prediction of response to hormone manipulation than measurement of ER alone (Table 13.3). PR positivity is also correlated with a longer disease-free interval.

Table 13.3 Response to endocrine therapy.

Receptor status	Response (%)
ER −ve PR −ve	<10
ER −ve PR +ve or ER +ve PR −ve	35
ER +ve PR +ve	70

The site of metastatic disease may well influence responsiveness to hormonal treatment. Bone metastases are relatively likely to respond, although the ultimate outcome for such patients is poor, with a mean survival time of only about 12–15 months. Nevertheless, some patients with bone metastases from breast cancer do survive very much longer (sometimes several years) provided they are sufficiently hormone-responsive.

In general, most premenopausal patients with recurrent disease, if known to be ER-positive, are treated either by LHRH therapy (goserelin is often preferred) or by radiation-induced menopause or laparoscopic oophorectomy in the first instance. Postmenopausal patients are more usually treated with tamoxifen if they have not already received it as adjuvant therapy (see below). In each case at least 30% of patients can be expected to respond, the exogenous hormone continued indefinitely while the patient's response persists. Further hormone therapy should be reserved for patients who responded to the initial hormonal procedure. An important new group of agents—the oral aromatase inhibitors, such as anastrozole—block the formation of oestrogen precursors and their conversion to oestrogen in peripheral tissues (pp. 92–4). Tolerance and acceptability to anastrozole and other similar compounds is generally excellent, and these agents have become rapidly established as second-line agents after tamoxifen failure in ER-positive postmenopausal patients. The recommended dose of anastrozole is 1 mg daily.

When relapse occurs following these initial measures, other useful agents include anabolic steroids, progestogens and glucocorticoids. Anabolic steroids are more effective in postmenopausal women and seem particularly helpful for bone metastases. Twenty per cent of untreated patients will respond, but side-effects of virilization can be troublesome. A convenient preparation is nandrolone decanoate (Deca-Durabolin) 50–100 mg given intramuscularly every 3–4 weeks. Progestational agents can be used if there has been a previous hormone response. The most commonly used drug is medroxyprogesterone acetate (MPA, Provera), which is often given at a dose of 100 mg three times daily by mouth, though weight gain may limit the tolerability. Another frequently used progesterone, megestrol acetate (Megace), is equally effective.

The question of whether hormone manipulation should still be preferred to cytotoxic chemotherapeutic treatment of first relapse has been widely debated. Although, in quantitative terms, the choice lies between hormonal manipulation (which has a 30% likelihood of response) and combination chemotherapy (with a response rate of double this figure), this is an oversimplification of what is often a complex decision. Hormone-induced responses tend to be more durable and are usually accompanied by minimal toxicity to the patient. Chemotherapy-induced responses tend to be of shorter duration and are accompanied by a wider spectrum of physical and psychological difficulties. In the UK there is no doubt that most clinicians prefer hormone manipulation first. The increasingly wide availability of ER assay makes this decision more straightforward; hormone therapy should be limited to the ER-positive group.

Chemotherapy

Chemotherapy in breast cancer is firmly established as one of the major therapeutic modalities. Although introduced much more recently than other treatments, chemotherapy has assumed increasing importance, both in primary management (as adjuvant therapy) and for patients with metastatic disease. Responses have been documented to many classes of drug, including alkylating agents, antimetabolites, spindle poisons, antitumour antibiotics, taxanes and several others. The observation of objective tumour response, coupled with frequent improvement in subjective well-being, makes these agents well worth considering in the management of metastatic disease. In general, skin, lymph node, and soft-tissue metastases respond more readily than deposits in the liver or lung, which in turn are more likely to respond than bone metastases. Previous responsiveness to hormone therapy does not appear to predict the probability of response to chemotherapy. Over the past few years, it has become clear that taxane agents such as paclitaxel and docetaxel have marked activity in breast cancer and may be particularly useful in treating recurrent or metastatic tumours that are no longer responsive to traditional agents [37].

Following successes with combination chemotherapy in Hodgkin's disease and acute leukaemia, it is now usual to employ cytotoxic drugs in combination in breast cancer, rather than as single agents. Early work using a five-drug regimen of vincristine, methotrexate, cyclophosphamide, prednisolone and 5-fluorouracil

Table 13.4 Examples of combination chemotherapy regimens for advanced breast cancer.

Regimens	Dose and route
CMF	
Cyclophosphamide	100 mg/m^2 p.o. days 1–14
Methotrexate	40 mg/m^2 i.v. days 1 + 8
5-FU	600 mg/m^2 i.v. days 1 + 8 (repeated every 28 days) (many variants)
VAP	
Vincristine	2 mg i.v. days 1 + 8
Doxorubicin	40–50 mg/m^2 day 1
Prednisolone	30 mg/day for 7 days (repeated every 21 days)
AC	
Cyclophosphamide	1 g/m^2 i.v. day 1
Doxorubicin M-M-M	40 mg/m^2 i.v. day 1 (repeated every 21 days)
Melphalan	10 mg p.o. per day for 3 days
Methotrexate	50 mg i.v. bolus day 1 (every 21 days)
Mitomycin C	15 mg i.v. bolus (given every alternate course, i.e. every sixth week)

i.v., intravenously; p.o., by mouth.

(5-FU), suggested that very high response rates could be obtained, but greater experience showed that the response rate was nearer 50%. Since that time a variety of different combination regimens have been used, and some of the commenest are shown in Table 13.4.

The most effective combination of drugs is uncertain. Many include doxorubicin, probably the most active single agent for breast cancer and is often still used as a single agent, both at relapse and as part of adjuvant regimens (see below). Treatment with intermittent combination chemotherapy has how largely replaced low-dose continuous administration. Toxicity is largely predictable, but usually no worse than would be expected from the additive use of the single agents chosen. For CMF, for example, the major problems are nausea, stomatitis and cystitis, and for VAP (vincristine, doxorubicin and prednisone) the commonest side-effects are neuropathy and alopecia. Treatment with the taxane group has emerged as an important additional class agent in patient resistant doxorubicin.

Despite impressive response rates, the expected lifespan for patients with metastatic breast cancer has changed little, if at all, as a result of the more widespread use of these drugs. More intensive chemotherapy regimens may possibly be associated with higher response and survival rates, and it has even been claimed that high-dose chemotherapy with stem cell support may be justifiable, although recent results have been disappointing. Complete responders to chemotherapy certainly have a better prognosis than partial responders, but the adverse effects in non-responders must be weighed against these benefits. This may be one reason for the failure of combination chemotherapy to improve overall survival in patients with metastatic disease. Other reasons are that the responses are often short-lived (sometimes only a few months), and probably occur in patients with an intrinsically better prognosis than non-responders. A central problem, as with so many areas of cancer chemotherapy, is to select those who are likely to respond well, and avoid overtreating patients unlikely to be helped. Chemotherapy responses are more likely to be achieved in patients who are fit, have soft-tissue rather than bone metastases, have a small number of metastatic sites and have received no previous chemotherapy. Oestrogen receptor status has little predictive value for chemotherapy response.

An important study comparing the addition of a humanized monoclonal antibody, trastuzumab ['Herceptin'], to chemotherapy was recently published [38]. All patients were known to have tumours expressing the growth factor receptor gene, human epidermal growth factor receptor (*HER*-2), an adverse risk factor in breast cancer. Responses and survival were increased, with an improved progression-free interval from 4.6 to 7.4 months, though at the cost of increased cardiotoxicity. The improvement may be small but the study probably represents a real step forward in application of specific target-directed biological therapy.

A final additional beneficial type of treatment of metastatic disease involves the pamidronate and other bisphosphonates for patients with bone metastases [39]. Most studies show that pamidronate infusion (90 mg) given monthly, together with hormonal or chemotherapy, reduces skeletal complications and gives useful palliation of pain.

Treatment of special problems in metastatic disease

Radiotherapy is the treatment of choice for patients with painful bone metastases, offering relief of symptoms in over three-quarters of all cases, although objective radiological evidence of recalcification is much less common. Some sites are particularly problematic, such as large cortical deposits in the femur or other weight-bearing bones, in which case it is often necessary to combine radiotherapy with internal orthopaedic fixation before a fracture occurs. Sternal metastases should be treated promptly since, if left untreated, the thoracic cage is unstable, leading to a mid-dorsal vertebral fracture which can be life-threatening.

Brain metastases occur in about 15% of all patients with breast cancer. Radiotherapy is beneficial in approximately two-thirds, often with control of symptoms until the patient's death. Spinal cord compression is also common, and its treatment is discussed in Chapter 8.

Pelvic irradiation to a relatively modest dose leads to complete and lasting amenorrhoea in premenopausal patients, and radiation-induced menopause has therefore been used as an alternative to oophorectomy—particularly in patients whose general condition makes surgery inappropriate. The probability of total amenorrhoea is dose-dependent and fractionated treatment (12–15 Gy, five fractions over 1 week) is usually given. Radiation-induced menopause appears as successful as oophorectomy for relief of symptoms. Clinical problems from metastases at other sites, such as skin, lymph node, pelvic or painful hepatic deposits, can often be alleviated by local radiotherapy even when systemic treatments have failed.

When local recurrence occurs after mastectomy, radiotherapy is undoubtedly the treatment of choice if not previously given. However, local recurrence often occurs in the context of systemic metastases, and if there is evidence of more widespread disease systemic treatment is often more appropriate. Even under these circumstances radiotherapy may be the best treatment for a troublesome local recurrence. If postoperative radiotherapy has previously been given it may be difficult to give further treatment because of the radiation tolerance of local structures such as brachial plexus, skin and lung. Treatment by electron beam irradiation or hyperthermia can be helpful in this difficult situation [40].

Prognosis of breast cancer

Five- and 10-year survival rates do not give a true picture since relapses may occur well beyond this point (Fig. 13.7), with a few additional deaths from relapse beyond 25 years. Prognosis is dependent on tumour stage, size of the primary (Fig. 13.8) and tumour grade but probably independent of the extent of initial surgery (see also Fig. 4.2).

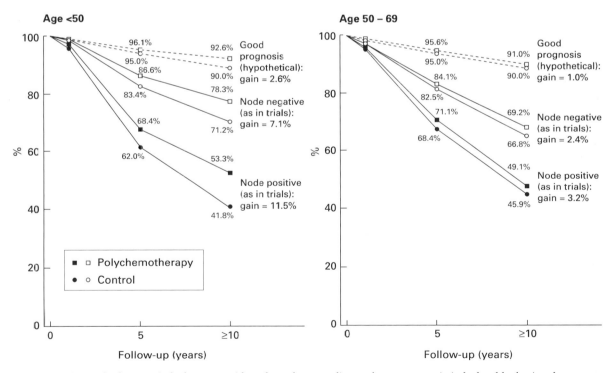

Fig. 13.7 Estimate absolute survival advantages with prolonged polychemotherapy for populations of women with good, inter-mediate and poor prognosis (calculated by having the proportional risk reduction unaffected by prognosis). From [28].

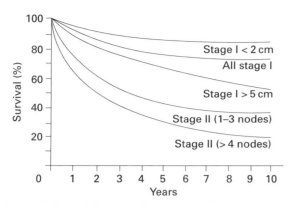

Fig. 13.8 Survival in stages I and II operable breast cancer. In stage I disease tumour size is an important prognostic determinant, as is degree of involvement of axillary nodes in stage II.

Axillary lymph node involvement is particularly important: of patients with stage I disease ($T_{1-2} N_0$) 80% are alive at 10 years whereas with stage II disease ($N_{1-3} M_0$) 10-year survival is only 35%. Biopsy of a single sentinel node within the lower axilla (identified by radiographic scintigraphy) may provide reliable information on axillary node involvement, without axillary node dissection [41], a finding which could dramatically reduce the need for axillary dissection.

The significance of the age of the patient at diagnosis is uncertain, but young patients do face an exceptional lengthy period at risk, and appear to have more to gain from adjuvant chemotherapy [34]. Pregnancy in patients with breast cancer does not appear to have any adverse effect. Complete sequencing of the *p53* gene appears to provide useful prognostic information—mutations in certain regions of the gene carrying a significantly worse prognosis [42]. As far as a genetic predisposition is concerned, a recent study of *BRCA1* patients showed no evidence of a different prognosis as compared with sporadic cases [43]. Finally, there is increasing evidence that specialist breast cancer centres offer a standard of care which leads to an improved outcome—including survival [44,45]. Breast cancer should no longer be regarded as the province of the general surgeon.

Cancer of the male breast [46]

Breast cancer in men is at most, only 1% as common as in women (Fig. 13.1). Little is known of the aetiology, although a few family clusters have been reported, and it may be more common in patients who have had bilharzia with consequent liver damage and hyperoestrogenism. It has been reported in patients with Klinefelter's syndrome, in which gonadotrophin levels are characteristically elevated, and in patients with gynaecomastia.

Most patients present with a tender indurated nipple, often with crusting or discharge, sometimes bloodstained. The disease involves the chest wall early. Routes of spread are similar to the disease in women, as is the pattern of metastasis. Most of the tumours are ER-positive.

Treatment is usually by mastectomy. Many surgeons prefer radical mastectomy because of the paucity of breast tissue in males and the possibility of early direct invasion, coupled with the lesser mutilation of this operation in men. Local irradiation should be given when axillary lymph nodes are involved.

For recurrent disease orchidectomy is generally considered the treatment of choice, with responses in 60% of cases. The value of other endocrine manoeuvres is uncertain, but treatment with tamoxifen, progestogens, cyproterone or hypophysectomy have all been employed. There have been few trials of chemotherapy, but it is often used when hormone treatments have failed and responses may be seen. Overall, the prognosis appears to be worse than in women [47].

References

1 McPherson K, Steel CM, Dixon JM. Breast cancer. epidemiology, risk factors and genetics. *Br Med J* 2000; 321: 624–8.
2 Haber D. Roads leading to breast cancer. *N Engl J Med* 2000; 343: 1566–8.
3 Kauff ND, Satagopan JM, Robson ME *et al.* Risk-reducing salpingo-oophorectomy in women with a *BRCA1* or *BRCA2* mutation. *New Engl J Med* 2002; 346: 1609–15.
4 Writing Group for the Women's Health Initiative Investigators. Risks and benefits of estrogen plus progestin in healthy postmenopausal women. *JAMA* 2002; 288: 321–33.
5 Hunter DJ, Spiegelman D, Adam H-O *et al.* Cohort studies of fat intake and the risk of breast cancer—a pooled analysis. *N Engl J Med* 1996; 334: 356–61.
6 Marsden J. Hormone-replacement therapy and breast cancer. *Lancet Oncol* 2002; 3: 303–11.
7 Collaborative Group on Hormonal Factors in Breast Cancer. Breast cancer and breastfeeding collaborative reanalysis of individual data from 47 epidemiological studies in 30 countries including 50 302 women with breast cancer and 96 973 women without disease. *Lancet* 2002; 360: 187–95.
8 Coleman MP. Trends in breast cancer incidence, survival and mortality. *Lancet* 2000; 356: 590–3.
9 Hedenfalk I, Duggan D, Chen Y *et al.* Gene-expression

profiles in hereditary breast cancer. *N Engl J Med* 2001; 344: 539–48.

10 Elston CW, Ellis IO, Pinder SE. Prognostic factors in invasive carcinoma of the breast. *Clin Oncol* 1998; 10: 14–17.

11 Wärnberg F, Yuen J, Holmberg L. Risk of subsequent invasive breast cancer after breast carcinoma in situ. *Lancet* 2000; 355: 724–5.

12 Julien JP, Bijker N, Fentiman IS *et al*. Radiotherapy in breast-conserving treatment for ductal carcinoma in situ: first results of the EORTC randomised phase III trial 10 853. *Lancet* 2000; 355: 528–33.

13 Fisher B, Dignam J, Wolmark N *et al*. Tamoxifen in treatment of intraductal breast cancer: NSABP B-24 randomised controlled trial. *Lancet* 1999; 353: 1993–2000.

14 Lourisch C, Jackson J, Jones A *et al*. Relationship between tumor location and relapse in 6871 women with early invasive breast cancer. *J Clin Oncol* 2000; 18: 2828–35.

15 Armstrong K, Eisen A, Weber B. Assessing the risk of breast cancer. *N Engl J Med* 2000; 342: 564–71.

16 Gøtzsche PC, Olsen O. Is screening for breast cancer with mammography justifiable? *Lancet* 2000; 355: 129–34.

17 Eisinger F, Geller G, Burke W *et al*. Cultural basis for differences between US and French clinical recommendations for women at increased risk of breast and ovarian cancer. *Lancet* 1999; 353: 919–20.

18 Lidbrink E, Elfving J, Frisell J *et al*. Neglected aspects of false positive findings of mammography in breast cancer screening: analysis of false positive cases from the Stockholm trial. *Br Med J* 1996; 312: 273–6.

19 Hakama M, Holli K, Isola J *et al*. Aggressiveness of screen-detected cancers. *Lancet* 1995; 345: 221–4.

20 Krag D, Weaver D, Ashikaga T *et al*. The sentinel node in breast cancer: a multicenter validation study. *N Engl J Med* 1998; 339: 941–6.

21 Woodman CBJ, Threlfall AG, Boggis CRM *et al*. Is the three-year breast screening interval too long? Occurrence of interval cancers in the NHS screening programme's north western region. *Br Med J* 1995; 310: 224–6.

22 Early Breast Cancer Trialists' Collaborative Group. Favourable and unfavourable effects on long-term survival radiotherapy for early breast cancer: an overview of the randomised trials. *Lancet* 2000; 355: 1757–70.

23 Fisher B, Bauer M, Margolese R *et al*. Five years' results of a randomized clinical trial comparing total mastectomy and segmental mastectomy with or without radiation in the treatment of breast cancer. *N Engl J Med* 1985; 312: 665–73.

24 Overgaard M, Hansen PS, Overgaard J *et al*. Postoperative radiotherapy in high-risk pre-menopausal women with breast cancer who receive adjuvant chemotherapy. *N Engl J Med* 1997; 337: 949–55.

25 Cancer Research Campaign Working Party. Trial for early breast cancer. A detailed update at the tenth year. *Lancet* 1980; ii: 55.

26 Tobias JS. Radiotherapy and breast conservation. *Br J Radiol* 1986; 59: 653–66.

27 Calle R, Pilleron JP, Schlienger P, Vilcoq JR. Conservative management of operable breast cancer. Ten years' experience at the Foundation Curie. *Cancer* 1978; 42: 2045–53.

28 Early Breast Cancer Trialists' Collaborative Group. Polychemotherapy for early breast cancer. an overview of the randomised trial. *Lancet* 1998; 351: 1451–67.

29 Early Breast Cancer Trialists' Collaborative Group. Tamoxifen for breast cancer. An overview of the randomised trials. *Lancet* 1998; 352: 930–42.

30 The ATAC (Arimidex, Tamoxifen, alone or in combination) Trialists' Group. Anastrozole alone or in combination with tamoxifen versus tamoxifen alone for adjuvant treatment of post-menopausal women with early breast cancer. *Lancet* 2002; 359: 2131–9.

31 Nissen-Meyer R, Kjellgren K, Malmio K *et al*. Surgical adjuvant chemotherapy. Results with one short course with cyclophosphamide after mastectomy for breast cancer. *Cancer* 1978; 41: 2088–98.

32 Recht A, Come SE, Henderson IC *et al*. The sequencing of chemotherapy and radiation therapy after conservative surgery for early stage breast cancer. *N Engl J Med* 1996; 334: 1356–61.

33 Dixon JM, Hortobaggi G. Treating young patients with breast cancer: evidence suggests that all should be treated with adjuvant therapy. *Br Med J* 2000; 320: 457–8.

34 Jakesz R, Hausmaninger H, Samonigg H. Current perspective: chemotherapy versus hormonal adjuvant treatment in premenopausal patients with breast cancer. *Eur J Cancer* 2002; 38: 327–33.

35 Brinkley D, Haybittle JL. The curability of breast cancer. *Lancet* 1975; ii: 95–7.

36 Wiseman H. *Tamoxifen. Molecular Basis of Use in Cancer Treatment and Prevention*. Chichester: John Wiley, 1994.

37 Seidman AD, Reichmann BS, Crown JP *et al*. Paclitaxel as second and subsequent therapy for metastatic breast cancer: activity independent of prior anthracyclene response. *J Clin Oncol* 1995; 13: 1152–9.

38 Slamon DJ, Leyland-Jones B, Shak S *et al*. Use of chemotherapy plus a monoclonal antibody against HER-2 for metastatic breast cancer that overexpresses HER-2. *N Engl J Med* 2001; 344: 783–92.

39 Lipton A, Theriault RL, Hortobaggi GN *et al*. Pamidronate prevents skeletal complications and is effective palliative treatment in women with breast carcinoma and osteolytic bone metastases. *Cancer* 2000; 88: 1082–90.

40 Vernon C. Hyperthermia in the treatment of cancer: current techniques and future prospects. In: Tobias JS, Thomas PRM eds. *Current Radiation Oncology*, Vol. II. London: Arnold Publications, 1996: 343–462.

41 Veronesi U, Paganelli G, Galimberti V *et al*. Sentinel-node biopsy to avoid axillary dissection in breast cancer with clinically negative lymph nodes. *Lancet* 1997; 349: 1864–7.

42 Bergh J, Norberg T, Sjogren S *et al*. Complete sequencing

of the p53 gene provides prognostic information in breast cancer patients, particularly in relation to adjuvant systemic therapy and radiotherapy. *Nature Med* 1995; 1: 1029–34.

43 Verhoog LC, Brekelmans CTM, Seynaevy C *et al.* Survival and tumour characteristics of breast-cancer patients with genetic mutations of *BRCA1. Lancet* 1998; 351: 316–21.

44 Basnett I, Gill M, Tobias JS. Variations in breast cancer management between a teaching and a non-teaching district. *Eur J Cancer* 1992; 28A: 194–550.

45 Gillis CR, Hole DJ. Survival outcome of care by specialist surgeons in breast cancer: a study of 3786 patients in the West of Scotland. *Br Med J* 1996; 312: 145–8.

46 Joshi MG, Lee AK, Loda M *et al.* Male breast carcinoma: an evaluation of prognostic factors contributing to a poorer outcome. *Cancer* 1996; 77: 490–8.

47 Ravandi-Kashani F, Hayes TG. Male breast cancer. A review of literature. *Eur J Cancer* 1998; 34: 1341–7.

14 Cancer of the oesophagus and stomach

Carcinoma of the oesophagus

Incidence and aetiology

Oesophageal cancer is commoner in males, with a male : female ratio of over 2 : 1 and a peak incidence in the 60–80 age group (Fig. 14.1). In the UK it has become more prevalent in the last 10 years. In some Scandinavian countries, carcinoma of the oesophagus is as common in women as in men. There are marked geographical variations in incidence, with very high levels near the Caspian Sea, central Asia and the Far East (Fig. 14.2), and in the USA it is commoner in less advantaged socioeconomic groups, diagnosed three times as frequently in black as in white people. Aetiological factors include cigarette smoking, excessive alcohol intake and malnutrition. Repeated oral infection, development of benign oesophageal stricture or achalasia and a history of syphilis, are also thought to be contributory. The Plummer–Vinson (Paterson–Kelly) syndrome of a congenital web in the upper oesophagus, with glossitis and iron-deficiency anaemia, is a known predisposing factor, more common in women. There is a 7% incidence of oesophageal carcinoma in long-standing achalasia. Barrett's oesophagus should be regarded as a potentially premalignant condition, particularly in patients with dysplasia. Surgical excision is now frequently recommended as a prophylactic measure in this condition. Finally, oesophageal cancer is reportedly more common in breast cancer patients who have received radiation therapy (relative risk for squamous oesophageal cancer 5.42 and for adenocarcinoma 4.22) — presumably due directly to radiation carcinogenesis [1].

Pathology

The oesophagus can be conveniently divided into three sections: the cervical oesophagus (distal limit 18 cm from upper incisors), mid third (distal limit 30–31 cm from incisors) and lower third (distal 10 cm of oesophagus). The most frequent sites for oesophageal cancer are the narrowed areas in the cricopharyngeal region, adjacent to the bifurcation of the trachea, and in the lowest part of the oesophagus near the sphincter. Lower third lesions are commonest (40–45%), followed by mid third (35–40%) and cervical oesophageal cancers (10–15%). Both squamous carcinomas and adenocarcinomas occur, the histology varying with the level in the oesophagus. Cervical oesophageal and upper third lesions are always squamous cell in origin. Adenocarcinomas are occasionally seen in the mid third and are increasingly common in the lower third, though many of these are strictly speaking of gastric origin. Adenocarcinoma of the oesophagus is rising in incidence [2] and now accounts for over a quarter of oesophageal cancer, compared with under 7% in the 1960s. This five-fold increase in adenocarcinoma of the oesophagus remains unexplained, the only known predisposing features being Barrett's oesophagus and duodenal ulcer (and occasionally in previously irradiated patients — see above). Other tumour types are very rare and include melanoma and leiomyosarcoma.

Tumour spread (Fig. 14.3) occurs chiefly by direct extension and by lymphatic metastases. Direct extension occurs early, both intramurally in the craniocaudal direction and circumferentially. Insidious submucosal spread is almost universal and carries important implications

215

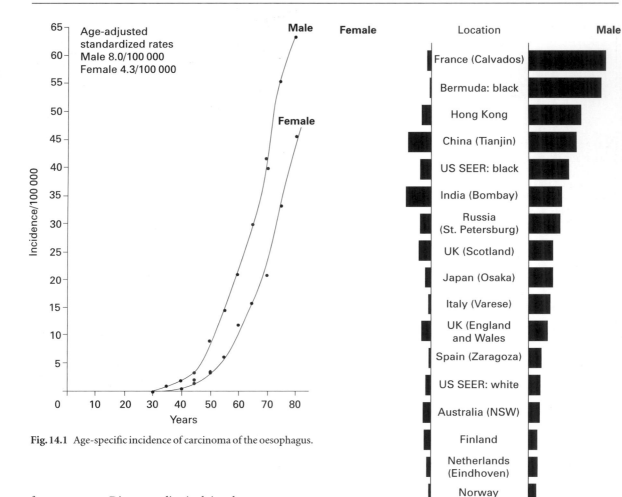

Fig. 14.1 Age-specific incidence of carcinoma of the oesophagus.

Fig. 14.2 Incidence of oesophageal cancer, 1983–87. Directly standardized rates per 100 000 (world population). These international comparisons show a high incidence stretching from the Caspian Sea across Mongolia and Northern China. European rates are generally low, with the remarkable exception of the Calvados region in northern France.

for treatment. Direct mediastinal involvement occurs, usually later in the disease, by penetration of the muscular coat. Fistulous connection to the trachea may occur.

Cancers of the upper or cervical oesophagus chiefly drain to the deep cervical nodes either directly or via paratracheal or retropharyngeal lymphatics. Mid and lower third lesions drain to the posterior mediastinal nodes and abdominal nodes, sometimes traversing the diaphragm. Haematogenous spread characteristically occurs later, though unexpected hepatic metastases may be encountered at laparotomy in cases thought to be suitable for radical surgery. The liver is much the commonest site of haematogenous spread, though bone, lung and brain deposits also occur.

Clinical features

The risk of oesophageal adenocarcinoma is almost eight times higher in persons with symptoms of gastro-

oesophegeal reflux (heartburn, regurgitation)—even higher if the reflux symptoms occur predominantly at night [3]. When the disease becomes established, dysphagia is the commonest symptom, almost always accompanied by weight loss, often amounting to 10% or more of body weight. The dysphagia is more pronounced for

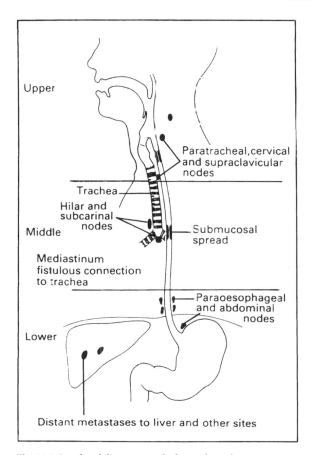

Fig. 14.3 Local and distant spread of oesophageal cancer.

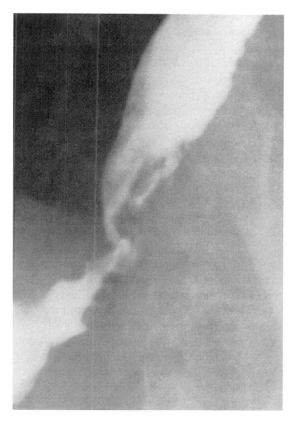

Fig. 14.4 Barium swallow showing carcinoma of distal oesophagus. A long irregular stricture is shown, with dilation above.

solids than liquids, and patients have often discovered for themselves that a soft or liquidized diet is the only means of securing a regular intake of food. Typically the dysphagia becomes more severe, and some patients progress to complete dysphagia with inability even to swallow their own saliva. Many are able to point to the site at which the food lodges. Pain is a relatively late symptom, usually felt retrosternally. Spillover or aspiration of oesophageal contents into the larynx or lung may cause coughing, and involvement of the recurrent laryngeal nerve may lead to hoarseness. Haematemesis and melaena are unusual.

On examination there may be no abnormality apart from obvious weight loss and malnourishment. Occasionally, patients present with metastatic symptoms—usually from liver metastases—with only minimal dysphagia. Evidence of metastases may be found on examination, with enlarged supraclavicular nodes or hepatomegaly.

Investigation and staging

Patients with dysphagia should be investigated with a barium swallow and meal. The characteristic appearance is of an obvious area of irregular narrowing (Fig. 14.4). Unlike patients with achalasia of the cardia, there is usually rather minimal dilatation of the proximal oesophagus, presumably because little time has intervened for dilatation to take place. The narrowed segment may be surprisingly long, often with an irregular 'shoulder'. Patients with severe dysphagia may be difficult to investigate because of the danger of aspiration of contrast material into the lungs. Paratracheal or other mediastinal node enlargement—usually well displayed on chest X-rays and thoracic computed tomography (CT) scanning—are common, and an absolute contraindication to radical surgery. The cause of the dysphagia is sometimes due to secondary mediastinal lymphadenopathy.

Direct oesophagoscopy and biopsy are mandatory in all patients who are fit enough to undergo the procedure, though this carries a small risk of oesophageal perforation, with mediastinitis and surgical emphysema which is often fatal.

No satisfactory staging system has been developed, possibly because of the inaccessibility of this tumour and difficulty in assessing the regional node involvement. About two-thirds of patients have lymphatic involvement at the time of diagnosis. The extent of the primary tumour may be impossible to determine even under direct vision, and it may sometimes be difficult or dangerous to pass the endoscope so the lower border may be inaccurately determined. Intraluminal endoscopic ultrasonography gives additional internal anatomical detail and is extremely useful in delineating mediastinal lymphadenopathy.

Treatment

It is generally agreed that adenocarcinoma of the oesophagus (almost always lower third lesions) is best treated by surgery if the lesion is technically operable. In most other cases, particularly those of the upper third and cervical oesophagus, combinations of chemotherapy and radiotherapy are probably the treatment of choice [4]. Before embarking on local treatment, the surgeon or radiotherapist must be clear as to whether the philosophy of treatment is radical or palliative.

Radical treatment

When radical surgical treatment is contemplated in patients who are generally fit and with no evidence of distant disease, it is important to determine the extent of the lesion before definitive resection is attempted. Exploratory laparotomy is often advocated and is a routine part of many operations when reconstruction is to be achieved by colonic transposition, creating a viable conduit between pharynx and stomach. Radical removal of the oesophagus, first attempted over 100 years ago by Czerny, is nowadays usually performed as a single-stage procedure with oesophagogastric anastomosis or colonic interposition. Formerly, operations were performed in which a permanent feeding gastrostomy was left as the means of providing nutrition.

Only a minority of patients with oesophageal cancer are suitable for radical surgery, and the commonest indication is a mid or lower third lesion, particularly where the histology is adenocarcinoma, in a fit patient with no demonstrable evidence of metastases. Until recently there was little, if any, evidence that preoperative radiotherapy or chemotherapy influences resection rate, operative mor-

tality rate or overall survival, but a recent large-scale study from the UK has shown a striking improvement using a preoperative combination of chemotherapy (cisplatin and fluorouracil) with radiation therapy [5]. The two-year survival rates were 43% and 34% (with or without chemotherapy); median survival rates were 16.8 months compared with 13.3 months. Previous studies had proven disappointing [6].

In patients with carcinoma of the *upper third of the oesophagus*, radiotherapy is usually considered to be the treatment of choice, though surgical treatment is preferred by some. No randomized comparison has been made. Combinations of chemoradiotherapy are increasingly recognized as more effective than radiation therapy alone [4,7]. Radiotherapy (with or without concomitant chemotherapy) has several advantages over surgery, including wider applicability (most patients are elderly and poorly nourished), avoidance of laryngectomy, and significant palliation of dysphagia in most patients, with cure in at least 10% of patients who are able to tolerate high doses: 60 Gy minimum in daily fractions over 6 weeks. In addition, surgical treatment (Fig. 14.5) carries a mortality of about 10% and, unlike radiotherapy, is inappropriate in patients with locoregional spread of disease. Indeed, in a major review of world series, a 29% mortality rate was described, in patients treated during the 1970s [8,9], though surgical mortality has fallen with better patient selection, surgical technique and supportive care. Despite poor

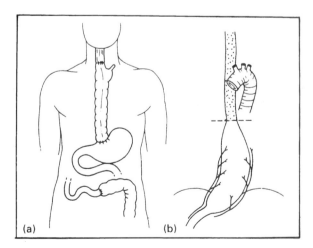

Fig. 14.5 Surgery for oesophageal cancer: (a) colonic interposition following total oesophagectomy; (b) gastric mobilization and pull-through for carcinoma of the lower third.

overall results, surgery has the advantage that palliation can be excellent and that, like radiotherapy, it may sometimes be curative.

The upper third of the oesophagus is technically a difficult area to irradiate because of the length of the treatment field, and the proximity of the spinal cord. Radiation fields should ideally extend for at least 5 cm above and below the known limits of disease, in order to treat adequately the presumed submucosal extension. As with postcricoid carcinomas, sophisticated planning techniques are often required, using twisted, wedged, oblique, multiple fields, often with compensators, and careful radiation planning at two or three levels so that a cylinder of tissue is irradiated to a uniform high dose without over-irradiation of the adjacent spinal cord (Fig. 14.6).

For tumours of the *mid third of the oesophagus*, radiotherapy is increasingly used as definitive treatment, or in combination with surgery; some surgeons feel that the operation is easier and the long-term results better when preoperative irradiation is given. For preoperative or radical radiotherapy of tumours of the mid third of the oesophagus, treatment is technically simpler than with tumours of the upper third. As with upper third tumours, synchronous chemoirradiation is now widely employed; at our own centre, a combination of mitomycin C and 5-FU is now regarded as standard treatment.

For cancer of the *lower third of the oesophagus*, surgery is often preferable and reconstruction, usually employing mobilized stomach (Fig. 14.5), less difficult.

With cancer of the lower third of the oesophagus there is a risk that the stomach will be involved with tumour, making it unsuitable for reconstruction. Radiotherapy can be useful for inoperable tumours.

At all sites, complications of treatment can be troublesome or even severe, both for radiotherapy and surgery. Radical radiotherapy is often accompanied by radiation oesophagitis, requiring treatment with alkaline or aspirin-containing suspensions to act locally on the inflamed oesophageal mucosa. Potential later complications include radiation damage to spinal cord (see Chapter 11) or lung, leading to radiation pneumonitis and occasionally dyspnoea, cough and reduction in respiratory capacity, though in day-to-day practice these are rarely seen. Oesophageal fibrosis and scarring can lead to stricturing of the oesophagus which may require dilatation to retain oesophageal patency. Despite these concerns, most patients tolerate this treatment surprisingly well, even when chemotherapy is used.

Surgical complications include oesophageal stricture and anastomotic leak, resulting in mediastinitis, pneumonitis and septicaemia, which can be fatal.

Palliative treatment [10]

Palliative treatment can be very valuable in oesophageal cancer, using either a Celestin or other indwelling prosthesis, by radiotherapy or laser treatment (or both), or occasionally by bypass surgery in which no attempt is made to resect the primary site, but an alternative conduit is created. Patients unsuitable for radical surgery or radiotherapy should always be considered for palliative treatment, particularly if the dysphagia is severe. Modest doses of radiation can result in impressive clinical improvements. In experienced hands, passage of a Celestin or expandable metallic mesh endo-oesophageal tube is relatively safe and effective, and can be combined with radiation therapy. Common problems associated with tube insertion include migration of the tube, gastro-oesophageal reflux (sometimes associated with lung aspiration of gastric contents) and retrosternal pain or discomfort. Complications from palliative irradiation should be minimal since dosage is low: treatment to a dose of 30 Gy in daily fractions over a 2-week period is usually beneficial, provided the dysphagia is not total, and high doses are rarely warranted. Endo-oesophageal brachytherapy offers a simple and rapid alternative, widely used at our own centre.

Since the early 1990s, laser therapy has assumed an increasingly important role [9] and can be used in conjunction with radiotherapy. It can promptly restore

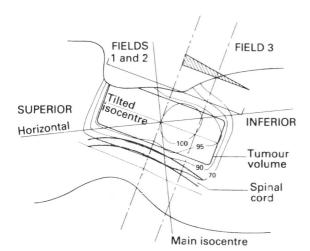

Fig. 14.6 Radical radiotherapy for carcinoma of the cervical oesophagus. The irregular anatomy necessitates a complex multifield treatment plan.

swallowing capacity, even sometimes after a single session, and is easily repeatable. For patients with unresectable tumours it may offer the best and least traumatic form of palliation.

An interesting addition to the use of laser therapy is the concept of photodynamic therapy, in which phthalocyamine derivatives are given to the patient prior to laser therapy and taken up preferentially by the tumour, thereby adding to the specificity of the treatment [11,12].

Prognosis

Results of treatment for oesophageal cancer are very poor (Table 14.1). In at least one series preoperative irradiation followed by surgical resection appeared to improve the prognosis [13] but with the dismal survival statistics currently reported, there is an urgent need for careful comparison of competing methods of treatment.

Earlam and Cunha-Melo [8,9] have reviewed the results of treatment in 90 000 patients with carcinoma of the oesophagus and arrived at an overall 5-year survival rate of 6% for radiotherapy and 4% for surgery. However, the case selection for surgery and radiotherapy differs [14] and the true advantage of radiotherapy may be greater, since, in general, fitter patients with more localized lesions are likely to have been treated surgically. More recent results employing combined chemoradiation have confirmed a 3-year survival rate of 30% (median duration of survival 17.2 months [3]).

Table 14.1 Survival in oesophageal cancer*.

Results of surgery
58% of all patients considered operable
39% of total were resectable
29% resection mortality
18% lived 1 year
9% lived 2 years
4% lived 5 years

Results of radiotherapy
51% of all patients offered palliative radiotherapy
18% lived 1 year
8% lived 2 years
6% lived 5 years

*Modified from [7,8]. Although more than 10 years old, these data are still representative.

Carcinoma of the stomach

Incidence and aetiology

Cancer of the stomach is declining in incidence but still remains an important cause of mortality worldwide; it is the second most common cancer after lung, with an estimated 755 000 new cases occurring annually. High incidence rates (30–80 per 100 000) occur in the Far East, Russia and eastern Europe. The overall incidence in the UK is 29 per 100 000 (men) and 19 per 100 000 (women). Incidence rises steeply with age, to over 200 per 100 000 men aged over 80. In both the UK and USA, there has been a gradual reduction of death rate in the last 20 years. In other countries the incidence is far higher, for example 80 per 100 000 in Japan and 70 per 100 000 in Chile (Fig. 14.7). Environmental causes are suggested by the fact that Japanese migrants to the USA show a reduction in incidence but still retain a higher risk than the indigenous population. The likelihood of developing gastric cancer is also related to socioeconomic class, the disease being twice as common in classes 4 and 5 as in classes 1 and 2 (Fig. 14.8).

The causes of carcinoma of the stomach are unknown, but genetic, environmental, dietary, infective and premalignant factors have been implicated. Gastric carcinoma is three to six times as common in patients with pernicious anaemia, which is itself an inherited disorder. The cancer is slightly more common in persons who have blood group A than in the general population, and possibly in patients who have had a Polya partial gastrectomy. Patients with inherited hypogammaglobulinaemia have a greatly increased risk of gastric cancer.

There is an increased incidence of carcinoma of the stomach in patients with chronic atrophic gastritis. The increased risk in patients with pernicious anaemia and atrophic gastritis is approximately three-fold. Gastric atrophy may be followed by intestinal metaplasia and it has been postulated that dietary carcinogens might provoke this change. Dietary characteristics of populations at high risk for gastric cancer include: high intake of salt, dietary nitrates, starches and carbohydrates; and low intake of raw vegetables, salads, fresh fruit and animal protein [14]. A hypothesis for the stepwise causation of gastric carcinoma is shown in Fig. 14.9 together with a summary of known aetiological features. It is likely that gastric atrophy leads to a rise in pH in the stomach and subsequent bacterial colonization which cannot occur at low pH. Gastric atrophy appears to relate to malnutrition in countries where there is a high risk of gastric cancer. Bacterial colonization of the stomach is much more common below 50 years of

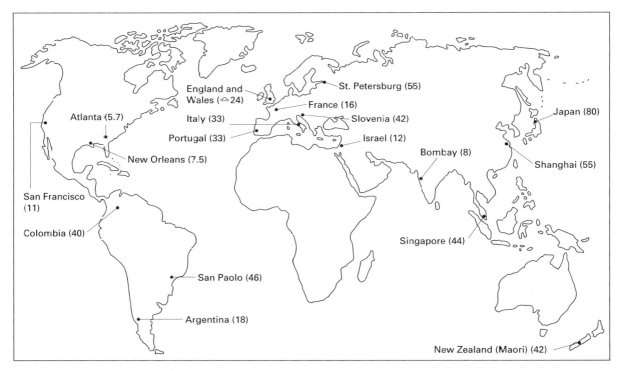

Fig. 14.7 Geographical incidence of stomach cancer figures indicate incidence per 100 000 male population. American figures are for the white population only; rates are approximately double in the black population. Stomach cancer probably remains the second commonest cancer worldwide, despite the recent decline in incidence.

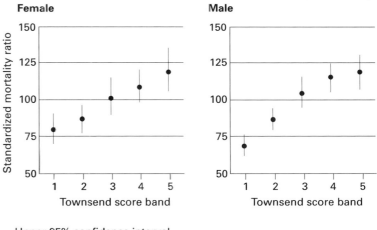

Fig. 14.8 Gastric cancer mortality related to socioeconomic class. Figures are for men aged 15–64 for the years 1970–72 in England and Wales. (Figures from data from the Office of Population Censuses and Surveys, 1978.) Values for each social class are in proportion to 100 which represents all social classes combined.

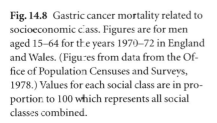

Upper 95% confidence interval
SMR
Lower 95% confidence interval

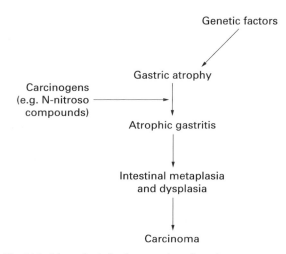

Fig. 14.9 A hypothesis for the causation of gastric cancer.

age in these regions. Pernicious anaemia is also accompanied by gastric atrophy, and hypoacidity may occur following Polya partial gastrectomy—both being situations where the risk of gastric cancer may be increased. The result of bacterial colonization may be to reduce dietary nitrates (present in water, vegetables and cured meats) to nitrites, which in turn react with amino acids to form *N*-nitroso compounds. These are carcinogens in animals (causing intestinal metaplasia of the gastric mucosa in rats) and may be so in humans.

The recently described association of gastric cancer with the *Helicobacter pylori* infection is exciting great interest [15,16]. Evidence is accumulating that it is an important risk factor for gastric carcinoma, and it has been formally recognized by the International Agency for Research on Cancer as a definite aetiological factor [17]. The preventive implications of this association, if confirmed, are of great potential importance, since the infection affects 30–50% of European adults and over 80% in parts of the developing world [15]. These figures do not explain the worldwide male preponderance of gastric cancer.

The association between gastric cancer and peptic ulceration remains uncertain [18] as is the relationship between gastric polyps and malignancy. Gastric polyps are relatively common and 10% show evidence of carcinoma *in situ*. This change has doubtful prognostic significance, and the lesion which seems most likely to be premalignant is the villous adenoma.

Pathology

Over 95% of gastric carcinomas are adenocarcinomas.

Carcinoid tumours, squamous carcinoma, adenoacanthoma and leiomyosarcoma make up the rest. *Early gastric cancer* [19] is defined as a tumour confined to the mucosa and submucosa, irrespective of lymph-node invasion. Histological differentiation from 'precancerous' lesions can be difficult, even with gastric biopsy. Symptoms are minimal and the diagnosis is often made at endoscopy for screening (see below) or for an unrelated symptom. The lesions are usually adenocarcinomas with features similar to those for advanced cancers.

The commonest type of gastric cancer is a diffuse infiltrating lesion which varies in size from 1 cm to a tumour which may occupy most of the stomach. It often invades through the stomach wall, spreading into the pancreas and omentum, metastasizing to regional lymph nodes, liver and peritoneal cavity. Some tumours exhibit a polypoid growth with projection into the lumen of the stomach, later invading the stomach wall and adjacent tissues. Others spread superficially through the mucosa, sparing regional lymph nodes until late in the disease and with a better prognosis. In other cases there is a diffuse sclerosis involving the whole of the stomach wall (*linitis plastica*). The stomach is small and contracted and will not distend. This tumour has a particularly poor prognosis. Cancers tend to arise in the antrum or lower third of the stomach and are more common on the lesser curvature. Some of these tumours are multicentric. The location of these tumours appears to be changing with time, with an increase in proximal tumours and a decline in those in the antrum, both in the West and in Japan.

Microscopically, the most useful division is made between those carcinomas where the cells resemble intestinal cells and there is intestinal metaplasia surrounding the tumour (intestinal type) and those which tend to infiltrate the gastric wall and are surrounded by normal mucosa (diffuse type). Tumours of the intestinal type are associated with a better survival, tend to occur in older patients and are more likely to be preceded by atrophic gastritis. In high-risk populations (such as Japan) most tumours are of this type. Diffuse carcinomas occur more frequently in women, are associated with blood group A and have a worse overall survival. Parietal cell tumours are an uncommon variant.

In Japan, screening programmes have resulted in many tumours being diagnosed early, and the term 'early gastric cancer' has been introduced for tumours limited to the mucosa or submucosa. These can be of the intestinal or diffuse types with varying degrees of differentiation. At this stage the prognosis is excellent [19], with over 90% of patients alive at 5 years. Lymphatic spread of the tumour

(Fig. 14.10) is via the superficial lymphatic networks into nodes in the left gastric chain and the splenic and hepatic chains along the lines of major vascular supply to the stomach. Spread is then to nodes in the coeliac plexus, the splenic chain and into the hepatic chain around the porta hepatis. There is sometimes enlargement of nodes in the left supraclavicular region deep to the sternomastoid insertion (Virchow's node). Cancer of the stomach also spreads locally through the stomach wall into the omentum, liver and pancreas. Portions of tumour can break off and seed widely through the peritoneal space, causing malignant ascites and Krukenberg tumours on the surface of the ovary. Blood-borne metastases are particularly common in the liver but pulmonary metastases also occur. Bone metastases are uncommon and central nervous system metastases are rare.

Clinical features

One of the great difficulties in diagnosis lies in the fact that the initial symptoms are often mild and indefinite. These include anorexia, nausea and vague upper abdominal pain, but many patients are only diagnosed at a time when a large epigastric mass is palpable (sometimes with ascites), making curative resection clearly impossible. Other symptoms include dysphagia (particularly with proximal tumours) and vomiting if there is outflow obstruction. Massive gastrointestinal bleeding does occur but is unusual. Low-grade bleeding is common and presentation with iron-deficiency anaemia not infrequent. Non-metastatic manifestations of malignancy are unusual, with the exception of acanthosis nigricans (see Chapter 9).

Clinical signs are minimal except in the late stages. The patient will usually appear to have lost weight, and may be anaemic. Virchow's node may be palpable in the left supraclavicular region and there may be an epigastric mass or hepatomegaly from metastases. Tumour masses may be felt on abdominal or pelvic examination and ascites may be present. All of these signs indicate advanced cancer which is inoperable and incurable.

Diagnosis

The standard diagnostic investigation has been the double-contrast barium meal examination. Typically, the malignant gastric ulcer shows elevated irregular borders and crater (Fig. 14.11) with abnormal mucosal folds. In antral lesions the resting volume of gastric juice may be large and in linitis plastica the stomach appears small and contracted. Infiltrating lesions give the stomach areas of rigidity which can be seen on screening during the examination. It is sometimes difficult to distinguish benign from malignant ulceration and small carcinomas can be missed.

Endoscopy has led to a great improvement in accuracy of diagnosis. If the diagnosis is suspected in a patient with persistent anorexia and weight loss, endoscopy should be performed in addition to the barium meal. At endoscopy, cytological washings are taken and multiple biopsies from the ulcer or tumour. A positive biopsy or cytology is obtained in around 90% of patients, except in the infiltrative forms of gastric carcinoma where the diagnosis can be missed both on endoscopic appearance and on cytological examination. Liver function tests, full blood count and chest X-ray should always be carried out. Computed tomography scanning and hepatic ultrasound may help to define nodal or hepatic metastases and extent of local spread such as involvement of the lesser sac or liver. Carcinoembryonic antigen is sometimes elevated but the relationship to tumour mass is too indefinite to be helpful either in diagnosis or in monitoring therapy.

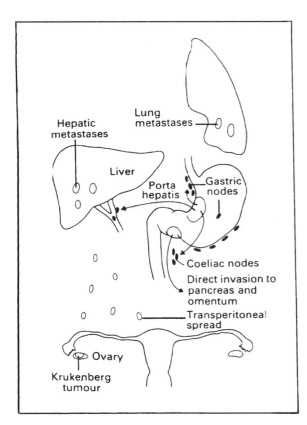

Fig. 14.10 Common paths of spread in gastric cancer.

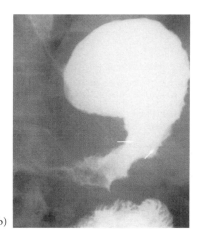

(a)

(b)

Fig. 14.11 Barium meal appearances in carcinoma of the stomach: (a) carcinoma at cardio-oesophageal junction showing tumour infiltration with mucosal irregularity; (b) linitis plastica. The tumour infiltrates extensively (arrowed).

A tumour node metastasis staging system has been developed and is shown in Table 14.2. In the UK, the majority of patients present at stages III and IV.

Early diagnosis of gastric carcinoma

Because so many patients present with inoperable disease, programmes have been devised to screen for the disease in countries such as Japan where there is a very high incidence. A high incidence (31%) of early carcinomas has been found, with an excellent survival following surgery. It is not clear if early gastric cancer will always develop into advanced disease but it is reasonable to assume that this will usually occur. Unfortunately in the UK, late diagnosis is the rule, only 20% of patients proving surgically operable with any serious prospect of cure [20]. Screening asymptomatic populations, especially in low-risk countries, has not proved cost-effective, though screening of patients with upper abdominal symptoms has been suggested as a compromise since 50% of cases of early gastric cancer diagnosed by screening had such symptoms. In countries such as the UK, such an approach is the only practical possibility in view of declining incidence. One study [21] showed that gastric cancer is detectable in 5% of such patients and 63% of these had early operable lesions. In addition, 75% of all patients had an identifiable cause of dyspepsia (including other cancers), adding to the value of endoscopy.

Treatment

Surgical treatment of gastric carcinoma

Surgical resection is the only curative treatment for gastric

Table 14.2 TNM staging system far gastric carcinoma.

T stage		
T_1	Limited to mucosa or submucosa	
T_2	Extension to serosa	
T_3	Extension through serosa	
T_4	Invasion of local structures	
N stage		
N_0	No nodes	
N_1	Local node involvement within 8 cm	
N_2	Node involvement more than 3 cm, but resectable	
N_3	Distant node involvement	
M stage		
M_0	No metastases	
M_1	Distant metastases	
Stage grouping		
Stage	I	$T_1 N_0 M_0$
	II	$T_{2-3} N_0 M_0$
	III	$T_{1-3} N_{1-2} M_0$
		$T_{4a} N_0 M_0$
	IV	$T_{1-3} N_3 M_0$
		$T_{4a} N_{1-3} M$

carcinoma. A variety of procedures can be performed, depending on the localization of the tumour and the degree of local extension. The most radical surgery involves total gastrectomy (Fig. 14.12), although for relatively localized tumours a partial gastrectomy can be performed. Some form of subtotal gastrectomy is the most generally employed surgical procedure. Total gastrectomy, if required, involves removal of the entire stomach, the greater omentum, usually removal of the spleen and occasionally of the lower portion of the oesophagus if the tumour is proximal. In a radical subtotal gastrectomy 80% of the

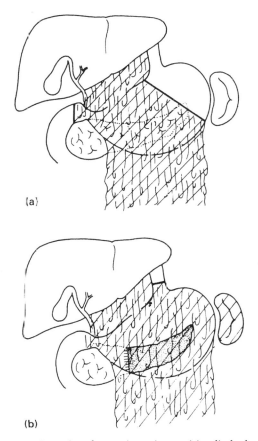

Fig. 14.12 Operations for gastric carcinoma: (a) radical subtotal gastrectomy; (b) extended total gastrectomy.

Table 14.3 Response to cytotoxic agents in gastric carcinoma.

Drug	Response rates (%)
Single agents	
Doxorubicin, epirubicin	15–25
5-FU	15–20
Mitomycin C	25–30
Nitrosoureas	5–15
Alkylating agents	10–15
Cisplatin	20
Combination chemotherapy	
5-FU, doxorubicin, mitomycin (FAM)	30
5-FU, doxorubicin, cisplatin	35–40
5-FU, doxorubicin, methotrexate (FAMTX)	35–45
5-FU (infused), epirubicin, cisplatin (ECF)	50–60

stomach is removed with the omentum and part of the duodenum. The extent of regional lymphadenectomy has been the subject of intense debate over the past few years [22]. A large Dutch group recently reported additional operative complications and mortality with the more radical Japanese approach of regional node dissection — though this procedure is performed routinely in Japan — without necessarily adding to overall survival.

The morbidity of total gastrectomy is considerable, with difficulty in maintaining body weight and, if the patient survives, the inevitable production of iron- and vitamin B_{12}-deficient anaemia requiring lifelong treatment.

Patients presenting with a large intra-abdominal mass, malignant ascites, demonstrable nodal deposits, fixity of the tumour, or liver metastases are generally inoperable. In inoperable cases, bypass procedures are usually unrewarding.

The results of surgery are poor [22,23]. In European studies only 60% of patients undergoing surgery prove to have resectable tumours. Of these, only 20–25% will be alive at 5 years. This gives an overall 5-year survival rate of 10–15% in all operated cases. European mortality rates vary from a high level of 26 per 100 000 (Portuguese males) to a low of 8.5 per 100 000 (Denmark). Female rates are somewhat lower — approximately one-half in each country (1990 data). In Japan the results are much better, with a higher surgical resectability rate (70–75%). Of those resected, 55% are alive at 5 years, and the 5-year postoperative survival rate is about 30%. In Japanese studies 15% of cases have early gastric cancer, compared with 2.5% in the West.

Radiation treatment

Palliation of some of the symptoms of gastric carcinoma can occasionally be achieved with radiation. Treatment is difficult since there are numerous radiosensitive organs in the upper abdomen, namely the small intestine, liver, spinal cord and kidneys. A dose of 40 Gy can usually be administered safely in 4–5 weeks. Anorexia and nausea are frequent and patients usually lose weight during the procedure. The intention is palliative, although occasional long-term survival has been noted.

Chemotherapy for cancer of the stomach

Cancer of the stomach is the gastrointestinal adenocarcinoma which is arguably most sensitive to cytotoxic drugs. In advanced gastric cancer some drugs are able to produce response rates of greater than 30% (Table 14.3). Most responses are partial, lasting for only a few months. There is no evidence that survival is prolonged by the use of chemotherapy either as single agents or in combination, even though responders will live longer than non-responders, as in most other tumours.

The single most effective agent appears to be doxorubicin and the usual dose is $60\,mg/m^2$ every 3 weeks. 5-Fluorouracil has been widely used but the response rate is relatively low. There has been extensive experience with mitomycin C in Japan, and some trials from that country have reported response rates of 40%, though most trials suggest a lower response rate. Nitrosoureas and alkylating agents are less useful. Cisplatin is active but nausea and vomiting may be a problem.

In advanced gastric cancer several combination chemotherapy regimes have been used and some of these are shown in Table 14.3. One of the most widely used has been the combination of 5-FU, doxorubicin and mitomycin (FAM) with a response rate of about 40%, but more intensive regimens have produced response rates as high as 62% [24]. Epirubicin is now more frequently used instead of doxorubicin, often in combination with cisplatin and infusional 5-FU. It has been suggested that this type of chemotherapy may improve resection rates when used preoperatively. There is, however, no convincing evidence that patients are ever cured by chemotherapy, though useful palliation can sometimes be achieved.

Treatment effectiveness may possibly be improved by use of long-term intravenous 5-FU infusion with addition of cisplatin and/or epirubicin. Ambulatory infusion has been made practicable by battery-driven infusion pumps. Response rates are high and the toxicity appears acceptable.

Adjuvant chemotherapy

There has been recent interest in the use of chemotherapy as an adjuvant to surgical removal of the tumour [25,26]. So far, most studies have failed to show an improved survival in the chemotherapy-treated group compared with surgery alone. However, a recent randomized study from the USA provided a remarkably positive result in adjuvant chemoradiotherapy used postoperatively for high-risk adenocarcinoma of the stomach or gastro-oesophageal junction [27].

References

1 Ahsan H, Neugut AL *et al.* Family history of colorectal adeno-matous polyps and increased risk for colorectal cancer. *Ann Intern Med* 1998; 128: 114–17.

2 Powell J, McConkey CC. Increasing incidence of adenocarcinoma of the gastric cardia and adjacent sites. *Br J Cancer* 1990; 62: 440–3.

3 Lagergren J, Bergstrom R, Linogren M, Nyren O. Symptomatic gastroesophageal reflux as a risk factor for esophageal adenocarcinoma. *N Engl J Med* 1999; 340: 825–83.

4 Al-Sarraf M, Martz K, Herskovic A *et al.* Progress report of combination chemoradiotherapy versus radiotherapy alone in patients with esophageal cancer: an intergroup study. *J Clin Oncol* 1997; 15: 227–84.

5 MRC Oesophageal Cancer Working Party. Surgical resection with or without preoperative chemotherapy in oesophageal cancer: a randomised controlled trial. *Lancet* 2002; 359: 1727–33.

6 Kelson DP, Ginsberg R, Pajak TF *et al.* Chemotherapy followed by surgery compared with surgery alone for localized oesophageal cancer. *N Engl J Med* 1998, 339: 1979–84.

7 Herskovic A, Martz K, Al-Sarraf M *et al.* Combined chemotherapy and radiotherapy compared with radiotherapy alone in patients with cancer of the esophagus. *N Engl J Med* 1992; 326: 1593–8.

8 Earlam R, Cunha-Melo JR. Oesophageal squamous cell carcinoma. I. A critical review of surgery. *Br J Surg* 1980; 67: 381–90.

9 Earlam R, Cunha-Melo JR. Oesophageal squamous cell carcinoma. II. A critical review of radiotherapy. *Br J Surg* 1980; 67: 457–61.

10 Tobias JS, Bown SG. Palliation of malignant obstruction — use of lasers and radiotherapy in combination. *Eur J Cancer* 1991; 27: 1350–2.

11 Hopper C. Oncological applications of photodynamic therapy. In: Tobias JS, Thomas PRM, eds. *Current Radiation Oncology*, Vol. 2. London: Edward Arnold, 1996: 107–20.

12 Barr H. Gastrointestinal tumours: Let there be light. *Lancet* 1998; 352: 1242–4.

13 Reed PI. Changing pattern of oesophageal cancer. *Lancet* 1991; 338: 178.

14 Chung SC, Stuart RC, Li AK. Surgical therapy for squamous-cell carcinoma of the oesophagus. *Lancet* 1994; 343: 521–4.

15 Anonymous. *Helicobacter pylori* and gastric cancer. *Drug Therapeutics Bull* 1998; 36: 57–9.

16 Eurogast Study Group. An international association between *Helicobacter pylori* infection and gastric cancer. *Lancet* 1993; 341: 1359–62.

17 Webb PM *et al.* Relation between infection with *H. pylori* and living conditions in childhood: evidence for person to person transmission in early life. *Br Med J* 1994; 308: 750–3.

18 Hansson LE, Nyren O, Hsing AW *et al.* The risk of stomach cancer in patients with gastric or duodenal ulcer disease. *N Engl J Med* 1996; 335: 242–9.

19 Everett SM, Axon ATR. Early gastric cancer: disease or pseudo-disease? *Lancet* 1998; 351: 1350–2.

20 Ellis P, Cunningham D. Management of carcinomas of the upper gastrointestinal tract. *Br Med J* 1994; 308: 834–8.

21 Hallisey MT, Allum WH, Jewkes AJ *et al.* Early detection of gastric cancer. *Br Med J* 1990; 301: 513–15.

22 Bonenkamp JJ, Hermans J, Sasako M, van de Velde CJ. Extended lymph-node dissection for gastric cancer. *N Engl J Med* 1999; 340: 908–14.

23 Allum WH, Powell DJ, McConkey CC *et al.* Gastric cancer: a 25-year review. *Br J Surg* 1989; 76: 535–40.

24 Cascinu S, Labianca R, Alessandroni P *et al.* Intensive weekly chemotherapy for advanced gastric cancer using fluorouracil, cisplatin, epi-doxorubicin, GS-leucovorin, glutathione and filgrastim: a report from the Italian Group for the Study of Digestive Tract Cancer. *J Clin Oncol* 1997; 15: 3313–19.

25 Neri B, de Leonardis V, Romano S *et al.* Adjuvant chemotherapy after gastric resection in node-positive cancer patients: a multicentre randomized study. *Br J Cancer* 1996; 73: 549–52.

26 Grau JJ, Estape J, Alcobendas F *et al.* Positive results of adjuvant mitomycin C in resected gastric cancer: a randomised trial on 134 patients. *Eur J Cancer* 1993; 39: 340–2.

27 Macdonald JS, Smalley SR, Benedetti J *et al.* Chemoradiotherapy after surgery compared with surgery alone for adenocarcinoma of the stomach or gastroesophageal junction. *N Engl J Med* 2001; 345: 725–30.

Cancer of the liver, biliary tract and pancreas

Primary liver cancer

There are four types of primary carcinoma which arise in the liver. The most frequent is hepatocellular carcinoma which, in the UK, is about 10 times more common than cholangiocarcinoma of the intrahepatic bile ducts which in turn is 10 times more frequent than angiosarcoma. Hepatoblastoma is a rare tumour of childhood. The importance of hepatocellular carcinoma is disproportionate to its incidence in the West, because there are now many clues about its aetiology and pathogenesis.

Hepatocellular carcinoma (hepatoma)

Incidence

There are about 1 million cases a year worldwide. In the UK and the USA the incidence is approximately 1.8 per 100000 for men and 0.7 for women (Fig. 15.1). The tumour can arise in childhood. Worldwide the incidence (per 100000) varies greatly: 104 in Mozambique, 29 in South Africa and 12 in Nigeria.

Aetiology

In the West, most cases of hepatocellular carcinoma (about 90%) arise in cirrhotic livers. When the disease arises in a non-cirrhotic liver the patient is usually younger than when there is associated cirrhosis. The causes of cirrhosis with the highest risk of developing a hepatoma are chronic hepatitis associated with hepatitis B, hepatitis C and haemochromatosis. Hepatoma is much more common in alcoholic cirrhosis where there is evidence of previous hepatitis B infection, and is infrequent in patients who have not been infected. Patients with primary biliary cirrhosis and hepatitis B surface antigen (HBsAg)-negative chronic active hepatitis are less at risk (although more likely to develop the cancer than the non-cirrhotic population). The carcinoma is more likely to develop in men (male : female ratio is 11 : 1) and in patients with long-standing cirrhosis over the age of 50. The association with cirrhosis is found in both high- and low-incidence areas. The duration of the cirrhosis is more important than the aetiology. The risk of development of hepatocellular carcinoma in a cirrhotic liver after 20 years is about 5% in women and 20% in men. In studies in patients with well-compensated cirrhosis the yearly incidence rate is about 3–5% [1]. The tumour is more likely to develop in patients with persistently elevated levels of α-fetoprotein (AFP). Few of these patients have operable tumours.

The geographical variations in incidence may reflect different causal factors. Cirrhosis from any cause is associated with hepatoma [2]. In low-incidence areas (Europe and North America) alcoholic cirrhosis is a more frequent association than in high-incidence areas where macronodular cirrhosis associated with hepatitis B virus (HBV) is the main association. Exposure to aflatoxin, derived

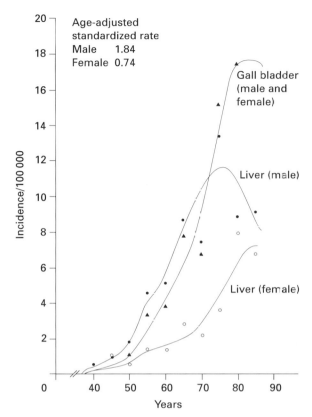

Fig. 15.1 Age-specific incidence of cancer of the liver and gall bladder (UK figures).

from the *Aspergillus flavus* mould on stored grain, is more frequent in high-incidence areas. The toxin may be one of the factors which act as tumour promoters.

There is a strong causal association with HBV. In high-incidence areas 80% of cases are associated with serological evidence of HBV, with a risk of 230:1 in HBsAg-positive individuals. In the West 15–20% are HBsAg-positive. Viral DNA sequences have been demonstrated in the genome of liver cells of HBsAg-positive individuals [3]. Hepatitis C virus (HCV) is an RNA virus which is not incorporated into the host DNA, but HCV proteins activate cell genes. Like HBV it is associated with hepatocellular carcinoma. Recently it has been shown that treatment of HCV chronic hepatitis with interferon X reduces the risk of hepatocellular carcinoma [4]. The carrier rate of hepatitis C is 0.2% in Northern Europe and 5% of the population in the Far East. It can be transmitted by parenteral inoculation. Hepatitis C appears to be the most important causal association in the USA, Europe and Japan.

Pathology

In 60% of cases the liver contains multiple nodules of cancer. In 30% of cases there is a large single mass of cancer often with surrounding lesions and, in the remaining cases, the liver is diffusely infiltrated. In 80% of cases the surrounding liver is cirrhotic. In the group of patients where it is not, the sex ratio is equal and the average age is lower. In a small subgroup of the patients without cirrhosis, the tumour forms cords with collagen strands (fibrolamellar carcinoma). In cholangiocarcinoma of the intrahepatic ducts the tumour cells form a tubular pattern, usually with extensive fibrosis.

Clinical features

The usual presentation is with right upper quadrant pain, weight loss and a palpable liver mass. In a cirrhotic patient this is often accompanied by a rapid deterioration in liver function. Usually, the cirrhosis is advanced and long standing. Presentation may therefore be accompanied by ascites. Ascites may be due to cirrhosis, or to the sudden onset of the Budd–Chiari syndrome due to hepatic vein occlusion.

On examination the patient with cirrhosis is usually ill, with evidence of cirrhosis and liver failure. The liver is enlarged with a palpable mass over which there may be a bruit. There may also be a moderate fever.

Diagnosis

Liver function tests have no diagnostic pattern or value but are always abnormal. The tumour may produce erythropoietin and secondary polycythaemia may therefore be present. Other non-metastatic manifestations include hypoglycaemia, hypercalcaemia, gonadotrophin production, ectopic adrenocorticotrophic hormone (ACTH) and elevated plasma calcitonin (see also Chapter 9).

The malignant hepatocytes in most hepatomas produce AFP which can be detected in the serum. With sensitive methods the serum AFP can be of diagnostic help. Levels below 10 ng/ml make the diagnosis very unlikely in a cirrhotic patient, although over half of non-cirrhotic patients do not have an elevated serum AFP. Levels from 10 to 500 ng/ml make the diagnosis probable, but cirrhosis due to chronic hepatitis may be associated with levels of this magnitude (as may metastases from the gastrointestinal tract). In the West, levels above 500 ng/ml in a cirrhotic patient make the diagnosis of hepatocellular carcinoma almost certain.

Computed tomography (CT) scans and ultrasound liver scans usually show a large lesion or multiple lesions, but in the presence of cirrhosis the appearances may not be diagnostic and care must be taken in interpretation. CT angiography may show a tumour circulation but is usually carried out only if there is diagnostic doubt or if there is a possibility of surgical resection or intra-arterial chemotherapy or embolization.

A biopsy of the lesion will help in diagnosis but may not be possible if liver function has deteriorated. If the prothrombin time is prolonged by more than 4 s, the procedure is unsafe since the tumours are vascular. Even with a biopsy, the histological distinction from metastatic tumours (such as hypernephroma) may be difficult.

Treatment [5]

Resection of the tumour offers a chance of cure. It must be considered particularly in a non-cirrhotic patient because the liver will regenerate even if three-quarters of the organ is removed. In a cirrhotic patient resection will usually precipitate a deterioration of liver function. Resection is therefore applicable to less than 10% of patients (Table 15.1). Good results have been claimed following liver transplantation for highly selected cirrhotic patients with small carcinomas generally under 5 cm in diameter [6].

Embolization or ligation of the hepatic artery has been used, but these procedures also cause deterioration of function in the cirrhotic patient. Selective hepatic artery embolization may be attempted in a cirrhotic patient if the tumour is localized. The value of this technique has not been adequately assessed, but pain may be relieved and survival may possibly be improved [7].

Chemotherapy may produce tumour regression, and the single most useful agent is doxorubicin. This is usually given at 50–70 mg/m^2 every 3 weeks, but the dose should be halved if the bilirubin is twice normal since the drug is detoxified by the liver. The response to chemotherapy can be assessed by pain, AFP levels and ultrasound or CT scan. As in gastric cancer, there is increasing interest in infusional intravenous chemotherapy. Intra-arterial treatment may produce considerable shrinkage but is more complex.

Table 15.1 Indications for surgery in hepatocellular carcinoma.

No extrahepatic spread
No vascular invasion
Adequate liver function

The liver does not tolerate radiotherapy to high dose. Fatal hepatic damage occurs when the dose to the whole liver is above 38 Gy. Locoregional radiotherapy may produce regression with less toxicity. Recently a small trial has suggested that ^{131}I-labelled lipiodol, given through the hepatic artery, may delay recurrence after surgery.

Prognosis

When a hepatoma arises in a cirrhotic liver the prognosis is very poor; 50% of all patients are dead in 3 months, with no survivors at 12 months. Without cirrhosis only 10% will be alive at 2 years. The prognosis is better in patients with small tumours, those who are suitable for complete surgical resection or who show a complete response to chemotherapy. Overall 5-year survival after surgical resection is 15%, although if the tumour is less than 3 cm the figure rises to 50%. These figures have suggested that the results might be improved if patients with cirrhosis are screened regularly with ultrasound and AFP measurement. The impact of such a policy on survival is not known.

Angiosarcoma

These malignant vascular tumours arise in normal livers. They are rare, but of interest since they are known to occur in workers who have had chronic exposure to polyvinylchloride (PVC). The tumours develop 15–20 years after exposure to PVC. They have also been reported in patients who received thorotrast (a radioactive contrast agent used diagnostically in 1930–50). The presentation is of a painful hepatic mass, and diagnosis is made by biopsy. Surgical resection may be possible.

A very rare, indolent, vascular tumour termed *epithelioid haemangioendothelioma* may occur in the liver. Treatment is by local excision if possible.

Hepatoblastoma

This rare tumour occurs in childhood. The tumour is associated with anomalies such as hemihypertrophy, and with storage diseases and the Fanconi syndrome. The pathological features are of immature hepatic epithelial cells or a mixture of these cells with mesenchymal elements.

It usually arises in the right lobe and presents with a visible asymptomatic mass which later causes pain and weight loss. Like hepatocellular carcinoma (which can also occur in children over 5 years of age) the tumour produces AFP. It can be demonstrated by isotopic ultrasound and CT scanning but arteriography gives the best localization and is essential if resection is to be attempted.

The tissue diagnosis is usually made at operation when an attempt at resection is made. The chance of cure is greater if there is complete surgical excision. Up to 75% of the liver can be removed but haemorrhage can be severe and great skill is necessary.

Postoperative chemotherapy is usually given. Doxorubicin is the most effective agent but responses also occur with alkylating agents, 5-fluorouracil (5-FU) and cisplatin [8]. It is now clear that unresectable cases can be made to respond to chemotherapy so that surgery can be performed, and there is growing interest in preoperative chemotherapy in this disease. Combinations of doxorubicin and cisplatin have increased response rates. Although in such a rare disease randomized trials are almost impossible, there is increasing evidence that chemotherapy may be increasing the likelihood of surgical care. Serum AFP can be used to assess response.

Cancer of the gall bladder and biliary tract

Incidence and aetiology

Cancer of the gall bladder and biliary tract has an equal incidence in men and women, most cases occurring after the age of 65 (Fig. 15.1), when it is commoner than hepatocellular carcinoma. Gall stones are a predisposing cause, but the incidence of gall bladder cancer in patients with untreated cholelithiasis is probably not more than 2%, which does not justify surgery for asymptomatic gall stones. Worldwide, liver flukes are the major predisposing cause (*Clonorchis sinensis, Opisthorchis felineus*). These flukes produce a chronic sclerosing cholangitis which appears to be premalignant. Bile duct cancer is also associated with ulcerative colitis, occurring in approximately 0.5% of cases [9].

Pathology

Carcinoma of the gall bladder, which is the commonest cancer of the biliary system, usually arises in the body and only rarely in the cystic duct (4% of cases). The tumours are usually adenocarcinomas (85%) but anaplastic (6%) and squamous (5%) histologies occur.

Half of all bile duct cancers develop in the distal common duct, with carcinoma of the ampulla of Vater being the second commonest biliary cancer. The cancers arise in the proximal duct in 30% of cases and proximal to the porta hepatis in a further 20%. They are almost always adenocarcinomas, usually well differentiated and sometimes with a fibrous stroma.

All these tumours spread locally and to regional lymph nodes and there may be multiple primary bile duct tumours. From these nodes, lymphatic spread is to the coeliac and aortic nodes. Hepatic metastases are common. Gall bladder cancer may seed into the peritoneum, and both types of cancer may directly invade the liver. Carcinoma of the ampulla is usually slow growing and causes obstructive jaundice early before it has spread widely. The tumour often ulcerates and sometimes bleeds, and the jaundice may fluctuate if the tumour sloughs. This form of biliary tract cancer has the best prognosis.

Clinical features

Cancer of the gall bladder usually presents with right upper quadrant pain, later with nausea, vomiting, weight loss and obstructive jaundice. Because of pre-existing gall stones the symptoms may be attributed to this cause at first and the diagnosis delayed.

Cancer of the biliary tree presents similarly but usually causes obstructive jaundice. At this stage the tumour is often advanced. The gall bladder may be enlarged and palpable if the distal duct is obstructed.

Diagnosis

The diagnosis of early gall bladder carcinoma is difficult because the symptoms suggest gall stone disease. By the time a mass is palpable surgical resection may be impossible. A cholecystogram is often unhelpful, because the gall bladder is non-functioning. Ultrasound and CT scanning may show a mass, but in the majority of cases the diagnosis is only made at a laparotomy for presumed gall stone disease. In carcinoma of the extrahepatic bile ducts, obstructive jaundice leads to investigation. Percutaneous transhepatic cholangiograms may give an outline of the proximal ducts, and endoscopic retrograde cholangiopancreatography (ERCP) may demonstrate the lower end of the block and provide material for cytological examination (Fig. 15.2), as well as permitting a stent to be inserted. The transhepatic route may also allow a catheter to be placed past the lesion with relief of jaundice either preoperatively or as a palliative procedure.

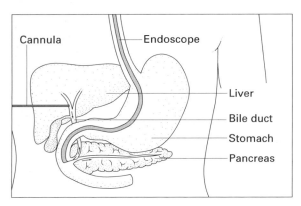

Fig. 15.2 Percutaneous cholangiography and ERCP.

Treatment

Surgery

When a gall bladder carcinoma is found at laparotomy the surgeon must decide if it can be resected. The experience of the surgeon is an important factor in this decision. The results of simple cholecystectomy are not good since the tumour may be locally extensive. Portions of the liver may have to be removed for complete excision. Distant lymph node spread may have occurred and surgical excision deemed unwise, and a palliative procedure is then undertaken, if possible with biliary decompression.

In the surgical management of bile duct cancer it is of great value to have the extent of the tumour defined preoperatively by radiographic means. Diffuse intraductal spread cannot be resected. Spread into the intrahepatic ducts, invasion of blood vessels and distant lymph nodes, and peritoneal and hepatic metastases are also indications of unresectability. Microscopic examination of bile duct carcinomas often reveals intramural spread. In spite of formidable surgical difficulties, tumours at the junction of the right and left hepatic ducts can sometimes be removed, as can mid and distal duct tumours, the latter by radical pancreaticoduodenectomy (Fig. 15.3).

In all, only 15% of bile duct cancers will be operable, and major resections have a high mortality (10–15%).

Palliative relief of obstruction may be obtained by bypass operation but internal bile duct drainage by non-surgical procedures is now becoming a preferred method of palliation. Carcinoma of the ampulla has the most favourable prognosis with a 5-year survival of 25–30% after radical pancreaticoduodenectomy.

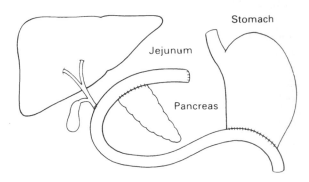

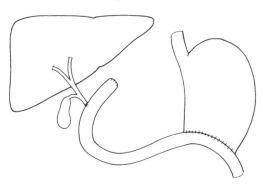

Fig. 15.3 Surgical operations for cancer of the bile ducts and pancreas.

Radiotherapy

Many patients with biliary tract cancer have a localized but unresectable tumour. In these cases effective control can for a time be achieved with radiotherapy. The dose is usually 40–50 Gy in daily fractions, but the treatment details depend on the volume and site of the irradiation. Relief of pain and obstructive jaundice may be achieved.

Chemotherapy

There has been little systematic study of the role of chemotherapy in biliary tract cancer. Responses have been reported with 5-FU, mitomycin and doxorubicin, but are usually short-lived. Newer approaches include long-term infusion therapy using 5-FU as for cancer of the stomach (pp. 225–6).

Cancer of the exocrine pancreas

Incidence and aetiology

Globally, the incidence of carcinoma of the pancreas is slowly rising, although in many parts of the UK this increase seems to have levelled out over the past decade. At present it is 15 per 100 000 in men and 13 per 100 000 in women (Fig. 15.4). The condition has a high mortality, less than 1% of patients surviving 5 years. The disease is twice as common in diabetes mellitus. It also appears to be a smoking-related cancer, with about 40% of cases in men, and 25% in women, attributable to smoking. There is possibly an increased incidence in patients with calcific or chronic pancreatitis [10] which, in turn, is associated with excess alcohol consumption. An increased risk has also been reported in metal, mine, chemical and sawmill workers [11]. Wide variance in incidence has been noted across the world, from 2.2 cases per 100 000 in India, Kuwait and Singapore to 12.5 per 100 000 in parts of Scandinavia (Fig. 15.5). Urban and socioeconomically disadvantaged populations have a higher incidence in the developed world.

Pathology

The great majority of histologically verified tumours are adenocarcinomas (Table 15.2), though in many patients a histological diagnosis is never established. The adenocarcinomas are thought to arise from the ductular epithelium and those arising in large ducts tend to be more often mucin-producing than those originating in ductules. An intense fibrotic reaction often accompanies the tumour. Cystadenocarcinoma (1%) has a particularly good prognosis. Acinar cell tumours constitute 5% of the total. Sarcoma of the pancreas is a rare disease, usually occurring in childhood.

The exocrine pancreas has an extensive lymphatic drainage along blood vessels. Spread to local nodes has usually occurred by the time of presentation in tumours of both the body and tail.

The head of the pancreas is the site of the tumour in 65% of cases, the body and tail in 30% and the tail alone in 5%. Local spread occurs and accounts for many of the clinical features (Fig. 15.6). Tumours in the head spread into the duodenum, obstruct the bile duct, and spread back into the retroperitoneal space and forward into the lesser sac and peritoneal cavity. The portal vein may be infiltrated, and tumours of the body and tail may occlude the splenic vein and extend into the transverse colon and spleen. Metastatic spread to the peritoneum, liver and lung is frequent.

Pain and weight loss are the most frequent symptoms [11,12]. With tumours of the head the pain is usually epigastric, and with the tail it may be in the left upper quadrant. The pain gradually becomes severe and unremitting, is often nocturnal and extends into the back as retroperitoneal structures are invaded. The patient may obtain relief by bending forwards. Acute exacerbations may be due to episodes of pancreatitis. Left-sided abdominal pain and altered bowel habit may be caused by infiltration of the colon by tumours of the body or tail. Mental depression is said to be common, but it is not clear if this is more

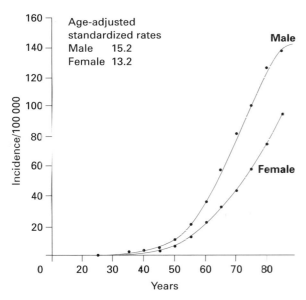

Fig. 15.4 Age-specific incidence of cancer of the exocrine pancreas (UK figures).

Table 15.2 Pancreatic tumours.

	Malignant (%)
Tumours of exocrine pancreas	
Adenocarcinoma	
Acinar cell tumour	
Sarcoma	
Tumours of endocrine pancreas	
Islet cell tumours	20
Gastrinoma	70
Glucagonoma	60
Vipoma	90
Carcinoids	Not known
Somatostatinoma	90

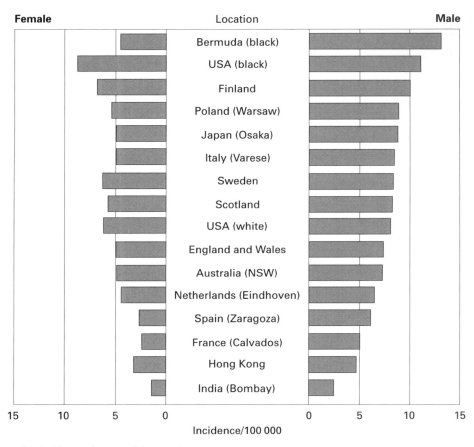

Fig. 15.5 Geographic incidence of cancer of the exocrine pancreas.

marked in pancreatic cancer than in other causes of serious illness. Acinar cell carcinoma may be accompanied by a syndrome of patchy inflammation and necrosis of subcutaneous fat with polyarthralgia and eosinophilia. There are high levels of lipase in serum. The syndrome resembles relapsing panniculitis (Weber–Christian disease). Another non-metastatic manifestation of pancreatic carcinoma is superficial migratory thrombophlebitis (see Chapter 9). Oesophageal varices may develop if the portal vein is occluded and may lead to gastrointestinal bleeding. Diabetes mellitus may be the presenting feature and carcinoma of the pancreas must be kept in mind in elderly patients developing glycosuria.

Obstructive jaundice is frequent and eventually occurs in 90% of patients with tumours of the head. It is usually progressive, although fluctuations may occur if the tumour sloughs. It is much less common in tumours of the body and tail. Fever may occur due to cholangitis. The gall bladder is not usually palpable — unlike a bile duct or ampullary carcinoma. Peritoneal dissemination leads to malignant ascites, which is present in 15% of cases at diagnosis.

Investigation and diagnosis

It is difficult to diagnose early pancreatic carcinoma at the stage before obstruction of the bile duct or infiltration of the duodenum. It should be considered in any patient with unexplained continued upper abdominal pain. Barium examinations are usually helpful only when the tumour is large. There may be enlargement of the duodenal loop and displacement of the gastric antrum and posterior wall. The tumour may have infiltrated the duodenal and gastric mucosa and this may be seen as an abnormal pattern on the barium meal.

In recent years diagnosis of smaller tumours and of tumours of the body and tail has become somewhat easier with the use of ultrasound and CT scanning. Ultrasound

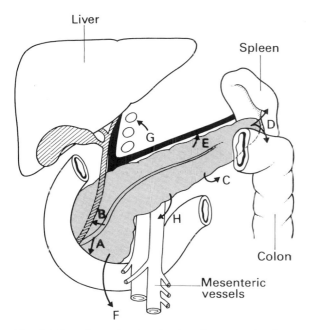

Fig. 15.6 Sites of spread and production of symptoms in adeno-carcinoma of the pancreas: (A) to duodenum, with pain, vomiting, obstruction; (B) to bile duct and pancreas, with jaundice, pancreatitis; (C) to retroperitoneum, with back pain; (D) to spleen and colon, with left upper quadrant pain; (E) to portal and splenic vein, with varices, splenomegaly, hepatic disorders; (F) to peritoneal cavity, with ascites; (G) to lymph nodes, with obstructive jaundice; and (H) to bloodstream, with distant metastases.

examination of the pancreas is, however, a procedure requiring considerable experience on the part of the radiologist and false negative results are not infrequent. Endoscopic ultrasonography has proven extremely valuable in selected cases [13]. Computed tomography scanning may show a pancreatic mass or extension of the pancreas into the fat space surrounding it, and there may also be evidence of metastatic spread to adjacent nodes and the liver (Fig. 15.6). If a mass is found, fine-needle aspiration may give a cytological diagnosis. Selective coeliac and superior mesenteric artery angiograms may be of diagnostic value but have seldom been performed since the advent of CT scanning.

When the disease presents with obstructive jaundice, transhepatic cholangiography and ERCP will usually be performed (Fig. 15.2). The transhepatic approach will show the proximal site of obstruction and help to distinguish the tumour from carcinoma of the gall bladder, ampulla or bile ducts. ERCP may show stenosis of the main

pancreatic duct or compression of the common bile duct by tumour. Specimens for cytology can be taken from the pancreatic duct. ERCP has a high diagnostic accuracy (75–85%), but early diagnosis, before biliary obstruction has occurred, remains the clinical problem because symptoms are often late or non-specific. Carcinoembryonic antigen (CEA) is present in the serum of most patients but is also found in other gastrointestinal diseases and in acute pancreatitis. CA-19-9 and pancreatic oncofetal antigen may be present in serum but are not specific for the disease.

Treatment

Surgery

Radical surgical resection offers the only hope of cure [14]. Radical pancreaticoduodenectomy and total pancreatectomy are formidable surgical procedures (Fig. 15.3). Preservation of part of the pancreas is desirable but there are considerable problems with fistula formation at the anastomotic site. Total pancreatectomy leads to major problems with diabetes and lack of exocrine function.

Few patients are suitable for surgery, because at the time of diagnosis there are often nodal or distant metastases or a large infiltrating mass which is clearly inoperable. Careful definition of the extent of the tumour preoperatively is essential. In general, only tumours involving the body or tail will prove to be operable. In operable cases the mortality is 15–20% and 5-year survival not greater than 15%.

If the tumour cannot be removed, the obstruction can be relieved by a biliary bypass procedure. This is usually performed surgically, but recently it has become possible to place catheters in the biliary tree by the percutaneous transhepatic route or via the ampulla of Vater.

Radiotherapy [15]

Palliation, especially of pain, can be achieved by radiotherapy. With external beam irradiation the dose required is high (50–60 Gy). Some reports have suggested that a few patients may achieve long-term remission and occasionally cure. The synchronous administration of 5-FU as a radiation sensitizer appears to improve local control and possibly even survival, though overall results remain unimpressive [16]. Interstitial radiation using ^{125}I implants has also been used, sometimes supplemented with external beam irradiation. Ultrasound and CT imaging are of great help in planning treatment.

Chemotherapy

Few cytotoxic drugs are effective in pancreatic cancer (Table 15.3). Responses occur with 5-FU, nitrosoureas, mitomycin C and alkylating agents. The criteria for response differ in the various studies and most responses are small in degree and short in duration. Combination chemotherapy has improved the response rate a little [17] but complete responses are rare and patients are never cured. The toxicity of treatment makes chemotherapy unsuitable for the majority of patients because of ill health and advanced disease at presentation. Intravenous infusional chemotherapy is under investigation.

Palliative treatment and prognosis

Pain may be relieved by analgesics, but radiotherapy may be helpful in preventing the need for opiates for several months. Chemical block using alcohol into the coeliac plexus is difficult but sometimes very helpful in relieving pain. Percutaneous drainage of the biliary tree may relieve itching and steatorrhoea due to obstructive jaundice. Steroids may help improve appetite for a while. Overall, the prognosis is very poor, with treatment making a minor long-term impact. For both men and women, the median survival time is well under 1 year, and less than 2% of all patients survive for 5 years.

Neuroendocrine tumours of the gastrointestinal tract [18]

These are rare tumours which can be divided into carci-

Table 15.3 Chemotherapy of pancreatic cancer.

Approximate response rate	(%)
Single agents	
5-FU	20
Alkylating agents	10
Streptozotocin	12
Mitomycin C	25
Doxorubicin	10
Nitrosoureas	10
Ifosfamide	10
Drug combinations	
5-FU, mitomycin, doxorubicin	40
5-FU, streptozotoxin, mitomycin	35
5-FU, BCNU	30

noid tumours largely affecting the small bowel (with an incidence of one per 100 000) and pancreatic neuroendocrine tumours (0.4 per 100 000). Carcinoids are divided into their site of origin from the fore-, mid- or hindgut. The endocrine pancreatic tumours are classified according to the hormonal syndrome they produce. The carcinoid syndrome is produced by tumours of the fore- and mid-gut especially in the presence of hepatic metastases. Not all pancreatic tumours produce a functional hormone and only 20% are malignant.

Carcinoid tumours

The curious name of these tumours was coined in 1907 to emphasize the benign course which they follow, although a proportion are malignant at the outset and others become so with time.

Pathology

Localized intestinal carcinoids are present in 0.5% of autopsies, usually near the appendix or along the small bowel or descending colon. There are, however, many other sites at which carcinoids may occur — bronchus, thymus, pancreas as well as any part of the gastrointestinal tract, ovary and testis.

Appendiceal carcinoids are usually near the tip. The tendency to metastasize is related to size; tumours less than 1 cm in size are rarely associated with metastases, while 80% of those greater than 3 cm have metastasized. Metastases are much more common with small-bowel carcinoids than with appendiceal tumours.

Macroscopically, carcinoid tumours are often yellow or orange in colour. Microscopically, they consist of densely packed epithelial cells which stain with silver nitrate. Mid-gut carcinoids are derived from enterochromaffin cells in the small-bowel mucosa but the cell of origin of many of the pancreatic tumours is not known. The cells contain synaptophysin and chromogranin which can be used to identify the tumours. Most patients have elevated levels of chromogranin A in the serum, which can be an aid in diagnosis. The hormones produced by the tumours are responsible for the carcinoid syndrome. Both primary and secondary tumours are often slow growing. The commonest metastatic site is the liver. Lung and bone are less frequently involved. Carcinoid tumours are associated with multiple endocrine neoplasia (MEN-1). There is an associated gut adenocarcinoma in 15% of patients.

Clinical features

LOCAL SYMPTOMS

The patient may present with local symptoms due to metastases. Pain in the right upper quadrant, due to distension of the liver by metastases, is a frequent symptom; weight loss, anorexia and malaise occur later as liver function deteriorates. Primary intestinal carcinoids are seldom diagnosed during life unless they cause obstruction, intussusception or pain in the right iliac fossa leading to appendicectomy.

THE CARCINOID SYNDROME

This syndrome occurs in about 50% of all patients with hepatic metastases from carcinoid tumours. A variety of chemicals are produced by the tumour and their release is accompanied by symptoms which may dominate the clinical picture. The syndrome is particularly likely to occur with bronchial carcinoid even without hepatic metastases, since the venous drainage is into the systemic circulation and not via the liver, which metabolizes the pharmacological mediators liberated by intestinal carcinoids.

In normal individuals tryptophan is converted into nicotinic acid. In carcinoid, 5-hydroxytryptamine (5-HT) is produced instead and, occasionally, pellagra occurs due to nicotinic acid deficiency. A metabolite of 5-HT, 5-hydroxyindoleacetic acid (5-HIAA) is excreted in the urine. When present in excess it confirms the diagnosis. 5-HT is quickly inactivated in the lungs and liver, so large quantities must be produced to cause symptoms. The release of 5-HT is probably responsible for diarrhoea. The diarrhoea is typically episodic, watery and may be explosive, leading to incontinence. It is often accompanied by noisy borborygmi and cramping pains. Excess 5-HT is probably responsible for endocardial fibrosis which can lead to tricuspid incompetence, which in turn may cause right-sided heart failure with ascites, and deep cyanosis in the flushed face. Bradykinin is produced by some tumours and may be partly responsible for the flushing which is characteristic of the syndrome. The flush is at first intermittent, often being precipitated by emotion and alcohol. The face and neck become red and the patient may perspire. It lasts a few minutes and is reminiscent of the flushing of menopausal women. Later the flushing becomes more frequent and some patients become almost permanently flushed. Telangiectases occur on the face, and skin may become thickened. Prostaglandins are liberated from some tumours and may contribute to both the flushing and the diarrhoea. Bronchospasm occurs and has been variously attributed to histamine, bradykinin and prostaglandins. It is episodic at first but permanent wheezing dyspnoea may develop. Episodes of hypotension are sometimes seen and are thought to be caused by 5-HT. A carcinoid crisis is a combination of hypotension, wheezing and flushing. It is treated by intravenous octreotide.

OTHER CLINICAL FEATURES

The tumours are slow growing and the diagnosis is often missed or delayed for months or years. If all the symptoms are present the diagnosis is easy to make, but if the complaint is of diarrhoea alone, negative investigations may lead to the diagnosis of 'irritable bowel syndrome'. Bronchial carcinoids usually present with unilateral airways obstructions and haemoptyses. Carcinoids in the bronchus, thymus and pancreas occasionally cause Cushing's syndrome, due to production of ACTH by the tumour bilateral adrenal hyperplasia. The primary tumour may be small. They may also secrete antidiuretic hormone and growth hormone-releasing peptide.

Diagnosis

The tumours can be visualized preoperatively by CT and magnetic resonance imaging Scintigraphy using labelled octreotide (which demonstrates the somatostatin receptor) is positive in 70–80% of patients, and is especially useful in demonstrating distant metastases.

In patients without the carcinoid syndrome the diagnosis is made by the primary tumour in the bowel causing abdominal symptoms leading to laparotomy or, in the lung, symptoms of a bronchial adenoma leading to bronchoscopy or thoracotomy. Secondary deposits in the liver are usually diagnosed by liver biopsy.

In patients with the carcinoid syndrome the 24-h urinary 5-HIAA is usually elevated. False positive results can be obtained with 5-HT containing foods (bananas contain 4 mg 5-HT). In some patients the urinary 5-HIAA excretion may vary from day to day and this leads to false negative results and makes 5-HIAA excretion an unreliable guide to treatment. Foregut carcinoids may produce 5-HT and not 5-HIAA. About 60% of tumours take up meta-iodobenzylguanidine, especially if the tumours are of foregut origin and produce 5-HT. The value of scanning is mainly to localize sites of metastasis.

Management [19]

Localized intestinal, bronchial or foregut carcinoids should be removed surgically. In metastatic carcinoids, surgery should be considered if liver secondaries are found which are well localized and which are resectable. This may relieve symptoms for months or years because the tumour is slow growing. Another effective means of reducing the tumour mass is hepatic artery embolization. These surgical approaches may result in a sudden release of large quantities of pharmacologically active agents, resulting in hypotension and bronchospasm. Some patients with hepatic metastases may be suitable for liver transplantation.

In patients with metastatic carcinoid syndrome which cannot be treated surgically, the usual approach is to attempt to block the pharmacological effects of the tumours in the first instance. However, this is usually only partially successful since each symptom may be produced by more than one agent and pharmacological antagonists are partially effective against some tumour products and do not exist for others.

The somatostatin analogue octreotide is the single most effective agent. It controls flushing and diarrhoea in 70% of patients. The starting dose is 50 µg t.d.s. increasing to 200 µg. There may be tumour regression. Lanreotide is a useful slow-release form.

Diarrhoea may be mitigated by simple measures such as codeine phosphate, diphenoxylate or loperamide. Cyproheptadine antagonizes 5-HT and also blocks the histamine (H1) receptor. It may be effective in controlling diarrhoea and, interestingly, may occasionally cause tumour regression. The drug may cause dry mouth and drowsiness.

Flushing due to bradykinin may be partially antagonized by phenothiazines and, since catecholamines can provoke bradykinin release, α-adrenergic blockade with phentolamine may also have some effect. Prostaglandin effects may occasionally be partly alleviated by indomethacin.

Bronchospasm may be helped by agents that block histamine (cyproheptadine) or bradykinin (phenothiazines) can be tried, as can conventional bronchodilators, but the results are often disappointing.

Cytotoxic chemotherapy is usually ineffective. It is the only direct treatment for widespread liver metastases and may be indicated if the carcinoid syndrome is uncontrollable by other means. In this situation sudden destruction of the tumour may lead to release of tumour products with severe asthma, diarrhoea and flushing.

The agents with activity are streptozotocin, 5-FU, doxorubicin, dacarbazine and cisplatin. Streptozotocin is the most effective drug. In combination with 5-FU or with doxorubicin, response rates of 30% are reported. The so-matostatin analogue octreotide is effective in producing control of the symptoms of carcinoid. The dose range is 200–1500 µg/day. Ten per cent of tumours show reduction in tumour size. Response duration is of the order of 6 months.

Alpha-interferon has been used alone or with chemotherapy. Some of the responses have been very durable. About 50% of cases show improvement biochemically, although tumour shrinkage occurs in less than 15%. The toxicity of α-interferon is considerable but symptoms of carcinoid syndrome may be greatly relieved. Further progress may be achieved by combinations of octreotide interferon and chemotherapy.

Endocrine tumours of the pancreas

A variety of endocrine tumours may develop in the pancreas (Table 15.2). Although they are uncommon, they are of importance both because they present with symptoms due to the excess hormone production and can therefore be difficult to diagnose, and because they shed light on the normal function of the endocrine pancreas. It has been postulated that there is a system of cells derived from neural crest of neuroectoderm which have particular biochemical characteristics, namely uptake and decarboxylation of amines such as dopa and 5-hydroxytryptophan. The amine precursors uptake and decarboxylation (APUD) system was proposed as the cell of origin in medullary carcinoma of the thyroid, carcinoid tumours, small-cell lung cancer, endocrine tumours of the pancreas, phaeochromocytoma, neuroblastoma and others. There is debate as to whether the concept can be used to account for the origin of these tumours. The hypothesis does, however, help to explain the syndromes of MEN. About 70% of the tumours are malignant and a similar proportion produce hormone. Metastases are usually to liver and adjacent nodes.

Multiple endocrine neoplasms

These inherited syndromes have been the subject of intense genetic studies in recent years. The locus of the MEN-1 gene is on the long arm of chromosome 11 (11q13) and tumour development is associated with loss of heterozygosity at this site. Multiple endocrine neoplasia-2 syndromes are associated with a germline mutation in the *ret* proto-oncogene which codes for a tyrosine kinase. The mutation is dominant.

Three syndromes are recognized.

1 *MEN-1 (Wermer's syndrome)*. This consists of hyperplasia or adenomas of parathyroids and tumours of islet cells, pituitary, adrenal cortex and thyroid (in order of frequency). Patients usually present with hypercalcaemia. Hypoglycaemia and pituitary tumours are less common. The pancreatic islet cell tumour may be malignant. It is usually an insulinoma but gastrinoma, glucagonoma or vipoma may occur (see below). The condition is inherited as an autosomal dominant, and usually presents at age 20–60. The gene maps to chromosome 11q.

2 *MEN-2 (Sipple's syndrome)*. This consists of medullary carcinoma of the thyroid, phaeochromocytoma and parathyroid hyperplasia. The phaeochromocytoma is often bilateral. About 10% of all cases of medullary carcinoma of the thyroid are part of the MEN-2a or MEN-2b syndrome. The syndrome usually presents with symptoms of a phaeochromocytoma or with a lump in the neck. It can occur at any age. The plasma calcitonin is elevated if medullary carcinoma of the thyroid is present and since C-cell hyperplasia precedes the development of malignancy, siblings of patients should have their plasma calcitonin measured. DNA analysis of potential carriers of MEN-2a provides unequivocal identification prior to symptoms [20]. Treatment of these tumours is discussed in Chapter 20. The condition is also autosomal dominant.

3 *MEN-2b (mucosal neuroma syndrome)*. In this condition phaeochromocytoma and medullary carcinoma of the thyroid also occur (as in MEN-2a) but the patients also have neuromas of the lips, tongue, mouth and entire gut. The underlying genetic abnormality is a mutation in the *RET* proto-oncogene which codes for a tyrosine kinase receptor. There may be hyperextensible joints, pes cavus and soft-tissue prognathism. The management is of the thyroid carcinoma and phaeochromocytoma as in MEN-2a. Parathyroid hyperplasia is less frequent than in MEN-2a. The disease presents earlier than MEN-2a. It is also due to a mutation in *RET*.

Insulinoma

Pathology

These are tumours of the α-cells of the islets. They produce proinsulin which is converted to insulin. The insulin is secreted with its connecting C peptide (which joins the two chains). The tumours are often small and arise with equal frequency in head, body and tail, and 20% are multiple and an equal number malignant. About 5% are associated with MEN-1 syndrome. The diagnosis of malignancy is difficult histologically but metastases occur to liver and adjacent nodes in about 10% of cases.

Clinical features

The patient presents with symptoms of excess insulin production: loss of consciousness, dizziness, episodic mental confusion and weakness. As the condition progresses the mental confusion is present most of the time and irreversible dementia may occur. It usually presents in midlife but can occur at any age. Other symptoms of MEN-1 may be present. The vagueness of the presentation often leads to considerable diagnostic delay.

Diagnosis

A fasting blood sugar of below 2.8 mmol/l is the characteristic finding. The fasting test must be carefully controlled, and blood is taken for both sugar and insulin measurements. In a normal person, fasting lowers the blood sugar (but seldom less than 2.8 mmol/l) but the plasma insulin then falls. By contrast, with insulinoma the plasma insulin is either very high or inappropriately raised or maintained while the blood sugar falls. The main differential diagnosis is from self-induced (factitious) hypoglycaemia, which should be suspected particularly in medical staff. Exogenous insulin is, however, associated with a low C-peptide level while insulinoma is not. Surreptitious taking of a sulphonylurea can also cause diagnostic difficulty.

Selective arteriography is helpful in determining whether the lesions are single or multiple. Computed tomography and ultrasound scanning are sometimes useful.

Treatment

After localization a partial pancreatectomy is performed, leaving the head of the pancreas wherever possible. When the tumour has not been localized preoperatively, it may none the less be palpable at operation. The plasma insulin is monitored during the operation. If no tumour is found, a subtotal pancreatectomy is usually performed. Chemotherapy is discussed below.

Metastases are uncommon but if they occur they may respond to streptozotocin, 5-FU or doxorubicin. A combination of all three has also been used, with response rates of 50–60%. Diazoxide can be used to treat hypoglycaemia. Glucagon is of little value.

Gastrinoma (Zollinger–Ellison syndrome)

Incidence and pathology

These tumours are uncommon. They probably arise from the delta or D cells of the islets and are often malignant [21]. They usually present at age 20–45 and probably account for 0.1% of all peptic ulcer disease. Ninety per cent occur in the pancreas, 5% in the duodenum and others occur in the stomach and, very rarely, in the thyroid and ovary. They may be single or multiple and vary greatly in size (less than 5 mm to 15 cm). Gastrinomas are most common in the body or tail and microscopically resemble carcinoids. This resemblance and the fact that occasionally other peptide hormones are produced (ACTH, vasoactive intestinal polypeptide (VIP), glucagon) lend weight to the hypothesis that their origin is from APUD cells. In 60% of patients metastases have occurred at diagnosis usually to adjacent nodes and liver, but more distant spread is not uncommon.

Most of the gastrin produced in the tumour is a peptide of 17 amino acids (G-17) but a larger molecule (G-34) is also formed. Circulating gastrin is mainly G-34. The constant stimulation of the gastric parietal cells leads to a great increase in their mass. In some patients other features of the MEN-1 syndrome are present — usually hyperparathyroidism.

Clinical features [22]

The dominant symptom is peptic ulceration. Usually the ulcer is in the first part of the duodenum or in the stomach. Occasionally there are multiple ulcers which extend down in the proximal duodenum. Recurrence soon after medical treatment, perforation and haemorrhage all occur. The symptoms of ulceration are severe and response to medical treatment is limited, although H2 receptor antagonists are effective for a while.

Diarrhoea occurs in 30–50% of cases, due to the large volume of acid produced by the stomach. Pancreatic lipase is inactivated at low pH, leading to steatorrhoea. The low pH also interferes with bile salt function and with the activity of intrinsic factor.

Investigation and diagnosis

The history of recurrent severe peptic ulceration with diarrhoea in a young person should point to the possible diagnosis. There is occasionally a family history of endocrine neoplasia. Acid output is raised, but not necessarily to levels above that found in some patients with duodenal ulcer. The diagnosis is confirmed by finding an elevated plasma gastrin level. Most radioimmunoassay antibodies will detect all types of gastrin molecule produced by gastrinomas.

When the diagnosis has been made, attempts are usually made to locate any tumour. CT scanning and ultrasound may be helpful in showing metastases but usually fail to demonstrate the primary, and angiography is little better. Laparotomy is usually required to assess operability.

Management

Pancreatectomy is seldom practicable. The tumours are often multifocal and have frequently metastasized. Histamine antagonists have greatly improved medical management. Before their introduction total gastrectomy was the preferred treatment for intractable ulceration. Death is more a consequence of the complications of ulceration than of malignancy, though this may change with the use of cimetidine. About 60% of patients are alive 5 years after diagnosis.

Vipoma (Verner–Morrison syndrome)

This rare syndrome of profuse watery diarrhoea, facial flushing, hypokalaemia, hypochlorhydria and hypertension is caused by the secretion of VIP by tumours of the pancreatic islets [23]. VIP (and the syndrome) can be produced by phaeochromocytomas, ganglioneuroblastomas and bronchogenic (small-cell) carcinoma. Hyperglycaemia and hypercalaemia may also occur and can be caused by VIP.

The tumours are usually solitary and can sometimes be shown angiographically. Treatment is by surgical removal. There is a high risk of malignancy.

Glucagonoma

These are tumours of the pancreatic α cell and usually affect postmenopausal women. The clinical syndrome is characterized by a severe skin eruption with migratory erythema, bullous ulceration and scabbing on the legs, trunk, genital area and face (migratory necrolytic erythema). In addition, there is normochromic anaemia, stomatitis, diarrhoea and hypokalaemia. Most of the tumours are in the body and tail and are often malignant (60%) but with a slow growth rate. Metastasis is usually to the liver.

The diagnosis is made by the typical rash and the raised plasma glucagon levels. Glucagon causes gluconeogenesis and glycogenolysis, elevating the blood sugar. The mechanism of production of the skin rash is not known. Treatment is by surgical removal wherever possible.

Somatostatinoma

This rare islet cell tumour is usually malignant. The syndrome consists of steatorrhoea and diarrhoea due to suppressed pancreatic exocrine function, gall stones due to decreased gall bladder contractility, diabetes from suppression of insulin, and hypochlorhydria from suppression of gastrin.

Plasma somatostatin and calcitonin are elevated. Diagnosis is late because the symptoms are not specific. The tumours should be removed if metastases have not yet occurred.

Chemotherapy of advanced endocrine tumours of the pancreatic islet cells

There are few controlled trials of the value of chemotherapy in these diverse tumours. Streptozotocin has been widely used. It produces tumour regression in 30% of advanced cases. Both doxorubicin and 5-FU produce responses in patients who have been treated with streptozotocin and those who are untreated. Chlorozotocin, which like streptozotocin is a nitrosourea-containing agent, has a similar level of activity.

In a trial of the Eastern Cooperative Oncology Group [24], streptozotocin appeared to have superior activity when combined with doxorubicin than when combined with 5-FU. Both combinations were superior to chlorozotocin alone when judged by response rate. The doxorubicin-containing combination produced responses in 70% of patients and may have prolonged their survival. Streptozotocin produces severe nausea which chlorozotocin does not, so the latter drug may replace streptozotocin in combination. Octreotide is a somatostatin analogue with a longer half-life, it binds to the cell receptor and inhibits hormone release and downregulated cell growth. Biochemical parameters improve in 30% of patients but only 10% show reduction in tumour size. Subjective improvement is common. Side-effects are mainly of gastrointestinal disturbance. It can potentiate hypoglycaemia, but is none the less of value in islet cell tumours. Alpha-interferon (in doses of 3–9 MU 3–7 times a week) produces biochemical response in 50% of cases and objective shrinkage in 10%. Trials are now in progress and combinations of α-interferon and octreotide are being assessed.

References

1 Colombo M, de Franchis R, del Ninno E *et al.* Hepatocellular carcinoma in Italian patients with cirrhosis. *N Engl J Med* 1991; 325: 675–80.

2 Adami O, Hsing AW, McLaughlin JK *et al.* Alcoholism and liver cirrhosis in the etiology of primary liver cancer. *Int J Cancer* 1992; 51: 898–902.

3 Patterlini P, Gerken G, Nakajima E *et al.* Polymerase chain reaction to detect hepatitis B virus DNA and RNA sequences in primary liver cancers from patients negative for hepatitis surface antigen. *N Engl J Med* 1990; 323: 80–5.

4 Effect of interferon α on progression of cirrhosis to hepatocellular carcinoma: a retrospective cohort study. Report of the International Interferon α Hepatocellular Carcinoma study group. *Lancet* 1998; 351: 1535–9.

5 Hussain SA, Ferry DR, El-Gazzaz G *et al.* Hepatocellular carcinoma. *Ann Oncol* 2001; 12: 161–72.

6 Mazzaferro V, Regalia E, Doci R *et al.* Liver transplantation for the treatment of small hepatocellular carcinomas in patients with cirrhosis. *N Engl J Med* 1996; 334: 693–9.

7 Williams R, Rizzi P. Treating small hepatocellular carcinomas. *N Engl J Med* 1996; 334: 728–9.

8 Senzer NN, Terrell W, Pratt CB. Evaluation of a chemotherapeutic regimen for primary liver cancer in children. *Cancer Treatment Rep* 1978; 62: 1403–4.

9 Levin B, Ridder RH, Kirsner JB. Management of precancerous lesions of the gastrointestinal tract. *Clin Gastroenterol* 1976; 5: 827–53

10 Lowenfels AB, Maisonneuve P, Cavallini G *et al.* Pancreatitis and the risk of pancreatic cancer. *N Engl J Med* 1993; 328: 1433–7.

11 Wanebo HJ, Vezeridis MP. Pancreatic carcinoma in perspective: a continuing challenge. *Cancer* 1995; 78: 580–91.

12 Coutsofides T, McDonald J, Shibata HR. Carcinoma of the pancreas and periampullary region: a 41-year experience. *Ann Surg* 1977; 186: 730–3.

13 Rösch T, Lorenz R, Braig C *et al.* Endoscopic ultrasound in pancreatic tumour diagnosis. *Gastrointest Endosc* 1991; 37: 347–52.

14 Edge SB, Schmieg RE Jr, Rosenlof LK *et al.* Pancreas cancer resection outcome in American University centers in 1989–90. *Cancer* 1993; 71: 3502–8.

15 Harter WK. Pancreatic cancer: radiotherapeutic approaches. In: Ahlgren JD, McDonald JS, eds. *Gastrointestinal Oncology*. Philadelphia: JB Lippincott, 1992: 215–25.

16 Kalser MH, Ellenberg SS. Pancreatic cancer: adjuvant combined radiation and chemotherapy following curative resection. *Arch Surg* 1985; 120: 899–903.

17 Smith FP, Schein PS. Chemotherapy of pancreatic cancer. *Semin Oncol* 1978; 6: 368–77.

18 Öberg K. Neuroendocrine gastrointestinal tumours. *Ann Oncol* 1996; 7: 453–63.

19 Caplin ME, Buscombe JR, Hilson AJ *et al*. Carcinoid tumour. *Lancet* 1998; 352: 799–805.

20 Eng C. The RET Proto-oncogene in multiple endocrine neoplasia type 2 and Hischsprung's disease. *N Engl J Med* 1996; 335: 943–52.

21 Martin ED, Potet F. Pathology of endocrine tumours of the GI tract. *Clin Gastroenterol* 1974; 3: 511–32.

22 Regan PT, Malagelada JR. A reappraisal of the clinical, roentgenographic and endoscopic features of the Zollinger–Ellison syndrome. *Mayo Clin Proc* 1978; 53: 1923.

23 Verner JV, Morrison AB. Non-beta islet cell tumours and the syndrome of watery diarrhoea, hypokalaemia and hypochlorhydria. *Clin Gastroenterol* 1976; 3: 595–608.

24 Moertel CG, Lefkopoulo M, Lipsitz S *et al*. Streptozotocin-doxorubicin, streptozotocin-fluorouracil, or chlorozotocin in the treatment of islet-cell carcinoma. *N Engl J Med* 1992; 326: 519–23.

16 Tumours of the small and large bowel

Tumours of the small bowel

Incidence, aetiology and pathology

Even though the small bowel includes 90% of the surface area of the gastrointestinal tract, small-bowel tumours account for well under 5% of all gastrointestinal tumours; only half of them are malignant [1]. Although malignant lesions occur most frequently in the duodenum and jejunum, benign adenomas and fibromas are more common in the ileum. The incidence of adenocarcinoma is more common in patients with familial adenomatous polyposis, Peutz–Jeghers syndrome and Crohn's disease, and generally diagnosed over the age of 60 years. Long-standing coeliac disease predisposes to the development of small-bowel lymphoma (see Chapter 26).

The commonest malignancies are adenocarcinomas (45%), carcinoid tumours (30%), lymphomas (10%) and sarcomas (mostly leiomyosarcomas). Metastatic deposits (most frequently from ovary or pancreas) are at least as common as primary tumours.

Adenocarcinoma of the small bowel metastasizes to the liver and regional nodes. Characteristically these are raised ulcerating neoplasms; histologically they are usually mucin-secreting adenocarcinomas. Small-bowel lymphomas are usually diffuse and poorly differentiated. The small bowel is an important site of non-Hodgkin's lymphoma in childhood. The management of small-bowel lymphoma is discussed in Chapter 26.

Carcinoid tumours arise principally in the ileum, caecum, appendix and duodenum. They appear as small yellowish nodules in the bowel wall, arising from the chromaffin cells which probably belong to the amine precursors uptake and decarboxylation system and which secrete small polypeptide hormones and amine. The management of the carcinoid syndrome is discussed in Chapter 15.

Clinical features

Clinical diagnosis is difficult and not usually achieved before surgery. Patients often present with abdominal obstruction or intermittent pain, often with melaena. Intussusception may be the cause of the obstruction and pain.

Chronic anaemia, weight loss, diarrhoea and steatorrhoea may occur, particularly with lymphomas. Some patients develop a palpable abdominal mass, with abdominal distension if there is intestinal obstruction. Commonly, there are no abnormal physical signs. Perforation is rare with adenocarcinoma, but common with lymphoma.

Diagnosis

Contrast X-ray studies are essential but not always helpful. In proximal tumours a barium follow-through is required, whereas in distal lesions causing ileocolic intussusception the barium enema is usually more useful. Hypotonic duodenography may give better visualization of duodenal lesions and small-bowel enemas are helpful with lower tumours. Occasionally an ultrasound or computerized tomography (CT) scan is helpful to delineate a mass. Duodenal lesions can usually be seen

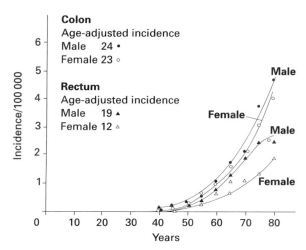

Fig. 16.1 Age-specific incidence of carcinoma of the large bowel.

endoscopically, and biopsy and cytological specimens can be obtained.

Treatment and prognosis

Surgical removal is the most important method of treatment. Benign tumours can usually be removed by simple resection, but adenocarcinomas require wider excision including, if possible, removal of the lymph node drainage area since lymphatic invasion is common. Only 70% of tumours are resectable. For duodenal cancers, pancreatico-duodenectomy may be required.

Lesions of the terminal ileum are often best treated by hemicolectomy, in order to achieve an adequate resection of regional lymphatics. With leiomyosarcomas, regional node involvement is less frequent and removal of the lymph node drainage area may not be necessary.

For lymphomas of the small bowel, a particularly careful search of the abdomen is mandatory since multiple-site involvement, including liver or spleen is common. Wide resection of the involved area is necessary, with removal of adjacent nodes. Further treatment with chemotherapy or radiotherapy is usually necessary (see Chapter 26).

In resecting small-bowel carcinoids, the site and size of the tumour are helpful guides. Carcinoid tumours of the appendix are unlikely to metastasize, and simple appendicectomy is probably sufficient. In any lesion larger than 2 cm a more widespread excision seems justified because of the risk of spread beyond the primary site.

Only 20% of patients with small-bowel adenocarcino-mas survive 5 years. For localized carcinoid tumours, 5-year survival rates of up to 90% have been reported. The prognosis for metastatic disease is discussed in Chapter 15. Leiomyosarcomas are discussed in Chapter 23.

Tumours of the appendix

These are uncommon, and 90% are carcinoids which are treated by local resection. The remainder are either adeno-carcinomas or mucocoeles which contain a gelatinoid mucoid material and can undergo malignant change to become papillary mucinous cystadenocarcinomas. Rupture of these lesions leads to the condition of *pseudomyxoma peritonei*, a gelatinous, ascitic, implanting tumour which can coat the entire peritoneal surface resulting in progressive abdominal enlargement, often mimicking ovarian carcinoma. Treatment of pseudomyxoma involves surgical evacuation, though repeated operations are usually required. Both whole-abdominal irradiation and intraperitoneal or systemic chemotherapy have been advocated, although their effectiveness is uncertain. Cisplatin or carboplatin are the drugs normally used intraperitoneally.

Tumours of the large bowel

Incidence and aetiology

Cancers of the large bowel (colon and rectum) are among the commonest of malignant tumours (third in the UK after lung and breast), and represent the second largest cause of death from cancer in the Western world. In the UK, over 30 000 people develop colorectal cancer each year. Cancers of the colon outnumber rectal carcinomas by 3:2 (Fig. 16.2), and the two sites together constitute 10–15% of all cancers, the number of cases gradually rising due to population growth and increasing age. The disease is uncommon in Africa, Asia and South America, suggesting a possible dietary aetiology. High intake of animal fat increases the risk of colon cancer [2], possibly explaining the high incidence of colorectal carcinoma (30–60 per 100 000) in North America, western Europe and Australia. Substitution of chicken or fish for high-fat red animal meat now seems justified by current data [3]. Other dietary components of aetiological importance include vegetables, fibre and vitamin C (all of which probably lower the risk) whereas high alcohol consumption appears to increase it. A colonic breakdown product of dietary fibre, the fatty acid butyrate, appears to inhibit

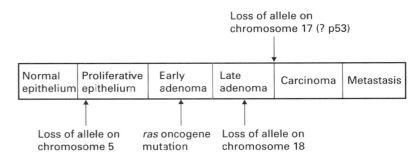

Fig. 16.2 The genetic changes in the development of the adenoma–carcinoma sequence.

carcinogenesis by activating the cell cycle inhibitor *p21*. A number of reports have suggested that regular use of aspirin and/or non-steroidal anti-inflammatory agents may be protective [4] but recent studies of high-fibre supplements have been disappointing [5].

In the USA, the incidence rate among black people increased by 50% between 1947 and 1969, which may reflect an increasingly 'Westernized' diet in this group. Epidemiological data largely supports this view. Western diets, containing high proportions of meat and animal fats but little fibre, are quite unlike the typical African diet. Africans have a more rapid stool transit time, which may lead to a reduced exposure to any carcinogen passing down the alimentary canal. Japanese immigrants to the USA show an increasing incidence of colorectal cancer in succeeding generations. Close relatives of patients with carcinoma of the colon have a slightly higher incidence themselves, suggesting a common genetic factor operating within a background of high dietary risk. Western diet favours a gut bacterial population which produces enzymes capable of converting sterols to carcinogens in the bowel. The enzyme 7-α-dehydroxylase converts bile acids to deoxycholic and lithocholic acid. In animal models, bile acids can act as carcinogenic promoters in tumours initiated by agents such as dimethylhydrazine.

Several conditions predispose to the development of large-bowel cancers. In ulcerative colitis, the risk increases with length of history and extent of involvement [6]. In the past some physicians recommended total colectomy if the disease had been active for more than 10 years since these patients often develop multicentric or poorly differentiated carcinomas. Recent studies suggest that a careful 'watch' policy is satisfactory.

Familial adenomatous polyposis coli (FAPC) also predisposes to malignant change. Siblings and parents of patients with adenomatous polyps are clearly at increased risk of colorectal cancer, especially when the adenoma is diagnosed below the age of 60 years [7]. The distal colon

tends to be most severely involved and the similarity of symptoms of familial polyposis and true carcinoma makes diagnosis of the development of malignancy extremely difficult. Most surgeons now recommend restorative proctocolectomy (in which a 'pouch' is fashioned from small bowel to replace the rectum), a procedure now considered safe, generally well tolerated, and with a good prognosis (see p. 248).

Non-familial (sporadic) adenomatous polyps are also premalignant. Most cancers apparently arise from them, though in contrast, not all adenomas become cancerous. Such lesions are found increasingly with age, and residual evidence of an adenomatous polyp occurs in a small percentage of patients with bowel cancer. The risk of malignant change increases greatly with increasing size of the polyp [8]. Many surgeons advocate routine removal of polyps found at sigmoidoscopy, particularly since two-thirds of large-bowel cancers are found in the rectum and sigmoid colon (see below). Vinous adenomas at any site in the bowel are premalignant. The risk relates to size and histology; villous lesions are more likely to become malignant than tubulovillous or tubular adenomas. They present with diarrhoea, rectal bleeding or a characteristic picture of fluid and electrolyte loss, often with severe hypokalaemia. The incidence of malignant change is at least 15% and possibly higher, and these lesions should always be removed even if this necessitates an extensive operation. Other familial syndromes known to be associated with an increased incidence of colorectal carcinoma include Gardner's, Turcot's, Peutz–Jeghers and Lynch syndromes.

The last few years have seen a major advance in our understanding of chromosomal changes in familial adenomatous polyposis. The familial polyposis gene is located on chromosome 21 (5q). Loss of an allele at this site has been found in 40% of cases of sporadic carcinoma of the colon, implicating the FAP gene in the pathogenesis of the disease. Allele loss has also been found for the *p53* gene on chromosome 17 and another gene on 18q—called *DCC* (deleted in colorectal carcinoma). A model of the genetic changes in the development of the adenoma–carcinoma sequence is shown in Fig. 16.2.

A hereditable non-polyposis predisposition occurred in some families which showed a striking excess of death from colon cancer and, in some families, other adenocarcinomas.

Mismatch repair genes are the genetic basis for hereditary non-polyposis colon cancer. The genes are *hMSH2* on chromosome 2p, *hMLH1* on 3p, *hPMS1* on 2q and *hPMS2*. Thus four separate genes have now been located, mutations of which predispose to colonic cancer by decreasing the efficiency of mismatch repair in DNA, presumably allowing defects induced by carcinogens to cause genetic damage [7]. At present there is no simple way of screening for the genetic abnormality which may occur at many different locations in each of the genes.

Screening for colorectal cancers

Since early or precancerous lesions can be resected if identified, prompt management should lead to reduced incidence and mortality from bowel cancer [8]. The high prevalence of colorectal cancer in the Western world is sufficient for screening to be a realistic proposition, using relatively inexpensive and reliable investigations—faecal occult blood testing, digital rectal examination and sigmoidoscopy [9]. As the disease is strongly age-related, with 94% of all cases in patients over 50 years, a high-risk group should not be difficult to identify. Patients with a strong family history or those with FAPC would also be candidates for screening, although the costs and benefits of these methods still remain uncertain. The present position is that screening may be feasible, and that randomized controlled trials have shown that screening by faecal occult blood testing every 2 years has the potential to reduce mortality by up to 20% [10]. The technique clearly has a sufficiently high sensitivity to warrant further study.

Pathology and surgical staging

The distal part of the large bowel is the commonest site of malignancy: approximately 20% occur in the sigmoid colon and 40% in the rectum (Fig. 16.3). The typical lesion is either polypoid with a fleshy protuberance on a narrow base, or sessile with a broader base and a generally flatter appearance. The most characteristic form is a well-demarcated polypoid mass with ulceration in its centre, involving part or all of the bowel circumference. The tu-

mour may have breached the full thickness of the bowel wall, although lateral spread beyond 3 cm is unusual. Local lymphatic invasion is common and about one-third of these patients have evidence of nodal metastases at presentation. Blood-borne metastases are usually via the portal vein and the liver is much the commonest site of distant spread. Systemic haematogenous dissemination to the lung, brain and skeleton occurs less frequently. Local recurrence can be a major problem, often leading to intestinal or ureteric obstruction, or fistula formation.

Surgical staging is of great importance since there is no better guide to prognosis. Although well-localized tumours carry a high probability of surgical cure, over half of all large-bowel cancers ultimately prove fatal.

The Dukes staging system is widely employed and is easy to apply. It is a valuable predictor of survival in both colonic and rectal lesions (Table 16.1); extensive regional node involvement has a particularly adverse prognosis. Tumour grade and depth of penetration are also important. Some of these factors are interdependent since the higher the tumour grade, the more likely the risk of local nodal metastasis.

Clinical features and diagnosis

The symptoms of colorectal cancer vary with the site of the tumour (Fig. 16.4). In the caecum and right side of the

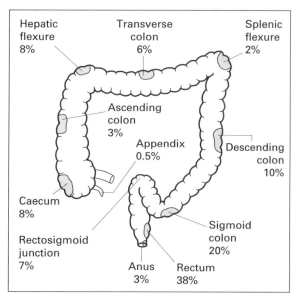

Fig. 16.3 Cancer of the large bowel: proportion of all cases arising at each site.

Table 16.1 Dukes staging system for rectal cancer (with percentage of 5-year survival).

Stage	Description
A	Confined to bowel wall, i.e. mucosa and submucosa, or early muscular invasion (80%)
B	Invasion through the muscle wall but no lymph node involvement (50%)
C1	Lymph node involvement but not up to highest point of vascular ligation (40%)
C2	Nodes involved up to highest nodes at the point of ligation (12%)

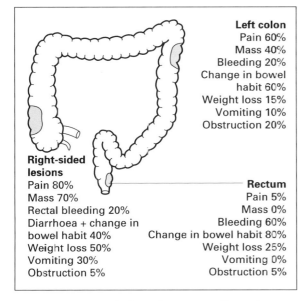

Left colon
Pain 60%
Mass 40%
Bleeding 20%
Change in bowel habit 60%
Weight loss 15%
Vomiting 10%
Obstruction 20%

Right-sided lesions
Pain 80%
Mass 70%
Rectal bleeding 20%
Diarrhoea + change in bowel habit 40%
Weight loss 50%
Vomiting 30%
Obstruction 5%

Rectum
Pain 5%
Mass 0%
Bleeding 60%
Change in bowel habit 80%
Weight loss 25%
Vomiting 0%
Obstruction 5%

Fig. 16.4 Symptoms of colorectal cancer according to site.

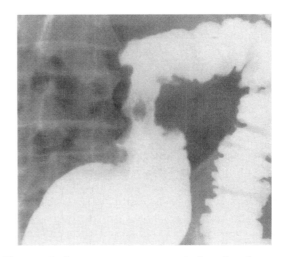

Fig. 16.5 Barium enema appearances in large-bowel cancer showing carcinoma of the rectosigmoid.

colon, the main complaint is of ill-defined abdominal pain which may be mistaken for gall bladder or peptic ulcer disease. Chronic iron-deficiency anaemia from occult blood loss is common and may be the presenting feature. Frank melaena may occur, and episodes of diarrhoea are not uncommon. An abdominal mass may sometimes be felt.

In left-sided colonic lesions the pain is usually cramping and suggestive of intestinal obstruction. Abdominal distension may be present. Constipation, occasionally alternating with diarrhoea, is a frequent complaint and symptomatic rectal bleeding occurs in 20% of patients. Rectal carcinoma is often accompanied by passage of bright red blood. However, this is a common symptom in

the normal population since haemorrhoids are very frequent. Change in bowel habit with tenesmus and constipation are later symptoms.

Rectal examination is the most important single procedure for diagnosing large-bowel tumours since three-quarters of all rectal lesions are within reach. Sigmoidoscopy allows examination of up to the distal 25 cm of large bowel, and the majority of rectal tumours can be diagnosed in this way. The introduction of flexible sigmoidoscopy and colonoscopy gives a more accurate preoperative diagnosis of the majority of large-bowel cancers, although their use is not yet routine. Radiologically, the double-contrast enema has improved diagnostic accuracy, giving better resolution of small tumours. The characteristic appearance is of a narrowed or strictured segment, or a mass indenting the contrast medium (Fig. 16.5). On the right side of the colon, the tumour is more easily missed, particularly in the caecum, which may be poorly demonstrated by the examination. In doubtful cases, the investigation should be repeated or colonoscopy performed. Use of CT scanning with air-contrast CT pneumocolon has also become widespread and is probably the radiological method of choice for assessing operability. 'Virtual colonoscopy', a newer technique employing helical CT with fine slice imaging, has also been claimed to provide high concordance with conventional colonoscopy [11], though as yet it remains inadequately evaluated.

Carcinoembryonic antigen (CEA) is a tumour marker often produced by these carcinomas, but is insufficiently specific to be a reliable indicator of disease since it can also be elevated in pancreatitis, inflammatory bowel disease, and in people who are heavy smokers or have a high intake of alcohol. It can be useful in monitoring disease in patients with a preoperatively raised CEA which has fallen following successful surgery, in whom a rise in CEA may be the first sign of recurrence. The question of what to do when recurrence is suggested by a rise in CEA has not yet finally been answered since a postoperative elevation may be due to unresectable metastasis [12].

The differential diagnosis of large-bowel cancer includes diverticular disease, ulcerative or ischaemic colitis and irritable bowel syndrome. Other causes of rectal bleeding, such as haemorrhoids and polyps, may cause diagnostic difficulty. Abdominal pain may suggest biliary tract disease or peptic ulceration. Radiologically, it may be difficult to distinguish left-sided neoplasms from diverticular disease, and benign tumours such as lipomas and neurofibromas may occur at any site, though these are extremely rare.

Prognostic factors

Approximately one-half of all patients with colorectal cancer will die of locally advanced, recurrent or metastatic disease, with most recurrences occurring within 2–3 years following initial surgery [13]. Well-known adverse factors include high pathological stage, degree of penetration of the primary tumour, lymph node involvement and age below 40 years. Undifferentiated tumours, heavy mucus secretion or 'signet ring' forms, inadequate resection margins, vascular or lymphatic invasion or large-bowel obstruction are also prognostically important. Preoperative CEA above 5 mg/ml indicates a high risk of recurrence, though CEA levels are usually related to stage and histology. Normal levels in node-positive patients do not obviate the need for consideration of adjuvant therapy (see below). Five-year survival figures are shown in Table 16.1.

Management

Surgery

Surgery remains the cornerstone of treatment. Radical surgical resection is usually preferred to simple excision, because of the risk of unsuspected node metastases as well as the possibility of multicentric tumours. Wide removal of the involved segment should include resection of the local lymphatic drainage area (Fig. 16.6). Even in patients with hepatic or peritoneal metastases, surgical resection

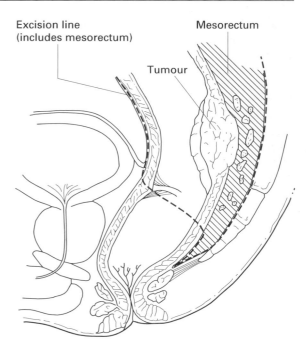

Fig. 16.6 Mesorectal excision.

may offer the best means of palliation. The operative procedure should rest firmly on a knowledge of the anatomy of the vascular supply and lymphatic drainage of the affected bowel segment, and care must be taken to avoid tumour implantation into the operative field. Anastomotic recurrences have become extremely uncommon, provided that an adequate operation has been undertaken. They are increasingly regarded as a failure of surgical technique.

In rectal cancer the type and extent of the excision depend on the site of the tumour. Far lower and middle rectal lesions, the classic abdominoperineal resection introduced by Miles is still widely performed (Fig. 16.6). Sphincter-preserving surgery, first performed in the late 1930s, is now performed on over 50% of surgically resectable rectal cancers. Local resection is sometimes performed for small, mobile polypoid lesions of favourable histological grade. Patients who are unwell through obstruction, cachexia or perforation may benefit from an initial defunctioning colostomy before tumour removal is attempted. Even in totally unresectable lesions, a colostomy should generally be performed since this will at least allow a reasonable quality of life and makes high-dose radiotherapy for the primary tumour a feasible proposition (see below).

Surgical mortality has rapidly diminished in recent years and is now below 3% in experienced hands. Complications include anastomotic leaks, postoperative infection and urinary dysfunction, particularly if nerve damage has occurred during the operation. Despite radical segmented bowel excision, the incidence of local recurrence is about 10%. Excision of the mesorectum undoubtedly reduces local recurrence, and is now widely performed (Fig. 16.6). High-grade rectal lesions are particularly likely to recur locally, especially where regional node metastases have been demonstrated. Detailed pathological description of the surgical specimen is extremely important and should include the gross and microscopic extent of surgical margins, depth of penetration, number of nodes removed (and involved) and, in particular, whether the apical node (highest level) is positive. Characteristics such as venous or lymphatic invasion, perineural invasion, histological subtype and grade should also be documented.

In familial polyposis, colectomy with an ileorectal anastomosis has improved median survival from 35 years of age to 65 years. The persistent excess mortality is due to the occurrence of upper gastrointestinal (duodenal and gastric) cancers and intra-abdominal desmoid tumours.

Radiotherapy

This modality of treatment has become widely employed in rectal cancer [14], especially in carcinomas below the mid-sigmoid region. Local lymph node involvement is clearly less common in surgical specimens of rectal carcinomas obtained from preoperatively irradiated patients, suggesting that radiation therapy may be capable of producing histological resolution of lymph node involvement ('down staging') [15]. Radiotherapy can also be useful for inoperable or recurrent cancers. Troublesome symptoms of pain or rectal bleeding can usually be palliated and long survival occasionally achieved. Perineal, anastomotic or wound recurrences can be extremely painful, particularly if ulceration occurs. In such cases, and indeed when the surgeon cannot achieve complete operative removal of the primary lesion, radiotherapy is likely to be the most effective treatment. Doses in the range of 40–50 Gy in 4–5 weeks are usually recommended. As a result of this experience, studies of preoperative irradiation, usually to modest doses, have also been carried out.

Several large prospectively randomized trials have now provided powerful evidence to support its use as a surgical adjunct (Dukes' stages B and C) [15,16]. In the UK, the current Medical Research Council study aims at randomization between preoperative radiotherapy (as per the Swedish study published in 1997) and selective postoperative radiotherapy for patients with involved margins following surgery.

In mobile cancers of the lower rectum, Papillon [17] was the first to develop elegant endocavitary techniques using high-dosage radiation therapy to a limited volume, avoiding the need for surgery. In a carefully selected group of 133 patients, he demonstrated a 5-year survival rate of 78%, often in patients whose general condition was poor.

Chemotherapy

5-Fluorouracil (5-FU) has been widely used in patients with *recurrent* or *metastatic large-bowel* cancers for almost 20 years. This relatively non-toxic monochemotherapy sometimes produces impressive symptomatic improvement, although objective responses are usually incomplete and transient, and occur in not more than 20% of all patients. There is little evidence as yet to suggest that such treatment prolongs survival in the whole group, though prolongation of life has been claimed in responding patients. Treatment with 5-FU can be given in a variety of ways, though intermittent infusional intravenous therapy is preferred. The response to 5-FU in metastatic colorectal cancer can be increased by concomitant administration with folinic acid (see Chapter 6) and a synergism with an interferon has been suggested. Other agents, although active, are either less effective or have greater toxicity. Nitrosoureas—*bis*-chloroethyl nitrosourea (BCNU), *cis*-chloroethyl nitrosourea (CCNU) and methyl-CCNU —and mitomycin C have been extensively tested and produce objective responses in about 10–20% of patients. Of the newer agents, the most promising appears to be irinotecan, an S phase specific derivative of camptothecin which interferes with DNA replication as a topoisomerase I inactivator, thus inhibiting cell division (see Chapter 6), which has no cross-resistance with 5-FU. Oxaliplatin, a platinum derivative, has also been claimed to have a significant response rate in patients with metastatic disease.

Various combinations of these and other agents have been employed but with limited success. Other studies have shown a greater increase in responsiveness to combination chemotherapy. Despite a significant improvement in response rate for patients receiving combination chemotherapy, there is unfortunately only a small survival benefit, though treatment-related toxicity is greater. In *metastatic disease* pain may be relieved and with combination therapy regressions do occur [18]. With intra-arterial infusion, responses may occur even in tumours resistant to intravenous chemotherapy. The complexity of the treatment and the lack of survival advantage reduces the value of this approach. Long-term intravenous infusion of 5-FU at a daily dose of $300\,mg/m^2$ (often given over 12 weeks) is now widely employed for clinically evident metastases. Treatment of hepatic metastases is discussed further in Chapter 8.

Treatment with chemotherapy has been recommended postoperatively as a *surgical adjuvant* and there is increasing evidence that this may be valuable [19–21]. It must be appreciated that survival gains of only 5% would save very large numbers of lives in this common disease. Trials to demonstrate these small differences have to be very large (see Chapter 2, pp. 13–16), for example the recently published QUASAR study of 4927 patients [20]. Small trials (thus far the majority) are likely to be misleading. Nevertheless, the traditionally nihilistic view of colorectal carcinoma as a non-responsive solid tumour clearly has to be revised [22].

For patients with rectal carcinoma, in contrast to those with colonic carcinoma, there is a significant risk of locoregional failure as the only or first site of recurrence following a curative surgical procedure. The best adjuvant therapy for rectal carcinoma (Dukes' stage B or C) is probably postoperative radiotherapy plus chemotherapy. The large-scale prospectively randomized trial data from Krook *et al.* [19] suggested that both radiotherapy and adjuvant chemotherapy may play an important role in the management of high-risk rectal cancer, with improvement in 5-year recurrence-free survival from 41.5% (radiation alone) to 62.7% (radiation plus chemotherapy with 5-FU and methyl-CCNU). It may also be possible to achieve equally good results with less toxic chemotherapy. The value of the 'immunoadjuvant' levamisole was tested in the QUASAR study and appeared totally ineffective.

Hepatic metastases from colorectal cancer can be treated by infusion of 5-FU into the hepatic vein and the use of this technique is at present under study in a very large-scale trial in the UK as an adjuvant to surgery in colorectal cancer in patients without visible metastases. Other techniques for attempting control of hepatic metastases include partial hepatectomy, interstitial laser ablation, and photodynamic therapy for selected patients with relatively limited-volume disease [23].

Living with a colostomy

Patients faced with the prospect of a permanent colostomy need sympathetic support. Quite apart from worrying about its appearance and the possibility of spillage and odour, most patients are concerned that they will find it impossible to manage the colostomy themselves without skilled help. They may need reassurance that the presence of the colostomy does not imply that residual cancer has been left behind and also that it will be possible to return to a normal active life. Despite enthusiastic help, many patients will develop depressive symptoms and in a proportion, agoraphobia or fear of social contact may become a disability. The value of a skilled stoma therapist cannot be overestimated, and the same is true of the well-informed self-help groups such as the British Colostomy Association.

It is often valuable for the patient with cancer of the large bowel to meet a colostomy patient before the definitive surgery is performed. In many instances this has been crucial in persuading a hesitant patient to undergo what subsequently proves to be curative surgery.

Screening

Secondary prevention (the identification of high-risk groups and early detection of the disease) has been the subject of much investigation. The three methods used have been plasma CEA, sigmoidoscopy and faecal occult blood testing. Carcinoembryonic antigen has proved an insensitive test for early cancer and is no longer used. Studies using sigmoidoscopy have suggested a higher survival rate for those thus diagnosed, and flexible sigmoidoscopes may make the procedure more acceptable to patients. Occult blood testing of stools (using the guaiac test which turns blue with red cell pseudoperoxidase) has also been used in controlled trials [10, 24]. In one study the rate of positive slide tests was 2.4%, and of those who were then investigated 9% had cancer of the colon or rectum, 80% of which were Dukes' stage A or B. The effect of occult blood testing in the general population on mortality from colorectal cancer is still uncertain, and a longer follow-up period is needed. In high-risk groups such as patients with FAPC, family histories suggestive of hereditary non-polyposis cancer of the colon (HNPCC); screening with flexible sigmoidoscopy and faecal occult blood testing is recommended. The frequency with which sigmoidoscopy should be carried out is not yet known.

Carcinoma of the anus [25]

Pathology and clinical features

Fortunately these tumours are rare, accounting for about 2% of all large-bowel cancers. They are slightly more common in women and may occur in association with carcinoma of the cervix or vulva. Carcinoma of the anus is reportedly more common in anoreceptive male homosexuals and is recognized as an acquired immune deficiency syndrome (AIDS)-related (though not AIDS-defining) malignancy. It is also commoner in immune-suppressed organ allograft transplant recipients. There is increasing evidence to suggest an infectious aetiology [26], most likely via human papilloma virus (HPV), notably HPV16, which is generally considered causative for cancer of the cervix as well. In the study from the Danish group [26] there were consistent and statistically significant associations between measures of sexual activity and the risk of anal cancer for both men and women. For example, the risk in women with 10 or more sexual partners was nearly five times that of women with only one lifetime partner. Strong associations with a variety of venereal diseases were also confirmed. Screening for anal carcinoma in high-risk populations (homosexual and bisexual males, using exfoliative cytology) has been suggested as being cost-effective (comparable to cervical screening in females) [27].

The tumour may present as small firm nodules which may be confused with haemorrhoids, the true nature of the lesion becoming apparent only after histological review of the surgical specimen. Rectal bleeding and pain are common symptoms. The diagnosis is often delayed since the symptoms are attributed to haemorrhoids or fissure *in ano*. Other lesions producing occasional diagnostic confusion include leucoplakia, Bowen's disease or Paget's disease of the anus. Local invasion of the anal sphincter and rectal wall is not uncommon, with more advanced local spread involving the prostate, bladder or cervix. Although mostly squamous carcinomas, other histological types occur including basal cell carcinoma and melanoma. It is important, if possible, to distinguish tumours above the pectinate line from those below since the latter tend to have a better prognosis.

Treatment

Surgical resection is now no longer appropriate as first-choice therapy since non-surgical sphincter-conserving treatment with radiotherapy and chemotherapy is generally curative and has become standard treatment [18,28,29]. This represents an important and exciting change from traditional teaching. Surgery may, however, be required for postradiation recurrence.

In cases initially treated by surgery or radiotherapy but subsequently developing inguinal node metastases,

block dissection of the nodes is usually required, though additional postoperative irradiation can be useful if the dissection is incomplete. Prophylactic block dissection of the inguinal nodes is not usually recommended. Chemoradiotherapy is clearly superior to radiation therapy alone, particularly in terms of local recurrence; overall survival may also be improved. In a large-scale multicentre UK study of nearly 600 patients randomly assigned to treatment by radiation therapy alone or with synchronous fluorouracil and mitomycin, the local failure rate was reduced from 61 to 39% [29], resulting in a fall of almost 50% in the number of patients requiring radical salvage surgery with permanent colostomy. Radiation fields should be generous, to include local lymph node drainage sites as well as the primary carcinoma with an adequate margin, all irradiated to a minimum dose of 50 Gy.

Prognosis

Prognosis in carcinoma of the anus depends on the location and tumour grade. The 5-year survival rate in patients undergoing abdominoperineal resection is 30–50%. Results from radical radiochemotherapy are at least as good, reportedly as high as 67% (5-year survival rate), with excellent functional preservation in the majority of cases. In the recent UK-based multicentre randomized study, 5-year survival was 58% for the radiotherapy group and 65% for the combined modality group [29]. For tumours of the anal verge, the 5-year survival rate is of the order of 60%. If inguinal nodes are involved at diagnosis, 5-year survival falls to 15%.

References

1 Di Sario JA, Burt RW, Vargas H *et al.* Small bowel cancer: epidemiological and clinical characteristics from a population-based registry. *Am J Gastroenterol* 1994; 89: 669–701.

2 Willett WC, Stampfer MJ, Colditz GA, Rosner BA, Speizer FE. Relation of meat, fat and fiber intake to the risk of colon cancer in a prospective study among women. *N Engl J Med* 1990; 323: 1664–72.

3 Cummings JH, Bingham SA. Diet and the prevention of cancer. *Br Med J* 1998; 317: 1636–40.

4 Logan RFA, Little J, Hawtin PG *et al.* Effect of aspirin and non-steroidal anti-inflammatory drugs on colorectal adenomas. *Br Med J* 1993; 307: 285–9.

5 Shatzkin A, Lanza E, Corle D *et al.* Lack of effect of a low-fat, high-fibre diet on the recurrence of colorectal adenomas. *N Engl J Med* 2000; 342: 1149–55.

6 Ekbom A, Helmick C, Zack M *et al.* Ulcerative colitis and colorectal cancer—a population-based study. *N Engl J Med* 1990; 323: 1228–33.

7 Marra G, Boland CR. Hereditary non-polyposis colorectal cancer: the syndrome, the genes and historical perspectives. *J Natl Cancer Inst* 1995; 87: 1114–25.

8 Mulcahy HE, Farthing MJG, O'Donoghue DP. Screening for asymptomatic colorectal cancer. *Br Med J* 1997; 314: 285–91.

9 Ransohoff DF, Sandler RS. Screening for colorectal cancer. *N Engl J Med* 2002; 346: 40–4.

10 Atkin W. Implementing screening for colorectal cancer. *Br Med J* 1999; 319: 1212–13.

11 Fenlon HM, Nunes DP, Schroy PC *et al.* A comparison of virtual and conventional colonoscopy for the detection of colorectal polyps. *N Engl J Med* 1999; 341: 1496–503.

12 American Society of Clinical Oncology: 1997 update of recommendation for the use of tumour markers in breast and colorectal cancer. *J Clin Oncol* 1998; 16: 793–5.

13 Berman JM, Cheung RJ, Weinberg DS. Surveillance after colorectal cancer resection. *Lancet* 2000; 355: 395–9.

14 Colorectal Cancer Collaborative Group. Adjuvant radiotherapy for rectal cancer: a systematic overview of 8507 patients from 22 randomised trials. *Lancet* 2001; 358: 1291–304.

15 Swedish Rectal Cancer Trials Group. Improved survival with preoperative radiotherapy in resectable rectal cancer. *N Engl J Med* 1997; 336: 980–7.

16 Kapiteijn E, Marijnen CA, Nagtegaal ID *et al.* for the Dutch Colorectal Cancer Group. Preoperative radiotherapy combined with total mesorectal excision for resectable rectal cancer. *N Engl J Med* 2001; 345: 638–46.

17 Papillon J, Bérard P. Endocavitary irradiation in the conservative treatment of adenocarcinoma of the low rectum. *World J Surg* 1992; 16: 451–7.

18 Maughan TS, James RD, Kerr DJ *et al.* Comparison of survival, palliation and quality of life with three chemotherapy reimens in metastatic colorectal caner: a multicentre randomised trial. *Lancet* 2002; 359: 1555–63.

19 Krook JE, Moertel CG, Gunderson LL *et al.* Effective surgical adjuvant therapy for high risk rectal carcinoma. *N Engl J Med* 1991; 324: 709–15.

20 QUASAR Collaborative Group. Comparison of fluorouracil with additional levamisole, higher-dose folimic acid, or both, as adjuvant chemotherapy for colorectal cancer: a randomised trial. *Lancet* 2000; 355: 1588–96.

21 Moertel CG, Fleming TR, MacDonald JS *et al.* Levamisole and fluorouracil for adjuvant therapy of resected colon carcinoma. *N Engl J Med* 1990; 322: 352–8.

22 Slevin M. Adjuvant treatment for colorectal cancer: no more room for nihilism. *Br Med J* 1996; 312: 392–3.

23 Taylor I, Gillams AR. Colorectal liver metastases: alternatives to resection. *J Roy Soc Med* 2000; 93: 576–9.

24 Mandel J, Church T, Ederer F, Bond J. Colorectal cancer mortality: effectiveness of biennial screening for fecal occult blood. *J Natl Cancer Inst* 1999; 91: 434–7.

25 Ryan DP, Compton CC, Mayer RJ. Carcinoma of the anal canal. *N Engl J Med* 2000; 342: 792–800.

26 Frisch M, Glimelius B, van den Brule AJC *et al.* Sexually transmitted infection as a cause of anal cancer. *N Engl J Med* 1997; 337: 1350–8.

27 Goldie, SJ, Kuntz KM, Weinstein MC, Freedberg KA, Palefsky JM. Cost-effectiveness of screening for anal squamous intraepithelial lesions and anal cancer in human immunodeficiency virus-negative homosexual and bisexual men. *Am J Med* 2000; 108: 634–41.

28 Tanum G, Tveit K, Karlsen K *et al.* Chemotherapy and radiation therapy for anal carcinoma: survival and later morbidity. *Cancer* 1991; 67: 2462–6.

29 UKCCCR Anal Cancer Trial Working Party. Epidermoid anal cancer: results from the UKCCCR randomised trial of radiotherapy alone vs. radiotherapy, 5-fluorouracil and mitomycin. *Lancet* 1996; 348: 1049–54.

17 Gynaecological cancer

Introduction

Gynaecological cancers account for approximately one-quarter of all malignant disease in women, with striking differences in incidence for each of the major primary sites (Fig. 17.1). Worldwide incidence rates differ greatly (Fig. 17.2). Endometrial carcinoma has become more prevalent with increasing average body weight and is now both the commonest and most frequently cured of gynaecological malignancy [1]. Tumours of the female genital tract are important not only because of their high incidence, but also because many can be diagnosed while still relatively localized. Standard screening techniques can detect both early and even premalignant stages of disease (see below). Management requires the combined skills of surgeons, radiotherapists and medical oncologists; many women with gynaecological cancer are best treated with a combination of these approaches.

The overall incidence rates of carcinomas of cervix, corpus uteri and ovary are approximately equal, but because curative treatment is much less likely in ovarian carcinoma, the mortality from this disease now exceeds the combined death rate from carcinomas of the cervix and corpus [1,2]. There are a number of known aetiological factors for gynaecological cancer. Epidemiological studies have shown, for example, that the low incidence of carcinoma of the ovary in Japanese women rapidly rises within a generation or two when they emigrate to the USA—a six-fold increase which strongly suggests environmental factors predominating over genetic ones. The importance of family history in ovarian cancer is increasingly recognized; a meta-analysis of 15 cohort and case–control studies gave a relative risk of 3.8 for sisters, and 6.0 for daughters of cases [3]. In addition, the daughter's social behaviour is also important as a risk factor: good examples also include the high risk of ovarian cancer among nulliparous or subfertile women and the close relationship between in situ invasive carcinoma of the cervix, and early sexual experience and social class (Fig. 17.3). Screening programmes have undoubtedly helped to reduce the frequency of invasive carcinoma of the cervix [4], which has fallen sharply during the 1990s.

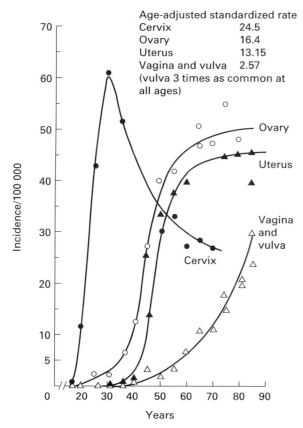

Fig. 17.1 Age-specific incidence of gynaecological cancers. The high incidence of carcinoma of the cervix below the age of 40 is chiefly due to *in situ* cases.

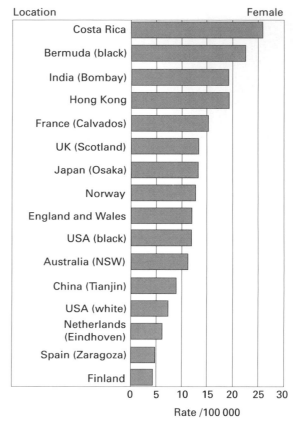

Fig. 17.2 Geographic variation in incidence of carcinoma of the cervix per 100 000 (excluding *in situ* cases). Total new cases annually: 370 000.

Carcinoma of the cervix

Incidence and aetiology

The aetiology of carcinoma of the cervix remains a subject of great interest. The disease is clearly related to sexual intercourse and multiple partners.

More women with cervical cancer have been sexually active under age 20 than matched controls. Race and social class may not be independent factors since sexual behaviour may differ in these groups. It has frequently been suggested that the low incidence of carcinoma of the cervix among Jewish women may be the result of male circumcision, though more recent studies suggest that circumcision of the male partner may be less important than was previously thought. It is likely that such women start intercourse later in life and have fewer partners. There is some evidence that the peak age of onset is falling, possi-

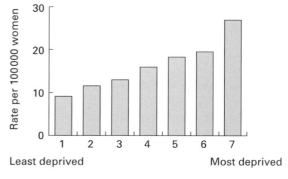

Fig. 17.3 Age-standardized incidence rates by Carstairs deprivation category. From CRC CancerStats: Cervical Cancer—UK, Cancer Research Campaign (1999), p. 5.

bly because of changes in social habits (see below). In recent years there has been a significant reduction in invasive carcinoma of the cervix, coupled with an increase in microinvasive or *in situ* disease. Just over 3000 new cases are diagnosed annually in the UK, and in 1998 there were 1340 deaths.

The aetiology has been linked to sexually transmitted infection by the human papilloma viruses (particularly types 11, 16 and 18) which have been shown to produce morphological changes in human vaginal cells [5]. Apart from the known link with sexual activity and deprivation score, important additional factors include smoking, and a history of cervical dysplasia. Women in developing countries also have a much higher risk. In addition, there is a substantial incidence in women over age 65 years who are not routinely screened in most Western countries. Older women often present with late stages of disease, and a more active screening programme in older women in the UK would result in hundreds of lives saved every year.

Pathology and spread

Routine Papanicolaou screening cytology has taught us a great deal about precancerous lesions in the cervix. These changes, collectively known as cervical intraepithelial neoplasia (CIN), can be graded according to the degree of cytological abnormality. Carcinoma *in situ* (CIN III) represents the most severe of the preinvasive intraepithelial changes, and a large proportion (possibly 30–40%) will develop into true invasive carcinomas if left untreated.

The usual invasive lesion is a squamous carcinoma (85% of all cases). Microscopically, these are arranged in nests and sheets, invading the cervical stroma. Adenocarcinomas account for a further 5–10%, and the remainder are much rarer lesions including mixed adenosquamous tumours, adenoacanthomas, small-cell cancers and sarcomas. The majority of adenocarcinomas of the cervix arise from the endocervical canal.

The major routes of spread are predictable, forming the basis of standard surgical and pathological staging (Table 17.1; Fig. 17.4). Direct and lymphatic spread occur much

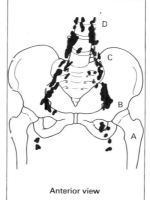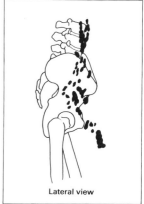

Anterior view   Lateral view

Fig. 17.4 Lymphatic drainage of the cervix. Lymphatic involvement in carcinoma of the cervix generally occurs in an orderly progression. The sequence is: (A) obturator; (B) internal, external and common iliac; (C) lateral sacral; (D) para-aortic.

Table 17.1 Clinical staging in carcinoma of the cervix.

Stage	Description
Pre-invasive carcinoma	
Stage 0	Carcinoma *in situ*
Invasive carcinoma	
Stage I	Disease confined to the cervix
Ia	Microinvasive carcinoma
Ib	All other cases of stage I
Stage II	Disease beyond cervix but not to the pelvic wall. Upper 2/3 of vagina may be involved
IIa	No parametrial involvement evident
IIb	Parametrial involvement
Stage III	Extension to pelvic side wall and/or lower third of vagina. Includes cases with hydronephrosis or non-functioning kidney (unless other known cause exists)
IIIa	No extension to pelvic side wall
IIIb	Extension to pelvic side wall and/or hydronephrosis or non-functioning kidney
Stage IV	Carcinoma beyond true pelvis or involving mucosa of bladder or rectum
IVa	Spread to local organs
IVb	Spread to distant organs

earlier than haematogenous dissemination. The most important direct routes of spread are downwards into the vaginal vault (often extending microscopically beyond the limits of visible disease) and laterally beyond the paracervical tissues to the parametria, resulting in extension to the lateral pelvic wall.

Lymphatic spread is via the paracervical lymphatics, to pelvic and para-aortic groups which follow the course of the major vessels. There is a high incidence of nodal spread even in patients with localized disease, and lymph node involvement occurs in almost 20% of these 'early' cases. Sites of blood-borne metastases include the lungs, liver and bone (rarely, and chiefly by local extension).

Clinical features

Women with dysplasia or CIN of all grades are asymptomatic but coexisting other conditions such as cervical erosion may produce incidental symptoms.

Invasive cancers present with vaginal bleeding (80%) and/or discharge, often offensive and discoloured. Some women consider these symptoms a normal feature of their lives and fail to seek advice for many months. Vaginal bleeding often follows intercourse. Abdominal pain, dyspareunia or low back pain also occur, and suggest a bulky or advanced lesion. Urinary and rectal symptoms suggest locally extensive disease. The tumour is usually visible with simple speculum techniques. *Exophytic* lesions are bulky, often forming large friable polypoid growths, making them easy to diagnose. *Infiltrative* tumours show little in the way of visible ulceration as the abnormal growth is often directed inwards towards the body of the uterus, often replacing the cervix and upper vagina by a large confluent malignant ulcer. If the disease recurs following treatment, a characteristic clinical syndrome usually occurs, with pelvic, back and buttock pain, bowel disturbance, and unilateral leg oedema due to lymphatic and venous obstruction.

Staging

Careful staging is essential, yielding important prognostic information and allowing comparison of results in centres using different approaches. The International Federation of Gynaecology and Obstetrics (FIGO) staging system is in common use (Table 17.1), and the current tumour node metastasis (TNM) system is less popular. Staging is based on colposcopy, inspection, palpation, curettage and biopsy, together with investigations such as chest X-ray and computed tomography (CT) or magnetic resonance imaging (MRI) scanning. Colposcopy is indispensable, capable of diagnosing stage 0 and Ia cancers which might otherwise escape detection. Wherever possible, examination is performed under anaesthesia. Using these criteria, the reproducibility of assessment is excellent. There is an increasing incidence of nodal metastases with advancing stage, with involvement in almost 20% of patients with stage Ib disease, and over 60% of patients with stage III disease.

Management

For patients with CIN III, therapeutic cone biopsy usually results in complete excision and cure, with preservation of reproductive function. However, newer approaches, particularly laser surgery or cryotherapy, can be expected to cure 70% of cases without cone biopsy [7]. Occasionally, hysterectomy is performed in women beyond childbearing age or in those who have no wish for further children.

For patients with frankly invasive disease, the most important modalities of treatment are surgery and radiotherapy. Management details vary from one institution to another, and it would be unrealistic to deny that local expertise and facilities play an important part in these decisions. Most centres rely on the FIGO staging system to provide guidelines for management.

Stage Ib and IIa cancers now account for over half of all carcinomas of the cervix. In some patients, the invasive nature of the disease is more limited than was previously recognized. For this group, with microinvasive or non-confluent early invasive disease, therapeutic intervention may perhaps be more conservative. It is important to distinguish true microinvasive lesions from those with microscopic evidence of lymphovascular involvement. Surgery and radiotherapy are equally effective, with high 5-year survival rates (over 85–90% in patients with stage Ib disease) following either method. Although radiotherapy has become standard treatment in many institutions, few direct comparisons are available from the same source. Surgical series tend to be more highly selective—in some series, the operability rate of patients with stage Ib disease is not much more than half of all patients referred for consideration of surgery. In patients who are suitable, a radical (Wertheim's) hysterectomy is usually recommended. This involves total abdominal hysterectomy, with removal of a 2–3 cm cuff of vagina and all supporting tissues within the true pelvis. A complete pelvic lymphadenectomy is performed because 20% of patients have lymph node involvement. Bilateral oophorectomy is often performed but is not mandatory since the tumour rarely metastasizes to the ovary. Indeed, in young women, conservation of the ovaries is one of the advantages which surgery has over radical radiotherapy.

Care must be taken not to damage the ureters, and operations as extensive as this require great skill. It is better for a limited number of gynaecologists to maintain the technique and to practise it frequently than for all gynaecologists to perform this sort of operation infrequently. An important advantage of surgery is the definition of the true state of spread, to allow more accurate overall planning of treatment; the radiotherapist will never have such complete information. Although early surgical morbidity is greater than that from radiotherapy in the younger age group, there are undoubtedly fewer late complications. Surgery is certainly the treatment of choice for young women in whom avoidance of late radiation reactions is particularly desirable. It is often possible to conserve at least one ovary in an otherwise radical operation.

In older patients, there is little dispute that radical irradiation is the most appropriate form of treatment. A large randomized study from Italy confirmed identical results for both surgery and radical radiation therapy: 83% overall survival, and 74% disease-free survival at 5 years [8]. However, in these older patients, late or 'severe' morbidity was more frequent in the surgical group (28 vs. 12%).

For patients presenting with more *advanced stages of disease (IIb–IV)*, radiotherapy is clearly the treatment of choice. In some centres (mostly in North America), radical lymphadenectomy is performed in selected cases, but its therapeutic contribution is uncertain and it has no place in routine management. The claim that radiotherapy cannot deal with node-positive cases seems unfounded. The number of histologically positive nodes is as low as one-third of the expected number treated by surgery alone, suggesting that radiation therapy can successfully 'down stage' in individual cases. An extremely important recent finding, confirmed in several randomized studies, is the improved results from combined chemoradiation therapy [9]. Various chemotherapy regimens have been used, generally cisplatin-based, given synchronously together with radical radiation therapy. This has rapidly become standard therapy.

Radiation technique and dosage

Radiotherapy is the most important single treatment for carcinoma of the cervix, and can cure a large proportion of patients, even including some with advanced disease and those who relapse following surgery. Both internal (intracavitary) and external treatments are used. Intracavitary

radium treatment is of considerable historic importance in the evolution of modern radiotherapy techniques, but with improvements in equipment, external irradiation has assumed an increasing role. In general, intracavitary treatment is of greater importance in early disease and external beam treatment makes the greater contribution in advanced cases. Some patients with early disease are initially unsuitable for intracavitary treatment, particularly where there is distortion of local anatomy, where the vaginal vault is narrow or the cervical os is obliterated by tumour, making it impossible in the first instance.

Intracavitary treatment consists of placement of an intrauterine source (usually radioactive caesium rather than radium, because of its more suitable characteristics — see Chapter 5) together with radioactive sources adjacent to the cervix in the lateral vaginal fornices (Fig. 17.5). Most centres perform these insertions under general anaesthetic, though local or epidural anaesthetic may be sufficient. Radiotherapy departments now mostly employ after-loading techniques, whereby the plastic housing for both the intrauterine and vaginal fornix containers is introduced first and the active source inserted only when the geometrical placement is perfect. These techniques produce a typical pear-shaped isodose distribution (Fig. 17.6). In this way the uterus, cervix and upper vagina all receive a high dose of radiation, with a decreasing but significant dosage to the paracervical and parametrial tissues including at least some of the regional lymphatics.

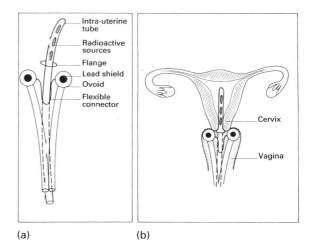

(a)　　　　　　　(b)

Fig. 17.5 Typical disposable after-loading system of intracavitary irradiation in carcinoma of the cervix: (a) components; (b) in position. After placement, these sources act as a single irradiation source, and the components are packed into position to retain their location.

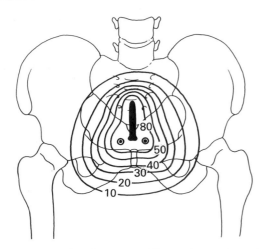

Fig. 17.6 Typical isodose curves following intracavitary placement of caesium sources for carcinoma of the cervix. The numbers refer to the dose in Grays.

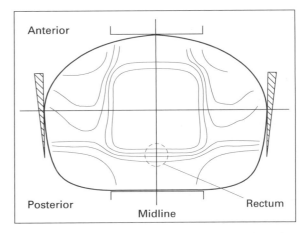

Fig. 17.7 Typical 'whole-pelvis' fields (external beam) used in carcinoma of the cervix. Megavoltage equipment is employed but techniques vary widely.

Traditionally, two points, designated A and B, are used as a guide to dosimetry. Though variability in gynaecological anatomy necessarily makes dosimetry based on these arbitrary points difficult, they are widely used as a basis for dose calculation. Point A is located 2 cm from the midline of the cervical canal and 2 cm superior to the lateral vaginal fornix. Point B is 3 cm lateral to point A (that is, 5 cm from the midline along the same lateral axis).

There is a great variety of applicators, some of which are now disposable. Most low-dose-rate techniques employ a treatment time of the order of 2–3 days, though a more popular alternative is the use of high-dose-rate equipment such as the Cathetron or micro-Selectron, which allow remote control after-loading of ^{60}Co or ^{192}Ir sources into manually placed applicators. This equipment certainly carries the advantage of a more rapid treatment with minimal inpatient care, without risk of radiation exposure for staff.

When external beam irradiation is employed in conjunction with intracavitary irradiation, the pelvis is usually treated to a dose of 40–50 Gy over 4–5 weeks (or equivalent) and supplementary treatment to the parametrial region may also be indicated. Some centres employ higher dosage. A multifield arrangement is usually better tolerated, and a typical field size of 15 × 15 cm is usually adequate to cover the primary tumour and local nodes (Fig. 17.7). Although some shielding may be possible, irradiation of significant volumes of small and large bowel (including rectum) is unavoidable. In general, it is irradiation damage to these organs which limits whole-pelvic

dosage. In advanced cases (stages III and IV), external irradiation is particularly valuable, often controlling pain, haemorrhage and discharge within days. Additionally, intracavitary treatment may become possible as a result of tumour shrinkage.

Combinations of intracavitary and external beam treatment are often employed, though the emphasis varies in different departments. For patients with early stages of disease, intracavitary irradiation is of the greatest importance and for more advanced cases, particularly with lateral spread to the pelvic side-wall, external radiation therapy to the whole pelvis contributes more to the final probability of cure. When both methods are employed — as in the majority of patients — some radiotherapists prefer the traditional approach of using intracavitary irradiation first, whereas an increasing number always use external beam treatment initially. Certainly there will be a few cases in whom the attempt to insert radioactive tubes at the outset is unsuccessful, because of tumour bulk which can to some extent be reduced by treating with external irradiation first.

Although the complications of irradiation have been substantially reduced by improved technique and understanding of radiation pathology, they cannot be avoided entirely. Early problems include diarrhoea, anorexia, nausea, erythema, dry and (less frequently) moist desquamation of the skin, mostly easily controllable with symptomatic measures. Intracavitary treatment may produce proctitis and/or cystitis. Late complications are more important and include chronic proctosigmoiditis, small-bowel damage and rectovaginal or vesicovaginal fistulae, which can require urinary or colonic diversion. Chronic skin changes (excessive fibrosis, depigmentation, telangiectasia) are common though rarely cause serious problems. After radiotherapy, the upper vagina usually becomes stenosed and dry. Sexual intercourse is certainly possible but additional lubrication is often required. Conversely, radical surgery leads to a short but normally lubricated vagina. The frequency of radiation sequelae is dependent on dose and technique.

Radiation damage occurs even in the most experienced hands since malignant tumours are only marginally more sensitive to radiation than normal tissues and radiation dosage is therefore limited by the tolerance of surrounding normal tissues such as bladder, bowel, kidneys and skin (see Chapter 5). Fortunately, with increasingly sophisticated planning and treatment techniques, severe complications such as fistulae and bowel necrosis are now seen far less frequently.

Treatment of recurrent disease

In patients with recurrent postirradiation local disease, without evidence of distant metastases, pelvic exenteration represents the only chance of cure. This is a major operation, with complete removal of the pelvic contents usually including the rectum and bladder, and with a permanent colostomy and ileostomy. Few surgeons are prepared to undertake this formidable procedure, and very careful selection of patients is essential.

Chemotherapy

The most important use of chemotherapy is clearly in conjunction with radiation for primary treatment [10]. Several agents have now been identified with significant response rates. For treatment of recurrent disease, multiagent regimens are preferred since the response rates are clearly higher—for example, the combination of bleomycin, ifosfamide and cisplatin has a response rate of over 70% in previously untreated patients with advanced disease [11]. Many patients do at least enjoy a subjective improvement, often including worthwhile relief of pain.

Prognosis

There has been a continuous fall in the overall death rate from carcinoma of the cervix between 1940 and 1990, partly due to the 100% curability of CIN III which, in recent years, has been diagnosed more frequently as a result of routine cervical smear testing. For *invasive* carcinoma there has also been a real improvement in overall survival, particularly in older women, in the period 1950–98 (Fig. 17.8). However, in the increasing proportion of young patients diagnosed during the 1970s and 1980s, the disease appears to be more aggressive.

Five-year survival rates reflect the final outcome in the majority of patients, since most will recur before 5 years or not at all. Tumour stage is the most important prognostic factor, and patients with stage I disease have a 5-year survival rate of 80–90%; the 10–20% who fail are probably those who have occult abdominal nodal disease. For patients with stage III disease, the 5-year survival rates are around 25% and stage IV disease has a particularly bad prognosis.

Cancer of the cervix and pregnancy

Diagnosis of cancer of the cervix complicates one in 2500 pregnancies. Moreover, in about 1% of cases of cervical cancer, the diagnosis is made during pregnancy, and this proportion will rise as the mean age of diagnosis of cervical cancer falls. Management depends on the stage of disease at diagnosis, and also the stage of the pregnancy and the mother's wishes regarding termination.

If carcinoma *in situ* is diagnosed in a young woman, it is usually safe to allow the pregnancy to continue, though regular cervical smears and colposcopy should be undertaken throughout the pregnancy. In older women, early

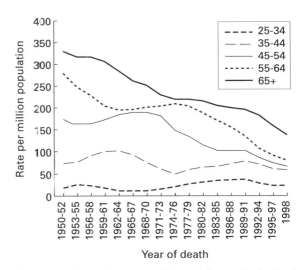

Fig. 17.8 Death rates for cancer of the cervix by age. England and Wales, 1950–98. From CRC CancerStats: Cervical Cancer—UK, p. 6. © The Cancer Research Campaign 2000.

surgical treatment (cone biopsy) has in the past been considered advisable though there is a 20% complication rate, particularly from haemorrhage. It is no longer considered necessary, providing regular colposcopy is undertaken.

For invasive carcinoma, treatment during the first and second trimester should generally be undertaken without regard to the fetus, providing the patient is prepared to accept termination. Pelvic irradiation causes fetal death and inevitable abortion within 6 weeks. Following evacuation of the uterus, intracavitary treatment can be undertaken in the usual way. If the diagnosis is made in the final trimester, treatment can safely be delayed, with elective caesarean section before the 38th week. Treatment is by surgery (sometimes performed at the time of the caesarean section) or by irradiation following healing of the surgical wound. Unfortunately, delayed treatment cannot always be recommended in the third trimester—for example, where severe haemorrhage presents a real threat to the mother's health. Provided that diagnosis and treatment are prompt, the results are as good as those obtained in non-pregnant patients.

Carcinoma of the uterus

Aetiology

Endometrial carcinoma is commonest among women 50–70 years of age, with a mean age at diagnosis of 63 years. Its incidence has risen slightly in the past 20 years, though the reasons are not entirely clear (see below). There are wide variations in incidence (Fig. 17.9), and it is common in Jewish women. The death rate is low since this is a relatively slow-growing and well-localized malignancy. Obesity, hypertension and diabetes have long been considered to be risk factors and are directly or indirectly associated with excess oestrogen exposure. It seems likely that there is peripheral conversion of oestrogen precursors in fat, which may account at least for the role of obesity. Diabetes and hypertension appear to be risk factors only by virtue of their association with obesity. A widely discussed aetiological factor is the presence of endometrial hyperplasia, particularly in relation to oestrogenic hormone replacement therapy at the menopause, which frequently produces such change. Of the two major types of hyperplasia, cystic glandular hyperplasia has a low rate of progression, while in the other type, atypical adenomatous hyperplasia, at least 10% of patients progress to develop endometrial carcinoma, and one study has suggested an incidence as high as 23% [12]. Late

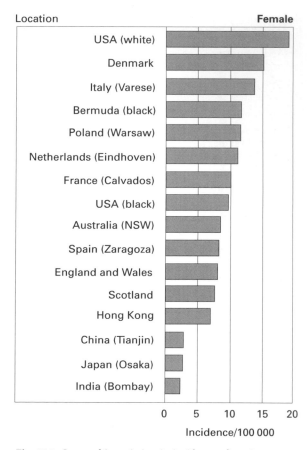

Fig. 17.9 Geographic variation in incidence of uterine cancer, 1983–87 per 100 000 (world population).

menopause is a risk factor because of excess and prolonged oestrogen exposure and also the frequency of late anovulatory (oestrogenic) cycles and the presence of metropathia.

A number of studies have suggested an increased incidence (up to five-fold) of carcinoma of the endometrium in patients taking exogenous oestrogens. However, there are a number of criticisms, including the frequency with which control cases and patients taking oestrogen were examined, as well as the possibility that hyperplasia can be difficult to distinguish from frank malignancy, even by experienced pathologists. Unopposed continuous oestrogen replacement is more dangerous in this respect than cyclical oestrogen used in conjunction with a progestogen. Low-dose oestrogen probably carries little risk. Tamoxifen is clearly associated with a small additional risk of endometrial carcinoma [13] (see Chapter 13), whereas

Table 17.2 Tumour grade, depth of myometrial invasion, and pelvic or para-aortic nodal metastasis in patients with uterine cancer*.

Depth of invasion	Grade 1 ($n=180$)	Grade 2 ($n=288$)	Grade 3 ($n=153$)	Grade 1 ($n=180$)	Grade 2 ($n=288$)	Grade 3 ($n=153$)
	Number (%) with pelvic nodal metastasis			Number (%) with para-aortic nodal metastasis		
Endometrium only ($n=86$)	0	1 (3)	0	0	1 (3)	0
Inner ($n=281$)	3 (3)	7 (5)	5 (9)	1 (1)	5 (4)	2 (4)
Middle ($n=115$)	0	6 (9)	1 (4)	1 (5)	0	0
Deep ($n=139$)	2 (11)	11 (19)	22 (34)	1 (6)	8 (14)	15 (23)

*Percentages represent the proportion of women who had metastases in each subgroup defined by both tumour grade and depth of invasion. Data from [14].

progesterone, the major component of most contemporary oral contraceptive agents, generally confers a protective effect against the development of endometrial cancer, persisting at least a decade beyond regular use.

Finally, uterine carcinoma is the commonest noncolonic type of malignancy in female patients with hereditary non-polyposis colorectal cancer (Lynch syndrome II), these patients also having a high incidence of breast and ovarian cancer.

Pathology and staging

By far the commonest of tumours of the body of the uterus is endometrial adenocarcinoma, which constitutes 95% of all endometrial neoplasms. The next largest group is adenoacanthoma, an adenocarcinoma with areas of benign squamous metaplasia. Mixed mesodermal tumours also occur, as well as adenosquamous carcinoma and a variety of soft-tissue sarcomas (chiefly leiomyosarcoma), arising from the muscle wall.

Three grades or histological differentiations are recognized. The commonest group is the well-differentiated (grade I) adenocarcinoma. Lymphatic spread is chiefly to pelvic nodes, particularly the external and common iliac groups (and thence to the para-aortic nodes), as well as the paracervical and obturator nodes. Lymph node 'skipping'—that is, with metastatic involvement of para-aortic nodes bypassing the pelvic node groups—is well described. Inguinal node metastases are also encountered. Both tumour grade and depth of myometrial invasion are predictors for nodal involvement (Table 17.2), and it seems clear that local nodal metastases are almost as common in endometrial carcinoma as in cancer of the cervix [14].

As the histological grade, depth of invasion, nodal involvement and likelihood of local recurrence are interrelated variables, it is difficult to assess the separate

Table 17.3 The 1988 system for surgical staging of carcinoma of the uterus. After [1].

Stage	Description
Stage IA	Tumour limited to endometrium
IB	Invasion of less than half the myometrium
IC	Invasion of more than half the myometrium
Stage IIA	Endocervical glandular involvement only
IIB	Cervical stromal invasion
Stage IIIA	Tumour invading serosa or adnexa, or malignant peritoneal cytology
IIIB	Vaginal metastasis
IIIC	Metastasis to pelvic or para-aortic lymph nodes
Stage IVA	Tumour invasion of the bladder or bowel mucosa
IVB	Distant metastasis including intra-abdominal or inguinal lymph nodes

contributions to prognosis. Histological grade does not form part of the current staging notation (Table 17.3). Myometrial invasion is important since its depth correlates closely with the incidence of recurrence. Patients whose tumour shows only superficial invasion have a local recurrence rate of well below 10%, whereas with deep invasion the recurrence rate is approximately 25%. Direct spread to the cervix and vagina also occurs, though vaginal 'satellite' metastases (that is, not as part of direct extension) are unusual at presentation. They are commoner in patients with recurrent disease, and occur predominantly in patients who have not been treated with radiotherapy. Local spread to other pelvic structures such as the broad ligament, fallopian tubes and ovaries also occurs.

Blood-borne metastases are unusual, though more common than with carcinoma of the cervix. Peritoneal involvement, pulmonary deposits and even ascites are features of advanced disease. Late metastases to para-aortic nodes, lung, bone and supraclavicular nodes are increasingly encountered with greater survival time.

Routes of spread and current staging systems are summarized in Fig. 17.10 and Table 17.3. The FIGO staging system developed from a clinical to a surgical/pathological (including cytological) assessment and was formalized in 1988. The large majority of patients with endometrial carcinoma have localized disease, potentially curable by surgery. The commonest clinical stage at presentation is Ia or Ib. Surgical staging at laparotomy is particularly important, often dictating which patients require additional treatment, using information which cannot be determined preoperatively.

Clinical features and treatment

Postmenopausal bleeding is the cardinal symptom and is an indication for dilatation and curettage even if the bleeding is mild. Twenty per cent of cases occur in peri-menopausal patients, so intermenstrual bleeding is also important. About 5% of all cases occur in patients below the age of 40. Other symptoms such as pain and vaginal discharge are uncommon and suggestive of more advanced disease. The uterus may be enlarged clinically—these patients should be investigated with particular urgency. The diagnosis is established by curettage, the differential diagnosis including postmenopausal bleeding from other causes, of which the most common is probably atrophic vaginitis.

Surgery is the most important treatment for endometrial carcinoma [1]. A total abdominal hysterectomy with bilateral salpingo-oophorectomy is the operation of choice. Because of the success of surgical treatment in localized cancers, the role of radiotherapy as a routine additional treatment has been questioned [15]. There seems little need for irradiation for localized well-differentiated tumours without evidence of myometrial invasion. Conversely, where the histology is poorly differentiated or anaplastic, radiation is often offered because of the risk of local recurrence, particularly with evidence of myometrial invasion beyond one-third of the thickness of the uterine wall. With myometrial penetration, or involvement of the cervix, the risk of node metastases is also high—at least 30% in a high-grade tumour.

Additional radiotherapy treatment can be either preoperative, usually by means of intrauterine radioactive caesium insertion, or by external beam irradiation to the true pelvis. Preoperative intracavitary irradiation reduces the volume of tumour and also reduces the probability of subsequent vaginal metastases. However, preoperative treatment may be technically difficult because of enlargement of the uterus and/or widespread intrauterine involvement by the tumour. It may be necessary to pack the uterus with several irradiating sources, rather than relying on the arrangement usually employed for carcinoma of the cervix. Our own practice is to recommend postoperative external irradiation in selected cases with adverse risk factors (see above). In most patients, a dose of 45–50 Gy in daily fractions over 4.5–5.5 weeks is well tolerated and effective. In patients with stage I disease it seems likely that long-term pelvic control can be achieved as effectively by external beam irradiation as by vaginal brachytherapy [16].

In patients with recurrent disease, the use of further irradiation, endocrine therapy with progestogens, or chemotherapy can all be worthwhile. Vaginal recurrences, usually seen in previously unirradiated patients, respond to local therapy with intravaginal caesium though some oncologists prefer interstitial radiotherapy (usually with ^{192}Ir). The most valuable form of systemic therapy is progestogen treatment, particularly valuable for patients with distant metastatic disease. About one-third of patients have an objective response, often remarkably durable. Conversely, progestogen as an adjuvant to surgery has not been shown to prolong survival. The most popular drug is medroxyprogesterone acetate, given by mouth at doses of the order of 100 mg three times per day. Pulmonary metastases seem particularly likely to respond.

In patients who fail to respond to progestogen therapy, chemotherapy has sometimes been of value. The most useful agents appear to be taxanes, 5-fluorouracil (5-FU),

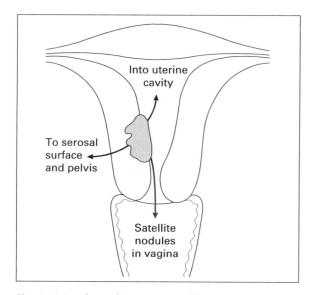

Fig. 17.10 Local spread in carcinoma of the corpus uteri.

cyclophosphamide, doxorubicin and cisplatin or carbo-platin. Combination chemotherapy produces more responses than treatment with single agents, but at the cost of increased toxicity. There is no place for chemotherapy in the routine treatment of early endometrial carcinoma [17].

For further discussion of uterine sarcomas and their management, see Chapter 23.

Prognosis

The age-adjusted death rate is 1.4 per 100 000, far below the incidence rate. About two-thirds of patients are cured by surgery (or occasionally radiotherapy in inoperable cases). Survival rates fall with extrauterine spread, poorly differentiated (high-grade) tumours and deep myometrial invasion. Taking together the large series of patients treated with preoperative radiotherapy and surgery, the 5-year survival rate is over 75%. Indeed, the results of radiotherapy alone have often surprised those who feel surgery to be essential. In Kottmeier's classic series of almost 1500 patients treated by radiation in Stockholm, the 5-year survival was 63%. The survival of 'operable lesions' (809 patients) was 79%, comparable to or better than many of the surgical series. These reports have been updated by Einhorn [18].

The relatively favourable prognosis of endometrial carcinoma is largely due to the preponderance of localized disease, itself probably a reflection of the slow-growing nature of the tumour and the early concern aroused by its major symptom, postmenopausal bleeding.

The increasing incidence of adenosquamous carcinomas is worrying since this group of tumours has a poor prognosis. The 5-year survival rate is less than 20%, compared to over 70% for well-differentiated adenocarcinomas and adenoacanthomas. Patients with sarcomas of the uterus also do far less well, with reported 5-year survival rates between 15 and 32%. If leiomyosarcoma is discovered as an incidental finding following removal of a uterine fibroid, the survival rate is over 80%; whereas in patients with invasive leiomyosarcomas, survival is very poor indeed.

Carcinoma of the ovary

Little is known of the aetiology of this disease. It is commoner in women carrying the *BRCA1* gene [19], and in nulliparous and subfertile women. An increasing number of pregnancies seem to be protective. There are wide demographic differences in mortality; for example, the rate in Denmark is six times as great as in Japan. There is both a familial incidence and an apparent link with breast cancer—perhaps related to nulliparity and *BRCA1*. Early menopause seems to reduce the risk. In addition there is a 10% risk of ovarian tumours in patients with Peutz–Jeghers syndrome. It has become the commonest pelvic malignancy in many Western countries, and is the sixth commonest female cancer in the UK, with a crude yearly rate of 17.3 per 100 000. Worldwide, it is the sixth commonest cancer in women with an estimated 162 000 new cases annually.

Clinical features

These tumours usually present late and only one-third are localized at the time of diagnosis. Early ovarian cancer is often asymptomatic. When symptoms occur they are often vague and are overlooked by patients, even when the tumour is locally advanced and abdominal distension has become obvious. Lower abdominal pain, bloating and anorexia are common, but often insufficient to raise suspicion. Signs such as ascites or palpable pelvic masses often indicate advanced disease. Even with more widespread use of cervical smear tests and annual examination, the proportion of early diagnoses has not risen. There is no evidence that routine screening uncovers a significant number of women with early disease. Possibilities for the future include pelvic ultrasound, which is rapidly improving in its resolving power, transvaginal aspiration with cytology of washings and also the increasing use of CA-125, a moderately specific tumour antigen detected by a simple blood test, and with a semiquantitative relationship with tumour response. So far, the rate of diagnosis in asymptomatic women is low, but screening may prove valuable in the future, particularly perhaps if these tests are used in combination [20].

Pathology, staging and prognosis

There is great histological variety and the World Health Organization lists 27 subtypes. About 90% of ovarian carcinomas originate from the epithelial surface of the ovary, the remainder comprising the much less common group of germ cell tumours (both teratomas and dysgerminomas), ovarian sarcomas, granulosa cell tumours, thecomas, and Leydig and Sertoli cell tumours. Of the epithelial carcinomas, the major types include serous cystadenocarcinoma, mucinous, endometrioid, clear cell (mesonephroid) and undifferentiated adenocarcinomas. The tumour grade, or degree of differentiation, is of great prognostic importance [21], at least in serous tumours, in which the grade can vary from barely malignant to highly undifferentiated invasive tumours. In general, tumours which are relatively well differentiated are more likely to be operable. Mucinous tumours appear to be associated with improved survival.

Clinical staging is of considerable importance and is the most important indicator of prognosis [22]. The FIGO staging system is widely accepted (Table 17.4), and Table 17.5 shows the relation between stage and prognosis. Patients with disease localized to the ovaries have an overall survival rate of 60%. However, even within this group, further risk factors have been identified. For example, intracystic tumours have a 5-year survival rate of almost 100%, whereas in those with adherence of the tumour to surrounding structures, the 5-year survival is reduced by half. When the disease has spread outside the ovary but still confined to the pelvis, there is an important distinction between tumours with minimal local spread to adjacent gynaecological organs (stage IIa, carrying a 5-year survival rate almost as good as stage I tumours), and those which have spread more widely (stage IIb), which carry a very much poorer prognosis.

Once the tumour has disseminated into the peritoneal cavity, the outlook is very much worse, particularly with bulky abdominal disease. Common sites include the omentum, peritoneal surface (often the site of multiple seedlings) and undersurface of the diaphragm, a particularly important area for inspection at the initial operation (Fig. 17.11). Beyond the peritoneal cavity, important sites include liver, lungs and occasionally the central nervous system. Lymph node spread is chiefly to pelvic and para-aortic nodes, and less commonly to supraclavicular, neck and inguinal nodes. Bone marrow dissemination is extremely unusual.

For women below the age of 65 years, ovarian cancer is a significant cause of death, particularly since the majority present with advanced stages (Table 17.5). Survival has improved little if at all in recent years, with over 4000 deaths per annum in the UK making it the fourth most lethal female cancer (after breast, lung and large bowel) and accounting for 1000 more deaths than all other gynaecological cancers combined. The average 5-year

Table 17.4 FIGO staging system in carcinoma of the ovary. From [22].

Stage	Description
Stage I	Growth limited to ovary (26%)*
Ia	One ovary involved
Ib	Both ovaries involved
Ic	Ascites present, or positive peritoneal washings
Stage II	Growth limited to pelvis (21%)
Iia	Extension to gynaecological adnexae
Iib	Extension to other pelvic tissues
Stage III	Growth extending to abdominal cavity—including peritoneal surface seedlings, omentum, etc. (37%)
Stage IV	Metastases to distant sites (including hepatic parenchymal disease) (16%)

*Figures in parentheses refer to proportion of total cases presenting with each particular stage.

Table 17.5 Relationship between FIGO stage and prognosis in carcinoma of the ovary. From [22].

Stage	Number of patients	5-year survival rates (%)
Stage I	751	61
Ia	528	65
Ib	130	52
Ic	80	52
Stage II	401	40
IIa*	40	60
IIb	205	38
Stage III	539	5
Stage IV	101	3

*The distinction between stages IIa and IIb is particularly important, as the 5-year survival with stage IIa is similar to stage I disease.

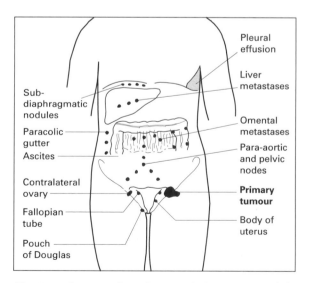

Fig. 17.11 Common sites of metastasis in carcinoma of the ovary.

survival is only of the order of 30%; overall, death from ovarian cancer accounts for 6% of all cancer deaths in women. The age-specific mortality increases from 0.8 (per 100 000) at ages 25–34, 17.7 at ages 45–54 and to 35.0 at ages 55–64.

Surgical management

Operative treatment has always been the cornerstone of successful management. The initial operation has a greater bearing on outcome than any subsequent therapy, and the success of postoperative treatment largely depends on careful operative assessment and adequate tumour removal.

Careful inspection of the whole of the abdominal cavity is essential before surgical resection. In particular, the infradiaphragmatic surfaces and paracolic gutters should be carefully assessed, since these are common but often overlooked sites of spread. Even when subdiaphragmatic seedlings are not visible, peritoneal lavage may reveal malignant cells from this and other sites. A substantial proportion of patients, initially thought to have localized disease, may have evidence of more widespread dissemination, making local treatment inappropriate.

For stage I disease, surgery is often adequate, and consists of total abdominal hysterectomy and bilateral salpingo-oophorectomy. Even with unilateral tumours, the opposite ovary is normally removed as there is a 20% frequency of bilateral tumours or occult metastases. In young women, particularly those anxious to retain one of the ovaries, conservative operations are occasionally performed. In tumours of borderline malignancy, conservative operations can be recommended with greater confidence, though most gynaecologists understandably prefer to perform a full operation unless the patient is particularly anxious to become pregnant.

In patients with more advanced disease (stages II–IV) the consensus of opinion favours excision of as much tumour as possible at the time of initial operation. Good palliation may be achieved by the reduction of a heavy tumour burden but there is little evidence that surgical debulking procedures substantially improve survival unless all or nearly all of the tumour can be excised. Many technically operable tumours are of relatively low grade, which will itself imply a more favourable prognosis. Nevertheless, the size of the largest postoperative residual tumour nodule is a good predictor of responsiveness to subsequent chemotherapy and also of the ultimate outcome [23]. Using a multiple linear regression equation with survival as the end-point, only histological tumour grade and size of the largest postoperative residual mass were factors of real importance; the operation itself contributed nothing, unless it reduced the size of the largest tumour mass to 1.6 cm (or less) in diameter.

Postoperative chemotherapy or radiotherapy in patients with residual palpable masses is extremely unlikely to be curative. For this reason a second operative procedure by an expert surgeon, at least in selected patients, may be needed. Lengthy operations—including removal of pelvic contents, omentectomy, bowel resection and excision of the entire parietal pelvic peritoneum—are now performed more frequently. A large-scale European cooperative study (319 patients prospectively randomized, after initial surgery and chemotherapy, to undergo further debulking or no additional surgery) confirmed the advantages of additional surgery [24]. Both progression-free interval and overall survival were lengthened in patients undergoing postchemotherapy surgical debulking (so-called 'second-look laparotomy').

Despite the advent of ultrasonography, CT and MRI scanning, there is no reliable guide to the effectiveness of treatment in advanced ovarian cancer short of a further exploratory procedure, so further surgery—even beyond the 'second-look'—is sometimes advocated. Laparotomy is often justifiable in cases where laparoscopic examination has failed to show residual disease and peritoneal washings are clear. It is difficult to demonstrate beyond doubt that second-look laparotomy has contributed to improved survival in ovarian cancer, but treatment decisions have become more logical as a result. It is now widely accepted that second-look laparotomy only has a role where it could reasonably be expected to influence further treatment.

The role of the gynaecological surgeon in the management of ovarian cancer has changed and continues to evolve. The initial assessment and operative procedure is critically important, both for localized and generalized disease. The surgeon has an important role in evaluation for treatment. Although second-look laparotomy is the most reliable means of judging response, there remains considerable doubt about its true therapeutic value.

Chemotherapy

After surgical excision, chemotherapy is the most important modality of treatment for ovarian cancer. It is essential for patients who present with disease outside the true pelvis (FIGO stages III and IV) and is increasingly offered to selected patients with more limited disease, notably with high-grade tumours, adherence or incomplete resection. Ovarian cancer is moderately sensitive to cytotoxic agents, but for most drugs, information regarding response rates was gained at a time when no attempt had been made to reduce tumour bulk before starting treatment. Since massive disease so clearly reduces responsiveness (see Chapter 6), the reported response rates may be lower than those which could be achieved under more favourable conditions. Nowadays response data should be based on careful pre- and post-treatment assessment of tumour size, including appropriate imaging techniques and, if appropriate, second-look laparotomy.

Single agents

At present, cisplatin, carboplatin and paclitaxel are regarded as the most active agents (with 50–70% response rates), but in the past alkylating agents were widely employed, including chlorambucil, cyclophosphamide and melphalan, with response rates of around 40%. Recent studies have not altered this figure. Of the antimetabolites, 5-FU and methotrexate have activity, but complete responses are rarely seen. Hexamethylmelamine is a drug with activity, though its side-effects are considerable (see Chapter 6) and it is not widely used at present. Cisplatin and its derivatives—notably carboplatin—have rapidly become established as the most important agents in ovarian cancer. Schedules of administration have varied widely and there is evidence that higher doses may be as-

sociated with increased response rates though with increased toxicity.

It is now clear that cisplatin and carboplatin are more effective agents than alkylating agents such as cyclophosphamide [25]. Cisplatin is a toxic drug, though advances in antiemetic therapy, particularly with 5-hydroxytryptamine-3 (5-HT$_3$) antagonists such as ondansetron and granisetron, have made it far more acceptable. Carboplatin has similar activity to the parent compound, but reduced toxicity (see Chapter 6) [24]. Unfortunately, despite the lesser degree of gastrointestinal toxicity, carboplatin is a more myelosuppressive agent than cisplatin and is less easy to use in combination regimens. Doxorubicin has some activity (30% response rate) but is not useful in patients who have relapsed after failure with alkylating agents. Paclitaxel (Taxol), the first in a group of taxane cytotoxic agents, clearly has activity in cisplatin-resistant disease [26]. The overall response rate, however, is under 25%, with few complete responders. It is now widely used as first-line treatment, generally in combination with cisplatin or carboplatin [27].

Combination chemotherapy

As in other malignancies, there has been an increasing tendency to use combinations of drugs for advanced ovarian cancer. In previously untreated patients, higher response rates have regularly been achieved than with single agents (Table 17.6). Most of these studies have not made any for-

Table 17.6 Novel and combination chemotherapy in advanced ovarian cancer*.

Drug	Dose	Response rate (%)
Paclitaxel	135 mg/m^2 by i.v. infusion over 24 h every 3 weeks	25†
Doxorubicin	40 mg/m^2 day 1	55
Cyclophosphamide	500 mg/m^2 day 1	
(A–C)	Every 4 weeks	
Hexamethylmelamine	150 mg/m^2 daily × 14	
Cyclophosphamide	150 mg/m^2 daily × 14	75
Methotrexate	40 mg/m^2 day 1, 8	
5-FU	600 mg/m^2 day 1, 8	
(Hexa-CAF)	Every 4 weeks	
Cyclophosphamide	300 mg/m^2 daily 1	
Doxorubicin	30–40 mg/m^2 day 1	
Cisplatin	50 mg/m^2 day 1	
(CAP)	Every 3 weeks	
Paclitaxel	135 mg/m^2 as 24-h i.v. infusion	70–75
Cisplatin	75 mg/m^2 i.v. at rate of 1 mg/min every 3 weeks	

*Schedules and administration vary widely. Reported response rates also differ and figures are approximate.
†In cisplatin-resistant patients.

mal comparison with a single agent so that an advantage in *survival* over simple alkylating agent therapy has been difficult to confirm. A large Italian study [28] suggested an improvement with combined use of cyclophosphamide and cisplatin (compared with cisplatin alone) although the addition of a third drug, doxorubicin, was unhelpful. A widely publicized study from the Gynecological Study Group in the USA concluded that cisplatin–paclitaxel is a superior combination to the widely used cisplatin–cyclophosphamide for patients with advanced disease [29]. Nevertheless, overall median survival remained disappointing at 38 months even for the cisplatin–taxane group (compared with 24 months for the remainder). The hope for improvement in survival rate for carboplatin–paclitaxel (probably the two most active agents) has not so far been realized.

In future studies of combination chemotherapy, it will be essential to compare newer combinations after 'debulking' surgery has been carried out. Studies which include a majority of patients with a poor prognosis (including those in whom the operation did not result in a worthwhile removal of bulk disease) may obscure the potential benefits of intensive chemotherapy in the others. For patients with a poor prognosis, the substantial toxicity of combination chemotherapy may not be justified by the few extra months of life. The current position is that surgical removal of as much of the tumour mass as possible, followed by an effective single agent, usually cisplatin or carboplatin, or a combination regimen including paclitaxel, will result in a minority of patients being free of tumour 1–2 years after the initial treatment, as judged by subsequent laparotomy or laparoscopy. The ultimate prognosis of these patients remains to be determined, but there is little doubt that cure is possible, albeit in a disappointingly small proportion [30].

Radiotherapy

Radiotherapy has historically been used as definitive therapy, as an adjuvant to surgery, for recurrent disease, and occasionally as preoperative treatment [31]. In the past it was sometimes recommended as postoperative treatment for patients with disease confined to the pelvis. Two main techniques have been used: first, pelvic irradiation (for patients with stage I or II disease) usually to a dose of 40–50 Gy over 4–5.5 weeks, using either anteroposterior or multifield techniques; and second, whole-abdominal irradiation. The latter is technically one of the most difficult techniques in clinical radiotherapy, always difficult to achieve, in view of the very large treatment volume.

Adequate irradiation, including the subdiaphragmatic areas, results in a treatment volume extending from the pelvic floor to the domes of the diaphragm. The dose rate has to be low (usually 1 Gy/day) for patients to be able to tolerate this treatment without developing severe nausea and myelosuppression. It is especially difficult to deliver after chemotherapy because of the risk of radiation nephritis and hepatitis. The kidneys and liver are shielded after doses of 15–20 Gy, and the total elsewhere has to be limited to doses of the order of 25 Gy (usually taking about 5 weeks of daily treatment) together with boosting of the pelvis alone to a dose of 40–50 Gy.

In FIGO stage I disease, retrospective studies of surgery alone compared to surgery with postoperative irradiation have suffered from the usual difficulty that the two study groups may not have been similar enough for valid comparison. In many of these retrospective studies, the group receiving postoperative radiotherapy did less well than the group receiving surgery alone, implying that patients selected for postoperative irradiation were, in general, a higher-risk group, because of cyst rupture at operation or other unspecified features. Five-year survival rates in patients with stage I disease vary from 50 to 65%, regardless of whether or not radiotherapy is given. Survival figures from prospective studies (surgery alone vs. surgery plus local irradiation) are beginning to emerge, though no clear differences have so far been demonstrated.

In stage II disease, it seems possible that there is a genuine benefit from the use of postoperative pelvic irradiation [22] although chemotherapy is now much more commonly used and is clearly the treatment of choice. In almost all series, admittedly retrospective, the 5-year survival rate was improved, particularly where adequate surgery had already been undertaken (see p. 265). Since these studies were performed before careful operative staging was a routine part of the initial assessment, many of these patients would in fact have had stage III disease. In patients with more advanced disease (stages III–IV) the value of postoperative irradiation is unconvincing. Although postoperative whole-abdominal irradiation has been claimed to produce modest improvement in 5-year survival from about 5 to 10%, this was largely before the era of more effective chemotherapy. In the 1970s, work from Toronto reawakened interest in radiation therapy for ovarian carcinoma. There was a clear survival advantage for patients receiving abdominopelvic irradiation (stages IIa–III), despite the difficulties in achieving more than a low dose of irradiation to such a large area. There seems little doubt that the superior results from this study largely reflected the adequacy of initial surgical treatment, with a highly significant survival difference in favour of patients without palpable postoperative tumour, regardless of whether chemotherapy or radiotherapy was used postoperatively. Clearly, with increased emphasis on surgical debulking at the initial operation and, if necessary, after chemotherapy, the role of pelvic or abdominal irradiation has diminished. Moreover, the incidence of recurrent bowel obstruction appears to be increased by the use of abdominal radiation therapy.

An alternative form of radiotherapy is the use of intraperitoneal radioactive colloids such as gold (^{198}Au) or phosphorus (^{32}P). Originally used for treatment of malignant effusions, this has also largely been replaced by systemic treatment with chemotherapy.

Unresolved controversies in epithelial ovarian cancer

Several important issues in management remain extremely contentious.

1 The contribution (and timing) of debulking surgery both to improving response rates to chemotherapy, and to overall survival [32].

2 The contribution from second-look laparotomy to treatment [24]. It seems unlikely that there is any major therapeutic benefit, though its value as a staging procedure remains uncertain. In selected cases, where further treatment decisions might depend initially on the presence of microscopic disease, it may still be valuable. It can also be justified within the context of prospective clinical trials.

3 The definition of the place of combination chemotherapy compared with the best single-agent therapy, and further assessment of the role of new platinum and taxane analogues in combination.

4 Is second-line chemotherapy of real value in patients who fail to achieve complete remission or who relapse after treatment? What are the most useful agents?

5 Might paclitaxel or analogues (as single agents or in combination) be more effective than standard regimens for primary treatment?

Germ cell tumours of the ovary

A pathological classification of these unusual tumours is shown in Table 17.7. Benign dermoid cysts are relatively common and cured by surgical excision. Occasionally, they consist largely of thyroid tissue, *struma ovarii*, which may even be functioning. Less than 5% of strumas are malignant—so-called *monomorphic* or *monodermal teratomas*. Very rarely they develop secondary malignant change, most commonly squamous carcinoma.

Of the malignant tumours, *dysgerminoma* is much the commonest; histologically it is a uniform clear cell tumour resembling seminoma in males. Lymphocytic infiltration is common. The endodermal sinus tumour (*yolk sac tumour*) is a highly malignant tumour which produces α-fetoprotein (AFP), demonstrable in the tumour and detectable in the blood. Rupture of the tumour occurs early. *Embryonal carcinoma* consists of glandular and papillary masses, often with trophoblastic elements which secrete human chorionic gonadotrophin (HCG). It may occur in childhood and produce sexual precocity. α-Fetoprotein

Table 17.7 Germ cell tumours of the ovary.

Tumour	Percentage of all malignant germ cell tumours
Benign (20% of all ovarian tumours) Dermoid cyst—mature cystic teratoma	
Malignant (3% of all ovarian tumours)	
Dysgerminoma	50
Endodermal sinus tumour or yolk sac tumour	20
Embryonal carcinoma	3
Malignant (immature) teratoma (includes malignant monodermal teratomas and carcinoids)	20
Mixed germ cell tumours	7
Choriocarcinoma	Rare
Gonadoblastoma	Rare

may also be produced by yolk sac elements. *Immature teratoma* is a mainly solid tumour containing a multiplicity of different tissues. Primitive neuroectoderm often predominates, but monomorphic forms consisting of thyroid tissue or malignant carcinoid also occur. Even when the tumour has not metastasized, carcinoid syndrome may occur because of the large size. The *mixed germ cell tumour* contains mixtures of the previous histological types. *Gonadoblastoma* is a small tumour arising in childhood, usually composed of several of the elements of the developing gonad. It may calcify, rarely metastasizes, but might cause virilization as it sometimes contains functioning Leydig cells.

Clinical features

In dysgerminoma, as with other malignant ovarian tumours, the presentation is with an abdominal mass and pain, but the mean age is far lower; 75% of patients are between 10 and 30 years old (median 20 years). They do not usually produce marker hormones unless teratomatous elements are present, and they not infrequently present during or shortly after pregnancy. Other germ cell tumours (yolk sac, endodermal sinus tumours, teratoma, mixed germ cell tumour) also occur in adolescents and young women. Many of these patients have precocious puberty, menstrual disturbance and a positive pregnancy test (with pregnancy as a differential diagnosis of the pelvic mass!). These tumours usually grow rapidly, causing abdominal pain.

Management

In dysgerminoma, management depends on stage. Ninety per cent of patients with FIGO stage I are cured by unilateral oophorectomy, but the recurrence rate is higher with large tumours, positive peritoneal washings at operation, or if the tumour contains mixed germ cell elements. If recurrence occurs, or if there are metastases, patients are usually treated with chemotherapy as for teratoma (see below), or by whole-abdominal irradiation. Yolk sac, endodermal sinus and mixed germ cell tumours have a much worse prognosis with surgical treatment than dysgerminoma, even in stage I disease. The use of serum AFP and β-HCG as markers has greatly improved the monitoring of chemotherapy, which is now an essential part of treatment for most patients (exceptions are discussed below).

The use of platinum-based regimens has followed the outstanding success achieved in testicular teratoma. Since the tumours are unilateral they can be managed by unilateral salpingo-oophorectomy followed by chemotherapy, with the possibility of preservation of fertility. Exceptions to the use of chemotherapy include teratomas which contain low mitotic activity, those with no embryonal or trophoblastic elements and where there are no detectable tumour markers after surgery. Such patients can be treated by surgery alone, but do need careful follow-up. Ovarian choriocarcinoma is usually treated with chemotherapy as for other non-dysgerminomatous ovarian germ cell tumours. Combinations of cisplatin, etoposide and bleomycin are used, in regimens identical to those used for testicular non-seminomatous germ cell tumours (see Chapter 19). The efficacy of modern chemotherapy is well illustrated by a series of 59 patients with metastatic disease treated at a single large centre in London [33]. Overall survival of 88% was achieved using the POMB/ACE regimen (see Chapter 19), with no relapses occurring more than 3 years after treatment.

Ovarian carcinoid tumours and struma ovarii are treated by unilateral oophorectomy.

Granulosa cell tumours of the ovary

These tumours account for 3–5% of malignant ovarian tumours. The cell of origin is unclear. They are frequently hormone-producing. The granulosa–theca tumour is composed of cells which resemble the normal granulosa cell of the follicle. It may be difficult to decide whether the tumour is malignant or not because it often lacks the typical cellular features of malignancy. Capsular invasion and cellular atypica are the most reliable signs of malignancy, and influence prognosis. Granulosa–theca cell tumours produce oestrogen (mainly from theca cells), androgens and progesterone. Oestrogen-related symptoms include postmenopausal bleeding, menorrhagia and breast tenderness. Virilizing symptoms, which are rarer, include hirsutism and oligomenorrhoea. The prognosis is excellent as they are mostly cured by conservative surgery (unilateral salpingo-oophorectomy). Responses to chemotherapy have been recorded in patients with recurrence.

Sertoli–Leydig cell tumours of the ovary

These rare tumours, representing 0.5% of ovarian cancers, are seen at age 20–40 and are sometimes termed *arrhenoblastomas*. Eighty per cent of them are associated with virilization. The histological appearance varies and some are poorly differentiated, though all contain Leydig cells identical to the male testicular cell. Occasionally, teratomatous elements are present.

Following surgical removal, the prognosis is excellent and over 90% of patients are alive at 10 years. The tumours are rarely bilateral so unilateral oophorectomy is usually adequate.

Carcinoma of the fallopian tube

This uncommon gynaecological malignancy is sometimes considered as a 'variant' of ovarian carcinoma since the two diseases share the common aetiological feature of low fertility or nulliparity, with adenocarcinoma (solid, cystic or mixed) as the commonest histological type. Clinical symptoms include pelvic pain and vaginal discharge, which is sometimes profuse and often blood-stained. Other symptoms, similar to those found in ovarian carcinoma, include abdominal distension, altered bowel habit or, in occasional cases, dyspareunia.

Staging and treatment are similar to the recommendations for ovarian cancer (see above). Where a carcinoma of the fallopian tube is encountered at the initial laparotomy, it is much more likely to be due to secondary involvement from a carcinoma of the ovary than a true primary fallopian tube cancer. As for ovarian cancer generally, stage is an important prognostic determinant.

Carcinoma of the vulva

This uncommon tumour accounts for about 5–6% of all gynaecological cancer (1% of all cancer), with about 1000 new cases annually in the UK, chiefly affecting the older age group. Invasive carcinoma is distinctly uncommon in patients under 50 years of age (Fig. 17.1) while carcinoma *in situ* (now generally referred to as vulval intraepithelial neoplasia (VIN) III, analogous to CIN III), typically occurs in younger women (median age 50).

Aetiology, pathogenesis and diagnosis

Leucoplakia and other dystrophic changes in vulval skin can predispose to carcinoma. These can be hypoplastic, including lichen sclerosus and atrophic vulvitis, or hyperplastic, including leucoplakia as well as hypertrophic vulvitis. The hypoplastic form of dystrophic change is not usually regarded as premalignant, although there are certainly instances on record where this appears to have been the case. These are distinct from true intraepithelial neoplasia, which is a group including carcinoma *in situ* (often multifocal), and Paget's disease. Most vulval cancers are squamous cell carcinomas, though other types are occasionally seen, including adenocarcinoma (usually arising in a Bartholin's gland), melanoma, basal cell carcinoma, fibrosarcoma and adenoid cystic carcinoma. Diabetes is not infrequently associated with carcinoma of the vulva.

Pruritus vulvae, pain, ulceration, bleeding or discharge, are the usual symptoms, although some patients are unaware of a vulval problem and seek advice about a lymph node in the groin. The most common sites are the labia majora, although the labia minora and clitoris can be primary sites. All thickened, fissured, ulcerated or sloughing lesions should be viewed with great suspicion, particularly in elderly patients, and biopsied. Histological distinctions between leucoplakia, lichen sclerosus et atrophicus and frank invasive carcinoma can be difficult, particularly since intraepithelial cancer can occur in areas of hypertrophic leucoplakia. Vulval carcinomas are almost always visible, so careful follow-up of suspicious lesions should not be difficult. Clinical photographs are useful to document slowly evolving changes.

Benign lesions can cause diagnostic confusion. These include chronic vulvitis, vulval condylomas of tuberculous, syphilitic, viral or unknown aetiology, lymphogranuloma inguinale, lymphogranuloma venereum (chiefly in younger patients) and vulval abscesses. The vulva is occasionally a site of secondary spread from carcinoma of the endometrium, cervix and large bowel.

Patterns of spread and clinical staging

The FIGO system is widely used (Table 17.8) and is based on the predictable behaviour of vulval carcinoma. Dissemination is chiefly via direct and lymphatic routes, and

Table 17.8 FIGO staging in carcinoma of the vulva.

Stage	Description
Stage 0	Carcinoma *in situ*
Stage I	Tumour confined to vulva (<2 cm) No palpable nodes
Stage II	Tumour confined to vulva (>2 cm) No palpable nodes
Stage III	Tumour spread to urethra, vagina, or perineum Palpable mobile nodes
Stage IV	Tumour infiltrates bladder or rectum Fixed nodes

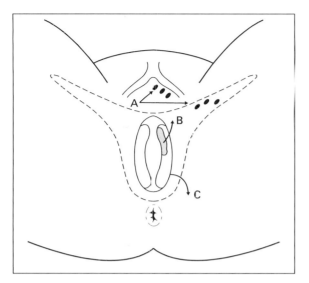

Fig. 17.12 Local and nodal spread in carcinoma of the vulva. (A) Nodal involvement: inguinal, femoral, deep pelvic and common iliac nodes. Bilateral spread is common. (B) Anteriorly to contiguous parts of the vulva, clitoris, vagina, urethra and bladder. (C) Posteriorly to posterior vulva and rectum. Dotted line shows incision and resection in radical vulvectomy.

haematogenous spread is very unusual. Local spread occurs to contiguous areas of the vulva, vagina and urethra, or to the perineum and/or anus (Fig. 17.12). Local pubic tenderness results from infection and periostitis, though malignant bone erosion has been described. Nodal involvement may be uni- or bilateral, first to the inguinofemoral group, then more deeply (including contralateral node sites). Clitoral lesions may spread to either groin but do not directly involve deeper node groups without superficial node involvement in the first instance. Overall, nearly half of all vulval cancers have evidence of local lymphatic involvement.

Investigation and management

Routine investigation should include full blood count, chest X-ray and electrolyte estimation. MRI is useful in delineating pelvic and para-aortic nodes, particularly in patients where there is doubtful clinical evidence of involvement and the gynaecologist is uncertain whether to proceed with surgery. Needle aspiration of enlarged superficial nodes may occasionally help to decide whether surgery is appropriate.

Treatment

Treatment is by surgical excision, preferably of the primary carcinoma and lymphatic drainage *en bloc*. Even in patients who are elderly or have advanced local disease, surgery is generally the treatment of choice. Wide excision of vulval skin has traditionally been considered necessary since contiguous subdermal lymphatic spread is common; however, many gynaecologists are now less radical in their approach. Removal of the lower part of the urethra may also be necessary in more advanced stages. Because of the laxity of skin and subcutaneous tissue in this area, primary closure is usually possible despite the wide excision. Although postoperative infection is not uncommon and is the major surgical complication, most patients rehabilitate well. Surgical excision is generally regarded as the treatment of choice although a few patients are unfit for these procedures, and palliative local irradiation can be extremely valuable, particularly in those with pain and ulceration. Radiation tolerance in these elderly patients is limited by bladder, bowel and other local structures. It is usually possible to achieve a total dose of at least 45–55 Gy in 4–5.5 weeks, to the perineum and/or nodal sites. Treatment to a radical dose of 60 Gy should be attempted in younger, fit patients. In some patients with extensive nodal disease, a combination of primary resection with groin exploration and postoperative radiotherapy (to the nodal areas) represents the best means of achieving local control. The role of chemotherapy remains to be defined, though recent reports using synchronous chemoradiation therapy in selected patients have been encouraging, and radical chemoirradiation has been suggested as a serious alternative to surgery [34].

Prognosis

The survival rate depends largely on whether or not there is nodal involvement. About 75% of operable patients without lymphatic metastases are alive disease-free at 5 years, whereas the 5-year survival of patients with inguinal or femoral node deposits is 30–40%, and less than 20% in patients with pelvic node involvement, even where pelvic lymph node dissection has been performed. Very occasionally further surgery (including pelvic exenteration) may be considered for patients with recurrent disease, though the end-results are generally poor.

Carcinoma of the vagina

This is a rare tumour, accounting for less than 1% of all gynaecological malignancy (i.e. about one-fiftieth as common as carcinoma of the cervix) and chiefly occurring in the 50–70 year age group. Little is known of the aetiology, but prolonged irritation from a vaginal ring pessary sometimes appears to predispose to malignant change. Vaginal carcinoma is almost invariably a squamous cell carcinoma, most frequently arising in the upper vagina, sometimes extensively involving the vaginal wall. Clear cell adenocarcinoma of the vagina has been reported in girls and young women whose mothers were taking exogenous stilboestrol in pregnancy—an example of a transplacental carcinogen with a latent period of 15–30 years. Secondary deposits are occasionally encountered in the vagina, usually as a result of lymphatic spread from endometrial carcinoma (often thought to occur at operation); vaginal deposits from malignant melanomas are also well recognized, and on rare occasions the vagina is the primary site of a melanoma. Direct extension may occur from carcinoma of the cervix or bladder.

Symptoms, diagnosis and staging

A painless blood-stained vaginal discharge is the commonest symptom. In view of the typical age group, vaginal bleeding, when it occurs, is usually postmenopausal. Urinary complaints (frequency, nocturia and haematuria) or rectal discomfort occur with advanced disease. As with carcinoma of the cervix, spread of the disease tends to take place chiefly by direct and lymphatic invasion (Fig. 17.13), to the parametria, pelvic side-wall and bladder. The lymphatic route varies with the site of the lesion. Lymphatic drainage of the upper part of the vagina is similar to that of the cervix—i.e. via external, internal and common iliac nodes. Lesions situated lower in the vagina drain to pelvic, inguinal and femoral nodes. Posteriorly placed lesions may spread towards the rectum because the lymphatic drainage of the posterior vaginal wall is to deep pelvic nodes (sacral, rectal and lower gluteal). As with carcinoma of the cervix, haematogenous spread is uncommon, and local control of disease tends to be the major clinical problem.

Careful vaginal examination should always be performed in patients presenting with vaginal bleeding and discharge, with direct inspection using a vaginal speculum. Colposcopy and biopsy can be extremely valuable, particularly where the speculum examination is inconclu-

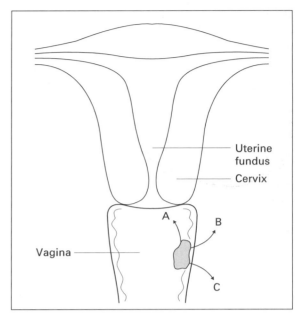

Fig. 17.13 Local and lymph node spread in carcinoma of the vagina. (A) Submucosal spread to adjacent parts of vagina and cervix. (B) Parametrial tissues, bladder, rectum and eventually to pelvic side-wall. (C) Lymphatic spread: upper vagina as for cervix (Fig. 17.4). Posterior vagina as for rectal lymphatics. Anterior wall: towards lateral pelvic wall nodes. Lower vagina: to pelvic and inguinofemoral nodes.

sive. Cytology of vaginal smears can be diagnostic. Where there is no obvious visible lesion, but definite cytological abnormalities are present, carcinoma *in situ* (now often termed vaginal intraepithelial neoplasia or VAIN) of the vagina must be suspected. This condition should also be considered where cervical cytology has yielded malignant cells but colposcopy-directed biopsy of the cervix has proved negative—particularly where subsequent high vaginal smears are still abnormal. Although an annual smear test is often performed after hysterectomy for benign disease—particularly in the USA—this method of screening for vaginal carcinoma is unrewarding and cannot be recommended.

Important investigations for symptomatic patients include examination under anaesthetic with cystoscopy, cervical dilatation and biopsy, and uterine curettage to exclude a primary carcinoma of the cervix. CT or MRI scanning, sigmoidoscopy and peritoneal cytology may help to confirm the extent of spread in doubtful cases.

Table 17.9 FIGO staging of carcinoma of the vagina.

Stage 0	Carcinoma *in situ*
Stage I	Vaginal wall only
Stage II	Subvaginal tissue involved
Stage III	Extension to pelvic side wall
Stage IV	Spread beyond true pelvis —
IVa	to adjacent organs
IVb	to distant organs

A FIGO staging system is generally used. This clinical staging system (Table 17.9) has been in use for over 10 years.

Treatment

Surgery and radiotherapy can both be effective, though surgical resection has to be very radical to stand a real chance of success and is not often employed as a primary procedure. Total vaginectomy, pelvic lymphadenectomy and abdominal hysterectomy would be necessary, with reconstruction of the perineum and vagina where possible. This operation is only suitable for early lesions (stage I) or in a few highly selected cases following radiation failure. For most patients, radiotherapy is considered to be the treatment of choice.

Vaginal intraepithelial neoplasia

For stage I tumours, surgery is sometimes recommended, particularly in younger patients with more distal lesions (lower third of vagina). For the large majority of patients, however, treatment by intracavitary caesium insertion is combined with external beam irradiation as for carcinoma of the cervix (see above), particularly with tumours of the upper part of the vagina. Irradiation of the whole pelvis, using external beam multifield techniques, may be the best means of achieving homogeneous treatment to the primary and local node groups. In patients with more advanced disease (FIGO stages II–IV), a dose of 45–50 Gy, given in daily fractions over 4.5–5 weeks, is usually well tolerated and generally considered adequate for sterilizing microscopic direct or local lymphatic extension, though it is essential to give additional irradiation to the primary site and to any area which is obviously clinically involved. This is achieved either by intracavitary treatment or by additional external beam radiotherapy to encompass the whole of the vagina, treating the primary site if possible to a total of 60 Gy in daily fractions over 6 weeks.

Side-effects include acute proctitis in a substantial pro-portion of patients. Late radiation-induced rectal stricture may follow. Other complications include increased urinary frequency with cystitis and in the longer term, local fistula formation, proctitis or sigmoid colitis, which may require bowel diversion, although local intrarectal steroid preparations may be adequate if the bowel is sufficiently viable. In view of the poor results and high complication rate with very advanced (stage IV) disease, treatment of these patients is usually palliative and lower doses, consistent with symptom relief, are generally more appropriate. Overall, the results of treatment are disappointing. Even with a radical approach, the 5-year survival rate falls from 75% with stage I disease, to 25% with stage II and less than 5% for patients with stage IV tumours.

Carcinoma *in situ*

The whole of the vaginal mucosa is usually irradiated using a vaginal applicator containing radioactive sources (often termed Dobbie applicators after their originator). The intravaginal mould can be differentially loaded to treat the area at greatest risk to a higher dose, but irradiation of the whole mucosa is usually advised as there may be more than one neoplastic site. Complications of treatment include vaginal stenosis, lack of lubrication and proctitis. A radical dosage of at least 60 Gy mucosal dose is usually recommended.

Alternatively, laser therapy with colposcopy may be adequate for well-localized lesions. Occasionally, treatment by topical chemotherapy (generally with 5-FU) may be valuable, sometimes in conjunction with local irradiation.

Choriocarcinoma

This rare tumour has received considerable attention because of its extreme chemosensitivity, placing it in the small group of solid tumours which can be cured even when metastatic [35]. In addition, the secretion of a tumour marker, HCG (see Chapter 4) in 100% of cases of choriocarcinoma, permits a logical treatment approach based on a reliable index of tumour bulk.

The tumour most frequently follows pregnancies which have resulted in a complete or even a partial hydatidiform mole (occurring in approximately one in 1400 normal pregnancies in the UK), though it may rarely accompany a normal or ectopic pregnancy, or even a termination. It seems increasingly probable that most, or even all, carcinomas following an apparently normal pregnancy are, in reality, metastases from an undetected small intraplacental carcinoma, easily overlooked unless the placenta is minutely examined [36]. It is more common in Asia than in Europe or the USA, and following pregnancy in 'elderly' subjects (that is, over 40 years).

Pathology

Histopathologically, the tumour consists of malignant syncytio- or cytotrophoblast cells, which can be shown immunocytochemically to contain HCG. Following successful evacuation of a hydatidiform mole, sequential determination of plasma HCG provides reliable information as to the completeness of the evacuation [37]. In some cases, the HCG level falls more slowly to normal than would be predicted by the half-life of HCG (24–36 h), suggesting that spontaneous regression of a tumour may have occurred. In others, local or distant invasion of tumour supervenes and the HCG level remains elevated.

The traditional classification of trophoblastic tumours — into *hydatidiform moles, invasive moles* and *true choriocarcinomas* — was based on morphology. However, the availability of the quantitative HCG assay has largely supplanted these terms, since the diagnosis is made as a result of persistently raised HCG and tissue is now rarely available. It is probably better to use the term 'gestational trophoblastic tumour' instead. Abnormalities such as mitotic activity, degree of cellular atypia and local invasiveness appear to correlate fairly closely with prognosis.

Although the tumour may remain localized within the uterus, local extension into the myometrium or even the serosal surface or vagina may take place, sometimes causing severe intrauterine or intraperitoneal bleeding. More distant blood-borne secondary deposits occur, chiefly to lung, liver and brain, with a frequency which depends on the antecedent history: possibly as many as one in 20 molar pregnancies, but very rarely following normal or ectopic pregnancy.

Diagnosis and staging

Vaginal bleeding during or after pregnancy should be regarded with suspicion. Some patients appear to suffer from particularly marked symptoms of pregnancy, or preeclampsia. Ultrasound examination may lead to an almost certain diagnosis of a molar pregnancy before delivery. In the UK, evacuation of a hydatidiform mole and/or persistent elevation of postpartum HCG levels should result in registration of the patient at a reference centre (Charing Cross Hospital, London, in the South and Sheffield in the North). The patient will then be followed closely, sending regular samples of blood and/or urine to the designated centre. Staging investigations include repeat estimations of β-HCG, with chest and abdominopelvic CT scanning. Pelvic ultrasound may also be valuable.

Risk classification is important since optimal treatment is different for patients at varying risk of drug resistance [35]. Important prognostic factors include age (older patients do worse), interval between antecedent pregnancy and start of chemotherapy, initial HCG level, number and sites of metastases (the brain is a particularly adverse site) and previous administration of chemotherapy.

Treatment

Patients with *low-risk* disease are treated either by chemotherapy (generally single-agent chemotherapy with methotrexate) or by hysterectomy in patients who have no wish for further children. Where surgery is performed, it is often recommended that the hysterectomy be 'covered' by administration of methotrexate. If methotrexate is the definitive method of treatment it is usually given daily or every other day for 1 week, the treatment repeated until the HCG marker has been undetectable in the serum for 6–8 weeks. Patients should be advised to avoid further pregnancy for at least 1 year.

Patients with more advanced *moderate-risk* disease are treated with combination chemotherapy, once again using serial HCG assays as a means of monitoring response. Surgery (hysterectomy) may be necessary if vaginal bleeding is troublesome.

Most drug regimens include methotrexate, actinomycin D and an alkylating agent (cyclophosphamide or chlorambucil). Newer regimens include vinca alkaloids, cisplatin and etoposide. One hundred per cent of patients in this category respond to combination chemotherapy, usually resulting in cure, and high-risk patients or those with drug resistance to 'conventional' regimens respond to newer drugs [38]. In patients with pulmonary metastases but no other adverse features, single-agent chemotherapy with methotrexate and folinic acid remains the treatment of choice.

Prognosis

Before chemotherapy was available, patients with localized disease were treated by surgery and/or pelvic irradiation and the cure rate was 40%. Patients with advanced disease were virtually never cured. With current treatment, 100% of patients with localized disease should be cured, and over 70% of patients with more advanced stages. Even with stage IV disease, the majority survive, and the number of tumour deaths in England and Wales is now under 10 per annum. For the most part, fertility of choriocarcinoma survivors is well maintained.

References

1 Rose PG. Medical progress: endometrial carcinoma. *N Engl J Med* 1996; 335: 640–9.

2 Parker SL, Tong T, Bolden S *et al.* Cancer statistics, 1996. CA. *Cancer J Clin* 1996; 46: 5–27.

3 Stratton JF, Pharoah P, Smith SK, Easton D, Ponder BA. A systematic review and meta-analysis of family history and risk of ovarian cancer. *Br J Obstet Gynaecol* 1998; 105: 493–9.

4 Quinn M, Babb P, Jones J *et al.* Effect of screening on incidence of and mortality from cancer of cervix in England: evaluation based on routinely collected statistics. *Br Med J* 1999; 318: 904–8.

5 Ferenczy A, Franco E. Persistent human papillomavirus infection and cervical neoplasia. *Lancet Oncol* 2002; 3: 11–16.

6 Castellsagué X, Bosch FX, Muñoz N *et al.* Male circumcision, penile human papilloma virus infection, and cervical cancer in female partners. *New Engl J Med* 2002; 346: 1105–12.

7 Cox JT. Management of cervical intraepithelial neoplasia. *Lancet* 1999; 353: 857–90.

8 Landoni F, Maneo A, Colombo A *et al.* Randomised study of radical surgery versus radiotherapy for stage Ib–IIa cervical cancer. *Lancet* 1997; 350: 535–40.

9 Rose PG, Bundy BN, Watkins EB *et al.* Concurrent cisplatin-based radiotherapy and chemotherapy for locally advanced cervical cancer. *N Engl J Med* 1999; 340: 1144–53.

10 Thomas GM. Improved treatment for cervical carcinoma—concurrent chemotherapy and radiotherapy. *N Engl J Med* 1999; 340: 1198–9.

11 Blackledge F, Buxton EJ, Mould JJ *et al.* Phase II studies of ifosfamide alone and in combination in cancer of the cervix. *Cancer Chemotherapy Pharmacol* 1990; 26 (Suppl.): 512–16.

12 Kurman RJ, Kaminski PF, Norris HJ. The behavior of endometrial hyperplasia: a long-term study of 'untreated' hyperplasia in 170 patients. *Cancer* 1985; 56: 403–12.

13 Bergman L, Beelen ML, Gallee MP *et al.* Risk and prognosis of endometrial cancer after tamoxifen for breast cancer. *Lancet* 2000; 356: 881–7.

14 Creasman WT, Morrow CP, Bundy BN *et al.* Surgical pathologic spread patterns of endometrial cancer. *Cancer* 1987; 60 (Suppl.): 2035–41.

15 Creutzberg CL, Van Putten WL, Koper PC *et al.* Surgery and postoperative radiotherapy vs surgery alone for patients with Stage 1 endometrial carcinoma: multicentre randomised trial. *Lancet* 2000; 355: 1404–11.

16 Rush S, Gal D, Potters L *et al.* Pelvic control following external beam radiation for surgical stage I endometrial adenocarcinoma. *Int J Radiation Oncol Biol Physics* 1995; 33: 851–4.

17 Steere C, Harper P. Is there any place for chemotherapy in endometrial cancer? In: *Best Practice and Research, Clinical Obstetrics and Gynecology.* Harcourt, 2001: 447–67.

18 Einhorn N. Role of radiation therapy in carcinoma of the endometrium. In: Tobias JS, Thomas PRM, eds. *Current Radiation Oncology*, Vol. 2. London: Edward Arnold, 1996.

19 Ford D, Easton DF, Bishop DT, Norad SA, Coldgar DE. Risks of cancer in BRCA1-mutation carriers. *Lancet* 1994; 343: 692–5.

20 Jacobs IJ, Skates SJ, MacDonald N *et al.* Screening for ovarian cancer: a pilot randomised controlled trial. *Lancet* 1999; 353: 1207–10.

21 Vergote I, de Brabanter J, Fyles A *et al.* Prognostic importance of degree of differentiation and cyst rupture in Stage 1 invasive epithelial ovarian carcinoma. *Lancet* 2001; 357: 176–82.

22 Tobias JS, Griffiths CT. Management of ovarian carcinoma: current concepts and future prospects. *N Engl J Med* 1976; 294 (818–23): 877–82.

23 Griffiths CT. Surgical resection of bulk tumor in the primary treatment of ovarian carcinoma. *Natl Cancer Inst Monogr* 1975; 42: 101.

24 Van der Burg MEL, van Lent M, Buyse M *et al.* The effect of debulking surgery after induction chemotherapy on the prognosis in advanced epithelial ovarian cancer. *N Engl J Med* 1995; 332: 629–34.

25 The ICON Collaborators. ICON 2 randomised trial of single-agent carboplatin against 3-drug combination of CAP in women with ovarian cancer. *Lancet* 1998; 352: 1571–6.

26 Trimble EL, Adams JD, Vena D *et al.* Paclitaxel for platinum-refractory ovarian cancer: results from the first 1000 patients registered to NCI treatment referral center 9103. *J Clin Oncol* 1993; 11: 2405–10.

27 Berek JS, Bertelsen K, du Bois A *et al.* Advanced epithelial ovarian cancer: 1998 consensus statements. *Ann Oncol* 1999; 10: 91–6.

28 Gruppo Interregionale Cooperativo di Oncologia Ginecologica. A randomized comparison of cisplatin with cyclophosphamide/cisplatin and with cyclophosphamide/doxorubicin/cisplatin in advanced ovarian cancer. *Lancet* 1987; ii: 353–9.

29 McGuire WP, Hoskins WJ, Brady MF *et al.* Cyclophosphamide and cisplatin compared with paclitaxel and cisplatin in patients with stage III and stage IV ovarian carcinoma. *N Engl J Med* 1996; 334: 1–6.

30 Neijt JP. New therapy for ovarian cancer. *N Engl J Med* 1996; 334: 50–1.

31 Einhorn N, Lundell M, Nilsson B *et al.* Is there a place for radiotherapy in the treatment of advanced ovarian cancer? *Radiotherapy Oncol* 1999; 53: 213–18.

32 Hunter RW, Alexander NDE, Soutter WP. Meta-analysis of surgery in advanced ovarian carcinoma: is maximum cytoreductive surgery an independent determinant of prognosis? *Am J Obstet Gynecol* 1992; 166: 504–11.

33 Bower M, Fife K, Holden L *et al.* Chemotherapy for ovarian germ cell tumours. *Eur J Cancer* 1996; 32A: 593–7.

34 Wahlen SA, Slater JD, Wagner. *et al.* Concurrent radiation

therapy and chemotherapy in the treatment of primary squamous cell carcinoma of the vulva. *Cancer* 1995; 75: 2289–94.

35 Berkowitz RS, Goldstein DP. Gestational trophoblastic diseases. *Semin Oncol* 1989; 16: 410–16.

36 Fox H. Gestational trophoblastic disease: neoplasia or pregnancy failure? *Br Med J* 1997; 314: 1363–4.

37 Seckl M, Fisher RA, Salerno G *et al.* Choriocarcinoma and partial hydatiform moles. *Lancet* 2000; 356: 36–9.

38 Bower M, Newlands ES, Holden L *et al.* EMA/CO for high-risk gestational trophoblastic tumours: results from a cohort of 272 patients. *J Clin Oncol* 1997; 15: 2636–43.

18 Genitourinary cancer

Over a quarter of all cancers in males is due to tumours of the kidney, bladder, prostate. Testicular tumours are dealt with separately in Chapter 19. Other rare sites of cancer include the urethra, penis and epididymis. Although surgery has traditionally been the cornerstone of treatment, both radiotherapy and cytotoxic chemotherapy are assuming an increasing importance. Management approaches and guidelines have changed markedly during the past 25 years.

Tumours of the kidney

Incidence and aetiology

Tumours of the kidney account for about 2% of all cancers (Fig. 18.1). The incidence has increased by over 40% during the past three decades [1]. Clinical evolution is sometimes measured over many years, with apparent success followed by late recurrence, often several years later. In adults, the commonest type of renal tumour is the *renal cell carcinoma* (*hypernephroma*) which accounts for 75% of adult cases. Tumours of the renal pelvis are uncommon (10%) and are discussed later. In children, *nephroblastoma* (*Wilms' tumour*) is among the commonest of malignant paediatric tumours, and is discussed in Chapter 24.

Renal cell carcinoma is about twice as common in men (Fig. 18.1), aetiologically related to cigarette smoking, and with a median age at diagnosis of around 65 years. There is considerable variation in incidence throughout the world

(Fig. 13.2), and apart from cigarette smoking (which doubles the likelihood of renal cell carcinoma), obesity also appears to be a risk factor [2]. Although only a small proportion of patients have an affected family member, the risk is increased four-fold in first-degree relatives of patients. Little else is known about its pathogenesis, though it is common in patients with von Hippel–Lindau (VHL) syndrome (characterized by haemangioblastomas in the cerebellum and retina, associated with phaeochromocytoma), occurring in some 40% of all patients and frequently proving fatal. Stone formation in the renal pelvis, carcinogenic derivatives of aromatic amines or tryptophan, and phenacetin abuse are all thought to be important causes of renal pelvic tumours.

The VHL gene is a classic tumour suppressor gene whose inactivation leads to tumour development—often with bilateral involvement. The gene has been localized to chromosome 3p25. Other possible causative factors are listed in Table 18.1.

Renal cell adenocarcinoma (hypernephroma)

Pathology and staging

Stone formation in these tumours arise from the epithelium of the renal tubules themselves. For this reason, the term renal cell adenocarcinoma is now increasingly preferred to hypernephroma. A new histological classification was introduced in 1986, based on histological and morphological criteria and subsequently validated on a

Table 18.1 TNM classification of malignant tumours [3].

T—Primary tumour	
T_X	Primary tumour cannot be assessed
T_0	No evidence of primary tumour
T_1	Tumour 7.0 cm or less in greatest dimension, limited to the kidney
T_2	Tumour more than 7.0 cm in greatest dimension, limited to the kidney
T_3	Tumour extends into major veins or invades adrenal gland or perinephric tissues but not beyond Gerota's fascia
T_{3a}	Tumour invades adrenal gland or perinephric tissues but not beyond Gerota's fascia
T_{3b}	Tumour grossly extends into renal vein(s) or vena cava below diaphragm
T_{3c}	Tumour grossly extends into vena cava above diaphragm
T_4	Tumour invades beyond Gerota's fascia
N—Regional lymph nodes	
N_X	Regional lymph nodes cannot be assessed
N_0	Regional lymph nodes metastasis
N_1	Metastasis in a single regional lymph node
N_2	Metastasis in more than one regional lymph node
M—Distant metastasis	
M_X	Distant metastasis cannot be assessed
M_0	No distant metastasis
M_1	Distant metastasis

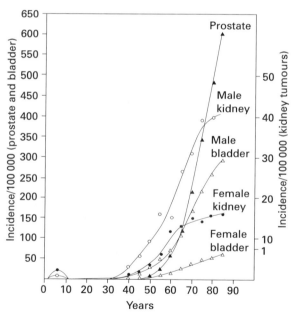

Fig. 18.1 Age-specific incidence of renal, bladder and prostatic cancer.

molecular basis. The commonest variety, clear-cell carcinoma, makes up three-quarters of all cases and is characterized by deletion or inactivation of the VHL gene. Most of the remaining cases are chromophilic (also called papillary) carcinomas (12% of the total).

Local, lymphatic and haematogenous spread are all relatively common, making surgery unwise or technically impossible in about one-third of all cases.

Direct invasion into perirenal tissues occurs in over 20% and local lymph node metastases in 8%. Renal vein invasion is also common, with cords of tumour cells sometimes growing directly into the inferior vena cava, although this is often undetectable preoperatively. Likelihood of dissemination correlates with histological differentiation. In patients with low-grade carcinoma the incidence of metastatic disease at presentation is very low.

The current tumour node metastasis (TNM) staging system chiefly relies on information obtained at operation (see Table 18.1). Prognosis is closely related to stage (see p. 282). About 2–3% of all renal cell carcinomas are bilateral at presentation.

Clinical features

These tumours present with a wide variety of symptoms. Approximately 50% of patients have haematuria, often very slight but occasionally sufficiently severe to produce anaemia. Loin pain and a palpable mass are classical features, and a large mass may be palpable. Fatigue and weight loss are common and many patients present with complaints resulting from metastases, such as pathological fracture through a bone deposit, dyspnoea and cough from mediastinal, hilar or lung metastases, or even epil-

Female Location **Male**

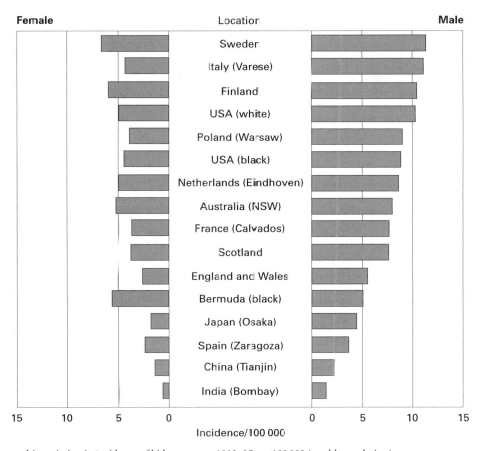

Sweden
Italy (Varese)
Finland
USA (white)
Poland (Warsaw)
USA (black)
Netherlands (Eindhoven)
Australia (NSW)
France (Calvados)
Scotland
England and Wales
Bermuda (black)
Japan (Osaka)
Spain (Zaragoza)
China (Tianjin)
India (Bombay)

15 10 5 0 0 5 10 15
Incidence/100 000

Fig. 18.2 Geographic variation in incidence of kidney cancer, 1983–87 per 100 000 (world population).

epsy from an intracerebral deposit. Approximately one-quarter of patients have evidence of distant metastases at presentation. Renal cell tumours are a well-known cause of pyrexia; fever without other symptoms is not uncommon. Hypertension, polycythaemia and hypercalcaemia also occur in about 5% of patients. About 2% of male patients present with a varicocoele, usually left-sided, due to obstruction of the testicular vein. Liver function tests may be abnormal even in patients without metastatic disease, although they are unreliable as tumour markers.

Even when a renal cell carcinoma is suspected, the diagnosis can be difficult. Intravenous urography (IVU), ultrasound or computed tomography (CT) scanning usually demonstrate a space-occupying mass in the renal cortex, often with distortion of the calyceal system (Fig. 18.3a).

Renal calcification, particularly if 'rim-like', is a common finding. Further radiological investigations using

magnetic resonance imaging (MRI) scanning may give additional information (Fig. 18.4). Before surgery, a chest X-ray is essential in case pulmonary metastases are already present, and CT scanning is advisable since pulmonary metastases have to be at least 2 cm in diameter to be visible on a standard chest X-ray. Isotope bone scanning may reveal unsuspected bone metastases particularly in patients whose primary lesion is palpable. Biochemical tests of renal and liver function are important, and it is also wise to perform isotope renography preoperatively, to assess the function of the contralateral kidney.

Management

Surgical resection is the most effective method of treatment, though over 25% of renal carcinomas are technically unresectable. *En bloc* resection of the kidney with as little disturbance as possible is probably the best

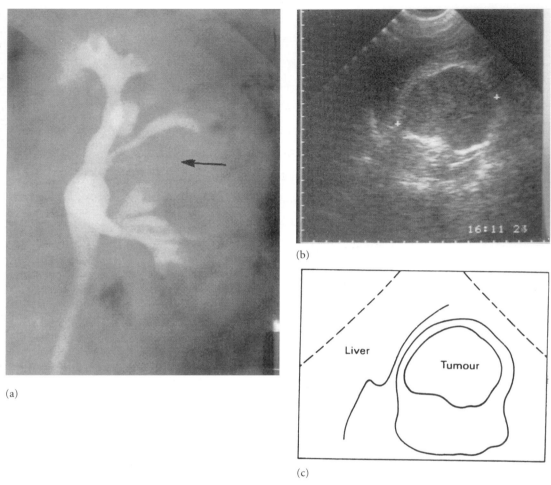

(a)

(b)

Liver

Tumour

(c)

Fig. 18.3 (a) Intravenous urogram in renal carcinoma. The left kidney contains a tumour (arrowed) which displaces the calyces. (b) Transverse ultrasound scan showing a large renal carcinoma below the liver. (c) Line drawing of (b).

approach, coupled with a dissection from the aortic bifurcation to the diaphragm, and with prevention of tumour dissemination by early ligation of the renal artery and vein. Although still controversial, lymph node dissection seems advisable since the incidence of regional lymph node involvement is around 15%. In cases where the tumour is large, or difficult to remove, it may be necessary to perform nephroureterectomy, with removal of part of the bladder if indicated. Radical surgery is usually the best way forward even where extension of the tumour to the renal vein or inferior vena cava (IVC) has occurred. Difficulties arise where a renal carcinoma occurs in a solitary or horseshoe kidney, and the commonest approach is to perform a partial nephrectomy. Occasionally, if the tumour is too large for a conservative resection, total nephrectomy is un-

avoidable, with transplantation of an allogeneic kidney (if available) at a later procedure.

In patients with obvious clinical or radiological evidence of metastases elsewhere, the choice of initial treatment is more difficult [4]. The primary lesion may be technically operable, and providing the patient's condition is reasonably good, nephrectomy is by far the most effective and simplest means of securing control of the primary, particularly when there are troublesome symptoms such as renal pain or haematuria [1]. Although there are sporadic case reports of regression of secondary lung deposits following resection of the primary tumour [5], this phenomenon is in fact very rare and the possibility of its occurrence should never be used as the sole rationale for surgery [6]. Since this capricious tumour can remain

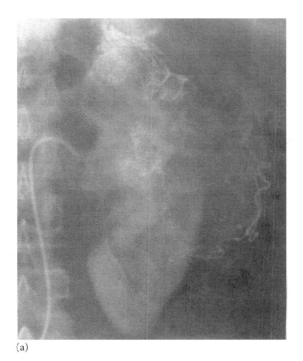

(a)

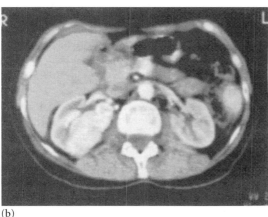

(b)

Fig. 18.4 Renal arteriogram (late arterial phase). (a) A tumour circulation is seen due to a large carcinoma occupying the upper two-thirds of the kidney. (b) CT scan of the abdomen (with contrast) in a patient with a carcinoma of the right kidney.

quiescent for many years (even decades) before metastases become apparent, it is sometimes recommended that solitary metastases should be surgically removed. In symptomatic patients with obvious widespread metastatic disease in whom nephrectomy seems unwise, renal artery embolism or occlusion is worth considering since it leads to partial or complete infarction of the kidney and offers a

reasonable chance of temporary control. It should probably be used only in symptomatic patients since it can be painful and hazardous, though some urologists use it routinely as a preoperative adjunct to nephrectomy. Several other methods of occlusion are currently in use, including intra-arterial balloon catheter occlusion, induction of autologous local thrombus, or insertion of foreign material such as gelatine sponge or polyacrylamide gel. Radiotherapy is no longer used in primary management [7].

SYSTEMIC TREATMENTS AND PALLIATIVE THERAPY

In spite of early reports of response to hormone preparations, the overall response rate to progestogens and androgens is very low, of the order of 5%. Despite this disappointing figure, these agents are non-toxic and therefore worth considering in patients with widespread metastases. Medroxyprogesterone acetate is widely used (100 mg three times per day by mouth). Other hormonal agents, such as flutamide and tamoxifen, probably have similar response rates [8]. Chemotherapy has had little success [9]. The most widely used agents are vinblastine, cisplatin *cis*-chloroethyl nitrosourea (CCNU), doxorubicin, cyclophosphamide and hydroxyurea. None of these has high activity on its own, and in combination the response rate is still very low (20% at best). Dissatisfaction with these poor results has led to the increasing interest in newer therapies in metastatic renal cancer, notably immunotherapy using cytokines and other agents [1,10,11]. In 1983 human interferon was first reported to show activity, although sadly the response duration is usually short and the experimental use of interferons together with chemotherapy does not appear promising. Use of interleukin-2, lymphokine-activated killer (LAK) cells and other types of interferon seems less encouraging despite the initial euphoria aroused by Rosenberg's contention [12] that metastatic renal cell carcinoma was frequently responsive. Although there are now more potentially valuable treatments available to such patients (for example, allogeneic peripheral blood stem cell transplantation as reported by Childs *et al.* [13]), the outlook in general remains bleak, with an overall median survival of approximately 9 months. Moreover, the toxicity of interleukin-2 (with or without LAK cells) remains considerable. No advantage was found in a comparative study (128 patients) using tamoxifen alone or tamoxifen plus interferon-α and interleukin-2 [14].

Although cytotoxic and cytokine drugs have no established role in palliation, treatment with radiotherapy may be helpful, particularly in the relief of bone pain. Bone metastases are very common and internal orthopaedic fixation of long bones is invaluable in prevention or treatment of pathological fractures, thereby allowing early mobility.

Prognosis

The prognosis in renal cell cancer depends on the stage and grade of the tumour, and the completeness of surgery (Fig. 18.5). The 5-year survival is approximately 55%, most of the loss of life occurring in the first 2 years after diagnosis. Improvements in imaging techniques have probably been responsible for a slight rise in cure rates over the past 20 years. For stage I tumours, the 5-year survival is over 65%, whereas if the regional nodes are involved this falls to 30%. For stage IV tumours, there are very few 5-year survivors. With high-grade tumours only 30% of patients are alive at 5 years, while with low-grade tumours 80% of patients survive.

Carcinoma of the renal pelvis [15]

These tumours are uncommon (about 7% of all renal carcinomas) and are usually transitional cell carcinomas (TCCs, 80%) or squamous cell carcinomas, which may be more common in women. Clinical symptoms include haematuria (90%) and loin pain due to obstruction of the renal pelvis. On examination, in advanced cases, there may be a palpable loin mass.

Investigation includes an IVU, which usually shows a filling defect in the collecting system and occasionally demonstrates non-function where there has been long-standing postrenal obstruction by tumour. Fifty per cent of patients have malignant cells in the urine, so cytological examination of the urine is essential.

Surgery is again the most important method of treatment. Nephroureterectomy is usually required; for transitional tumours a part of the bladder wall is also usually removed, as a wide area of epithelium is at risk. As the histology of the renal pelvic tumour is not usually known preoperatively, the operation is the same for both TCCs and squamous carcinomas. However, local ureteric stump recurrence is reportedly less frequent with squamous carcinomas.

Radiotherapy may be worth considering for inoperable or recurrent cases but there is little evidence that it is ever curative. It may, however, retard local progression of disease. In the follow-up period the possibility of a contralateral lesion must always be borne in mind. Repeated cystoscopy and cytological examination of the urine are both important since 50% of patients later develop a carcinoma of the bladder. About 10% of patients with TCC of the renal pelvis have a synchronous bladder carcinoma as well.

Carcinoma of the ureter

This rare tumour is usually a TCC, although sarcomas are occasionally encountered. Typically, the disease presents with frequency and dysuria. Ureteric colic is unusual. The diagnosis is usually made by IVU, which shows ureteric dilatation or distortion, or a non-functioning kidney. Retrograde pyelography demonstrates the site of the block. Urinary cytology may also be helpful.

Treatment is by nephro-ureterectomy, though occasionally the kidney may be preserved. In removing the ureter a cuff of bladder should be taken. Radiotherapy has occasionally been employed in patients with inoperable tumour, but with little success.

The prognosis depends largely on the cellular differentiation of the tumours. The 5-year survival rate is 80% with well-differentiated tumours, but only 10% with the most anaplastic forms.

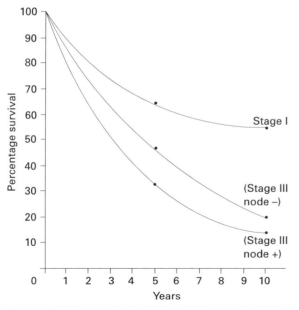

Fig. 18.5 Prognosis of renal adenocarcinoma related to stage and lymph node involvement.

Cancer of the urinary bladder

Aetiology and incidence

Predominantly a cancer occurring in males, bladder cancer is now the second commonest urological malignancy and has become the fifth most common cancer in men in Western countries, with 45 000 new cases in the USA annually, and of rising incidence. Global incidence rates are shown in Fig. 18.5. At the end of the 19th century it was recognized that workers in the aniline dye industry had a high incidence of bladder cancer, and the active carcinogen to which they were exposed was later identified as α-naphthylamine. Workers in the rubber industry form another group (see also pp. 20–2). Chronic bladder infection or infestation also predisposes to malignant change; worldwide, the most important of these causes is schisto-

somiasis. Cigarette smokers are at greatly increased risk, which partly explains its much higher incidence in males. At least 50% of cases in males and 25% in females are causally related to cigarette smoking, particularly to duration of smoking, and decreasing comparatively rapidly in ex-smokers. In the USA, the disease is reportedly four times as common in white men as in black and is commoner in urban areas. Other probable aetiological factors in bladder cancer include multiple urinary infections and previous exposure to cyclophosphamide [16].

Screening has increasingly been attempted; indeed, bladder cancer was probably the first solid tumour in males in which a systematic screening programme was seriously considered [17]. In low-risk groups (the general population) this has usually been done by dipstick testing for occult haematuria—a technique with high predictive accuracy but low yields (of the order of 2.5%) in un-

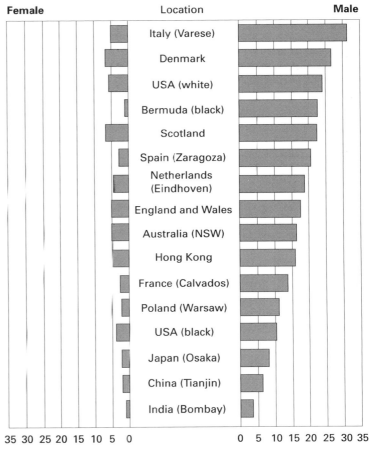

Fig. 18.6 Geographic variation in incidence of bladder cancer, 1983–87 per 100 000 (world population).

Incidence/100 000

selected males aged 21–72 years. In higher-risk groups the approach is clearly more logical, although even in men working in the rubber industry, it is nowadays difficult to confirm excess death rates, in contrast to studies performed in former years. At present the cost and low yield argue against the wide introduction of screening programmes, although careful investigation of even a single episode of haematuria (or occult haematuria) is mandatory.

Pathology and staging

Over 90% of bladder tumours are derived from transitional cell epithelium. In Western countries, TCC of the bladder is over five times as common as squamous cell carcinoma, although in Egypt, where schistosomal infestation is common, the squamous carcinoma is more frequent. Other histological types such as adenocarcinoma, leiomyosarcoma and rhabdomyosarcoma are rare. TCCs may be single or multiple, and are sometimes pedunculated, whereas squamous carcinomas are usually sessile and often necrotic in appearance. Multiple papillomatous tumours are often of low grade, but should be regarded as premalignant. Fortunately, the majority of patients (70%) with bladder cancer present with superficial disease only.

In TCC, pathological grading is of considerable importance, and well-differentiated tumours carry a better prognosis independently of tumour stage. Pathological

depth of infiltration of the bladder wall (P stage) directly correlates with survival.

The TNM staging notation (Table 18.2) allows a convenient shorthand description, based largely on the degree of local spread at presentation (Fig. 18.7). The most important distinction lies between T_2 and T_3 tumours, since over 50% of all patients with T_2 tumours will be alive at 3 years from diagnosis, whereas less than 25% of patients with T_3 tumours (that is, with invasion of the deep muscle of the bladder) will survive. The Union Internationale Contre le Cancer (UICC) staging criteria for bladder (and prostate) cancer now parallels the USA-based systems more closely. However, the resulting staging system takes far less account of clinical information, the previous, and TNM and P stage criteria, continue to be widely used.

Important prognostic factors are shown in Table 18.2. In addition to TNM stage, pathological grade and histological type, the size, location and number of bladder tumours all influence clinical management. Multiple bladder tumours are so frequently encountered that the whole of the transitional cell epithelial surface must be considered to be at risk, and in some instances where tumours are widespread throughout the bladder, total cystectomy may be required even though the local invasiveness of each one may be unimpressive. The major sites of distant metastasis are lymph nodes, lung, liver and bone.

Table 18.2 TNM and P staging for bladder cancer.

T_{is}	Preinvasive carcinoma (carcinoma *in situ*)
T_a	Papillary non-invasive carcinoma
T_0	No evidence of primary tumour
T_1	Tumour limited to the lamina propria (P_1). Bimanual examination may reveal a mobile mass which cannot be felt after transurethral resection
T_2	Tumour limited to superficial muscle (P_2). Mobile induration of the bladder wall may be present, but should be impalpable following transurethral resection
T_3	Invasion of deep muscle layer of the bladder wall (P_3). On bimanual palpation a mobile mass is felt which persists after transurethral resection
T_{3a}	Deep muscle invasion
T_{3b}	Invasion through the muscle wall
T_4	Invasion of prostate or other local structures (P_4); tumour fixed or locally extensive
T_{4a}	Tumour infiltrates prostate, uterus or vagina
T_{4b}	Tumour fixed to pelvic and/or abdominal wall
N_0	Regional lymph node involvement
N_1	Involvement of a single ipsilateral regional node group
N_2	Contralateral, bilateral or multiple regional node involvement
N_3	Fixed regional lymphadenopathy (i.e. a fixed space between this and the tumour)
N_4	Involvement of juxtaregional nodes
M_0	No distant metastases
M_1	Distant metastases

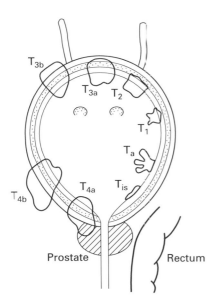

Fig. 18.7 T staging of bladder cancer: T_{is}, *in situ* carcinoma; T_a, non-invasive papillary carcinoma; T_1, limited to lamina propria; T_2, superficial muscle involvement; T_{3a}, deep muscle involvement; T_{3b}, full thickness of bladder wall; T_{4a}, invading neighbouring structures (prostate, vaginal); T_{4b}, involvement of rectum, fixed to pelvic wall.

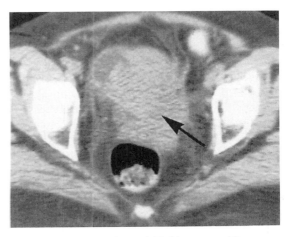

Fig. 18.8 CT scan in advanced bladder cancer. The tumour (arrowed) is shown extending posteriorly to the rectum and laterally to the side-walls of the pelvis. We are grateful to Professor Janet Husband for this photograph.

Patients with an abnormal chromosome complement have a poor prognosis. There appears to be a strong correlation between DNA content (ploidy) and level of invasion (pathological grade), depth of tumour invasiveness and response to certain types of therapy [15]. Tumours expressing A, B or H blood-group antigens have a better prognosis, though the reasons remain unclear. The development of a bladder cancer from normal or premalignant urothelial tissue may relate to the presence of transforming oncogenes, particularly those of the *ras* family which are known to be present on chromosomes 1, 11 and 12. There may be an association between *ras* expression and high histological grade.

Clinical features

The majority of patients with bladder cancer complain of haematuria, usually painless, although other symptoms such as urgency of micturition, nocturia and frequency or reduction of the urinary stream may also be present. Loin or back pain may occur if tumour obstruction has led to hydronephrosis or if large intra-abdominal lymph node metastases are present. Even single episodes of haematuria should be fully investigated by cystoscopy. Fortunately, the majority of patients with superficial tumours do not develop invasive disease; indeed, it is probably true that superficial and deeply invasive bladder carcinomas are distinctly separate disorders [1].

Definitive diagnosis requires cystoscopy with biopsy, which gives a clear indication of the site, size, general appearance and multiplicity of tumours. This procedure is normally performed under general anaesthesia, permitting a full examination including thorough rectal and bimanual palpation which are essential for accurate staging. Urinary exfoliative cytology is a valuable addition to diagnosis and is currently being evaluated as a means not only of diagnosis but also of monitoring response to treatment.

An intravenous urogram should be performed, giving essential information regarding the anatomy and functioning of the kidneys and ureters, and often further information as to the site and extent of the primary tumour. Renal function should be assessed by measurement of blood urea and creatinine clearance (or other form of assessment such as diethylenetriaminepenta-acetic acid (DPTA) clearance). To evaluate the degrees of extravesical spread MRI and CT scanning are extremely valuable (Fig. 18.8).

Management

Superficial bladder cancer

Management of superficial bladder tumours is almost entirely the province of the surgeon. Small papillary tumours can be repeatedly treated by cystodiathermy, often for many years, although other methods such as cryosurgery and laser treatment are becoming more widely used. Intravesical chemotherapy using thiotepa, mitomycin C, doxorubicin and other cytotoxics is sometimes able to prevent or treat small recurrences. Thiotepa is less used nowadays since it may cause considerable local discomfort. Although such tumours are rarely fatal, up to 10% of patients develop widespread intravesical recurrence after repeated cystodiathermy, necessitating further treatment either with radiotherapy or even by total cystectomy. In these, intravesical chemotherapy may prove helpful in avoiding or delaying such treatment, thereby improving the quality of survival.

Because superficial bladder cancers can progress to more deeply penetrating lesions, both external radiotherapy and intravesical chemotherapy have now been tested as means of preventing this. Bacille Calmette–Guérin (BCG) has been assessed in this way and also for recurrent carcinoma *in situ* [18]. No long-term benefit from these approaches has yet been shown. More recently, newer techniques such as intravesical interferon have shown promise. Photodynamic therapy has also been attempted, using haematoporphyrin derivatives taken up by the malignant urothelium followed by cystoscopy to reveal areas of fluorescence which correlate with areas of histologically proven tumour. The haematoporphyrin derivative can be used as a sensitizing agent for laser ablation.

Muscle-invasive disease

Treatment for invasive (T_2–T_3) bladder carcinoma has been considerably refined in recent years [19], with increasing emphasis on multimodal approaches including transurethral surgery, systemic chemotherapy, improved techniques for radiation therapy and advanced reconstructive techniques following surgical cystectomy. As Kaufman *et al.* pointed out, 'all have the potential to improve the quality of life and cure the disease' [19]. Choice of management for most patients usually lies between a surgical procedure, radiation therapy or a combination of both. In some patients with small lesions located in a mobile portion of the bladder, partial cystectomy is possible. An adequate cuff of normal bladder should be removed, and the procedure is only recommended where the initial capacity of the remaining bladder is likely to be greater than 300–400 ml. Scrupulous surgical technique is important in order to avoid implantation tumour nodules developing at the anastomosis, and the operation is less widely used than formerly. Interstitial irradiation is an alternative

to partial cystectomy in patients with T_2 and early T_3 lesions. A large study by van der Werf-Messing [20] gave a 5-year survival rate of 40% (T_2) and 25% (T_3), using interstitial (intravesical) irradiation with radium implants (sometimes with low-dose external irradiation), though her excellent results have proven difficult to replicate elsewhere.

The introduction of a satisfactory method of total cystectomy led to rapid acceptance of this operation as the treatment of choice for many patients with deeply invasive (T_3) tumours without extravesical or distant spread. This procedure involves complete removal of the bladder, prostate and seminal vesicles (or bladder and urethra in the female), although some surgeons prefer a still more radical approach which combines total cystectomy with a pelvic lymph node dissection. Urinary diversion is usually achieved by fashioning a conduit from a section of resected ileum into which the ureters are implanted and which opens on to the abdominal wall (ileostomy), or by implanting the ureters directly into the sigmoid colon or rectum (Fig. 18.9). Unfortunately, complication rates are substantial and reoperation is often necessary [21].

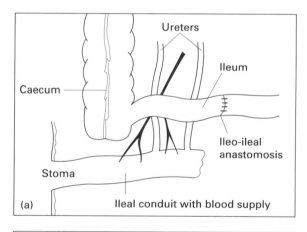

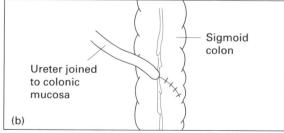

Fig. 18.9 Common procedures for ureteric diversion following total cystectomy: (a) formation of an ileal conduit; (b) implantation into sigmoid colon.

Furthermore, the quality of life in patients undergoing different types of bladder diversion has not been fully investigated [22] and retention of a normal bladder is clearly desirable whenever possible.

Combinations of surgery and radiotherapy seem to offer superior results to the use of total or radical cystectomy alone. Recent surgical advances have included more acceptable methods of urinary diversion including 'continent' types of stoma in which the patient can control the emptying of the urinary conduit by self-catheterization or other techniques, allowing more normal urinary function. A further important advance has been the possibility for the first time of continued sexual potency through careful sparing of critical neurovascular structures [23].

Radiotherapy or surgery?

In view of the effectiveness of radical radiotherapy for carcinoma of the bladder, it seems reasonable to ask whether cystectomy as primary management can be avoided altogether. Almost 20 years ago, a large UK co-operative study attempted to answer this question. Nearly 200 patients were allocated either to receive radical radiotherapy alone (60 Gy over 6 weeks) or preoperative irradiation (40 Gy over 4 weeks), followed by radical cystectomy a month later [24]. At 5 years, there was a trend in favour of the group undergoing both radiotherapy and surgery, with a survival rate of 38% compared with 29% for radical radiotherapy. Although the overall result did not achieve statistical significance, the combination of preoperative irradiation and surgery seemed more effective in younger patients and in males. The difference between the two groups may have been exaggerated because 20% of patients randomized to radiotherapy and surgery could not complete the treatment. After local recurrence with radiotherapy alone, it was possible to perform salvage cystectomy with the impressive result of a 52% 5-year survival postcystectomy. Similar results were later reported from centres in the USA and Denmark. More recently, several large groups have reported the results of treatment with radical radiotherapy alone, which increasingly seems closely comparable to those achieved by surgery [25].

The biological effectiveness of radiotherapy for bladder cancer is also shown by the phenomenon of postirradiation tumour 'down staging'. Several studies have shown that the P stage of the excised surgical specimen is frequently lower after radiotherapy than the initial tumour (T) staging would suggest. For example, in the Royal Marsden study, almost half (47%) of the bladder speci-

mens excised after radiotherapy demonstrated this effect [24]. Sterilization of locally involved lymph nodes can also be achieved by radiotherapy, the same study showing an incidence of node metastasis of 23% (the expected proportion would be 40–50% with unirradiated T_3 tumours). Only 8% of patients judged to be good responders to radiotherapy had histologically positive local nodes and required cystectomy, suggesting that preoperative irradiation may be particularly useful for those with limited or microscopic regional lymph node deposits. Perhaps the most important result of all was that where down staging occurred, the 5-year survival rate was 51%, whereas in patients who showed no such change the survival at 5 years was only 22%.

Although cystectomy remains a widely practised treatment for T_3 tumours, these and other data suggest that radiotherapy may be its equal, with considerable advantages in terms of morbidity. The quality of life with an ileal conduit is less satisfactory than for patients who micturate by the usual route. Common additional difficulties include odour, leakage, psychological adjustment to the stoma, and feelings of loss of sexual attractiveness. Many of these problems can be reduced by careful surgical technique but these patients naturally require a great deal of explanation and support pre- and postoperatively.

Radical external beam irradiation of bladder cancer requires supervoltage equipment and a multifield technique employing three or four fields (Fig. 18.10) and expert planning. There is considerable debate as to whether it is essential to treat the local pelvic nodes as well as the bladder itself. Although it is difficult to show an improved survival when the pelvic nodes are treated, the demonstration of down staging as described above certainly strengthens the case. Treatment-related morbidity is greater when the pelvis is treated, even to the relatively modest dose of 40 Gy. With nodal involvement, overall 5-year survival is below 10%, suggesting that the disease is usually disseminated at diagnosis in node-positive cases. Current studies (including studies from the Medical Research Council (MRC) and European Organization for Research and Treatment of Cancer (EORTC)) mostly favour the use of neoadjuvant chemotherapy programmes with small-volume irradiation — probably a more logical approach. Chemoresponders may well be the same type of patients who 'down staged' with pelvic irradiation. Chemotherapy is discussed more fully below.

Apart from the importance of radiation treatment with curative intent, symptoms such as pain, haematuria and frequency usually respond well, and radiotherapy is the most valuable palliative treatment even in advanced (stage

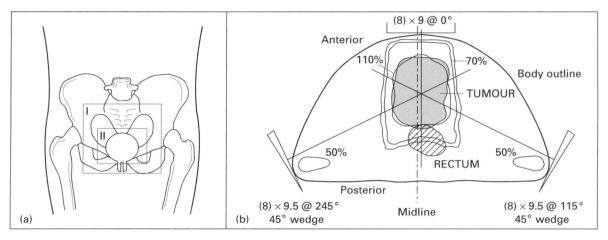

Fig. 18.10 Typical external irradiation treatment technique for invasive (T_3) carcinoma of the bladder. (a) Vertical representation of treatment volume. I: for first phase of treatment bladder and pelvic nodes are treated. II: for second phase of treatment the bladder is boosted to radical dose. Phase I is treated with the bladder full to minimize radiation damage to the small bowel. (b) Typical treatment plan in phase II of radical treatment (field sizes in cm).

IV) tumours where there is virtually no prospect of cure [26].

Role of chemotherapy

The value of systemic chemotherapy for metastatic or advanced bladder cancer remains controversial. It is increasingly used both for recurrent disease and also as an adjuvant to surgical or radiotherapeutic treatment, but its precise role remains unclear. In studies from the USA, patients with muscle-invasive bladder cancer have often been treated with bladder-conserving transurethral surgery, combination chemotherapy and radiation therapy with concurrent cisplatin administration [19,27]. In the Radiation Therapy Oncology Group (RTOG) study [27], 45% of the patients were alive and free of disease, the majority with functioning, tumour-free bladders (4 years follow-up data). Chemotherapy clearly increases complete remission rates in the adjuvant setting, but so far with only minimal detectable benefit in survival [28,29]. However, for many patients, conservative combination treatment will prove a more acceptable alternative to immediate cystectomy. Cisplatin, cyclophosphamide, doxorubicin, mitomycin C, 5-fluorouracil (5-FU) and methotrexate all produce responses of the order of 20–30%. Many groups have attempted to improve the results still further with combination regimes, but no clear-cut survival advantage has yet been demonstrated although there are recent encouraging early reports. Cis-platin is often regarded as the most active agent, yet the long-term survival results of combination regimes including cisplatin seem to be almost identical with those of cis-platin therapy alone. M-VAC (methotrexate, vinblastine, doxorubicin and cisplatin) is probably the most popular combination regimen in common use in the UK. Further studies will be required to determine whether any groups of patients really benefit from such intensive treatment. At present, chemotherapy for advanced bladder tumours cannot be considered as fully established therapy, particularly since these patients tend to be in poor health and often have impaired renal function.

There is considerable interest in the concept of neoadjuvant chemotherapy in carcinoma of the bladder. In one of the largest studies so far reported, 376 patients were treated by radiotherapy or cystectomy, with or without neoadjuvant and adjuvant methotrexate [30]. No benefit was seen, indeed the chemotherapy, though relatively simple, proved too toxic for many patients to tolerate. A further British study in patients prospectively randomized to receive neoadjuvant cisplatin (as opposed to no chemotherapy) was also disappointing [31]. However, the results of multimodal therapy (including concomitant cisplatin-based chemotherapy) for muscle-invasive disease are clearly encouraging [25]. In one recent study, for example, improved local control was seen in a cohort of 99 patients treated by concurrent cisplatin with preoperative or definitive radiation therapy [32]. With a mean follow-up of 6.5 years, the pelvic relapse rate was 25/48 (no chemotherapy) compared with 15/51 patients *with* chemotherapy; 3-year survival was 33% and 47%, respectively.

Prognosis

About 50% of all patients with invasive bladder cancer survive for 5 years. Important prognostic determinants include histological grade, tumour stage and presence of nodal spread. T_1 tumours have a 5-year survival of about 75% with surgery alone. In T_2 and early T_3 lesions the 5-year survival is 35%, while with more advanced disease, particularly where there is nodal involvement at diagnosis, only 10–15% will survive. There are virtually no long-term survivors when distant metastases are present at diagnosis. The use of adjuvant chemotherapy has not so far contributed to a significant improvement in these long-term results [33].

Carcinoma of the prostate

Incidence and aetiology

There are substantial worldwide variations in the incidence of carcinoma of the prostate (Fig. 18.11), which is among the commonest of all cancers in men (Fig. 18.1). In the UK it is the third largest cause of death from cancer in males (950 deaths each year), exceeded only by deaths from cancer of the lung and large bowel. From USA statistics, both incidence and mortality are considerably higher in black men than in white men. In the USA, England, Australia and Japan there is strong evidence to suggest an increasing incidence and mortality during the past 50 years [34] and the current death rate is 1520 per 100 000 men. The positive autopsy rate for unexpected prostatic cancer is of the order of 30% in men over 50 years.

Little is known of the aetiology of prostatic carcinoma [35]. Its incidence increases in first-generation males after migration from a less prevalent to a more prevalent area. Growth of prostate cancer is stimulated by androgens and the cancer does not occur in castrated men. It is also thought to be less common in hepatic cirrhosis which is accompanied by impaired oestrogen degradation. Susceptible families occur, though rarely; it has also been suggested that factors operating in prenatal life may have an important aetiological influence—both prematurity and pre-eclampsia being inversely associated with incidence [36].

Because of the frequency of prostatic carcinoma and its

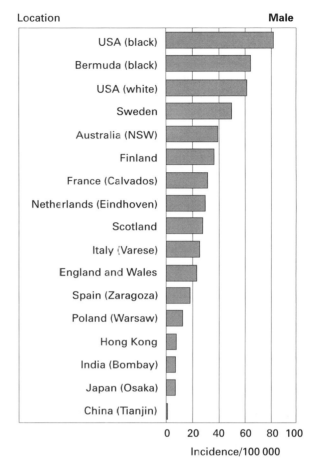

Fig. 18.11 Geographic variation in incidence of prostate cancer, 1983–87 per 100 000 (world population).

clear age relation, screening among unselected elderly males has increasingly been attempted, generally employing regular prostate-specific antigen (PSA) testing (see below) and clinical examination by digital rectal prostatic palpation [37]. The detection rate is of the order of 1%, but the majority of cases are confined to the prostate, strengthening the rationale. Regular testing for PSA [38] clearly increase the sensitivity although this is more costly. At present, despite the high incidence and detection rate, no series has convincingly shown a survival in screen-detected cases. Since the risk of developing prostate cancer is high, for example 0.37%/year×25 years=8% in a 50-year-old-male, further studies of screening are clearly warranted. Conversely, an important recent study has provided data suggesting that screening and early detection are difficult to justify at present [39]. Data from the

SEER (surveillance, epidemiology and end-result analysis) programme of the National Cancer Institute (NCI) were analysed, particularly with respect to assessment of national and regional trends. Incidence of prostate cancer rose dramatically during the two decades 1973–94, but at a far greater rate than mortality, suggesting that earlier detection is now frequently taking place. However, because of lead-time bias and other factors, the benefits of screening and early detection remain unproven, though the drawbacks are unequivocal, whereas the risk and harms of screening and resultant treatment are definite [40].

Pathology and staging

Adenocarcinoma is overwhelmingly the most common cell type, although TCC may arise in the large prostatic ducts. Other unusual types include squamous, mucinous, carcinoid and small-cell carcinomas. Three-quarters of all prostatic cancers arise in the posterior or peripheral part of the prostate, and about 10% are discovered during prostatectomy for apparently benign prostatic hypertrophy. These tend to be more localized than when the diagnosis of carcinoma is suspected clinically.

Histological grading is of considerable importance, though the majority of prostatic cancers are moderately well differentiated. The incidence of lymph node metastases increases with the degree of anaplasia and there is no doubt that patients with low-grade lesions survive substantially longer (60% 5-year survival, compared with 5% 5-year survival for patients with high-grade lesions).

No clinical or surgical staging system has yet found universal acceptance. The pattern of local invasion is shown schematically in Fig. 18.12. The TNM system is increasingly employed (Table 18.3), but can be difficult in practice, particularly in determination of the T stage of the tumour. For this and other reasons, the UICC TNM stag-

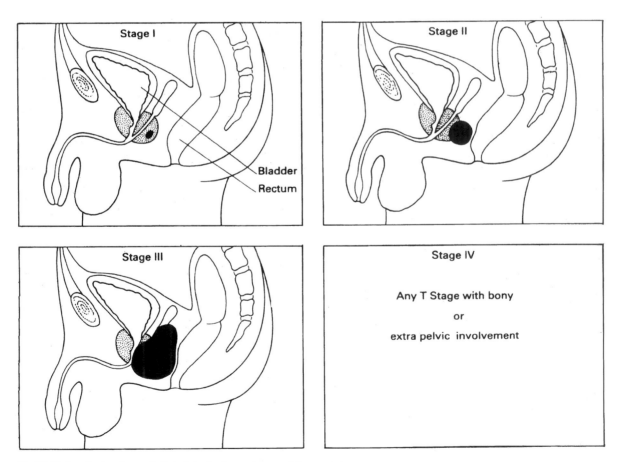

Fig. 18.12 Local extension and clinical staging in carcinoma of the prostate.

Table 18.3 Staging systems for carcinoma of the prostate.

UICC 1978/1982	AUS stage	UICC 1987
T_0 Occult carcinoma	A Occult carcinoma	T_1 Incidental
	A_1 One lobe	T_{1a} Three foci or less
	A_2 Multifocal or diffuse	T_{1b} More than three foci
T_1 Intracapsular tumour		
	B Confined to prostate	T_2 Clinically or grossly, limited to gland
	B_1 One lobe	$T_{1a} = 1.5$ cm
	B_2 Diffuse	$T_{2b} > 1.5$ cm/ $>$ one lobe
T_2 Tumour (?) but does not breach capsule		
T_3 Extraprostatic extension	C Extracapsular extension	T_3 Invades prostatic apex/beyond capsule/ bladder neck/seminal vesical/not fixed
T_4 Fixed invading adjacent organs		
T_4 Fixed or invades other adjacent structures		
N_1 Single regional node involved D_1	Pelvic node metastasis	N_1 Single $= 2$ cm
N_2 Multiregional nodes	N_2 Single, 2–5 cm, multiple $= 5$ cm	
N_3 Fixed node mass		
N_4 Juxta-regional nodes		
M_1 Distant metastasis	D_2 Distant metastasis	M_1 Distant metastasis

AUS, American Urological Society; UICC, Union Internationale Contre le Cancer.

ing criteria were revised in 1987. Even the more recent TNM system has not found wide acceptance. The widely used American system is simpler and correlates fairly closely with the TNM staging. Increasing attention is now paid to the pathological details of the prostatic specimen. The most widely used system is that of Gleason which was devised over 20 years ago for the USA-based Veterans' Administration Co-operative Urological Research Group (VACURG) [41]. The grades are as follows.

Grade 1: well-differentiated carcinoma with uniform gland pattern.

Grade 2: well-differentiated carcinoma with glands varying in size and shape.

Grade 3: moderately differentiated carcinoma with either (a) irregular acinae often widely separated; or (b) well-defined papillary/cribriform structures. This is the commonest pattern seen in carcinoma of the prostate.

Grade 4: poorly differentiated carcinoma with fused glands widely infiltrating the prostatic stroma. Neoplastic cells may grow in cords or sheets and the cytoplasm is clear.

Grade 5: very poorly differentiated carcinoma with no or minimal gland formation. Tumour cell masses may have central necrosis.

About half of all tumours exhibit more than a single pattern. The commonest pattern (the primary) and the less common pattern (the secondary) can be recorded separately or can be summed to produce an average pattern called the pattern score (often simply termed *the Gleason score* or *index*) which correlates well with mortality [42].

Clinical and pathological characteristics have proven to be a fairly accurate reflection of the true degree of spread. Where radical prostatectomy has been performed and the specimen carefully analysed, close agreement between surgical and clinical findings is discovered in about three-quarters of all cases, although sometimes with unsuspected local invasion—usually of the seminal vesicles. Invasion of pelvic lymph nodes may be clinically silent but is increasingly likely with advanced stages of disease as the prostate has an unusually rich lymph node network. Drainage is most commonly to the obturator-hypogastric group and then to the external and common iliac nodes. Distant metastases are predominantly osseous, particularly to the pelvic and lower lumbar vertebrae, though ribs, dorsal spine and skull are not uncommonly involved. The bone metastases are typically osteosclerotic, as a result of the relatively slow clinical evolution of disease, although the pattern may be chiefly lytic or mixed.

Clinical features and investigation

Prostatic carcinoma is often asymptomatic, and is increasingly diagnosed at routine rectal examination. The typical finding is a firm, indurated or craggy gland which is usually enlarged. There may be obliteration of the median sulcus or spread to the lateral pelvic walls.

patients, it is important to realize that in the irradiated prostate, subsequent biopsy may show evidence of persistent malignant cells for up to a year, without any supportive clinical suggestion that the treatment has failed. Up to 60% of patients with locally advanced disease may have positive biopsies up to 9 months after treatment, falling to only 24% at 12–30 months, without further treatment. A recent attempt at producing guidelines for treatment of clinically localized prostatic carcinoma concluded that outcomes from both surgery and radiotherapy were essentially similar, or at least that current data were inadequate to make a clear recommendation [55]. Patient preference was regarded as extremely important. Interestingly, and unlike the MRC report [53], surveillance for low- or intermediate-grade localized tumours resulted in 'only a marginal compromise of disease-specific survival at 5–10 years of follow-up'.

Complications of radical surgical treatment include an operative mortality rate of 1.5–5%, permanent impotence in a large majority of patients (unless treated by nerve-sparing procedures, see below), frequency of micturition and urinary incontinence of about 10–15%. Rectovesical fistula and ureteric damage may also occur. Important complications of radical radiotherapy include diarrhoea, dysuria and perineal skin reaction (sometimes severe), and long-term sequelae: subcutaneous fibrosis, urethral stricture and fibrotic reduction of bladder capacity. Treatment with a full bladder may help to keep the small bowel out of the irradiated volume. The lower level, relatively, of impotence as a side-effect is a valuable advantage since with either radical surgery or hormonal treatment for prostatic cancer, this is almost certain unless specific nerve-sparing surgical techniques are used. However, even with radical prostatic irradiation, impotence rates of up to 50% have been reported. The introduction of the nerve-sparing radical prostatectomy has led during the past decade to an enormous increase in the popularity of surgical treatment for localized carcinoma of the prostate, at least in the USA [34].

Hormonal therapy

In 1941, Huggins and Hodges discovered that prostatic cancers were almost always hormonally dependent [56]. Both oestrogen therapy and orchidectomy were found to be useful for palliation, particularly for bone metastases. Since the majority of patients are unsuitable for radical surgery, the use of oestrogen derivatives or orchidectomy was widely employed as a standard therapy both for early and advanced cases. Other oestrogen-related agents

such as estramustine (a combination of an oestrogen with a nitrogen mustard moiety at position C-17), became briefly popular but are probably no better than diethylstilboestrol.

Hormonal manipulation is used as definitive treatment for advanced disease (stages III and IV), although many oncologists offer local irradiation to patients with stage III disease who have no evidence of metastases elsewhere, if the clinical condition warrants an attempt at radical treatment.

The increasing availability of newer forms of androgen-ablating hormone therapy has widened the options and their side-effects and acceptability differ. However, it remains unclear whether the type of hormone therapy critically influences overall outcome, and also whether combined antiandrogen therapy is superior to single-agent or sequential treatment. Analogues of gonadotrophin-releasing hormone (called luteinizing hormone (LH) releasing hormone agonists) interfere with gonadotrophin release, leading to a fall in circulating testosterone. They initially lead to an increase in LH and follicle-stimulating hormone levels followed over a 1–2-week period by a down-regulation of surface receptors leading to chemically mediated castrate levels of testosterone. These include goserelin (Zoladex), a depot form of gonadotrophin-releasing hormone analogue, and flutamide, a pure antiandrogen compound which interferes with testosterone binding to the androgen receptor. Both of these, together with more traditional forms of hormone therapy (oestrogen derivatives, orchidectomy), appear to have similar response rates, though the analogue agents have fewer cardiovascular complications and are superior to diethylstilboestrol. Flutamide is probably similar in its mechanism of action to cyproterone acetate, which was introduced earlier (1973) and is also widely used. One advantage of treatment with flutamide and other non-steroidal pure antiandrogens over stilboestrol is the potential for preservation of potency, but side-effects can be troublesome and include gynaecomastia, disturbances of hepatic function and gastrointestinal toxicity; half-life is short so multiple daily doses are necessary. Unlike the progesterone-like cyproterone acetate, these agents do not lead to central inhibition of LH release. Since they block negative testosterone feedback, increased serum levels of testosterone occur.

Total androgen blockade, using combinations of hormonal agents in an attempt to block both testicular and adrenal output, has also been tested in randomized controlled studies [45,46,57,58]. In patients with advanced disease [58], there appears to be a very small benefit: combinations of a gonadotrophin-releasing hormone analogue together with an antiandrogen such as flutamide are generally employed. A recent large EORTC study has confirmed an improved disease-free and overall survival with total andragen blockade during (and for 3 years after) external irradiation in patients with locally advanced disease [59].

In palliative treatment of metastatic prostatic cancer, radiotherapy has an important role for painful bone metastases. These generally respond well to moderate doses of radiotherapy. In recent years, single-fraction hemibody irradiation has been increasingly used since widespread metastases in the lower spine are so common. Treatment of the lower half of the body to a single fraction dose of 7.5–10 Gy is well tolerated and often dramatically effective for pain relief.

In patients with widespread metastatic problems unresponsive to oestrogens or palliative irradiation, bilateral orchidectomy should be considered since worthwhile responses often occur. Patients with hormone-resistant prostatic carcinoma have particular problems [60] and long-term survival is unlikely, though it does seem important to keep the patient androgen-depleted. If antiandrogen treatment is withdrawn, testosterone levels may rise and survival may be shortened, especially in patients receiving gonadotrophin-releasing analogues.

Chemotherapy for prostatic carcinoma has been disappointing although a number of agents show modest levels of activity, including cyclophosphamide, methotrexate, 5-FU, mitozantrone, nitrogen mustard and cisplatin.

In patients with unresponsive widespread bone pain, treatment with radioactive phosphorus may be of value. Up to 75% of patients have been reported to benefit, though remissions tend to be short. ^{89}Sr has recently been marketed as a superior radionuclide for use in this way, and may possibly be preferentially taken up in metastases rather than treating the whole bone marrow.

Overall, it has been estimated that patients with carcinoma of the prostate lose, on average, almost a decade of life; the disease is now claiming 9500 lives annually in the UK [61,62].

Cancer of the urethra [58]

Male urethra

This very rare tumour may arise in the prostatic, bulbar or penile urethra, and is thought to be commoner in patients with a history of chronic inflammation or stricture. In the prostatic urethra the tumour is a TCC, but in the penile urethra squamous carcinomas are more common. The tumour spreads by direct invasion into the perineum and penile tissues.

The penile urethra drains to inguinal lymph nodes, and the prostatic urethra to pelvic nodes.

Urethral carcinomas present with a urethral mass, obstruction, fistula, pain and haematuria. The age range is 50–80 years. Prostatic urethral tumours are treated either by radical prostatectomy or cystoprostatectomy, or by radical radiotherapy. This latter method is increasingly employed, using doses of the order of 60–70 Gy to the prostate. Radiation technique is similar to that employed for carcinoma of the prostate. Distal carcinomas are usually treated by amputation of the distal part of the penis. Lesions of the bulbomembranous urethra are generally treated by radical excision.

Female urethra

The tumour is twice as common in females, and the histological pattern is more varied (squamous carcinoma in the distal two-thirds, and TCC in the proximal third). Adenocarcinoma may arise from the periurethral glands, and melanoma and sarcoma occasionally occur. Leucoplakia of the urethra is regarded as a premalignant change, as are urethral papillomas and polyps.

Presentation is usually with a mass, bleeding and offensive discharge. Lymphatic involvement occurs late, distal tumours draining to the inguinal nodes and those of the proximal urethra to the iliac nodes.

Tumours of the anterior urethra are sometimes treated by partial urethrectomy but there is a high risk of local recurrence, and nodal spread frequently occurs. Radical radiation therapy is increasingly used since surgical control of the more extensive tumours is hard to achieve and the results are very poor. Interstitial radioactive implants may be suitable for small tumours, and external beam radiation therapy for larger lesions. The usual tumour dose is of the order of 60 Gy, carefully fractionated to avoid stricture formation.

Cancer of the penis

Incidence and aetiology

Carcinoma of the penis is uncommon in Western countries, accounting for less than 0.2% of male cancer deaths. It is, however, much more frequent in South-east Asia, and in parts of India and Africa. General hygiene is thought to affect the incidence, and early circumcision is associated with a very low risk. Men with phimosis also appear to be at higher risk. At present, a viral origin seems likely to explain at least a proportion of cases [63]. At least one married couple have been described with coexistent penile and vulval carcinoma, and the viral hypothesis is strengthened by the observation that many patients with penile cancer also harbour condylomata acuminata. There is slight concordance between the incidence of penile and cervical carcinomas in sexual partners. In addition, there are several premalignant conditions which predispose to the development of the tumour. These include Bowen's disease (intraepithelial carcinoma), erythroplasia of Queyrat, leukoplakia and Paget's disease. Leukoplakia may coexist with an invasive carcinoma. These premalignant lesions should be treated by local excision. The carcinoma is almost always a squamous cell lesion although melanoma, basal cell carcinoma and Kaposi's sarcoma have all been described.

Clinical features

Presentation is usually with an exophytic, or occasionally an excavating, ulcerated lesion, most commonly arising in the glans or the inner surface of the prepuce. There is often wide surface extension before deeper invasion to the urethra and corpora cavernosa. Some carcinomas of the penis are clinically obvious with a circumferential exophytic necrotic tumour, whereas in other cases, careful inspection with retraction of the prepuce is necessary to allow the tumour to be visualized. Local invasion to the inguinal nodes is common, ulceration of inguinal node metastases often occurs. The superficial inguinal nodes drain the prepuce and most of the penile skin, whereas the glans and corpora cavernosa drain chiefly to the deep inguinal nodes. A biopsy should always be performed since non-malignant conditions, such as lymphogranuloma venereum, trauma, local infection, penile warts (condylomata) or leukoplakia can all cause diagnostic confusion.

A TNM staging classification has been proposed (Table 18.4), but can be difficult to apply in practice, particularly since palpable inguinal lymph nodes are often due to local infection. Though relatively unlikely to disseminate widely, the commonest sites of blood-borne metastases (M_1) are the skin (chiefly abdominal wall), lungs and bone, and a chest X-ray should always be performed as part of the investigation.

Table 18.4 TNM staging for cancer of the penis.

T_0	No evidence of primary tumour
T_{is}	Carcinoma *in situ* (includes Bowen's disease and erythroplasia of Queyrat)
T_1	Superficial tumour < 1 cm diameter
T_2	Larger tumour but remains superficial
T_3	Tumour invades underlying tissues
T_4	Tumour invades local tissues including corpora cavernosa, urethra or perineum
N_0	Regional lymphadenopathy
N_1	Unilateral regional node involvement
N_2	Multiple unilateral node groups involved, or bilateral nodes
M_0	No distant metastases
M_1	Distant metastases present

Treatment and prognosis

For very localized lesions, cryosurgery or laser excision may be adequate; for more extensive tumours wider excision has traditionally been considered the treatment of choice, although amputation of the penis has never been a popular method of treatment and radical local irradiation has increasingly been used as an alternative [64]. As the tumour is uncommon, few surgeons or radiotherapists have a large experience. Treatment is often individualized: a small non-infiltrating tumour, which can be surgically excised without amputation, is probably best treated by surgery, with local irradiation given wherever there is doubt about the adequacy of the resection edge of the specimen. Many oncologists are disinclined to offer radical irradiation in bulky lesions because of the probability of hypoxia within the necrotic part of the tumour which limits the prospect of radiocurability; such tumours are probably best dealt with surgically, particularly if partial amputation will suffice. More proximal lesions would require total amputation, and radical irradiation is often preferred in the first instance, with surgery if there is local recurrence.

A variety of radiotherapy techniques has been described, including superficial X-rays (with single or opposed direct fields), treatment by interstitial implantation or a radium mould, or by orthovoltage or supervoltage irradiation using photons or electrons. A wax block can be used to improve dose homogeneity. Interstitial implants often employ radioactive iridium. The total dose of external irradiation is usually 60 Gy in daily fractions over 6 weeks, or the equivalent over a shorter treatment period. With mould treatments using iridium wire or radium, the treatment can usually be completed within 1–10 days (the patient wearing the mould for 8–10 h per day), to a total dose of the order of 60 Gy. The major complications of radiation therapy for carcinoma of the penis include urethral stricture (10–12% of patients), fibrosis, ulceration and local recurrence (10–40% depending on the size of the tumour). For larger and more infiltrating tumours, surgery is probably the treatment of choice, particularly where the inguinal nodes are obviously involved by tumour. Where the inguinal nodes are mobile, block dissection is generally preferable to local irradiation, although it is wise to perform aspiration cytology to confirm that the nodes are indeed metastatic. Where the inguinal nodes are clearly fixed and surgery is not possible, local irradiation can be useful as a palliative procedure. Although remissions have been documented in such cases, survival is poor. The majority of patients with stage I (T_1 or T_2, N_0) tumours are free of inguinal metastases but the incidence in stage II (T_3, N_0 or N_{1a}) is well over 50%, and it is these patients who probably benefit most from block dissection.

Early carcinoma of the penis has an excellent cure rate with surgery and/or radiotherapy. Although few large series of patients have been reported, it seems probable that T_1 and T_2 N_0 cases are equally well treated by surgery or radiotherapy. In one recent series treated by ^{192}Ir, 25/31 patients had durable tumour control most of the failures were successfully treated by salvage surgery [64]. Patients with deep involvement of penile structures or inguinal node involvement do far less well, and the survival rate is approximately 50%. Where there are inoperable inguinal metastases or distant involvement, the 5-year survival rate is well under 10%.

References

1 Vogelzang NJ, Stadler WM. Kidney cancer. *Lancet* 1998; 352: 1691–6.

2 Chow WH, Gridley G, Fraumeni JF *et al.* Obesity, hypertension and the risk of kidney cancer in men. *N Engl J Med* 2000; 343: 1305–11.

3 Sobin LH, Wittekind, Ch. *TNM Classification of Malignant Tumours*, 5th edn. New York: Wiley-Liss, 1997; 181.

4 Bukowski RM, Novick AC *et al.* Renal cell carcinoma: molecular biology. In: *Immunology and Clinical Management.* New Jersey: Humana Press, 2000: 434.

5 Vogelzang NJ, Priest ER, Borden L. Spontaneous regression of histologically proved pulmonary metastases from renal cell carcinoma: a case with 5-year follow-up. *J Urol* 1992; 148: 1247–8.

6 Young RC. Metastatic renal-cell carcinoma: what causes occasional dramatic regressions? *N Engl J Med* 1998; 338: 1305–6.

7 Kjaer M, Frederiksen MD, Engelholm SA. Postoperative radiotherapy in stage I and II renal adenocarcinoma. A randomized trial by the Copenhagen Renal Cancer Study Group. *Int J Radiation Oncol Biol Physics* 1987; 13: 665–72.

8 Ahmed T, Benedetto P, Yagoda A *et al.* Estrogen, progesterone and androgen-binding sites in renal cell carcinoma. *Cancer* 1984; 54: 477–81.

9 Yagoda A, Abi-Rached B, Petrylak D. Chemotherapy for advanced renal-cell carcinoma, 1983–93. *Semin Oncol* 1995; 22: 42–60.

10 Gleave ME, Elhilahi M, Fradet Y *et al.* (Canadian Urology Group). Interferon gamma-1b compared with placebo in metastatic renal-cell carcinoma. *N Engl J Med* 1998; 338: 1265–71.

11 Amato R. Modest effect of interferon-α on metastatic renal-cell carcinoma. *Lancet* 1999; 353: 6–7.

12 Rosenberg SA, Lotz MT, Muul LM *et al.* Observations on the systemic administration of autologous lymphokine-activated killer cells and recombinant interleukin-2 to patients with metastatic cancer. *N Engl J Med* 1985; 313: 1485–92.

13 Childs R, Chernoff A, Contentin N *et al.* Regression of metastatic renal-cell carcinoma after non-myeloblative allogeneic peripheral-blood-stem-cell transplantation. *N Engl J Med* 2000; 343: 750–8.

14 Henriksson R, Nilsson S, Colleen S *et al.* Survival in renal cell carcinoma—a randomised evaluation of tamoxifen vs. interleukin 2, alpha-interferon and tamoxifen. *Br J Cancer* 1998; 77: 1311–17.

15 Hall MC, Womack S, Sagalowsky AI *et al.* Prognostic factors, recurrence, and survival in traditional cell carcinoma of the upper urinary tract: a 30-year experience in 252 patients. *Urology* 1998; 52: 594–601.

16 Wallace DMA. Occupational urothelial cancer. *Br J Urol* 1988; 61: 175–82.

17 Plail R. Detecting bladder cancer. *Br Med J* 1990; 301: 567–8.

18 Lamm DL, De Haven JI, Shriver J *et al.* Prospective randomized comparison of intravesical with percutaneous BCG vs. intravesical BCG in superficial bladder cancer. *J Urol* 1991; 144: 738–40.

19 Kaufman DS, Shipley WU, Griffin PP *et al.* Selective bladder preservation by combination treatment of invasive bladder cancer. *N Engl J Med* 1993; 329: 1377–82.

20 Van der Werf-Messing B. Cancer of the urinary bladder treated by interstitial radium implant. *Int J Radiation Oncol Biol Physics* 1978; 4: 373–8.

21 Hautmann RE, Miller K, Steiner U *et al.* The ideal neobladder: 6 years of experience with more than 200 patients. *J Urol* 1993; 150: 40–5.

22 Scher HI. New approaches to the treatment of bladder cancer. *N Engl J Med* 1993; 329: 1420–1.

23 Brendler CB, Steinberg GD, Marshall FF *et al.* Local recurrence and survival following nerve sparing radical cystoprostatectomy. *J Urol* 1990; 144: 1137–41.

24 Liu MCC, Zietman AL, Shipley WU. Organ preservation approaches with radiation therapy in muscle-invasive bladder carcinoma. *Ann Acad Med Singapore* 1996; 25: 441–7.

25 Bloom HJG, Hendry WF, Wallace DM, Skeet RG. Treatment of T3 bladder cancer: controlled trial of pre-operative radiotherapy and radical cystectomy vs. radical radiotherapy. Second report and review (for the Clinical Trials Group, Institute of Urology). *Br J Urol* 1982; 54: 136–51.

26 Duchesne GM, Bolger JJ, Griffiths GO *et al.* A randomised trial of hypofractionated schedules of palliative radiotherapy in the management of bladder carcinoma: results of MRC trial BA 09. *Int J Radiol Oncol Biol Physics* 2000; 47: 379–88.

27 Tester W, Caplan R, Heaney J *et al.* Neoadjuvant combined modality program with selective organ preservation for invasive bladder cancer: results of RTOG phase II trial 8802. *J Clin Oncol* 1996; 14: 11926.

28 Dunst J, Sauer R, Schrott KM *et al.* Organ-sparing treatment of advanced bladder cancer: a 10-year experience. *Int J Radiation Oncol Biol Physics* 1994; 30: 261–6.

29 McCaffrey JA. The role of chemotherapy in bladder cancer. *Cancer Topics* 1999; 11: 1–4.

30 Shearer RJ, Chilvers CED, Bloom HJG *et al.* Adjuvant chemotherapy in T3 carcinoma of the bladder: a prospective trial. *Br J Urol* 1988; 62: 558–64.

31 Wallace DMA, Raghaven D, Kelly KA *et al.* Neoadjuvant (pre-emptive) cisplatin therapy in invasive transitional cell carcinoma of the bladder. *Br J Urol* 1991; 67: 608–15.

32 Coppin CML, Gospodarowicz MK, James K *et al.* Improved local control of invasive bladder cancer by concurrent cisplatin and preoperative or definitive radiation. *J Clin Oncol* 1996; 14: 2901–7.

33 International collaboration of trialists (MRC, EORTC, NCI Canada, Norwegian and Spanish (CUETO) groups). Neoadjuvant cisplatin, methotrexate and vinblastine chemotherapy for muscle-invasive bladder cancer: a randomised controlled trial. *Lancet* 1999; 354: 533–40.

34 Lu-Yao GI, Greenberg ER. Changes in prostate cancer incidence and treatment in the USA. *Lancet* 1994; 343: 251–4.

35 Rowley KHM, Mason MD. The aetiology and pathogenesis of prostate cancer. *Clin Oncol* 1997; 9: 213–18.

36 Ekbom A, Hsieh C-C, Lipworth L *et al.* Perinatal characteristics in relation to incidence of and mortality from prostate cancer. *Br Med J* 1996; 313: 337–41.

37 Gerber FS, Chodak GW. Routine screening for cancer of the prostate. *J Natl Cancer Inst* 1991; 83: 329–35.

38 Schroder FH, Damhvis RA, Kirkels WJ *et al.* European randomized study of screening for prostate cancer—the Rotterdam pilot studies. *Int J Cancer* 1996; 65: 145–51.

39 Brawley OW. Prostate carcinoma incidence and mortality: the effects of screening and early detection. *Cancer* 1997; 80: 1857–63.

40 Neal DE, Donovan JL. Prostate cancer: to screen or not to screen? *Lancet Oncol* 2000; 1: 17–24.

41 Gleason DE, Mellinger GT, Veterans' Administration Co-operative Urological Research Group. Prediction of prognosis for prostatic adenocarcinoma by combined histological grading and clinical staging. *J Urol* 1974; 111: 58–64.

42 Gleason DF, Veterans' Administration Co-operative Urological Research Group. Histologic grading and clinical staging of prostatic carcinoma. In: Tannenbaum M, ed. *Urologic Pathology: the Prostate*. Philadelphia: Lea & Febiger, 1977.

43 Chan JM, Stampfer MJ, Giovannucci E *et al.* Plasma insulin-like growth factor-I and prostate cancer risk: a prospective study. *Science* 1998; 279: 563–5.

44 Emlyeaton M. What urologists say they do for men with prostate cancer. *Br Med J* 1999; 318: 276.

45 Mulley AG, Barry MJ. Controversy in managing patients with probable cancer. *Br Med J* 1998; 316: 1919–20.

46 Tyrell CJ. Controversies in the management of advanced prostatic cancer. *Br Med J* 1998; 316: 1919–20.

47 Chodak GW, Thisted RA, Gerber GS *et al.* Results of conservative management of clinically localised prostate cancer. *N Engl J Med* 1994; 330: 242–8.

48 Dearnaley DP, Khoo VS, Norman AR *et al.* Comparison of radiation side-effects conformal and conventional radiotherapy in prostate cancer: a randomised trial. *Lancet* 1999; 353: 267–72.

49 Duchesne GM. Radiation for prostate cancer. *Lancet Oncol* 2001; 2: 73–81.

50 Walsh PC, Partin AW, Epstein JI. Cancer control and quality of life following anatomical radical retropublic prostatectomy: results at 10 years. *J Urol* 1994; 152: 1831–6.

51 Ash DV. Management of localised carcinoma of the prostate: brachytherapy revisited. *Clin Oncol* 1997; 9: 219–21.

52 Johansson J-E, Holmberg L, Johansson S, Bergstrom R, Avami HO. Fifteen-year survival in prostate cancer: a prospective, population-based study in Sweden. *J Am Med Assoc* 1997; 277: 467–71.

53 MRC Prostate Cancer Working Party Investigators' Report. Immediate and deferred treatment for advanced prostate cancer: initial results of the MRC. *Br J Urol* 1997; 79: 235–46.

54 Eustham JA, Kattan MW, Groshen S *et al.* Fifteen-year survival and recurrence rates after radiotherapy for localised prostate cancer. *J Clin Oncol* 1997; 15: 3214–22.

55 Middleton RG, Thompson IM, Austenfeld MS *et al.* Prostate cancer clinical guidelines panel summary report on the management of clinically localized prostate cancer. *J Urol* 1995; 154: 2144–8.

56 Huggins C, Hodges CE. Studies on prostatic cancer. I. The effect of castration, of estrogen and of androgen injection on serum acid phosphatase in metastatic carcinoma of the prostate. *Cancer Res* 1941; 1: 293–7.

57 Crawford ED, Eisenberger MA, McLeod DG *et al.* A controlled trial of leuprolide with and without flutamide in prostatic carcinoma. *N Engl J Med* 1989; 321: 419–24.

58 Prostate Cancer Trialists' Collaborative Group. Maximum androgen blockade in advanced prostate cancer. an overview of the randomised trials. *Lancet* 2000; 355: 1491–8.

59 Bolla M, Collette L, Blank L *et al.* Long-term results with immediate androgen suppression and external irradiation in

patients with locally advanced prostate cancer (an EORTC study): a phase III randomized trial. *Lancet* 2002; 360: 103–8.

60 Ziotta AR, Schulman CC. Can survival be prolonged for patients with hormone-resistant prostate cancer? *Lancet* 2001; 357: 326–7.

61 Dearnaley DP. Cancer of the prostate. *Br Med J* 1994; 308: 780.

62 Moffat LE. Therapeutic choices in prostate cancer. *Prescriber's Journal* 1999; 39: 16–23.

63 Boon ME, Schneider A, Hoegewonig CJA *et al.* Penile studies and heterosexual partners: peniscopy, cytology, histology and immunochemistry. *Cancer* 1988; 61: 16529.

64 Kiltie AE, Elwell C, Close HJ, Ash DV. Iridium-192 implantation for node-negative carcinoma of the penis: the Cookridge Hospital experience. *Clin Oncol* 2000; 12: 25–31.

19 Testicular cancer

Although testicular tumours are uncommon, with a frequency of just over two per 100 000 males per year, they have an importance well beyond their low incidence: first, they represent the most common malignant solid tumours in young men between the ages of 15 and 34 years; second, they are exceptionally chemosensitive tumours with a high cure rate even with disseminated disease; and third, they often manufacture tumour markers which can be used to monitor treatment and to predict recurrence before it is clinically evident. Furthermore, their incidence has risen considerably over the past decade, particularly in the 15–19 age group (Fig. 19.1) [1]; in fact in industrialized countries the incidence increased 10-fold during the 20th century [2]. Worldwide incidence has doubled over the past 40 years. Some 1000 cases are now diagnosed annually in the UK, and over 7000 in the USA with far lower prevalence rates in Asia and Africa. During the same period there has been considerable progress in the management of these conditions, and death from testicular tumours is now extremely uncommon.

Germ cell tumours

Aetiology and incidence

Over 90% of testicular tumours are *germ cell tumours* which are believed to arise in the pluripotent germ cell. This cell, when malignant, can give rise to tumours which have either somatic or trophoblastic features or both. Somatic differentiation results in the mixture of tissues typically found in teratomas, while choriocarcinoma comes from trophoblastic differentiation. *Non-germ cell tumours* are described on p. 311 and include lymphomas, metasta-

tic deposits and Leydig and Sertoli tumours. Although most male germ cell tumours arise in the testis they may occasionally be *extragonadal* in origin, and these are briefly outlined on p. 310.

The presence of an undescended testis (cryptorchidism) is associated with a 10-fold increase in the incidence of testicular tumours [3]. About 10% of all patients with a testicular germ cell tumour have a history of maldescent. Orchidopexy reduces, but does not abolish, this risk. Data from North America suggest that testicular tumours are rarer in black than in white Americans (approximately 1 : 5 in incidence). Teratomas of the testis (about 50% of all germ cell tumours) present at an earlier age (peak age 20–30) than seminomas (peak age 30–50). The age-adjusted incidence in the UK is 3.8 per 100 000; incidence at different ages is shown in Fig. 19.2. There is a trend toward higher prevalence in the wealthier social groups, and early onset of puberty and sexual activity are both thought to operate as important aetiological factors. Bilateral testicular tumours occur in about 5% of all cases. Teratoma and seminoma are the usual tumours at 10–40 years, but in older age groups lymphoma is much commoner. Familial instances of testicular germ cell tumour have occasionally been described [4]. A second primary testicular germ cell tumour occurs in about 2% of patients.

What could be the mechanism of carcinogenesis [2,4]? Both chemicals and viruses are possible candidates for inducing the final common pathway of tumour development and clonal evolution, that is, gonadotropin-driven mitosis in spermatogonia [5]. It seems likely that atrophy of the germinal epithelium with loss of feedback inhibition of the pituitary may result in an increase in pituitary-driven hormonal stimulation of the remaining testicular

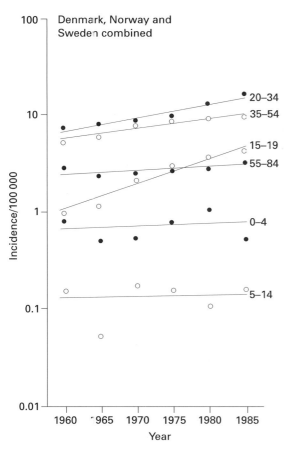

Fig. 19.1 Trends in incidence of testicular cancer in the age groups 0–4, 5–14, 15–19, 20–34, 35–54 and 55–84 years in the combined populations of Denmark, Norway and Sweden (1958–87).

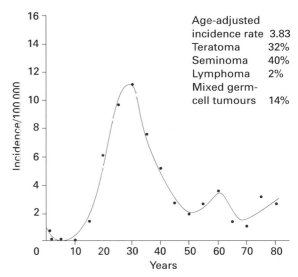

Fig. 19.2 Age-specific incidence of testicular tumours.

short arm isochromosome of chromosome 12 is the most frequent genetic marker in germ cell tumours (even including *in situ* cases).

Pathology

Several systems of classification are in current use (Table 19.1). In the UK, the commonest is the British Testicular Tumour Panel, while in the USA the Dixon and Moore classification is generally used [8]. Both are based on microscopic criteria, with an attempt to identify the predominant cell type. A major problem is that the tumours are often heterogeneous, the teratomas in particular displaying pleomorphism and a tendency to multiple cell types. Future classifications may depend increasingly on histochemical criteria, particularly in those which produce tumour markers.

Choriocarcinoma with any other cell type

Most testicular tumours are of germ cell origin (Fig. 19.3) and can usually be classified into seminomas (40%), teratomas (32%) or combined tumours with elements of both (14%). In the past 10 years there has been increased recognition that carcinoma *in situ* (also known as intratubular germ cell neoplasia) may occur in the testis, and may, after about 5 years of apparent dormancy, develop into an invasive carcinoma. This specific histological change is found in almost every case as precursors

germ cells, resulting in neoplastic change. There may even be a higher risk of relapse with total aspermia (the greatest degree of atrophy), perhaps even accounting for the worrying possible association with vasectomy—in which the risk of testicular neoplasia may possibly be higher, particularly in patients whose operation was complicated by haematoma or infection. Testicular atrophy following mumps orchitis may also result in neoplastic change via the same pathway. The role of testicular trauma has recently been more fully investigated and cannot confidently be excluded as a trivial factor [6] though it seems likely that genetic predisposition plays a far more important aetiological role—including both sibling and bilateral cases [2,4]. Germ cell tumours are almost always hyperdiploid [7]—often triploid or even tetraploid. A

Table 19.1 Pathological classification of testicular tumours.

British Testicular Tumour Panel
Seminoma
Malignant teratoma undifferentiated (MTU)
Malignant teratoma intermediate (MTI)
Malignant teratoma trophoblastic (MTT)
Teratoma differentiated

Dixon and Moore [8]
Pure seminoma
Embryonal carcinoma (pure or with seminoma)
Teratoma (pure or with seminoma)
Teratoma with embryonal carcinoma, choriocarcinoma or seminoma
Choriocarcinoma pure or with seminoma embryonal carcinoma (or both)

World Health Organization
1   Tumours of single-cell type
     Seminoma
     Embryonal carcinoma
     Teratoma
     Choriocarcinoma
2   Mixed histological appearances
     Embryonal carcinoma with teratoma
     Embryonal carcinoma with teratoma and seminoma
     Embryonal carcinoma with choriocarcinoma
     Teratoma with seminoma

of invasive germ cell tumours [9], and are particularly common in patients with a history of testicular maldescent [10]. The changes of carcinoma *in situ* are often widespread within the testis.

Although the precise histological type of germ cell tumour previously carried great prognostic significance, particularly in the distinction between seminoma and the teratomas (non-seminomas), dramatic improvements in treatment (particularly of teratomas) have reduced these disparities. Apart from the cell type, the most important prognostic feature, available from the operative specimen at orchidectomy, is the presence of tumour cells either at the cut end of the cord or within its vessels (intravascular invasion). Such tumours have an adverse prognosis. The level of initial tumour marker values (see below) also carries prognostic significance.

The relationship between *in situ* carcinoma and invasive testicular cancer is now increasingly well recognized, although testicular biopsy remains unacceptable to many. Nevertheless, a high-risk group can be recognized by presence of *in situ* change—of practical importance because low-dose irradiation of an affected testis can prevent the later development of an invasive tumour without lowering testosterone levels or affecting sexuality.

Chromosomal analysis has indicated a remarkable consistency in the finding of a single abnormality (isochrome 12p) which is almost as common in testicular tumours as the Philadelphia chromosome in chronic myeloid leukaemia. Other cytogenetic studies have suggested that seminomas may be an 'intermediate' step in the progression towards more malignant forms of testicular teratoma since the chromosome number for seminoma is intermediate between precursor *in situ* cell change and histologically more advanced disease [11].

Seminoma

Seminomas tend to be encapsulated, firm, with the cut surface pale grey and often featureless, and with little necrosis or haemorrhage. The microscopic appearance shows large round cells with distinct cell borders, clear cytoplasm, and large nuclei often with conspicuous nucleoli (Fig. 19.3). Lymphocytic infiltration is frequently seen. When spread beyond the testis occurs, it is almost invariably to pelvic and para-aortic lymph nodes later followed by involvement of mediastinal and supraclavicular nodes. Although chiefly testicular in origin, primary extragonadal seminomas are occasionally encountered in the retroperitoneal region, mediastinum, and suprasellar region or pineal area of the brain.

Teratoma (non-seminomatous germ cell tumours)

MALIGNANT TERATOMA UNDIFFERENTIATED (MTU, EMBRYONAL CARCINOMA)
This is the commonest non-seminomatous germ cell tumour. They are often firm and nodular, showing areas of haemorrhage and necrosis. Microscopically, large anaplastic cells are usually seen, with less distinct cell borders and an eosinophilic cytoplasm containing nuclei of widely varying shapes. Some form of differentiation may occur, often with a glandular pattern (Fig. 19.3).

TERATOMA DIFFERENTIATED
Occasionally, a fully mature or differentiated testicular teratoma is encountered, in which mature bone, bone marrow and cartilage, and other tissues may be present. Even these tumours should be regarded as 'potentially malignant'.

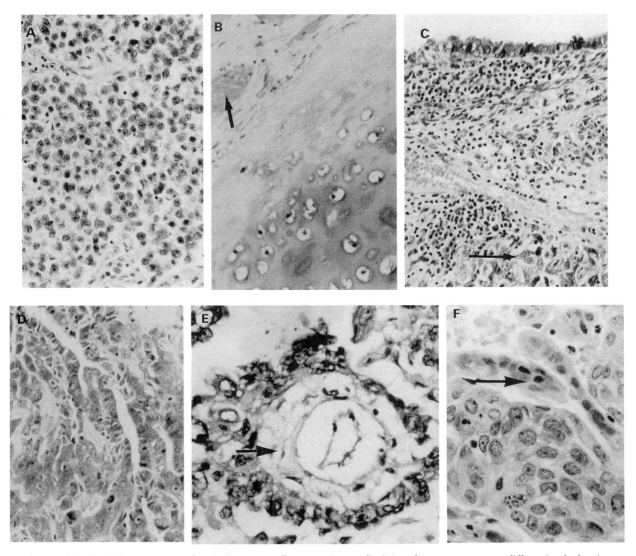

Fig. 19.3 Histological appearances of testicular germ cell tumours (original magnification ×200): (A) pure seminoma; (B) malignant teratoma differentiated, showing cartilage and smooth muscle (arrowed); (C) malignant teratoma intermediate, showing differentiated epithelium and embryonal carcinoma (arrowed); (D) malignant teratoma undifferentiated, showing embryonal carcinoma; (E) yolk sac tumour, showing a Schiller–Duval body (arrowed); (F) choriocarcinoma, showing syncytiotrophoblast (arrowed) and cytotrophoblast.

MALIGNANT TERATOMA INTERMEDIATE (MTI OR TERATOCARCINOMA)

This usually shows characteristic differences from MTU, with a nodular appearance which, on sectioning, frequently feels gritty because of the presence of cartilage and/or bone. There is often a wide variety of germ cell types, including cells derived from all three of the primitive germ cell layers, including bone, cartilage, connective tissue and smooth muscle as well as cells suggestive of respiratory or gastrointestinal epithelium.

MALIGNANT TERATOMA TROPHOBLASTIC (MTT, CHORIOCARCINOMA)

This is very much less common, and is histologically distinct because of the typical elements of cytotrophoblast and/or syncytiotrophoblast cells. They are highly malignant, metastasizing early and widely. It is extremely un-usual to encounter a true trophoblastic testicular tumour which is confined to the testis. Typically these are bulky tu-mours at presentation and are more often associated with brain metastases than other types of teratoma. Drug resis-tance often develops early, and a prognostic distinction can be drawn between MTT and the commoner teratoma types (MTI and MTU). MTU probably has a more rapid doubling time than MTI, more commonly presents with lung deposits, seems more responsive to chemotherapy and carries a somewhat better prognosis.

Patterns of metastases

Clinical staging is based on a relatively predictable pattern of progression (Fig. 19.4). The mode of spread is often lymphatic in the first instance, following the spermatic cord to the para-aortic nodes, thence to the retroperi-toneal and retrocrural nodes, thoracic duct, posterior me-diastinum and supraclavicular nodes (usually left-sided, although bifid or right-sided thoracic ducts occur in a small percentage of the population). Blood-borne spread frequently occurs, especially in MTT and MTU. In over 90% of cases this is associated with demonstrable nodal spread; in the remainder, metastases develop in the lungs in the absence of abdominal lymphatic disease. Liver in-volvement is unusual and exceptional in patients without lung deposits. Intracerebral and bone metastases are occasionally encountered. MTU is more commonly asso-ciated with locally invasive primary tumours and with haematogenous spread than MTI.

Clinical features

Patients typically present with a painless swelling of the testis, although pain occurs in about 25% of cases, partic-ularly with rapidly growing tumours. Some young men present with a tumour of only 2–3 cm while others are un-aware of the change until the testis is well over twice its normal size. Some insist that a traumatic injury to the testis preceded its enlargement. Although small hydro-celes are frequently present, invasion of the scrotal skin is extremely unusual and the tunica albuginea is rarely breached. Occasionally a spermatocele or varicocele may cause diagnostic difficulties.

The lymphatic drainage of the testis can be traced to the original embryonic site of origin in the abdomen (pelvic, common iliac and para-aortic nodes), rather than to adjacent nodes. Dissemination into these node groups is common and causes low back pain in about 10%. Patients

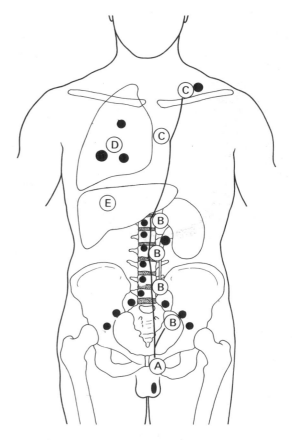

Spread

A Along lymphatics of cord
B Iliac and retroperitoneal (para-aortic) nodes
   including renal hilar nodes
C Mediastinal and supraclavicular nodes
D Lung
E Liver, brain and other sites
Sequence is usually A to E

Fig. 19.4 Pathways of spread of testicular germ cell tumours.

may also notice lymphadenopathy in other sites, particu-larly the left supraclavicular nodes. If there is a history of inguinal or testicular surgery (usually herniorrhaphy or orchidopexy), inguinal node involvement may occur due to interference with the normal lymphatic pathways. Occasionally, abdominal swelling may occur from mas-sive nodal deposits due to an unsuspected primary testic-ular tumour. The presenting symptoms will then be different—ureteric obstruction, acute abdominal pain or retrograde ejaculation as a result of pressure on the pre-sacral plexus.

When patients present with obvious abdominal involvement, it is sometimes the case that the only sign of the primary tumour is testicular atrophy rather than a mass. Gynaecomastia may also occur (in up to 25% of patients with advanced disease), presumably due to ectopic hormone production by the tumour. Rarely, patients initially present with symptoms due to secondary spread in lung, brain or other sites. Infertility, due to azoospermia, may be the presenting complaint and clinical examination of the testes should be a routine procedure in the infertility clinic.

When considering the diagnosis, other causes of testicular swelling may cause difficulty, including cystic swellings (hydrocele if involving the testis, varicocele if clearly separate) and solid masses such as a testicular torsion, haematoma or scrotal inguinal hernia. The commonest mistake, however, is to confuse epididymoorchitis in the young male, so often the cause of an important delay.

Tumour markers

These tumours often manufacture tumour markers; α-fetoprotein (AFP) and human chorionic gonadotrophin α (α-HCG) are the best known (see also Chapter 4). AFP is synthesized by the fetal yolk sac, and plasma levels are elevated in about 70% of patients with MTU or MTI. It is never raised in patients with pure seminoma, and detection of AFP in such cases must be assumed to be due to

foci of occult teratoma. Produced by trophoblastic elements in the tumour, β-HCG is detectable in the plasma of about 50% of patients with testicular teratoma and can also be modestly raised in patients with pure seminoma. With radioimmunoassay techniques it is possible to measure these hormones at nanogram levels. The marker levels vary independently, reflecting their differing cell of origin. This may be confusing since treatment may lead to a fall in one marker without affecting the other. If raised, repeat measurements give a quantitative indication of tumour responsiveness and are an established part of management. At presentation, it is essential to obtain a preoperative sample for measurements of tumour markers.

The levels will fall after orchidectomy to within the normal range provided the patient has no metastases (Fig. 19.5). If the preoperative levels of AFP and/or HCG are very high, the return of these values to normal may not be complete for several weeks since the half-life of AFP is 6–7 days (that of HCG is 16 h). The level of both AFP and HCG at diagnosis gives an indication of prognosis—patients with AFP levels above 500 ng/ml and/or HCG above 10 000 ng/ml clearly do worse.

Tumour markers are also of great importance in the early diagnosis of relapse (Fig. 19.5). Almost all patients with marker-producing tumours will develop elevated plasma levels as the first and most sensitive indication of relapse. Occasionally, patients with recurrent disease will develop a rise in only one marker even though both may

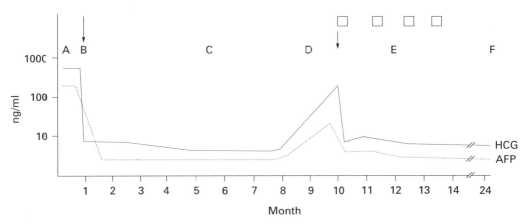

Fig. 19.5 Serum markers in testicular teratoma. **A** Presentation with left testicular swelling: HCG = 623 ng/ml, AFP = 246 ng/ml. **B** Orchidectomy: HCG falls in 6 days to 10 ng/ml, AFP falls more slowly (half-life 6 days) to 4 ng/ml. **C** No rise in markers, clinical remission. **D** HCG and AFP rise, CT scan confirms enlargement of para-aortic nodes. **E** Cyclical intermittent combination chemotherapy produces rapid fall in HCG and slower fall in AFP, both to normal values. **F** Two years after presentation: normal markers, clinical remission, probable cure.

previously have been elevated, due either to the differing sensitivity of components of the teratoma to chemotherapy or to a differential metastatic potential of the various elements of the primary. Tumour markers are particularly valuable in the diagnosis of extragonadal primaries since the differential diagnosis from other causes of a retroperitoneal, mediastinal or intracranial suprasellar mass is so wide.

Other tumour markers elaborated by testicular germ cell tumours include placental alkaline phosphatase (PLAP) and lactate dehydrogenase (LDH). Although they are of far less value for disease monitoring than AFP and α-HCG, LDH in particular can provide useful information and is useful in patients who are otherwise marker-negative. Although about 90% of cases of pure seminoma have elevated PLAP levels, it is an unreliable marker since it is also raised in other conditions and in smokers.

Staging

Clinical staging systems vary widely, but all depend on the anatomical extent of spread at diagnosis (Table 19.2). In the UK a simple system analogous to that used for Hodgkin's disease and other lymphomas (see Chapter 25) is often used. Greater detail can be incorporated, to take account of the importance of tumour volume in the abdomen and lungs, characteristics recognized as crucial to the outcome. Radiological techniques, such as lymphography, computed tomography (CT), magnetic resonance imaging (MRI) and positron emission tomography (PET) scanning have helped our understanding—for example, the frequency of spread to the mediastinum was not appreciated until the advent of CT scanning; it is now recognized that nearly 30% of patients with testicular teratomas have evidence of involvement. Other investigations include intravenous urography, and testicular ultrasonography, particularly helpful in seminoma where irradiation of the para-aortic nodes may still be an important part of treatment at some centres, so care must be taken to avoid irradiation of the kidneys. The staging notation in Table 19.2 is based on investigations including CT and MRI scanning.

In the USA, retroperitoneal lymph node dissection is still quite often performed, both for its value in staging and for possible therapeutic effect. The tumour node metastasis system is therefore partly surgically based (Table 19.2). In the UK, greater emphasis is placed on non-surgical approaches, and the accuracy of modern scanning methods is demonstrated by comparison with American data. These indicate that about 25% of lymph

Table 19.2 Staging of testicular tumours.

UK notation

Stage I	Tumour confined to testis (tumour markers not elevated after orchidectomy, all investigations negative)
Stage II	Tumour in pelvic and abdominal (retroperitoneal) nodes (tumour markers may be persistently elevated. Positive lymphogram or CT scan of abdomen)
I_{Ia}	Nodes < 2 cm diameter
I_{Ib}	Nodes 2–5 cm diameter
I_{Ic}	Nodes > 5 cm diameter
Stage III	Mediastinal and/or supraclavicular nodes
Stage IV	Distant metastases*
	L_1 < 3 metastases, maximum diameter < 2 cm
	L_2 > 3 metastases, maximum diameter < 2 cm
	L_3 maximum diameter > 2 cm

TNM staging notation

T_1	Confined to testis and adjacent spermatic cord
T_2	Tumour detected in spermatic cord at level of inguinal ring
T_3	Testicular capsule breached (or scrotal orchidectomy)
N_0	No pathological involvement
N_1	Normal size nodes, microscopic involvement
N_2	Enlarged nodes but no extranodal extension (A: < 2 cm and less than 5 nodes) (B: > 2 cm and more than 5 nodes)
N_3	Extranodal extension
N_4	Retroperitoneal nodes with residual disease after surgery
M_0	No distant metastases
M_1	Distant metastases

*The number and size of lung metastases should be noted, in view of the prognostic importance of this observation.

node dissection specimens in patients clinically thought to be free of extratesticular spread are, indeed, positive—a figure remarkably similar to British data from non-surgical series.

Management of testicular tumours

The last 25 years have seen major changes in management. Increased understanding of the importance of scrupulous staging, coupled with the advent of highly effective chemotherapy and routine use of tumour marker studies, has led to remarkable improvements and widespread acceptance that this is a tumour best treated by a multimodal approach. Expert surgeons, tumour pathologists, medical oncologists and radiation therapists all play an important and complementary role. Since these tumours are relatively uncommon and expert attention is so crucial, they are best treated in specialist units, or at the very least by study groups which will ensure uniformity of approach. For patients with a suspected testicular tumour, the correct surgical procedure is radical inguinal orchidectomy. Excision via the scrotal route, though still sometimes performed, should not generally be considered since trans-scrotal orchidectomy carries a real risk of scrotal recurrence or later development of inguinal node involvement. The spermatic cord should be excised as high as possible to provide information regarding the possibility of direct or intravascular spread of tumour, which has important implications for both management and prognosis. Before orchidectomy it is essential that the surgeon requests AFP and HCG levels, for the reasons described above.

Seminoma

If the tumour proves to be a pure seminoma, it is generally accepted that the surgeon has no further part to play, except perhaps for biopsy procedures if, for example, a supraclavicular node is discovered. Although American oncologists sometimes recommend surgery in seminomas with bulky abdominal lymph node metastases or where the HCG level is modestly raised, this is not usual practice in the UK. Radiotherapy alone will usually cure even bulky disease, and the addition of chemotherapy will increase this cure rate still further (see below).

Teratoma

For malignant teratomas there has in the past been an important difference of opinion between British and American authorities. For patients without abdominal involvement, or evidence of only minimal node deposits (usually detected at CT or MRI scanning), standard British practice has been to recommend treatment by irradiation (or more recently, by careful surveillance, see below).

In the USA most of these patients would have been treated by extended retroperitoneal lymphadenectomy, removing all lymphatic and connective tissues along the great vessels from the diaphragm to the level of the iliac vessels, a formidable surgical procedure. Many American urologists claim that a lymph node metastatic rate of 25% fully justifies radical lymphadenectomy in all cases. In the UK it is generally felt that combinations of radiotherapy and chemotherapy (or chemotherapy on relapse, if it

occurs) can effectively sterilize small-volume metastases in abdominal lymph nodes, and that the potential postoperative problems of aspermia (dry ejaculation) render such surgery unjustifiable.

Although it has been claimed that results of treatment by lymphadenectomy are superior to those in patients treated more conservatively, careful study of the literature does not bear this out. Comparisons are difficult since British patients are staged by clinical investigation, while most American urologists recommend lymphadenectomy as a staging as well as a potentially therapeutic procedure. It seems inescapable that many patients undergoing radical lymphadenectomy will have done so unnecessarily, in addition to having to face the undesirable sexual difficulties that the operation may bring. Reasonable comparison is possible between patients where lymphadenectomy confirms histologically positive para-aortic nodes and those from British series who have obviously positive CT or MRI scan appearances (stage II), where we see similar survival rates, regardless of treatment. In stage I disease, a large series from Indiana University, following almost 400 patients treated surgically, showed a 99% survival [12]; conversely, an equally large British multicentre experience gave a similar (98%) outcome [13]. Chemotherapy proved necessary in 18.5 and 27%, respectively, but infertility was greater in the surgical group.

Over the past 10 years, this debate has largely become historic since the recognition that many patients with early disease, well staged and without adverse features, can be safely followed up by postorchidectomy surveillance. This requires serial marker studies and CT scanning, but does not include immediate postoperative treatment. Although approximately 20% of these patients relapse, close monitoring ensures that the relapse is almost always of small volume, and 99% of patients are curable by modern chemotherapy. Almost 80% of stage I surveillance cases require no postorchidectomy treatment whatever — that is, they are cured by this simple operation. Surgery is, however, recommended quite often after initial chemotherapy in order to reassess residual intra-abdominal disease (discussed further on p. 309).

Radiotherapy

SEMINOMA

For patients with testicular seminoma radiotherapy can be curative, even in patients with advanced disease (although chemotherapy is increasingly preferred in this latter situation). For patients with stage I seminoma, modest dosage of irradiation to bilateral para-aortic nodes continues to be widely employed, since there can be no guarantee that orchidectomy alone will be curative. It seems unnecessary to include the lower pelvic or iliac nodes, as was previously traditional. Seminoma is among the most radiosensitive of all tumours; a dose of 30 Gy (anterior and posterior fields over a 3-week period) is normally considered adequate and leads to few acute or chronic side-effects. The need for adjuvant treatment in stage I seminoma was demonstrated in a Canadian trial comparing immediate radiation therapy with surveillance [14]. By 5 years, relapse had occurred in 18% of the patients undergoing close follow-up only, compared with only 5.5% after radiotherapy—the total series including over 170 patients. Well-tolerated single-agent carboplatin chemotherapy may prove to be as effective yet less toxic [5]. However, a recent study of 99 patients with stage II seminoma, mostly treated by orchidectomy and radiation alone (without chemotherapy), confirmed the excellent results achieved in patients with small-volume disease [15]. Those with stage IIa or IIb had a relapse-free survival (RFS) rate of 89%—virtually all cured. For more bulky cases, the RFS dropped sharply, with chemotherapy clearly the preferred option. Infertility is not normally a problem following adjuvant radiation therapy, provided that the contralateral testis is protected from scattered irradiation by means of lead shielding. Where a scrotal operation such as orchidopexy, trans-scrotal biopsy or scrotal orchidectomy has been performed, the scrotal sac and ipsilateral inguinal nodes must also be treated. Although preservation of fertility cannot be guaranteed, an attempt at shielding the contralateral testis should certainly be made.

In patients with abdominal node involvement at presentation, the relapse rate following radiotherapy was closely dependent on tumour bulk (less than 10% for small-volume disease, over 50% for bulky node involvement). For this reason, patients with bulky abdominal disease are now routinely treated with chemotherapy prior to (or even instead of) irradiation.

For stages III and IV disease, chemotherapy gives much the best opportunity of cure, although some centres have reported encouraging results with whole-body irradiation. Occasionally, patients with 'pure' seminoma have an elevated serum β-HCG, and HCG can be demonstrated immunocytochemically. This does not appear to be associated with a worse prognosis. An elevated serum AFP is usually regarded as an indication for treatment as for non-seminomatous germ cell tumours (see below).

Although seminoma is a highly curable tumour, many questions of management remain unanswered. Treatment of early stage disease by orchidectomy alone (without adjuvant radiotherapy) is becoming increasingly popular since the surveillance results from major treatment centres are holding up well. Conversely, this approach is more difficult for seminoma than with non-seminomatous germ cell tumours; useful marker elevations are generally unavailable. In the recent Canadian study, however, only one of the 364 patients died of uncontrollable disease [14] despite the higher relapse rate in patients not given immediate adjuvant radiation therapy.

TERATOMA

For non-seminomatous germ cell tumours, chemotherapy has become the dominant form of treatment and radiotherapy is now much less widely employed. In the first place, surveillance of patients with stage I disease is associated with a high cure rate—at least 75%. Even more important, chemotherapy is almost always curative in the minority who do require treatment. With bulky stage II disease, the case for chemotherapy as the treatment of choice is totally established [16]. Patients with stages III and IV disease are usually cured with chemotherapy, although radiotherapy may still have a possible adjunctive role in the control of bulky abdominal disease (see below), though surgical resection of residual masses is generally preferred.

Chemotherapy

The emergence of chemotherapy for testicular teratoma has been one of the most exciting advances in cancer medicine over the past 25 years. In the early 1960s one or two agents were available with known but limited activity. The next important step was the recognition of further agents of different classes, each with major activity. Vinblastine, bleomycin and cisplatin and its derivatives were all identified as independently effective.

These highly toxic regimens were a major advance, later replaced by a regimen which added cisplatin, a highly effective agent, the most powerful of all the cytotoxics for this condition, also relatively free from bone marrow toxicity, making it particularly suitable as part of a combination regimen. Over 20 years ago, Einhorn and colleagues at Indiana developed a combination of cisplatin, vinblastine and bleomycin (PVB) in patients with advanced disease [17]. This regimen is still sometimes used, although newer, less toxic combinations—particularly bleomycin, etoposide and cisplatin (BEP)—have now largely replaced it [16]. At major centres both in the USA and Europe, BEP is generally regarded as the 'gold standard' chemotherapy for testicular cancer.

Despite the remarkable results of modern therapy, the acute toxicity of all these regimens remains a serious problem, with gastrointestinal disturbance, granulocytopenia and infection, nephrotoxicity and pulmonary fibrosis as the major hazards. In Einhorn's earlier series (using PVB), four patients died in complete remission—two of these deaths were drug-related. Bleomycin is used in relatively large doses in these regimens, and, as haematological toxicity has diminished, pulmonary toxicity from bleomycin has become increasingly recognized (see Chapter 6). An important study from the USA-based Eastern Cooperative Oncology Group confirmed, however, that bleomycin remains an extremely important component of therapy; both RFS and overall survival were better in the BEP group (86 and 95%) than in the dual-agent etoposide/cisplatin group (69 and 86%) [18]. Although carboplatin is less toxic to the gastrointestinal tract than cisplatin, it is more myelotoxic and thus more difficult to use in combination with vinblastine and bleomycin. Later consequences of successful therapy are discussed in more detail below .

Some patients are now recognized as having a particularly poor prognosis. Adverse features include: presence of liver, bone or brain metastases; AFP at presentation of more than 1000 ng/ml; α-HCG more than 10 000 ng/ml; LDH above 10 times normal; mediastinal primary site; mediastinal node mass more than 5 cm; or more than 20 pulmonary metastases. Such cases are probably better treated by a still more intensive chemotherapy regimen, and about two-thirds of this group appear curable (see below).

Table 19.3 Chemotherapy regimens commonly used for testicular cancer (see text) [16].

Regimen	Component drugs	Dosage	Days given
BEP: four cycles at 21-day intervals			
	Bleomycin	30 mg	1, 8, 15
	Etoposide	100 mg/m^2 per day	1–5
	Cisplatin	20 mg/m^2 per day	1–5
EP: same regimen without bleomycin			
VIP: Day 1 = day 21			
	Vinblastine	0.11 mg/kg per day	1 and 2
	Ifosfamide	1200 mg/m^2 per day	1–3
	Cisplatin	20 mg/m^2 per day	1–5
VeIP: day 1 = day 21			
	Etoposide	75 mg/m^2 per day	1–5
	Ifosfamide	1200 mg/m^2 per day	1–5
	Cisplatin	20 mg/m^2 per day	1–5

There is rarely any justification for giving more than four courses of similar chemotherapy. Although most patients are cured, it is important not to assume failure if after this time there is radiological evidence of residual disease—for example, visible lung metastases, which sometimes fade radiologically over several months. For treatment of late recurrence, or of truly refractory disease, the introduction of ifosfamide-based or other intensive regimens has for the first time given durable responses and a small proportion of cures. The VIP regimen (containing vincristine, ifosfamide and cisplatin or carboplatin) is one example of a logical combination; with BEP as the primary choice, patients treated with VIP will not previously have been exposed to vinblastine. High-dose stem-cell supported procedures have also been increasingly employed [19]. The use of chemotherapy for patients with less advanced disease needs further exploration, particularly where there is modest para-aortic involvement (stages IIa and IIb).

It is also clear that seminoma is a highly chemosensitive disease. Most cases present early, at a radiocurable stage, but for the few who have advanced disease or later develop recurrence, there was little effective chemotherapy until the advent of cisplatin-based regimens. Current practice includes combinations of drugs similar to those used for teratoma, with radiotherapy sometimes still given to sites of bulk disease. However, single-agent cisplatin may be as effective for metastatic seminoma as the more complex combination regimens, and is still undergoing evaluation in this setting [16].

Long-term consequences of chemotherapy has been studied in considerable detail. One report from Germany assessed a group of 90 patients (median follow-up 58 months) of whom only 19% were totally symptom-free [20]. Thirty per cent reported Raynaud's phenomenon, 21% had tinnitus or hearing loss, and two-thirds had elevation of follicle-stimulating hormone. Other abnormalities included persistent hypomagnesaemia, reduced Leydig cell functioning, arterial hypertension and peripheral neuropathy. Fortunately, second cancers are extremely unusual [9].

Surgery after chemotherapy and radiotherapy

Surgery has an important role where there is residual disease after orchidectomy. Abdominal 'debulking' surgery, and even excision of pulmonary metastases by repeated thoracotomy, are frequently performed. Postponing surgery to the end of the chemotherapy programme gives an accurate histological picture of the effect of preceding

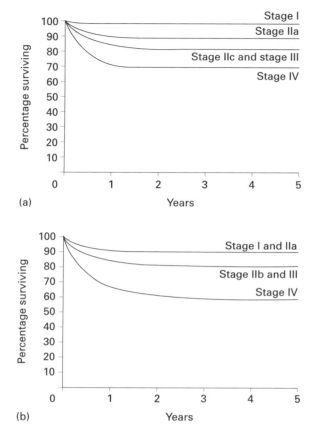

(a)

(b)

Fig. 19.6 Prognosis of testicular germ cell tumours related to stage: (a) seminoma; (b) teratoma (all types). These survival curves illustrate the dramatic improvement with advanced stages since the introduction of combination chemotherapy.

treatment, as well as removing tumour in patients with residual disease. Ideally, it should be performed only after tumour markers have fallen to undetectable levels and at least one additional course of chemotherapy has been given beyond this point. Many cases show clear evidence of treatment-induced differentiation into mature teratoma; although this observation is encouraging, its significance and implications for long-term survival are not entirely clear. Most appear to be cured, without relapse after several years' follow-up.

Prognosis of testicular tumours

Mortality from germ cell tumours continues to fall [16]. Stages I and II seminomas are nearly always curable by orchidectomy and radiotherapy (stage I, more than 95%;

stage II, 85–90%). The prognoses of bulky stage II (stage IIc) and stages III and IV have greatly improved with chemotherapy (Fig. 19.6a) and the majority are now cured even in these more advanced stages. It now seems clear that 80% of patients with stage I seminoma are cured by orchidectomy (surveillance alone), though adjuvant radiotherapy confers an even lower relapse rate [14].

In non-seminomatous germ cell tumours the prognosis is excellent for stage I and early stage II disease. In addition, well over 70% of all patients with stage III disease will be cured, but bulky disease and stage IV patients are still at risk of incomplete drug response and relapse. Nevertheless, the last decade has seen a great improvement even in this poor-prognosis group (Fig. 19.6b). Patients treated at specialist centres have a better prognosis with strict adherence to current treatment protocols. Results from large centres in the UK are among the best reported, with overall survival of 80–90% following treatment with regimens containing cisplatin, bleomycin, vinblastine, etoposide and/or other drugs. Poor-prognosis patients clearly require special attention and specialist referral [16,21]. An international germ cell consensus classification has been agreed, allowing metastatic cases to be reliably grouped as 'good', 'intermediate' or 'poor' prognosis [22]. The major effort in poor-prognosis patients lies in generating new chemotherapy programmes to improve on established regimens, and to ensure through public education that late initial presentation occurs as infrequently as possible [23].

Extragonadal germ cell tumours

Primary extragonadal germ cell tumours are extremely uncommon, but have been described in a variety of sites including the retroperitoneum, anterior mediastinum, suprasellar or pineal area and the presacral region. Although the pathogenesis is not entirely clear, it is possible that these tumours result from malignant change in primordial germ cells which have migrated incompletely (cell 'rests') or in cells displaced during embryogenesis. There appears to be a genetic predisposition at least in some cases, since Klinefelter's syndrome is a well-described predisposing feature.

The commonest sites are the anterior mediastinum (1% of all mediastinal tumours) and retroperitoneum. In occasional cases, an associated congenital or developmental abnormality is present. The largest group are mixed tumours, but pure seminomas are more common than pure teratomas or choriocarcinomas. Since primary testicular tumours can be small and impalpable, one should always be wary when diagnosing a germ cell tumour apparently arising from an extratesticular site, since metastases from an occult primary do occur. Acute leukaemia has been described in conjunction with mediastinal germ cell tumours.

Both teratomas and seminomas show the same radiosensitivity and chemosensitivity as for primary testicular tumours. For mediastinal seminoma, surgery followed by radiotherapy appears effective, with long-term survival rates of about 50%. However, in bulky disease chemotherapy can be extremely effective at reducing tumour volume (eliminating the need for wide-field irradiation of the lungs) and is increasingly preferred. Similar regimens are used, as for testicular primaries. For primary mediastinal non-seminomatous germ cell tumours, recent reports show good responses to modern chemotherapy, usually including cisplatin, vinblastine, etoposide, bleomycin and actinomycin D.

Primary germ cell tumours of the brain are treated somewhat differently. Most of these are pineal or suprasellar tumours; both teratomas and seminomas occur. These latter can sometimes be cured by wide-field irradiation, including full irradiation of the whole central nervous system. The 5-year survival rate in children with radiosensitive pineal tumours (usually not biopsied but assumed to be seminoma or the less common pinealoblastoma) is 50%. With proven pineal teratomas (biopsyproven or where the AFP or β-HCG are clearly raised) the outlook is less good, although response to chemotherapy can be dramatic.

The apparent rarity of extragonadal germ cell tumours may have to be revised in the light of recent reports describing patients originally thought to have undifferentiated carcinomas but with a clinical course and response to chemotherapy much more suggestive of extragonadal germ cell tumour. This has been described as the 'atypical teratoma syndrome' and in the majority of cases, serum markers (AFP and β-HCG) are raised, with subsequent staining of tissue sections by immunoperoxidase techniques showing intracellular AFP and β-HCG. Treatment with BEP or PVB is effective, with a high proportion of complete responders. In young men with mediastinal tumours which on biopsy prove to be 'poorly differentiated carcinoma' it is therefore essential to consider this diagnosis and to measure plasma β-HCG and AFP. Even if these are negative, it is so important not to overlook this potentially curable tumour that response to platinum-based regimens should be fully assessed.

Management of non-germ cell tumours of the testis

Orchidectomy alone is usually sufficient for Leydig and Sertoli cell tumours since these rarely metastasize. Lymphomas of the testis are usually large-cell centroblastic B-cell neoplasms. As they are frequently bilateral, irradiation of the contralateral testis is usually recommended even if the disease appears localized. These patients need careful staging as for other lymphomas (see Chapter 26). With paratesticular rhabdomyosarcomas, occult metastasis is so frequent that adjuvant combination chemotherapy is essential (see Chapter 24).

References

1 Moller H, Jorgensen N, Furman D. Trends in incidence of testicular cancer in boys and adolescent men. *Int J Cancer* 1995; 61: 761–4.
2 Harland SJ. Conundrum of the hereditary component of testicular cancer. *Lancet* 2000; 356: 1455–6.
3 Parker L. Causes of testicular cancer. *Lancet* 1997; 350: 827–8.
4 Oliver RTD. Testicular cancer. *Curr Opin Oncol* 1996; 8: 252–8.
5 Nicholson P, Harland SJ. Inheritance and testicular cancer. *Br J Cancer* 1995; 71: 421–6.
6 Swerdlow AJ, Huttly SRA, Smith PG. Testicular cancer and antecedent diseases. *Br J Cancer* 1987; 55: 97–103.
7 Chagant RSK, Rodriguez E, Bosl GJ. Cytogenetics of male germ-cell tumours. *Urol Clin N Am* 1993; 20: 55–66.
8 Dixon FJ, Moore RA. Testicular tumours: a clinicopathological study. *Cancer* 1953; 6: 427.
9 Bosl GJ, Motzer RJ. Medical progress: Testicular germ-cell cancer. *N Engl J Med* 1997; 337: 242–53.
10 Giwercman A, Grinsted J, Hansen B *et al.* Testicular cancer risk in boys with maldescended testis: a cohort study. *J Urol* 1987; 138: 1214–16.
11 Oliver RTD, Leahy M, Ong J. Combined seminoma/nonseminoma should be considered as intermediate grade germ cell cancer. *Eur J Cancer* 1995; 31A (13): 92–4.
12 Donohue JP, Thornhill JA, Foster RS *et al.* Primary retroperitoneal lymph node dissection in clinical stage A nonseminomatous germ cell testis cancer: review of the Indiana University experience 1965–89. *Br J Urol* 1993; 71: 326–35.
13 Read G, Stenning SP, Cullen MH *et al.* Medical Research Council prospective study of surveillance for stage I testicular teratoma. *J Clin Oncol* 1992; 10: 1762–8.
14 Warde P, Gospodarowicz MK, Panzarella T *et al.* Stage I testicular seminoma: Results of adjuvant irradiation and surveillance. *J Clin Oncol* 1995; 13: 2255–62.

15 Warde P, Gospodarowicz M, Panzarella T *et al.* Management of stage II seminoma. *J Clin Oncol* 1998; 16: 290–4.

16 Oliver RTD. Chemotherapy in testis cancer. In: *Comprehensive Urology* (ed. R.M. Weiss, N.J.R. George, P.M. O'Reilly). London: Mosby, 2000: 673–8

17 Einhorn L, Donohue JP. *Cis*-diamine-chloroplatinum, vinblastine and bleomycin combination chemotherapy in disseminated testicular cancer. *Ann Intern Med* 1977; 87: 293–8.

18 Loehrer P, Johnson D, Elson P *et al.* Importance of bleomycin in favorable prognosis disseminated germ cell tumors: an Eastern Co-operative Oncology Group Trial. *J Clin Oncol* 1995; 13: 470–6.

19 Lotz J-P, Andre T, Donsimoni R *et al.* High-dose chemotherapy with ifosfamide, carboplatin and etoposide combined with autologous bone marrow transplantation for the treatment of poor-prognosis germ cell tumors and metabolic trophoblastic disease in adults. *Cancer* 1995; 75: 874–85.

20 Bokemeyer C, Berger CC, Kuczyk MA, Schmoll H-J. Evaluation of long-term toxicity after chemotherapy for testicular cancer. *J Clin Oncol* 1996; 14: 2923–32.

21 Stiller CA. Non-specialist units, clinical trials and survival from testicular cancer. *Eur J Cancer* 1995; 31A: 289–91.

22 International Germ Cell Collaborative Group. International germ cell consensus classification: a prognostic-factor based staging system for metastatic germ cell cancers. *J Clin Oncol* 1997; 15: 594–603.

23 Steele JPC, Oliver RTD. Testicular cancer: perils of very late presentation. *Lancet* 2002; 359: 1632–3.

Thyroid and adrenal cancer

Cancer of the thyroid

Thyroid cancer is exceptional in many ways. First of all, some thyroid cancers are very indolent with a long natural history, often over many decades, even where complete control of the tumour has not been achieved. Second, because most thyroid cancers take up iodine, the use of oral radioactive iodine—a highly specific therapy—can destroy both normal and neoplastic thyroid cells, with total ablation of the tumour and excellent 20-year survival rates. Third, in the majority of patients with metastases from well-differentiated thyroid carcinomas, the metastatic lesions retain their important characteristic radioiodine uptake, so that even patients with metastatic disease at presentation can be treated successfully. If necessary, these treatments can be repeated several times, using whole-body isotope scanning for assessment of progress and to determine whether further therapy is required [1].

There are important histological and behavioural differences between the major types of thyroid cancer which help to determine treatment strategy (Table 20.1). Although these tumour subgroups are well defined, several types of thyroid carcinoma have been recognized only recently, and further histopathological refinements seem likely [2]. The clinician needs a complete histopathological description of the tumour which should include not only the tumour type but also the degree of differentiation, since tumour grading is now known to have important prognostic significance [3]. The degree of local invasion into blood vessels, local structures and adjacent lymph nodes should also be described.

Aetiology and incidence

There are about 14 000 new cases registered each year in the USA, and about 1100 deaths. In Britain the annual reported incidence is 2.3 (women) and 0.9 (men) per 100 000—about 900 new cases annually for England and Wales. A number of aetiological factors have now been described. Like other thyroid diseases, thyroid cancer is commoner in women than in men (Fig. 20.1), with a bimodal age distribution. The lower age peak of incidence is due to papillary and follicular tumours, and the rise in incidence in older patients is chiefly due to anaplastic cancers. Both thyrotoxicosis and Hashimoto's thyroiditis share a similar age distribution with well-differentiated thyroid carcinomas. About 90% of all cases of thyroid cancer are differentiated (papillary and follicular—see below) with, potentially, an excellent prognosis. It is clearly one of the radiation-related cancers, more frequent both in survivors of the atom bomb and following childhood irradiation of the neck (the latter with a 50-fold increased incidence), usually with a latent period of 10–30 years. The risk of carcinogenesis is higher in females, or where the radiation exposure occurred in very young children. Medullary thyroid carcinoma has both a familial and a sporadic incidence and may form part of the syndromes of multiple endocrine neoplasia (MEN; see Chapter 15).

Pathology

Papillary carcinoma

The commonest type of cancer is papillary carcinoma (Fig. 20.2), comprising about 60% of all thyroid cancers, with a slightly greater proportion of those occurring in childhood. In at least 20% of cases the tumour appears to be multifocal in origin, and in older patients tends to have a more aggressive clinical course, with correspondingly poorer survival. Papillary carcinomas are almost three times commoner in women, with a peak incidence in the

Table 20.1 Pathology of thyroid cancers.

Tumour	Epidemiology	Presentation	Macroscopic features	Microscopic features	Natural history: 10-year survival (%)
Papillary	60% of all thyroid cancers (Clinically overt) PI: 20–50 years W > M	Occult Clinically overt: clinically palpable palpablenodal metastasis	Well defined Non-encapsulated	Cuboidal or columnar cell with characteristic large pale nuclei with nuclei with an empty appearance (orphan Annie) Papillae: fibrovascular core Psammoma bodies: spherical, calcified, laminated glycoprotein bodies	95 Cure rate is high. In those not cured, the clinical course is indolent
Medullary	10% of thyroid cancers	Sporadic (80–90%) Hereditary: inherited in an autosomal dominant fashion. Can be assoc. with MEN syndrome type IIA or IIB	Sporadic tumours: single and unilateral Hereditary: multifocal and bilateral	Presence of amyloid in the tumour stroma	Sporadic 60 Hereditary 40
Anaplastic	10–15% of thyroid malignancies	Believed to arise from pre-existing, well-differentiated tumour. Hx of antecedent goitre	Invasive at time of presentation: thyroid and surrounding soft tissue	Variable: spindle cells to large squamoid epithelial cells	Worst prognosis: mean survival, 6–8 months after presentation

third and fourth decades. Any differentiated thyroid tumour that contains neoplastic papillae is by definition a papillary carcinoma, regardless of the presence of neoplastic follicles. The tumour is made up of cuboid cells and often contains psammoma bodies. A characteristic feature of papillary tumours is large empty nuclei—so-called 'orphan Annie' nuclei. Over 90% of these tumours appear to be encapsulated, but lymph node invasion is common, though not necessarily prognostically important. Occasionally, papillary microcarcinomas (even up to 1 cm in size) are discovered in thyroidectomy specimens where a neoplasm was not suspected preoperatively. These small clinically undetected tumours can generally be ignored (from the point of view of further treatment) unless adjacent to one of the resection margins. Larger tumours, with evidence of extrathyroid invasion and/or invasion of the thyroid capsule, are associated with a worse prognosis, though in general this is a slowly growing and fully resectable tumour, with a low overall mortality.

Follicular tumours

Follicular tumours (Fig. 20.2) are much less common (about 15% of all cases), often occurring in patients with a long history of goitre. They are unusual in children and are seen in a rather older age group than the papillary carcinomas, again with a slight female predominance. The mean age of diagnosis is about 10 years greater than for papillary cancer (52 compared with 41 years for patients with resectable disease [1]). Overall prognosis is good (Table 20.1). Lymph node involvement is uncommon, as the main route of dissemination is via the bloodstream

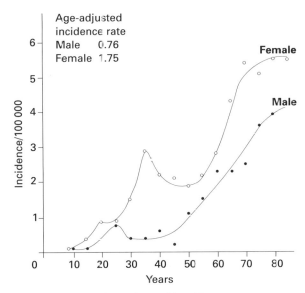

Fig. 20.1 Age-specific incidence of thyroid cancer.

with lung and bone as the commonest sites of metastasis. Histologically, microangioinvasion is a common feature even though, as with papillary carcinomas, over 90% of these tumours appear macroscopically encapsulated. The presence of tumour within the capsular venous sinusoids or permeation of extrathyroidal veins are both important adverse prognostic features. The tumour can be difficult to distinguish from atypical adenomas, since the presence of nuclear pleomorphism and even bizarre nuclear forms is not necessarily tantamount to true malignancy, in the absence of evidence of microangioinvasion.

Medullary thyroid tumours

Medullary thyroid tumours (Fig. 20.2) have a quite different derivation and are thought to arise from the parafollicular or C cells. The disease is often familial (see below). Typically, the stroma of the tumour has an amyloid appearance and the tumour itself may be bilateral. Medullary thyroid tumours have a high metastatic potential both to lymph nodes and to the bloodstream, and the extent of lymph node involvement is an important guide to prognosis [4]. The large majority secrete calcitonin, a particularly important tumour marker in view of the familial incidence of the disease and the obvious importance of identifying affected family members as early as possible [5]. Equally important is the use of the calcitonin assay for monitoring results of therapy. Familial medullary carcinoma of the thyroid is defined by the pres-

ence of the disease in four or more family members with no other evidence of MEN syndromes (see below) after careful screening. These cases tend to have a later onset than in MEN-2-associated cases, often behaving clinically in a more indolent fashion [5]. DNA testing can be particularly valuable in apparently familial cases, especially if the patient is under 40 years of age or has C-cell hyperplasia or multifocal tumours. If the test reveals no mutations in exons 10, 11, 13, 14 and 16 of the *RET* proto-oncogene, then the probability of the patient having MEN-2 is extremely low [6].

In the past, most patients reached the age of 30 years by the time of diagnosis. The mean age at diagnosis is expected to drop in the future, since the familial nature of the tumour is well understood and the use of the calcitonin assay has now become widespread.

Multiple endocrine neoplasia

Other abnormalities are sometimes present in familial cases, particularly phaeochromocytoma and hyperparathyroidism—the so-called MEN syndromes, which can occur with both sporadic or familial forms of medullary thyroid cancer. The disorders are inherited as an autosomal dominant with a high degree of penetrance but variable expression. The commonest variant of MEN, *Werner's syndrome*, can involve the thyroid and parathyroid glands, the pancreatic islets, pituitary or adrenal cortex (see Chapter 15). Two-thirds of patients have tumours of at least two of these endocrine glands. The second type of MEN, *Sipple's syndrome*, includes more patients with medullary thyroid carcinoma; approximately 95% of patients with MEN-2 will develop medullary carcinoma of the thyroid; 50% also have parathyroid hyperplasia and/or phaeochromocytoma. Mutations in the *RET* proto-oncogene, which codes for a tyrosine kinase receptor, have been implicated in over 90% of families with MEN-2, and predictive DNA testing of at-risk family members can now be performed [6]. Medullary thyroid cancer may be associated with ectopic hormone production from the thyroid tumour itself, and may produce adrenocorticotrophic hormone, vasoactive intestinal peptide and also prostaglandins and serotonin.

The gene for MEN-2a (medullary thyroid cancer, phaeochromocytoma and parathyroid hyperplasia) is inherited as an autosomal dominant trait with incomplete penetrance so that 40% of carriers do not present with symptoms until 70 years of age [7,8]. About 90% of patients with MEN-2 have type 2a disease; the less common 2b variety is usually clinically apparent at an earlier age be-

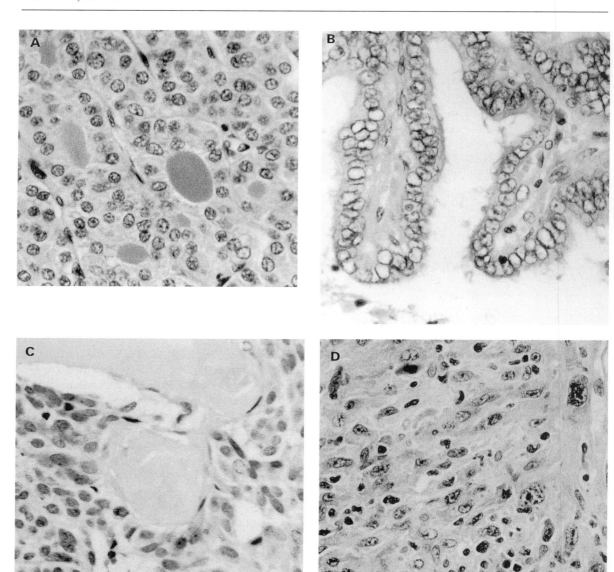

Fig. 20.2 Histological appearances in thyroid cancer: (A) follicular carcinoma showing follicle formation ($\times 200$); (B) papillary carcinoma showing characteristic 'empty' nuclei ($\times 200$); (C) medullary carcinoma showing small cells with masses of amyloid ($\times 200$); (D) anaplastic carcinoma ($\times 200$).

cause of a characteristic facial appearance. Detection of presymptomatic carriers by provocation of calcitonin release identifies 90% by the age of 25 years, but DNA analysis is more reliable still [9]. The gene is located in the pericentromeric region of chromosome 10, and studies using DNA restriction fragment polymorphism provide an accurate identification of the carrier state. A consensus statement from the European Community Medullary Thyroid Carcinoma Group has offered guidelines for a combined biochemical genetic MEN-2 screening, which should lead to rapid improvement in early detection and cure [6]. In patients at risk for MEN-2a and medullary carcinoma, prophylactic thyroidectomy is increasingly performed [10].

Anaplastic carcinoma

Anaplastic carcinoma of the thyroid (Fig. 20.2) is the predominant form in elderly people, with 75% of patients beyond 60 years of age at diagnosis. They form about 15% of all thyroid cancers, frequently occurring in women (3:2). Unlike well-differentiated thyroid cancer, they are generally rapidly growing tumours, often painful and with pressure symptoms as an early feature, apparently arising in a long-standing goitre. The course of these tumours is quite different from that of the more slowly growing varieties commoner in younger patients, and several histological subtypes have been recognized, including spindle and giant-cell carcinomas in which there may be areas of well-differentiated carcinoma, supporting the suggestion that they sometimes arise from transformation of pre-existing well-differentiated thyroid cancer.

A very small number of 'anaplastic' carcinomas are characterized by infiltration with small lymphocyte-like cells, and are generally known as *small-cell* carcinomas of the thyroid. These are typically found in elderly patients and are rapidly growing and locally invasive. *Thyroid lymphomas* are discussed in Chapter 26.

Diagnosis and investigation

Patients usually present with a firm mass in the neck, due either to the primary thyroid mass or to an involved cervical lymph node. It is sometimes possible to classify the thyroid mass on clinical grounds as obviously benign, suspicious of cancer or 'probable' [11,12], although only a minority of thyroid cancers present with symptoms or signs of real prognostic value, and most cases have a benign cause. In making these distinctions, useful clinical criteria include the size and position of the mass, its mobility and the presence of signs of compression of vital structures in the neck.

Non-malignant conditions can simulate thyroid cancer; these include benign adenomas and multinodular goitres, as well as less common causes such as thyroglossal or colloid retention cysts. These may cause particular difficulty since they also produce the 'cold' nodule on thyroid isotope scanning so characteristic of malignant neoplasms (Fig. 20.3). Ultrasound scanning will distinguish between cystic and solid lesions and is useful for monitoring and follow-up—for example, for a colloid nodule. The circulating thyroglobulin level may be elevated, but the test is still regarded by many as an unreliable marker of malignancy. Evidence of microcalcification in a soft-tissue X-ray, although rarely seen, is strongly suggestive of papillary

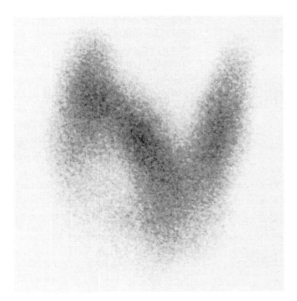

Fig. 20.3 ^{123}I scan of thyroid, showing a cold nodule in the enlarged right node.

carcinoma, and is due to the psammoma bodies. Apart from the mass itself, and the pressure effects such as stridor or recurrent laryngeal nerve involvement, patients with medullary carcinoma occasionally present with systemic endocrine symptoms from an associated MEN syndrome [6]. Most patients with thyroid cancer are clinically euthyroid. Autoimmune thyroiditis is associated with high levels of antithyroglobulin antibodies, low ^{131}I uptake and diffuse glandular enlargement—a syndrome quite different from de Quervain's subacute thyroiditis, in which the thyroid is often painful or tender.

In general, thyroid scans suggestive of a 'cold' nodule— one which fails to take up radioiodine—should be regarded as potentially malignant. Fine-needle aspiration cytology (rather than open surgical biopsy) is usually adequate as the initial investigation. In the first place, this will immediately identify a thyroid cyst, to the great relief of the patient. Furthermore, cytological testing generally reveals the nature of the malignant lesion, with accurate prediction of the neoplastic cell type, though one limitation is that with follicular carcinoma the distinction between benign and malignant may be impossible, in which case surgical biopsy is essential. At most, only 20% of these patients will prove to have a malignant neoplasm. Radionuclide scanning may be useful when the fine-needle aspiration specimen is 'suspicious' or indeterminate rather than clearly diagnostic, identifying 'hot' nodules which can be observed or treated medically [13]. In order to make an unequivocal diagnosis, hemithyroidectomy may sometimes be necessary or, in the case of larger lesions, partial or subtotal removal. For papillary (the largest single subtype), medullary and anaplastic cancers, needle aspiration may be sufficient, whereas in follicular carcinoma, important histological features may not be recognizable in such small specimens. With routine fine-needle biopsy, only about half as many patients require diagnostic thyroidectomy for thyroid nodules, and a far higher proportion of surgically treated patients do indeed have cancer [14].

Surgical management

A substantial thyroid resection may have been undertaken for diagnostic confirmation, consisting of unilateral thyroid lobectomy (hemithyroidectomy) with resection of the isthmus. However, there is no clear agreement, once the diagnosis has been established, as to whether the surgeon must then undertake a further operation to complete a total or near-total thyroidectomy. The risk of surgically induced hypoparathyroidism is low—probably about 3% in experienced hands. Repeat operations by inexperienced surgeons undoubtedly increase this hazard. In small cancers, completely enclosed by normal tissues, it may seem unjustifiable to advocate further surgery in view of the surgical risks. Nevertheless, routine total thyroidectomy is often recommended, even for *well-differentiated papillary tumours*, because of the high incidence of microscopic foci in the contralateral lobe [1,8]. A common recommendation in the UK is that a near-total or subtotal thyroidectomy be performed, though the use of serum thyroglobulin for follow-up has in recent years tended to modify this view. Younger patients under 40 years of age, with histopathology confirming a well-differentiated tumour, apparently completely removed, can be given suppressive thyroxine (T_4) to reduce thyroid-stimulating hormone (TSH) to an undetectable level (0.2 mU/l) on current highly sensitive immunoradiometric assays, with follow-up using serum thyroglobulin as a marker (see below). The availability of thyroglobin testing, coupled with a move towards more conservative surgery, has led to a controversy in selection of treatment options which has yet to be resolved.

For *follicular carcinomas* total thyroidectomy is usually best even in cases where metastases are present at the time of diagnosis, though this carries a risk of permanent hypoparathyroidism. In cases of papillary and follicular carcinomas, any obviously enlarged lymph nodes should be removed at the initial operation. *En bloc* resection of

the thyroid gland and pathological nodes should be attempted even if bilateral lymph nodes are present. Despite the high incidence of histologically confirmed malignancies in clinically impalpable lymph nodes (probably of the order of 50%), prophylactic lymph node dissection is not usually recommended since recurrence after subsequent postoperative treatment with radioiodine will occur in less than 30% of patients.

In *papillary carcinoma*, the presence of palpable lymph nodes at diagnosis does not appear to affect the prognosis. There is no difference in outcome between patients treated by prophylactic neck dissection in whom lymph node involvement is confirmed histologically, and those with a later nodal recurrence who are then treated by therapeutic lymph node dissection (and possibly other methods as well). This is particularly true of the largest group of low-risk patients: women under 40 years of age with well-differentiated tumours.

With *medullary carcinomas*, routine neck node dissection is sometimes recommended, in addition to total thyroidectomy [11], a view substantiated by the high local recurrence rate of the order of 25%. For *anaplastic carcinomas* surgical removal of the tumour should be attempted wherever possible, although this is often technically difficult since early direct extension is the rule and tissue planes may be hopelessly destroyed. These tumours are only partly responsive to external beam irradiation so surgical removal of as much tumour as possible is important, even where this involves cutting directly across tumour. Because of the frequency of compression of the oesophagus, pharynx and trachea, maintenance of the airway by tracheostomy is often required.

For true *small-cell carcinomas* and *lymphomas* of the thyroid, thyroidectomy is unnecessary although it is occasionally performed for biopsy purposes. Where these tumours are suspected, 'Tru-cut' or other needle biopsy procedures are more often employed in order to avoid thyroidectomy wherever possible. They are highly radiosensitive, and surgery plays a correspondingly small part in the management.

The role of radiotherapy

RADIOIODINE THERAPY (^{131}I)

Use of ^{131}I has been an integral part of treatment for well differentiated thyroid carcinoma for almost 50 years [15]. Postoperative management depends on histological findings, extent of disease and completeness of surgery. In most cases of *well-differentiated thyroid cancer* (both papillary and follicular), ablation of residual thyroid tissue, together with neck and whole-body scanning, should be carried out postoperatively, using oral radioactive iodine, particularly if there is any doubt as to the completeness of surgery. About half of all follicular carcinomas fall into this category, rather fewer in the papillary group. Treatment with ^{131}I is not necessary for all well-differentiated tumours [16] since occult and intrathyroid carcinomas have an excellent prognosis following surgery alone, and high doses of radioactive iodine can generally be avoided with safety in these predominantly young patients for whom radiation dose is an important consideration.

For patients in whom ^{131}I treatment is required, a moderately large dose should be given, of the order of 3 GBq (the becquerel has now replaced the curie; 1 Ci = 37 GBq) to ablate the residual thyroid tissue which always takes up iodine more avidly than the tumour, making therapeutic use of ^{131}I impossible in the presence of a significant volume of active residual thyroid tissue (Fig. 20.4). If thyroxine (T4) has been administered postoperatively, this must be discontinued 1 month before the radioiodine treatment, in order to ensure that the TSH rises. It is the rise in TSH rather than the hormone withdrawal that is important. After ^{131}I radioablation has been performed, a short 6-week course of triiodothyronine (T3) is then given (in preference to T4 which has a much longer duration of action and is therefore less flexible). After withdrawal of T3 for 10 days, neck and whole-body scanning is again performed; residual uptake in the neck or elsewhere provides evidence of metastatic or unresected primary cancer. If this is demonstrated a therapeutic dose of [131]I (5.5–7.0 GBq) is indicated. It is the most highly targeted type of radiation therapy in common use for human cancer treatment and can be repeated at approximately 3-monthly intervals (discontinuing exogenous T3 10 days beforehand) for as long as the repeat scans confirm residual active disease; that is, until the metastases are totally eradicated or treatment fails. An alternative to withdrawal of thyroid hormone therapy is the use of recombinant human thyrotropin [17].

Despite the dangers of significant radiation doses to the neck, marrow, gonads and other sites, it is important to realize that this specific and cytotoxic form of irradiation has produced many cures even in patients with widely metastatic disease. These patients (indeed most patients with thyroid cancer) need lifelong T4 replacement since all thyroid tissue will have been ablated long before the final therapeutic dose. In a proportion of patients no longer responsive to radioiodine, hormone replacement with T4 may produce further regression of disease (particularly in younger patients) because of the partial tumour dependency on TSH, which is suppressed by exogenous T4. Occasionally it is necessary to give therapeutic doses of ^{131}I when the patient has only just discontinued taking T3 or T4. In these cases TSH should be given for 2–3 days (by injection) before the ^{131}I is administered.

Although routine use of postoperative ^{131}I ablation is now regarded as overtreatment of many surgically treated cases of papillary carcinoma, the indications for use of radioiodine in selected patients were well demonstrated in classic studies by Mazzaferri and coworkers (Italy) [18] and by Tubiana and coworkers (France) [19]. Adverse features include age 40 years or over, a large primary tumour,

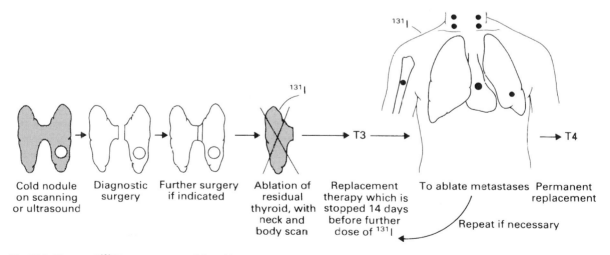

Cold nodule on scanning or ultrasound → Diagnostic surgery → Further surgery if indicated → Ablation of residual thyroid, with neck and body scan → Replacement therapy which is stopped 14 days before further dose of [131]I → T3 → To ablate metastases / Repeat if necessary → T4 → Permanent replacement

Fig. 20.4 The use of ^{131}I in management of thyroid cancer.

poorly differentiated histological features and extracapsular extension. Local recurrence is more than twice as common after subtotal as after total thyroidectomy and may result in increased mortality. Radioiodine ablation is indicated where adequate uptake can be demonstrated in patients with multiple, locally invasive, or large primary tumours, as well as those with distant metastases. Finally, the routine use of T4 is valuable even in patients who have not undergone total thyroidectomy and who do not require it for physiological replacement.

Follow-up investigation and examinations are particularly important as patients may develop recurrences many years after apparent cure. Follow-up should include careful clinical palpation of the thyroid, regular chest radiography (about once every 3 years since pulmonary metastases and mediastinal nodes are relatively common sites), together with serum thyroglobulin measurements. Radioiodine tests are now much less used, and serum thyroglobulin can and should be measured when the patient is taking T4 [20], yearly for the first 5 years after the patient is regarded as disease-free, and every second year of follow-up thereafter. Radioiodine testing (185 MBq is accepted as a safe outpatient dosage), with scanning 3–5 days afterwards, is increasingly used only in patients with an abnormal thyroglobulin level or in those known to have residual tumour postoperatively.

EXTERNAL IRRADIATION

In patients without adequate uptake of radioiodine, and particularly those which are locally unresectable (including almost all cases of anaplastic carcinoma and many medullary carcinomas), external irradiation has an important role. A radical dose is required, typically of the order of 65 Gy in 7 weeks [21], in order to delay local recurrence and prevent troublesome symptoms from local obstruction. It can be curative, though rarely in patients with anaplastic carcinoma. In patients with *thyroid lymphomas* and *small-cell tumours*, both of which are highly radiosensitive, external beam irradiation is the definitive treatment [22]. For these tumours a lower dose is adequate, of the order of 40–50 Gy in 4–5 weeks. Since the total volume treated can be very substantial and at a site where spinal cord damage is a real threat, radical irradiation of the thyroid is technically difficult, and several groups have developed sophisticated techniques using wedged field arrangements or arc rotation planning. Others prefer a more straightforward approach with a single anterior direct field, shaped by lead blocks in order to protect the larynx and, if necessary, the lungs. The radiation fields should cover the whole thyroid gland, and if possible the first-stage supraclavicular or cervical lymph nodes. The field may have to be extended inferiorly to include the upper mediastinal area if there is evidence of disease at this level. Intratracheal deposits, for example, are well described and can lead to haemoptysis.

RESULTS OF TREATMENT

For well-differentiated tumours the results of treatment are remarkably good. One substantial subgroup of patients—those below 40 years of age with well-differentiated papillary carcinoma—have a normal survival pattern equal to that of a comparable population. The prognosis is affected by the age at diagnosis (the lower the better) and by the sex of the patient. One large American Series, for example, confirmed a 10-year survival rate of 93% (papillary cancer) and 84% (follicular cancer) despite some patients developing local or even distant metastases [23]. Histological type also correlates with survival and, in general, the more well-differentiated the tumour the better the prognosis. For papillary carcinoma, evidence of extrathyroid disease reduces the 10-year survival to about 50%. For medullary carcinomas the survival is only about 40% [21,24], a reflection of its early metastatic potential and the ineffectiveness of ^{131}I therapy, itself a reflection of its different histogenesis. Worst of all, anaplastic carcinoma has a very poor prognosis with about 5% of patients surviving 5 years and essentially no 10-year survivors. It is important to distinguish small-cell carcinomas and thyroid lymphomas from the truly anaplastic group, since their prognosis is undoubtedly better, and thyroid lymphoma, though uncommon, has an extremely good prognosis. For anaplastic carcinoma even highly aggressive treatment including surgery, external irradiation (and sometimes chemotherapy) has failed to improve the outlook [25].

It is difficult to assess the separate contributions of surgery and radiation therapy since they are used in a complementary fashion, with radiotherapy only offered to patients with incompletely resected tumours—those with a higher risk of local recurrence and poorer ultimate survival. Nevertheless, Tubiana and coworkers' group [19] achieved a 10-year survival rate of over 70% in patients with papillary carcinoma who had undergone incomplete surgery. In follicular and medullary carcinoma the 10-year survival rates were 51 and 60%, respectively. For patients presenting with metastases, treatment with radioiodine (sometimes in combination with external irradiation to the primary tumour) may be very successful, with an overall survival rate of about 22% at 12 years. This reflects not only the effectiveness of ^{131}I therapy but also the indolent nature of this tumour, even when metastatic.

Chemotherapy for recurrent or metastatic thyroid cancer has been disappointing. The most active single agent is doxorubicin, with a response rate of about 30%, and with proven activity in all cell types. In addition, bleomycin has produced well-documented responses, and combinations of these and other agents have now been employed by several groups, reportedly with better response rates than with single agents alone. Duration of response is on the whole very short, quite apart from the fact that many of these patients are elderly and have rapidly advancing disease. Chemotherapy has only a limited role in the management of metastatic carcinoma of the thyroid, and treatment with external irradiation, radioiodine and exogenous T4 should always be considered first.

Overall, about 8–10% of patients with thyroid cancer die of their disease [26]. Despite the excellent overall result in many patients with well-differentiated cancers, follow-up should be lifelong because of the lengthy natural history [26].

Cancer of the adrenal gland

These rare tumours arise either from the adrenal cortex or the medulla, and in adults the ratio of adrenocortical carcinoma to malignant medullary tumours (malignant phaeochromocytoma) is approximately 2:1. Neuroblastoma, a common childhood tumour chiefly arising from the medulla, is discussed in Chapter 24.

Adrenocortical carcinoma

About a quarter of patients with adult Cushing's syndrome who have no obvious source of ectopic hormone production have an adrenal tumour, of which 30% are malignant [27]. Fewer than 30 cases are diagnosed in the UK per annum, most of which are hormonally active, presenting with features of Cushing's syndrome. In adrenal carcinoma patients, virilization, feminization or hyperaldosteronism (Conn's syndrome) are more common than in benign adenomas, although 30% of adrenocortical carcinomas are non-functional. The mean age at presentation is 45 years, with a female:male ratio of 2.5:1. Symptoms are usually present for 6–12 months before diagnosis, including glucocorticoid excess (45%), androgen excess (15%), both glucocorticoids and androgens (35%), and mineralocorticoids or oestrogens (5%). Benign adrenocortical tumours are typically yellowish in appearance and are adenomas often with lipid-laden large-cell or giant-cell patterns. Malignancy is likely if the mass is greater than 6 cm in diameter, characteristically with a more obviously necrotic or haemorrhagic appearance, with pleomorphic morphology and frequent mitoses. The distinction between adenoma and low-grade carcinoma can be difficult. Vascular invasion and distant dissemination (chiefly to bone, lung and liver) can occur.

At presentation 70% have locoregional disease and 30% have metastases. The diagnosis is usually made biochemically (persistent hypercortisolaemia with absent dexamethasone suppression and low plasma adrenocorticotrophic hormone), by computed tomography (CT) or magnetic resonance imaging (MRI) confirmation (Fig. 20.5) and, ultimately, tissue diagnosis following laparotomy or CT-guided biopsy. Adrenal hyperplasia is usually bilateral, so unilateral adrenal enlargement is strongly suspicious of a benign or malignant tumour. Other imaging techniques include ultrasound and selective angiography with venous sampling. Non-functional tumours are more difficult to diagnose preoperatively and generally occur in patients under 20 years of age. Clinical features include a palpable abdominal mass (often a substantial size because of the 'silent' nature of the tumour), weight loss or fever.

Treatment is primarily surgical, with wide resection usually via a substantial thoracoabdominal incision and preoperative steroid therapy with metastatic disease, systemic treatment with o,p'-DDD (a derivative of the insecticide DDT) can be beneficial, although side-effects can be extremely troublesome, often necessitating a reduction in dosage. In the majority of patients both a reduction in corticosteroid production and tumour regression can occur. Mitotane can often be given with little adverse effect, but

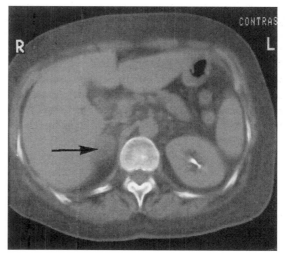

Fig. 20.5 CT scan of abdomen showing adrenal tumour (arrowed). Normal anatomy of other structures is also clearly shown.

the full daily dosage of 8–10 g may produce side-effects of anorexia, nausea, diarrhoea, confusion and lethargy, limiting treatment acceptability. These effects are largely due to contamination with DDT, and the pure drug is much better tolerated. Steroid replacement is usually necessary. Where there is failure of response to *o,p'*-DDD (or if side-effects are intolerable), palliation of the Cushing's syndrome may be achieved by agents such as metyrapone, aminoglutethimide or ketoconazole, which interfere with steroid synthesis. The new agent gossypol is under investigation and has been shown to produce responses [28]. Chemotherapy using cisplatin and etoposide occasionally produces responses. Surgical resection or embolization should also be considered, as well as palliative radiotherapy for patients with painful bone metastases. Overall, the prognosis is poor, with a median survival of 15 months, and only 20% of patients alive at 5 years. Adverse prognostic factors include age over 40 and metastases at presentation.

Adrenal medulla [29]

The cells of the adrenal medulla have a different derivation from those of the cortex, developing from neuroectodermal tissue and giving rise to both benign and malignant tumours. In adult life these include *phaeochromocytoma* (benign in 90% of cases), *ganglioneuroma* or *neuroblastoma*. In childhood, neuroblastoma is much the commonest of the adrenal medullary tumours (see Chapter 24).

Phaeochromocytomas can arise from the adrenal medulla (90%), organ of Zuckerkandl or adrenal medullary cell rests in the pelvis. Ten per cent are bilateral. They can occur sporadically or as part of a familial syndrome of MEN-2 (see Chapter 15). Other associated diseases include neurofibromatosis, von Hippel–Lindau and Sturge–Weber syndromes, cerebellar ataxia and tuberous sclerosis/astrocytoma. About 10% are histologically malignant, although conventional microscopic appearances are an unreliable guide to clinical behaviour and the diagnosis of malignancy must be made with caution.

Phaeochromocytoma can occur at any age but is commonest at 40–60 years. The annual incidence is one per 100 000 but it accounts for 0.1% of hypertension. Most patients are diagnosed as a result of investigation for sustained hypertension, but the secretion of catecholamines by the tumour may also cause paroxysmal symptoms (Table 20.2) (similar for both benign and malignant tumours) and include intermittent or paroxysmal headache, severe sweating attacks, postural hypotension, dysrhythmias and chest pain. Attacks may be precipitated by

Table 20.2 Symptoms caused by phaeochromocytoma.

Skin
Attacks of sweating, flushing, blanching

Cardiovascular
Hypertension, tachycardia, paroxysmal rhythm change, slow forceful beating chest pain, postural hypotension

Central nervous system
Headache, tremor, irritability, mood change, psychosis, anorexia

Metabolic
Weight loss, increased metabolic rate, glycosuria

certain foods, posture and micturition. Pregnancy may provoke attacks due to pressure. Some patients present primarily with an abdominal or pelvic mass. Patients may be thin and agitated (resembling thyrotoxicosis).

Confirmation of the diagnosis is made by demonstration of excess catecholamines (adrenaline, noradrenaline and metabolites) in both urine and blood. The paroxysmal nature of the disorder may lead to false negative plasma catecholamine measurement, so 24-h urine collections are essential. Measurement of vanillyl mandelic acid (VMA) in the urine will provide the diagnosis in 85% of patients. False positives may occur on diets high in vanillin (bananas, nuts, coffee).

In others it may be necessary to resort to provocative tests using pharmacological agents. Phentolamine in *very small doses* (0.5–1.0 mg) will produce a fall in blood pressure of 25 mmHg lasting from 5 min to 4 h. Histamine and tyramine provoke hypertension in these patients by liberating the excess catecholamines stored in nerve endings (but not in the tumour). The use of these drugs requires extremely careful monitoring. Provocative tests are now seldom necessary since the introduction of more sensitive tests. Indeed, the greater area of difficulty lies in distinguishing physiological hypersecretion.

Selective angiography and venous sampling may be necessary to localize the tumour, though CT or MRI scanning generally give excellent visualization of the adrenal. In most cases the diagnosis of malignancy can be made only when the resected specimen is examined histologically, but occasionally a patient may have clinically obvious metastases.

Treatment of malignant phaeochromocytoma is by surgical resection, with careful dissection and microscopical inspection of excision margins to ensure adequate clearance. Surgical excision of single metastatic deposits has also been recommended. Preoperatively the blood pressure is controlled by gradually increasing doses of phe-noxybenzamine (to produce α-receptor blockade). In patients with arrhythmia, a β-blocking agent is added after the blood pressure is brought under control (Fig. 20.6). Used alone they can precipitate severe hypertension. After good blood pressure control has been achieved for 10 days the resection is performed, with continuous intraoperative intra-arterial blood pressure monitoring, and careful use of phentolamine and β-blocking agents. A fall in blood pressure following removal can usually be controlled by blood transfusion.

The use of chemotherapy for metastatic disease is purely anecdotal but alkylating agents and doxorubicin have been reportedly effective. High-dose ^{131}I meta-iodobenzylguanidine has also been used therapeutically [30] and has a symptom improvement rate of over 60%. In patients with symptomatic inoperable phaeochromocytoma both α- and β-blockers are valuable in controlling symptoms, and may have to be maintained for several years in patients with slow-growing tumours. Although long-term survival has been recorded, the majority of patients with malignant phaeochromocytoma die of the disease; extra-adrenal primary sites are said to have a particularly poor prognosis.

Cancer of the parathyroid glands

This tumour is very rare, with fewer than 100 cases in the world literature. Under 5% of all parathyroid tumours are malignant. The disease has been reported following irradiation of the neck. Most parathyroid carcinomas secrete parathyroid hormone, causing hyperparathy-roidism, sometimes with a florid form of osteitis fibrosa cystica. The tumour tends to be slow growing, and long-term survival frequently occurs if complete surgical removal is performed. Local recurrence can lead to severe pressure symptoms in the neck, but can be surgically resectable. Distant metastases occasionally occur, chiefly to lung and liver.

References

1 Schlumberger MJ. Medical progress. papillary and follicular thyroid carcinoma. *N Engl J Med* 1998; 338: 297–306.
2 LiVolsi VA. Well differentiated thyroid carcinoma. *Clin Oncol* 1996; 8: 281–8.
3 Akslen LA, LiVolsi VA. Prognostic significance of histologic grading compared with subclassification of papillas, thyroid carcinoma. *Cancer* 2000; 88: 1902–8.
4 Machens A, Gimm O, Ukkat J *et al.* Improved prediction of calcitonin normalisation in medullary thyroid carcinoma patients by quantitative lymph node analysis. *Cancer* 2000; 88: 1909–15.
5 Saad ME, Ordonez MG, Rashid RK *et al.* Medullary carcinoma of the thyroid: a study of the clinical features and prognostic factors in 161 patients. *Medicine* 1984; 63: 319–42.
6 Eng C. The *RET* proto-oncogene in multiple endocrine neoplasia type 2 and Hirschsprung's disease. *N Engl J Med* 1996; 335: 943–51.
7 Mathew CGP, Easton DF, Nakamura Y *et al.* Presymptomatic screening for multiple endocrine neoplasia type 2A with linked DNA markers. *Lancet* 1991; 337: 7–11.
8 Calmettes C, Ponder BAJ, Fischer JA *et al.* Early diagnosis of the multiple endocrine neoplasia type 2 syndrome: consensus statement. *Eur J Clin Invest* 1992; 22: 755–60.
9 Lips CJM, Landsvater RM, Hoppener JWM *et al.* Clinical screening as compared with DNA analysis in families with multiple endocrine neoplasia type 2A. *N Engl J Med* 1994; 331: 828–35.
10 Wells SA Jr, Chi DD, Toshima K *et al.* Predictive DNA testing and prophylactic thyroidectomy in patients at risk for multiple endocrine neoplasia type IIa. *Ann Surg* 1994; 220: 237–50.
11 Clark L, Ibanez ML, White EC. What operation for carcinoma of the thyroid? *Arch Surg* 1966; 92: 23–6.
12 Thyroid cancer (leading article). *Br Med J* 1976; 1: 113–14.
13 Mazzaferri EL. Management of a solitary thyroid nodule. *N Engl J Med* 1993; 328: 553–9.
14 Gharib H, Goeliner JR. Fine-needle aspiration biopsy of the thyroid: an appraisal. *Ann Intern Med* 1993; 118: 282–9.
15 Chatal JF, Hoefnagel CA. Radionuclide therapy. *Lancet* 1999; 354: 931–5.
16 Sisson JC. Applying the radioactive eraser: I-131 to ablate normal thyroid tissue in patients from whom thyroid cancer has been resected. *J Nuclear Med* 1983; 24: 743–5.

Preoperative

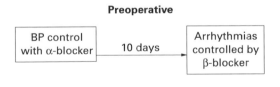

Perioperative

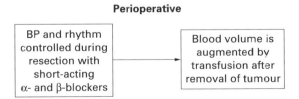

Fig. 20.6 Pre- and perioperative management of phaeo-chromocytoma.

17 Ladenson PW, Braverman LE, Mazzaferri EL *et al.* Comparison of administration of recombinant human thyrotropin with withdrawal of thyroid hormone for radioactive iodine scanning in patients with thyroid carcinoma. *N Engl J Med* 1997; 337: 888–96.

18 Mazzaferri EL, Young RL, Oertel JE *et al.* Papillary thyroid carcinoma: the impact of therapy on 576 patients. *Medicine (Baltimore)* 1977; 56: 171–96.

19 Tubiana M, Schlumberger M, Rougier P *et al.* Long term results and prognostic factors in patients with differentiated thyroid carcinoma. *Cancer* 1985; 55: 794–804.

20 Utiger RD. Follow-up of patients with thyroid carcinoma. *N Engl J Med* 1997; 337: 928–30.

21 Moss WT, Brand WN, Battifora H. The thyroid. In: *Radiation Oncology—Rationale, Technique, Results,* 5th edn. St Louis: Mosby, 1979: 233–42.

22 Souhami L, Simpson WJ, Carruthers JS. Malignant lymphoma of the thyroid gland. *Int J Radiation Oncol Biol Physics* 1980; 6: 1143–8.

23 Hundahl SA, Fleming ID, Freugen AM, Menck HR. A National Cancer Data Base report on 53,856 cases of thyroid carcinoma treated in the US, 1985–1995. *Cancer* 1998; 83: 2638–48.

24 Brooks JR, Starnes JF, Brooks DC *et al.* Surgical therapy for thyroid carcinoma: a review of 1249 solitary nodules. *Surgery* 1988; 104: 940–6.

25 Leeper RD. Symposium on thyroid cancer. *Med Clin N Am* 1985; 69: 1079–96.

26 Kendall-Taylor P. Managing differentiated thyroid cancer: better management can improve survival in this curable cancer. *Brit Med J* 2002; 324: 988–9.

27 Luton J-P, Cerdas S, Billaud L *et al.* Clinical features of adrenocortical carcinoma, prognostic factors, and the effect of mitotane therapy. *N Engl J Med* 1990; 322: 1195–201.

28 Flack MR. Oral gossypol in the treatment of metastatic adrenal cancer. *J Clin Endocrinol Metab* 1993; 76: 1019–24.

29 Modlin IM, Farndon JR, Shepherd A *et al.* Phaeochromocytoma in 72 patients: Clinical and diagnostic features, treatment and long-term results. *Br J Surg* 1979; 66: 456–65.

30 Bomanji J, Britton KE, Ur E *et al.* Treatment of malignant phaeochromocytoma, paraganglioma and carcinoid tumours with ^{131}I meta-iodobenzylguanidine. *Nuclear Med Comms* 1993; 14: 856–61.

Cancer from an unknown primary site

About 3% of all cancers, and 6% of cancer deaths, are cancers where the primary site is unknown after initial examination and investigation. In these cases the primary tumour is too small to be clinically apparent. Usually the histological diagnosis, obtained from a metastasis, is of an adenocarcinoma or poorly differentiated carcinoma.

There are few situations in medicine which are a greater test of clinical judgement. Multiple investigations may be undertaken designed to disclose the primary site, but these are frequently ineffective in disclosing the primary or changing management. A diagnosis is established in only 15% of cases. Postmortem a further 70% of diagnosis is attained.

Site of presentation [1]

The extent and nature of preliminary investigation will depend on the site of the metastasis. The common metastatic sites include lymph nodes, bone, brain, liver and skin. Table 21.1 shows the most frequent primary tumours presenting at these sites. With each metastatic site, investigation will have a different emphasis. For example, a squamous carcinoma in a cervical node indicates that the nasopharynx or lung is the likely primary site, and full examination, including the larynx, pharynx and postnasal space, will often give the diagnosis. Metastasis in an inguinal node or malignant ascites will necessitate gynaecological examination. Management will then be as for the underlying malignancy. When initial investigation has failed to give any clue to the primary cancer, the physician must ask 'If I find the primary, will there be any treatment which offers a reasonable chance of palliation or cure?'

A particularly important group of tumours are germ cell tumours which, it is increasingly recognized, may present as poorly differentiated carcinomas but are highly responsive to chemotherapy.

The sites of origin of metastasis from an unknown primary site

The distribution of cancers which present as metastases from an occult primary is not the same as the overall distribution of cancer. In Table 21.2 the frequency of presentation of metastasis from an unknown primary is shown compared with the frequency of cancers in general. The commonest tumours are pancreas, lung, liver, stomach and colorectal cancer. Common cancers such as breast and prostate are much less frequent causes of metastasis from an unknown primary. This is probably because primary tumours in the breast are relatively easily detected clinically, while prostatic cancer is associated with an elevation of the acid phosphatase or prostate-specific antigen (PSA).

Tumours where treatment may be curative or where prolonged palliation is possible are shown in Table 21.3. Investigation must therefore be directed towards the confident exclusion of these cancers.

Several studies have shown that the yield of investigation is low when applied routinely to all patients in this situation. In one report the primary site was identified in only 10% of cases, and in only 14 out of 266 cases was a treatable cancer detected [1]. In most cases therefore a primary will not be found at presentation and, even if it is, it is extremely unusual for a treatable disease to be discovered. A further problem in adopting an attitude of intensive investigation is that the studies may give false positive results. The patient may be subjected to a number of further investigations, often invasive, invariably expensive, and usually resulting in failure.

Table 21.1 Sites of metastases from an unknown primary site.

Site of metastasis	Likely primary site
High cervical nodes	Head and neck sites
	Thyroid, lung
Lower cervical nodes	Head and neck
	Lung
	Breast
	Gut (especially L. supraclavicular node)
Axillary nodes	Lung
	Breast
Skin	Breast
	Lung
	Melanoma
Bone	Myeloma
	Breast
	Kidney
	Prostate
	Lung
Brain	Lung
	Breast
	Prostate
	Melanoma
Inguinal nodes	Vulva
	Anorectal
	Prostate
	Ovary
Disseminated intra-abdominal adenocarcinoma (including liver metastasis)	Ovary
	Stomach
	Pancreas
	Gut

Table 21.2 Sites of origin of carcinomas presenting as metastases from unknown site.

	All unknown primary cases (%)	All cancers (%)
Pancreas	20	2
Lung	20	10
Unknown	15	–
Liver	10	2
Stomach	10	5
Colorectal	81	5
Breast	3	26
Thyroid	3	1
Renal	3	2
Prostate	3	18
Ovary	2	5
Other	3	14

Table 21.3 Treatable cancers which may present as metastases from an unknown primary.

Curable tumours which must not be missed
Germ cell and trophoblastic tumours
Lymphomas
Well-differentiated thyroid cancer

Tumours which can be palliated by chemotherapy
Breast
Ovary
Small-cell carcinoma of the bronchus

Tumours which can be palliated by hormone therapy
Breast
Prostate
Endometrial

Investigation and management [2]

The following is a guide to the management of this difficult problem. It must be emphasized that the degree to which investigation will be pursued will vary greatly with individual patients. The patient's age, fitness and degree of anxiety will all influence the decision as well as the possibility of finding a treatable tumour.

Review of histology

The most important first step is to discuss the biopsy with an experienced pathologist. The pathologist may have an idea where the primary site might be, but because of lack of clinical information, has left the diagnosis open. The usual appearance is of a poorly differentiated adenocarcinoma or an undifferentiated tumour. Special stains may be useful in providing further information, for example immunocytochemical staining for large-cell lymphomas. These tumours are often difficult to distinguish from anaplastic carcinoma, but are very responsive to chemotherapy. Mucin stains may demonstrate intracellular mucin and point to an origin in the gut, pancreas or stomach. Monoclonal antibodies reactive with membrane and cytoplasmic proteins may help to determine the cell of origin. It is important not to miss a large-cell lymphoma as a cause of an undifferentiated tumour, and antibodies to the common leucocyte antigen (see Chapter 26 and Fig. 3.12, p. 34) and to epithelial antigens such as cytokeratins can usually make this distinction.

Table 21.4 lists some of the more frequently used reagents. Some will work on paraffin sections, others require frozen tissue. Biopsy material should therefore not

Table 21.4 Further pathological investigation in diagnosis in metastasis from an unknown primary site.

Cellular structure	Investigation or reagent	Tumour types identified
Cytokeratins	Cam 5.2	Carcinomas
Oestrogen and progesterone receptor	Antibodies	Breast cancer and other gynaecological tumours
Epithelial membrane antigen (EMA)	Antibodies to EMA	Carcinomas (especially breast, gut, ovary, pancreas)
Prostate specific antigen (PSA)	Anti-PSA	Prostate cancer
Common leucocyte antigen (CLA)	Anti-CLA	Lymphomas (98% positive)
Desmin ⎫ intermediate Vimentin ⎬ filaments S100 ⎭	Antibodies	Some sarcomas
Melanoma-associated antigen	HMB-45	Melanoma
Thyroglobulin	Anti-thyroglobulin	Thyroid carcinoma
HCG	Anti-HCG ⎫	
AFP	Anti-AFP ⎬	Germ cell tumours
PLAP	Anti-PLAP ⎭	
Premelanosomes	EM	Melanoma
Dense core granules	EM	Neuroendocrine tumours (small-cell lung cancer)
Intermediate filaments	EM	Carcinoma

EM, electron microscopy.

be placed entirely in formalin when cancer is a possible diagnosis. Antibodies to epithelial membrane antigens are available which help to define epithelial tumours such as breast cancer or other poorly differentiated adenocarcinomas. Antibodies to prekeratin may be helpful in determining whether or not the tumour is of squamous origin; others react with melanoma-associated antigens. In a woman if the node is taken from an axillary or a supraclavicular site, oestrogen and progesterone receptor positivity may indicate breast origin for the tumour. Occasionally electron microscopy may help, for example in showing premelanosomes in malignant melanoma, or intercellular bridges in poorly differentiated squamous carcinoma. Undifferentiated germ cell tumours are curable cancers of young people which are easily overlooked. They may contain human chorionic gonadotrophin (HCG) and α-fetoprotein (AFP) and can be stained for the intracellular presence of these peptides by immunocytochemical techniques.

Biochemical and haematological investigation

Certain tests should be carried out as a routine. These include an acid phosphatase and/or PSA measurement in men over 40 years old to detect carcinoma of the prostate; and HCG and AFP determinations in young patients in case the tumour is of germ cell type. Hepatomas also produce AFP. Immunoelectrophoresis of plasma and examination of the urine for Bence-Jones protein is essential if myeloma is a possibility. The blood film may show leuco-erythroblastic anaemia, most commonly seen with breast cancer. Polycythaemia and thrombocytosis may occur with renal carcinoma and hepatoma.

Other investigations

A fresh urine sample should be taken to look for red cells, which may indicate an underlying renal carcinoma. A chest X-ray is an essential examination and may disclose a carcinoma of the bronchus or enlarged mediastinal lymph nodes suggestive of a lymphoma.

More invasive investigations are of more doubtful benefit. Computed tomography (CT) scans of the abdomen show the site of the primary tumour in 25% of cases. There is usually the pancreas if the metastasis is an adenocarcinoma. Treatment is unaffected by knowledge of the pancreatic primary. Mammography is essential if carcinoma of the breast is a differential diagnosis, since the presentation with a supraclavicular or axillary node does not rule out effective treatment of the tumour. The decision about further investigation is one which requires judgement and skill. In the main, the less experienced the physician, the greater the number of investigations performed. It requires considerable clinical authority and careful explanation to help the patient understand that further investigation is not needed (or likely to be helpful) after the metastasis has been discovered and treatable causes excluded.

Treatment [3]

The element of uncertainty in the situation and the serious nature and poor prognosis make management difficult for the patient and physician. If the diagnosis has been established as a germ cell tumour or other treatable condition as outlined in Table 21.3, then treatment is along the appropriate lines.

Approximately 80% of patients will have histological appearances of poorly differentiated adenocarcinoma or poorly differentiated carcinoma. Some of these patients may have a germ cell tumour and be curable by chemotherapy [4]. These patients often have a tumour located in the midline (in the mediastinum or para-aortic region), are usually less than 50 years old and sometimes have a rapidly growing tumour. In these cases, if the histology is poorly differentiated *adenocarcinoma*, the response rate to germ cell chemotherapy is low (about 30%) and usually short-lived. If the histology is poorly differentiated *carcinoma* the response rate approaches 80% in some series and some patients are cured [5]. These findings indicate that younger patients with poorly differentiated mediastinal carcinomas should receive platinum-based germ cell chemotherapy.

If the diagnosis is adenocarcinoma in an axillary lymph node treatment for breast cancer should be considered, even if the mammogram is normal. Although mastectomy will show an occult primary in 40–70% of cases, it is not clear that an immediate operation contributes to cure. A trial of hormone therapy as initial treatment is an appropriate step in postmenopausal women. Women with malignant ascites showing adenocarcinoma should be treated for ovarian cancer especially if CA-125 is elevated.

Some tumours may show neuroendocrine features (such as neurosecretory granules) on electron microscopy. A trial of chemotherapy for small-cell lung cancer might be considered for this group.

In many cases, however, no diagnosis will be reached, and the issue will then be to decide if chemotherapy should be used in an attempt to delay the progress of the disease. This depends very much on the clinical state of the patient and on the intensity of the patient's anxiety for treatment. Clinical pointers to responsiveness to chemotherapy (usually platinum-based) are tumours which are mediastinal or retroperitoneal, young age and tumours confined to the lymph nodes. Regressions can be induced with the use of drugs such as doxorubicin mitomycin, paclitaxel and 5-fluorouracil [6,7]. Such regressions are usually short-lived. Our practice is to use a combination including doxorubicin in those patients who are relatively fit, and have a strong desire for treatment. Often, there is a failure of response or only a short-lived response. Palliative treatment using radiotherapy to sites of pain or local swelling, and supportive measures (see Chapter 7) is then the mainstay of treatment.

Exceptionally, an isolated cerebral metastasis can be removed surgically. Removal of solitary brain secondaries (even when the primary site is known) is associated with less likelihood of recurrence in the brain and better quality of life than control with radiation alone [8].

Survival

Median survival is 3–5 months with 5–10% survival at 2 years. Response to chemotherapy is better if the histology is poorly differentiated carcinoma, if there are less than three metastatic sites, if carcinoembryonic antigen is not elevated and if the main location is retroperitoneal or peripheral nodes.

References

1 Altman E, Cadman E. An analysis of 1539 patients with cancer of unknown primary site. *Cancer* 1986; 57: 120–4.

2 Nystrom JS, Weiner JM, Wolf RM. Identifying the primary site in metastatic cancer of unknown origin. Inadequacy of roentgenographic procedures. *J Am Med Assoc* 1979; 241: 381–3.

3 Hainsworth JD, Greco FA. Treatment of patients with cancer of an unknown primary site. *N Engl J Med* 1993; 329: 257–63.

4 Greco FA, Vaughn WK, Hainsworth JD. Advanced poorly differentiated carcinoma of unknown primary site: recognition of a treatable syndrome. *Ann Intern Med* 1986; 104: 547–53.

5 van der Gaast A, Verweig J, Henzen-Logmans SC, Rodenburg CJ, Stoger G. Carcinoma of unknown primary: Identification of a treatable subset? *Ann Oncol* 1990; 1: 119–22.

6 Woods RL, Fox RM, Tattersall MHN, Levi JA, Brodie EN. Metastatic adenocarcinomas of unknown primary site. A randomised study of two combination chemotherapy regimens. *N Engl J Med* 1980; 303: 87–9.

7 Hainsworth JD, Erland JB, Kalman LA *et al*. Carcinoma of unknown primary site: treatment with 1-hour paclitaxel, carboplatin and extended schedule etoposide. *J Clin Oncol* 1997; 15: 2385–93.

8 Posner JB. Surgery for metastases to the brain. *N Engl J Med* 1990; 322: 544–5.

22 Skin cancer

Aetiology and pathogenesis

Over 40 000 new cases of skin cancer were reported in the UK in 1997 [1]. It is no surprise that skin cancers are the commonest of all malignancies since the skin is the largest and most accessible of our organs, directly exposed to environmental carcinogens. The earliest described and perhaps best-known example of a carcinogen-induced skin cancer, noted by Percival Pott in 1775, is the carcinoma of the scrotal skin affecting chimney sweeps who came into direct contact with soot in chimney flues. In the 19th century, an increase in incidence of skin cancers was reported following treatment with medicines containing arsenic: arsenical fumes had already been implicated in the causation of scrotal cancers of copper miners and smelters. Towards the end of the century it was suggested that strong sunlight might be a promoter of skin cancer; and shortly after the discovery of radium, Becquerel proposed that ionizing radiation might be the component of sunlight responsible for malignant change. The carcinogenic roles of ultraviolet (UV) radiation, X-rays and chemicals have now been confirmed; most important of all was the work of Yamagiwa and Ichikawa who demonstrated the carcinogenic properties of coal tar applied directly to skin of experimental animals [2], though it was Kennaway who isolated and identified the carcinogen as 3,4-benzpyrene. Over the past 40 years, the incidence of melanoma has doubled every decade, probably as a result of increased exposure to sunlight and the loss of our ozone layer, currently estimated to be decreasing by 0.2–0.8% annually.

Sunlight and occupational factors

Epidemiological studies have provided important clues to the aetiology of skin cancer, whose incidence varies directly in proportion to the intensity of sunlight, so that skin cancers are much more common in Australia (with the world's highest incidence rates) and South Africa than in more temperate areas [3]. A high proportion of skin cancers (particularly basal cell carcinomas) occur in sun-exposed areas of the body, and certain races such as fair-skinned Celts are particularly prone to developing skin cancer, probably due to a relative lack of protection by melanin pigment. By contrast, skin cancers are relatively uncommon in black races, presumably as a result of effective shielding by pigment in the superficial skin layers. Recent research into the epidemiology and genetics of basal squamous cell carcinomas suggest that they should be separately considered rather than, as previously, regarded collectively as a contrasting condition to melanoma but otherwise essentially similar to each other [4,5]. Public information programmes rightly emphasize the importance of avoiding overexposure to sunlight [3,6,7]. In black people, the distribution of skin cancers is much less determined by sunlight exposure than in Caucasians, and is almost as common in unexposed areas such as the trunk and lower limbs. The use of psoralens and UVA in psoriasis is associated with a risk of cutaneous malignancy, particularly on the male genitalia, and an association has been noted between skin carcinoma (predominantly squamous cell) and non-Hodgkin's lymphoma [8], with UV sunlight as the presumed aetiological linkage factor.

In the past, occupational carcinogens have been an important cause of skin cancer though increasing risk awareness has substantially reduced the hazard. However, industrial carcinogens such as petroleum derivatives, arsenicals and coal tar remain in common use, and protective clothing is still important. Even more critical is the need to keep radiation exposure to an absolute minimum, particularly for those working with X-rays, including medical, nursing and radiographic personnel who require regular monitoring of radiation exposure throughout their working lives.

Immunosuppression and viral causes

Recipients of renal allografts have an increased risk of cancer—up to as great as 100 times that of the general population. The most common malignancies are those of the skin including squamous and basal cell carcinomas, melanoma and Bowen's disease. Squamous carcinoma is more frequent than basal cell (a reverse of the usual pattern), sometimes multifocal and running an aggressive course.

Considerable interest has been aroused in the role of the wart viruses, *human papilloma virus* (HPV), and a pattern is now emerging in which HPV appear associated with the development of cancer in particular clinical settings. The genome of HPV type 5 has been found in squamous carcinoma of the skin in renal allograft recipients and also in the squamous cancers which occur in the rare inherited skin disorder *epidermodysplasia verruciformis*, in which patients develop multiple warts. Although HPV is now less widely regarded as the key aetiological agent, it seems extremely likely that it does indeed have carcinogenic properties.

Kaposi's sarcoma is discussed separately on pp. 341–2.

Premalignant lesions

A group of premalignant skin lesions has been recognized in which malignant change is sufficiently common to justify close surveillance. These include the following.

Inherited disorders

XERODERMA PIGMENTOSUM

This is an autosomal recessive disease characterized by increased sensitivity to UV light, with multiple solar keratoses, premalignant and ultimately malignant skin lesions on exposed surfaces. Melanoma squamous or basal cell carcinoma, all occur. The defect is due to UV-induced damage causing a deficiency in the excision repair mechanism for DNA.

NAEVOID BASAL CELL CARCINOMA SYNDROME (GORLIN'S SYNDROME)

This is a syndrome characterized by multiple basal cell carcinomas, particularly on the face and trunk, associated with cleft lip and skeletal abnormalities which include frontal bossing, mandibular cysts and bifid ribs [9]. It is inherited through a single autosomal dominant gene with complete penetrance but variable expression. About 40% of patients do not appear to have an affected parent.

There is also an increased tendency to other neoplastic changes, notably ameloblastoma and squamous cell carcinoma of, or around, the jaw, meningioma, melanoma and others. Management can be exceptionally difficult in view of the hundreds of naevi or invasive tumours these patients may develop, often in young adult life.

ALBINISM

This is a group of congenital diseases associated with defective skin pigmentation and an increased tendency to solar keratosis and squamous carcinoma *in situ.*

EPIDERMODYSPLASIA VERRUCIFORMIS

This is an autosomal recessive disease characterized by multiple flat warts. These and even non-affected skin may evolve into squamous carcinoma (see above).

GENETIC PREDISPOSITION TO MELANOMA

A melanoma predisposition gene, *CDKN2*, has now been identified, which maps to chromosome 9p21–p22 [10]. *CDKN2* mutations have been found in the germline of affected members of melanoma kindreds and there seems no doubt that in a minority of cases, familial melanoma genuinely occurs, such families having been reported from Europe, the USA and elsewhere.

Carcinogen-induced disorders

ARSENICAL KERATOSES

After exposure to inorganic arsenicals, keratotic lesions may develop 10 years or more later on the palms and soles. These lesions are premalignant, although overt cancer is uncommon. Bowen's disease (see below) is often present as well, together with superficial basal cell carcinomas at other sites.

SOLAR KERATOSES

Although histologically similar to arsenical keratoses, the

incidence of malignant change is much greater and the distribution also different, since these lesions chiefly occur on the face and dorsal aspect of the hands. Other changes of prolonged exposure to sunlight are present: furrowed elastic leathery skin, with wrinkling, atrophy and hyper- or depigmented patches.

RADIATION DERMATITIS

Following exposure to modest doses of superficial radiation (often given many years before for benign conditions such as ringworm, acne or hirsutism), the skin may assume a characteristic appearance, with depigmentation, atrophy of the skin, hair and sweat glands, and telangiectasia. These areas are more susceptible to malignant change. Basal cell carcinomas on the scalp are usually related to previous irradiation and may arise in skin without evidence of radiation change.

Miscellaneous disorders

BOWEN'S DISEASE

Often regarded as a premalignant skin disorder, this disease is in fact a superficial intraepidermal squamous cell carcinoma *in situ*, usually found on the trunk or limbs. Characteristically, it spreads laterally within the cutis, often at several sites, and evolving slowly from a small erythematous papule to a crusting lesion. Histologically, the basal layer is intact but the epidermis shows premature keratinization and is disrupted with homogeneous cells with basophilic cytoplasm, small nuclei and frequent mitoses. There is an important association with internal malignancies, as many as a quarter of all patients with Bowen's disease developing a deep-seated carcinoma during the 10 years following diagnosis.

LEUCOPLAKIA

These are indurated whitish plaques, often fissured with sharply defined borders, found on mucous membranes of the mouth. They may result from local irritation — ill-fitting dentures and smoking are frequently associated. The histology shows hyperplasia, hyperkeratosis and dyskeratosis; carcinoma *in situ* may arise, sometimes progressing to squamous cell carcinoma.

GENITAL CARCINOMA *IN SITU*

This disorder is now regarded as a form of intraepithelial neoplasia, presenting as a persistent red papule or plaque on the penis (and previously known as erythroplasia of Queyrat). The relationship with HPV remains contentious. Pathologically, there is an abnormal epidermis with an absent granular layer and small densely packed cells similar to those in Bowen's disease. Intraepithelial neoplasia may also be found on the vulva (see also Chapter 17).

Basal cell carcinoma

Basal cell carcinoma (rodent ulcer) accounts for over 75% of all cases of skin malignancy in the Western world. Its UK incidence has increased by well over 200% over the past 14 years. In parts of New England, USA, 40% of the population will have developed a basal cell carcinoma by the age of 85 years [11]. Age-specific incidence is shown in Fig. 22.1. They are epithelial tumours without histological evidence of maturation or tendency to keratinization, and arise from the undifferentiated basal cells of the skin which normally differentiate into structures such as hair or sweat glands. The tumour consists of uniform cells with darkly stained nuclei and little cytoplasm, often forming a

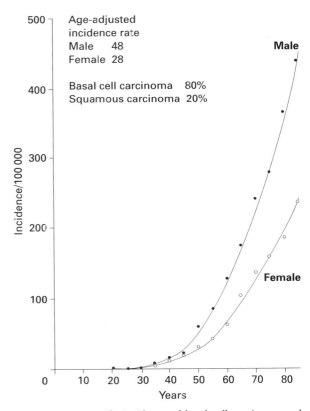

Fig. 22.1 Age-specific incidence of basal cell carcinoma and squamous carcinoma of the skin.

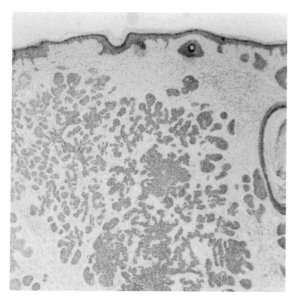

Fig. 22.2 Basal cell carcinoma of the skin, showing small nests of invading basal cells (×20).

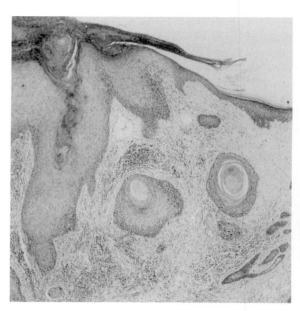

Fig. 22.3 Squamous cell carcinoma of skin, showing invading masses of squamous epithelium forming keratin pearls (×20).

characteristic palisade (Fig. 22.2). The tumour generally arises on exposed areas, particularly the skin of the face and most characteristically around the nose, forehead, cheeks and lower eyelid, although it may sometimes occur on the limbs. Macroscopically, the lesions are often described as either nodular, pigmented, sclerosing (morphoeic), cicatrizing, infiltrating or ulcerative. There is usually a firm pink papule with a distinct raised edge, often serpiginous, with a pearly and telangiectatic appearance and with a depressed or frankly ulcerated centre with or without a central crust. Although non-inflammatory and typically painless, it may irritate and will often bleed repeatedly if scratched.

Untreated, these tumours invade laterally or deeply with local destruction of cartilage or even bone. In the sclerosing variety the typical features may be absent and the margin indistinct, making diagnosis more difficult. Superficial basal cell carcinomas, often multiple, also have an unusual appearance and are more common on the trunk with a more plaque-like scaling patch configuration or a fine pearly edge.

Despite the highly malignant microscopic appearance of basal cell carcinomas, metastasis to local lymph nodes or distant sites is exceptionally rare [12], a remarkable fact in view of the large size that many of these cancers can achieve, and an important contrast with the behaviour of squamous cell carcinomas. Multiple primary tumours,

however, are not uncommon. In one American prospective study of 1000 patients with a basal cell carcinoma, 36% developed a second within 5 years. About 9% of Australian cases have multiple primary lesions [13].

Squamous cell carcinoma

Squamous cell carcinomas of the skin are less common than basal cell carcinomas (Fig. 22.1), though they share many characteristics. Sunlight or X-ray exposure, arsenic ingestion and occupational carcinogens are all aetiologically important. Multiple squamous cell carcinomas of the hand were common among radiation scientists in the early years of the 20th century until the hazard was recognized and methods of dosimetry improved. Histologically, these are typical keratinizing squamous lesions (Fig. 22.3), and to some extent the risk of local spread can be predicted from the histological appearance (more common with less well-differentiated tumours).

As with basal cell carcinomas, the commonest sites include sun-exposed areas of the head and neck, particularly the nose, temples, rim of the ear and lip, as well as the side and back of the neck, and the dorsal surfaces of the hand and forearm. The typical appearance is either a crusted scaly ulcer or a more nodular exophytic type which can fungate if untreated. The site of the tumour may be diagnostically helpful since squamous cell carcinomas, though commonest on the face, have a much more widespread distribution than basal cell carcinomas and a shorter history. A skin tumour of the hand or forearm is far more likely to be of squamous cell origin. Squamous cell carcinoma may be difficult to distinguish macroscopically from the usually benign condition *keratoacanthoma*, characterized by a locally rapidly advancing, discrete and often bulky papule on the face or neck, and typically with a central plug of keratin filling the ulcerated central area.

Squamous cell carcinomas arising in areas of radiation dermatitis are both clinically and histologically more aggressive than other varieties, though the mean latent interval is about 20 years. In one large series of nearly 400 patients, the mortality was as high as 10%. These tumours are now less frequent because of higher-energy radiotherapy equipment, and the infrequent use of radiotherapy for benign skin disorders and arthritic conditions. This is also true of squamous carcinomas arising from chronic burn ulcers, *Marjolin's ulcer*, though this used to be a common problem, typically with a lengthy period of quiescence terminated by a highly aggressive phase with metastases to the lungs and other sites. A similar type of squamous cell carcinoma occasionally develops in chronic sinus tracts of osteomyelitis or other chronic infections and in the dysplastic or scar areas of chronic skin diseases such as lupus vulgaris or lupus erythematosus.

Squamous carcinomas arising at mucocutaneous junctions such as the anus and vulva tend to be aggressive, as do those developing in areas of radiation-damaged skin, patches of Bowen's disease, or against a background of carcinoma *in situ*. Sweat gland carcinoma, an uncommon condition, may also behave unpredictably. These tumours most commonly arise in the axilla and anogenital regions, and should be distinguished from the rare sebaceous gland cancers. Finally squamous carcinomas are reportedly more common in areas of vitiligo, especially in black people.

Treatment of basal cell and squamous cell carcinoma

Because of their frequency and characteristic appearance, treatment without firm histological diagnosis is sometimes advocated. In general this is unwise and can be dangerous since the lesions most likely to metastasize are those least likely to have been correctly diagnosed. Elderly patients may be too unwell for biopsy but in all other cases, biopsy is essential. Benign conditions such as papillomas, sclerosing haemangiomas and keratoacanthomas can all be macroscopically confused with a basal or squamous cell carcinoma, and occasionally these two major types of skin cancer can themselves be difficult to distinguish from each other.

There are several effective methods of treatment, including electrocautery and curettage, cryosurgery, excisional surgery, chemosurgery, radiotherapy and topical chemotherapy. Since all of these have their strong adherents and each method yields a very high success rate, formal comparisons are difficult. In addition, approaches such as electrocautery and cryosurgery are in general confined to such small lesions (usually under 5 mm diameter) that the very high success rate of over 95% is not representative of an unselected group. Cryosurgery, usually using liquid nitrogen, is effective for small lesions, particularly for superficial tumours such as Bowen's disease and the most superficial of basal cell carcinomas. It can be extremely useful in elderly or immobile patients. Chemosurgery, an interesting technique first described by Mobs [14], employs a zinc chloride paste fixative which is applied to the tumour, partly destroying it and allowing easy removal from the underlying skin while preserving its histological pattern. Further paste is then applied to any area of residual tumour, and the whole process repeated. This technique can be useful even for fairly large tumours and at sites where radiotherapy may be hazardous (see below), though it is time-consuming and laborious, and demands great expertise and care. Despite these potential drawbacks, this approach, often termed as *micrographically controlled surgery*, has become popular.

For basal cell and squamous cell carcinomas too large for electrocautery, most dermatologists would agree that the real choice lies between excisional surgery and radiotherapy. Each has its advantages. Surgery is quick, does not require multiple visits to hospital, and is the only way to produce a complete specimen for the pathologist. Conversely, for large tumours a general anaesthetic is usually required, and skin grafting or flap rotation may well be necessary, with a less acceptable final cosmetic result as well as the risk of a higher postoperative complication rate. With tumours at difficult sites such as the inner canthus of the eye, surgery is probably best avoided since there is a risk of damage to the nasolachrymal duct, and surgical reconstruction can be very difficult. For squamous cell carcinomas, a wider excision is usually recommended because of the possibility of local lymphatic spread. There is no clear indication for routine lymph node dissection, although surgical excision is undoubtedly the treatment of choice for clinically involved regional nodes.

Radiotherapy is also highly effective, with a cure rate of over 90%. It is especially useful for tumours on the face, particularly around the eye, nose and nasolabial fold where tumours may infiltrate deeply and prove difficult to excise surgically without, in some cases, an unacceptable deformity. Both the columella of the nose and the ala nasae are difficult surgical sites, and radiotherapy is usually curative and gives excellent cosmesis. The radiation energy and effective depth-dose can be chosen to suit the individual tumour, and simple lead cut-outs can be tailor-made so that irregularly shaped tumours may be adequately treated without unnecessary treatment of large volumes of normal skin. For tumours of the lower eyelid and other sites where shielding of deeper structures is desirable (for example, gums, teeth and tongue in treatment of cancer of the lip), simple shielding can be introduced for each treatment session. Figure 22.4 shows a lead shield inserted under local anaesthetic into the lower conjunctival sac, protecting the eye while the lower lid is treated. Direct electron beams are often employed. The major disadvantage of radiotherapy is that in order to produce the best cosmetic result, fractionated regimes of treatment

over 2–3 weeks are required. For the elderly or infirm, the travelling may be tiring and a quick operation or treatment by a single large fraction of radiotherapy may be preferable.

A less highly fractionated course of radiotherapy (such as the Sambrook split course, in which two fractions of radiation are given some 6 weeks apart), has a very good cure rate but higher incidence of late skin changes—telangiectasia, atrophy and depigmentation. The aim of longer courses of radiotherapy is to reduce these late effects to a minimum, particularly important for facial skin cancers where a very high cure rate, coupled with a perfect cosmetic result, should be the aim. Acute skin changes consist of intense local erythema and inflammation, leading to early crusting, and resolution with healing which may take months to complete, particularly with larger lesions. Common fractionation regimens are shown in Table 22.1; they often reflect the capacity of the radiotherapy department to treat these common tumours, as much as the individual preference of the radiotherapist. Expressed in terms of the nominal standard dose (see Chapter 5), these treatments aim for a total of 1500–1900 ret. Squamous cell carcinomas require a wider treatment field than basal cell carcinomas, though most radiotherapists treat both lesions to the same doses and their radiocurability is probably identical [13]. Radiotherapy is unsuitable for the naevoid basal cell carcinoma syndrome, as it gives poor results with marked skin damage.

In an important randomized study from France, patients with basal cell carcinoma of the face (less than 4 cm) were treated either by surgery or radiotherapy [15]. Of 347 patients, the surgical group ($n=174$) had a 4-year failure rate of only 0.7% compared with a higher (7.5%) recurrence rate with radiotherapy ($n=173$). Cosmetically, the surgical group also appeared to show an advantage. Both forms of treatment were conducted by highly experienced teams, although the radiotherapy

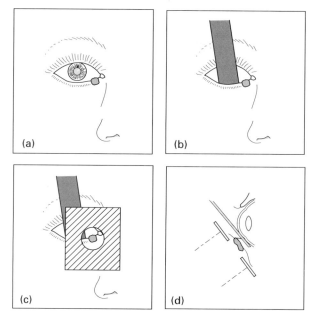

Fig. 22.4 Treatment of skin cancer on lower eyelid: (a) typical position of tumour; (b) lead spatula inserted into lower lid before each treatment, shielding cornea and lens; (c) lead cut-out in position; (d) lateral view.

Table 22.1 Fractionation regimens in basal and squamous cell carcinoma. Single-fraction or two-fraction policies are generally adopted in elderly patients for whom repeated visits may be difficult. In general, however, better cosmetic results are achieved with more prolonged fractionation.

20–22 Gy × 1
14 Gy × 2 (6-week gap)
7.5 Gy × 5 (7–10 days)
6.75 Gy × 6 (alternate days)
6 Gy × 9 (over 3 weeks)
4.5 Gy × 10 (over 3 weeks)

technique did vary widely among the four participating hospitals.

Topical chemotherapy, usually using 5-fluorouracil, has been increasingly employed in recent years, particularly for recurrent lesions where surgery and/or radiation therapy have already been used. Although its precise role has not yet been determined, advantages include the possibility of repeated use where necessary, as well as its value in premalignant lesions and large areas of carcinoma *in situ* where other approaches might be difficult. It is valuable in treatment of multiple lesions, particularly superficial basal cell carcinomas, but is not usually recommended for thick or infiltrating lesions. Topical cytotoxic therapy produces acute inflammation which is a disadvantage, although steroids are usually helpful.

Overall results of treatment of both basal cell and squamous cell carcinoma are excellent. Cure rates of 90–95% are regularly achieved by surgery or radiotherapy; for smaller tumours treated by curettage, cryosurgery or electrocautery the figures are claimed to be higher still. Sadly, the occasional tumour is encountered (particularly with basal cell carcinoma) which proves resistant to all methods of treatment, usually with multiple recurrences at the margins of the treated area, sometimes over a period of 10 years or more. These cases are characterized by relentless local invasion and destruction both laterally and deeply. Distant metastases to bone, lung or elsewhere are occasionally seen.

Malignant melanoma

Epidemiology and pathogenesis

Malignant melanoma is a far less common skin tumour than the cancers discussed above, but has a much worse prognosis. It accounts for about 3% of all skin cancers, with an annual incidence in the UK of about six per 100 000 population (Fig. 22.5), but it has become more common during the last four decades [3,16] — increasing at annual rates between 3 and 7% per year between the mid-1950s and the early 1980s. There is wide international variation: the disease is almost 10 times as common in Australia and New Zealand as in Europe, occurring most frequently in patients between 40 and 70 years old, with a slight female preponderance. This is in contrast to basal cell and squamous carcinoma (Fig. 22.1) implying a difference in the relative importance of external factors such as sunlight in aetiology in these types of skin cancer.

Like other skin cancers, melanoma is commoner in the

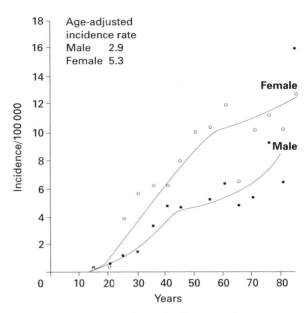

Fig. 22.5 Age-specific incidence of melanoma in the UK.

white population presumably because pigmented skin is effective in screening out solar UV light. The degree of sunburn, rather than sun exposure *per se*, may be an important aetiological feature [17]. About 75% of all malignant melanomas occur on an exposed site, chiefly affecting pale-complexioned white people, especially those with red hair and freckles [4]. The number of naevi on an individual's skin correlates quite closely with melanoma risk [18], and, melanoma families have been widely reported [19]. The amount of received sunlight, as measured by distance from the equator, also correlates well with incidence. The earth's ozone layer has an important protective effect, filtering out carcinogenic UV light.

Much can be done to inform the public of the dangers of over-exposure to the sun, and information about the value of early diagnosis is clearly worthwhile since the outcome is so dependent on stage (see below). Forceful advertising campaigns through public media and in medical waiting areas have become commonplace.

The major sites of melanoma in white people are the head and neck, trunk and limbs. In black people the bodily distribution is different, with a greater likelihood of primary sites on the palms of the hands, soles of the feet and mucous membranes.

Clinical and pathological features

Although more than half of all melanotic lesions arise

from a pre-existing benign naevus, some undoubtedly develop at sites of previously normal skin; in many cases the primary site is never discovered, the patient presenting either with lymphadenopathy or with more widespread involvement. Postmortem studies have shown that most of the organs of the body are capable of harbouring a primary melanotic focus: larynx, oesophagus, trachea, bronchus, gastrointestinal tract and leptomeninges have all been implicated. Certainly all these organs (and many more) contain clusters of melanocytes, but why these should undergo malignant change remains completely unknown.

Diagnosis of malignant melanoma is not always straightforward. Almost all of us have pigmented melanocytic naevi (approximately 12 in the average white person), and many innocent pigmented naevi appear to enlarge slowly over the years. They are maximal in number in the third decade of life and then slowly disappear. Those undergoing any form of rapid change, particularly with ulceration or bleeding, must be regarded with suspicion: most dermatologists will advise excision biopsy. Other important skin conditions may be difficult to distinguish from malignant melanoma unless a biopsy is obtained; these include pigmented basal cell carcinomas, solar keratoses, blue naevi, juvenile melanomas, pyogenic granulomas, sclerosing angiomas and benign pigmented melanocytic naevi.

Benign melanocytic naevi are derived from the intraepidermal melanocyte whose origin is from the neural crest. There are important differences between the various types of naevus, which may have a bearing on the pathogenesis of malignant melanoma. *Junctional naevi* are well circumscribed, small, flat, pigmented lesions arising from clumps of pigmented cells at the junction of dermis and epidermis. The normal skin lines are not distorted. Their proliferation and penetration into the true dermis result in a *compound naevus*. These are larger than functional naevi and may be raised. Coarse hair may develop and although the functional activity may then abate, the pigmented cells deep in the dermis may then continue to multiply, resulting in an *intradermal naevus*. Here the melanocytes are no longer in contact with the epidermis. Clinically, the lesion has very little pigmentation, usually presenting as a raised papule, commoner in the older age groups. Although functional naevi are certainly capable of malignant change, this happens only rarely. It is not clear how frequently melanoma arises in a common melanocytic naevus.

In the past decade there has been greater understanding of the importance of the *dysplastic naevus syndrome*, a condition originally recognized in familial melanoma but now regarded as more common in sporadic cases. The lesions tend to be larger than truly benign naevi, often irregular in outline and with more variable colour. The gene for familial dysplastic naevi has now been identified [20], located on chromosome 1. Despite the probable importance of the dysplastic naevus in the aetiology of malignant melanoma it should be recognized that the majority of these lesions appear stable or may even regress.

Enlargement of a pre-existing naevus occurs in 10–40% of patients with melanoma, though a more definite precursor, numerically less frequently encountered, is the *lentigo maligna*, or Hutchinson's melanotic freckle. This epidermal lesion results from maturation of atypical melanocytes thought embryologically to result from neural crest tissue. It is one of three well-recognized macroscopic varieties of malignant melanoma, accounting for up to 10% of all cases and, if suspected, demanding immediate surgical excision. Occurring on sun-exposed areas in elderly patients, there is initially a flat pigmented area on the skin which represents a radial growth phase of the tumour, expanding slowly over many years. Later an invasive vertical growth develops, visible as nodules within the lesion. Surgical excision in the radial growth phase is often curative. *Superficial spreading melanomas* are usually larger, often 2–3 cm in diameter, chiefly occurring in middle-age. They have an irregular edge, often with a pale central area. After 1–2 years the lesion may itch or ulcerate and may become nodular, due to vertical penetration of the lesion. In superficial spreading melanoma, about a third of patients have evidence of pre-existing dysplastic naevi. *Nodular melanomas* develop more rapidly still, almost always characterized by deep dermal invasion by the time of diagnosis. There is no recognizable radial growth phase, and areas of skin not exposed to light are often affected. Typically there is a raised nodule on the skin surface and the normal skin markings are disturbed. Ulceration occurs after 2–3 months and deep penetration occurs early. An association with a pre-existing naevi is less strong than in superficial spreading melanoma.

These three major types of melanoma account for almost 90% of all cases, the remainder arising from other types of naevus (congenital, blue, compound or intradermal), or from mucous membranes, meninges or other internal sites.

Stage of melanoma

The most important prognostic characteristics in malignant melanoma are the *level of invasion* (or microstage) and the *clinical stage of the tumour*. Clark *et al.* [21] described five separate levels of invasiveness (Fig. 4.1a), demonstrating that prognosis correlated well with depth of invasion. Subsequent work by Breslow suggests that vertical tumour thickness in millimetres may be an even better guide [22] and this method of pathological staging is now generally preferred. Tumours less than 0.75 mm in thickness very rarely metastasize. In addition, the *type* of primary may also influence the prognosis, nodular lesions in general having a worse prognosis stage for stage than the more common superficial spreading variety, reflecting the increased probability of nodal involvement with nodular lesions. Thinner melanoma can usually be diagnosed on simple histological criteria including nuclear atypic, asymmetry of the lesion, and the presence of single atypical melanocytes in the upper epidermis.

No single *clinical staging system* has been universally accepted, although patients with obvious lymphadenopathy undoubtedly do less well. A simple scheme is shown in Table 22.2. Involvement of regional nodes is usually judged clinically, but patients with palpable and histologically positive regional lymph nodes have a 5-year survival of less than 20%. Those with impalpable local lymph nodes but microscopical involvement have a 5-year survival of over 50%. In patients with melanomas up to 1.49 mm in depth, the survival rate is over 90%, reducing to 67% with tumours of 1.5–3.49 mm, and only 38% where the tumour is thicker still [16].

In reality, the problem of classification and case comparison is even more complex, since a surprising number of features are thought to have prognostic significance even in clinical stage I disease (Table 22.3). A diagnosis of regional lymphadenopathy or wider dissemination is of overriding prognostic significance. Important metastatic sites include liver, lung, spleen, bone, cardiac and central nervous system (particularly brain but also meningeal involvement). Clinical staging of melanoma naturally takes account of the routes of spread, and a full blood count, chest X-ray and liver function tests should be undertaken in all patients.

For those with small, thin stage I lesions, further investigation is not generally necessary [16], though liver and brain scanning will undoubtedly reveal an occasional case of unsuspected occult disease. Abdominal computed tomography (CT), magnetic resonance imaging (MRI) or whole-body positron emission tomography (PET) scanning may demonstrate unsuspected pelvic or para-aortic lymphadenopathy. Although these investigations are difficult (in terms of outcome) to justify as a routine, their increasing availability allows for better prognostic detail. Ultrasonography in skilled hands is a valuable, simple and non-invasive technique in melanoma since it provides reliable information for both hepatic and abdominopelvic staging. Recently the use of radiolabelled monoclonal antibodies (generally using ^{111}In or ^{123}I) for whole-body scanning has occasionally provided additional information, identifying previously unrecognized metastatic sites.

Treatment

Surgery

LOCAL EXCISION

For localized (stage I) malignant melanoma confined to the primary site, surgical excision remains the cornerstone of management. Because of the propensity of local lymphatic invasion, most surgeons recommend wide excision of the primary lesion, with a particularly generous clearance proximally, although recent approaches have become more conservative [23]. Wide excision usually requires split-skin graft coverage, and in relatively good prognoses (Clark's level 1 or 2 (Fig. 4.1a) and lentigo maligna lesions), less generous surgical excision with primary closure is probably adequate. A well-controlled study from the World Health Organization (WHO) Melanoma

Table 22.2 Clinical stage of malignant melanoma.

Stage I	Disease confined to local site (less than 1.5 mm in depth)
Stage II	Disease confined to local site (greater than 1.5 mm in depth)
Stage III	Regional lymph node metastases

Table 22.3 Prognostic factors in clinical stage I malignant melanoma.

Low risk
Radial (lateral) growth phase
Thickness < 0.76 mm or Clark's level 2

Intermediate risk
Level 3 invasion
Up to 1.5 mm thickness

High risk
Level 4 or 5
1.5–4.0 mm invasion
High mitotic rate
Satellite lesions
Ulceration
Axial location on hands or feet

Group has shown that with tumours 1 mm or less in depth, more conservative surgical excision is safe. The present view is that for each millimetre depth of tumour, a 1-cm margin is required, removing the need for surgical grafting in every case. Nodular lesions invade deeply usually as far as the papillary–reticular junction (Clark's level 3) or further and requiring deeper excision than primary lentigo maligna melanomas. Lesions of the hands and feet (for example, subungual melanomas) are generally best dealt with by partial amputation of the digit.

REGIONAL LYMPH NODE DISSECTION

Is it necessary to undertake local lymphadenectomy in all cases of malignant melanoma? In patients with stage I disease, lymphadenectomy undoubtedly gives useful prognostic information. The presence of microscopic disease worsens the 5 year-survival from 70% of cases (true stage I (node-negative) lesions) to only 50% with occult regional lymph node involvement (proven only by surgery).

Whether or not regional lymphadenectomy makes a therapeutic contribution to prognosis remains hotly contested. In general, for patients with good-risk melanoma—a small lesion of a limb, not nodular in character and of Clark's level 1—there is nothing to be gained by lymphadenectomy. For deeper lesions—for example, nodular and spreading melanomas of Clark's level 3, 4 or 5—lymphadenectomy is often recommended. Removal of the first node into which the primary melanoma drains—sometimes referred to as the 'sentinel node'—may be a reasonable compromise [23]. If negative for metastases, 'skip' lesions are unlikely. For melanoma of the trunk, early lymph-node dissection does seem to carry a small survival advantage [24].

Dissection is normally performed if there are clinically involved lymph nodes in the primary nodal drainage area, though it is doubtful whether it genuinely adds to survival. Only 10% of patients with clinically detectable lymphadenopathy confirmed at lymphadenectomy, are alive 5 years later. This unhappy situation is closely analogous to what we know from breast cancer studies, local node involvement generally reflecting disseminated but undetectable disease. In both of these illnesses, this prognostic information is gained by a procedure which is itself of doubtful benefit. Despite this dispiriting state of affairs, radical lymph node dissection for clinical stage II or III melanoma is the only practical means of therapy with any serious chance of success at present. For the highly selected group of patients with high-risk clinical stage II lesions of the distal portion of a limb, amputation may give the best chance of cure.

In the UK, few surgeons favour prophylactic lymph node dissection even in patients with high-risk lesions, even though it provides useful prognostic information. This view is borne out by careful analysis of a large group of Australian patients [25]. The extremely high incidence of this disease in Australia and New Zealand has led to special experience in the larger Australian centres, and the 5-year survival rates from Queensland appear better than for anywhere else in the world (Queensland 81%; England 61%; USA 37%). Although this might suggest particular expertise, it is also true that a higher proportion of Australian patients have primary melanotic lesions confined to the epidermis, with a relatively good prognosis. Further results from Australia suggest a possible benefit of prophylactic lymph node dissection with melanomas of intermediate thickness, though the majority of patients suffer side-effects without any obvious advantage. However, a recent multicentre, randomized, controlled study showed no obvious benefit for prophylactic regional node dissection—at least in terms of survival [26]; these were melanomas of intermediate, 1–4 mm thickness. Somewhat surprisingly, 5-year survival is only 20% better for patients with microscopic (non-palpable) nodal involvement than for patients who present with overt nodal disease (50 vs. 28%): there is clearly a limit to what can be achieved by surgical resection [22].

Radiotherapy

There are few reports of the use of radiotherapy as an alternative to surgery for primary melanomas, though it is known that melanoma cells *in vitro* are not completely radioresistant [27]. Despite the long-held clinical belief that radiation therapy is of no value, radiotherapy can in fact be quite useful for patients in whom surgery is unsuitable because the lesion is too advanced, particularly in lentigo maligna melanoma. Since many lesions are on the extremities, a high dose can usually be reached without danger to internal structures. Large infrequent fractions of treatment (greater than 5 Gy) are often used in an attempt to overcome the shoulder effect thought to be largely responsible for resistance (see Chapter 5).

Chemotherapy

Management of disseminated disease represents an almost insoluble problem. Median survival for patients with disease beyond the regional lymph is only 6 months, though patients with predominantly skin involvement have a median survival of almost a year. Although malignant melanoma is often cited as a tumour in which spontaneous regression occurs, the actual incidence of the phenomenon is no more than 1%, and lengthy survival is exceptionally rare. Nevertheless, with the demonstration in the early 1970s of some degree of sensitivity to chemotherapy, the use of *cytotoxic* drugs for disseminated melanoma became widely adopted although objective responses have been low (Table 22.4) and the overwhelming majority of these responses are less than complete. Furthermore, responses are usually seen in skin, but are very uncommon in liver, brain, bone and lung — sites which are the main cause of death. The most active agents are dacarbazine (DTIC) and vindesine, with response rates of 20–30%. It is not clear whether the use of drugs in combination offers genuinely superior results to treatment with single agents alone; other active agents include nitrosoureas (notably *bis*-chloroethyl nitrosourea and fotemustine) and cisplatin. Use of these, and also DTIC, has become more common with the advent of new-generation 5-hydroxytryptamine-3 (5-HT$_3$) antagonists such as ondansetron, which offer superior control of nausea and vomiting, but combinations such as bleomycin, lomustine, vincristine and DTIC have mostly failed to live up to their early promise. Another experimental approach has been the use of high-dose chemotherapy (generally with melphalan, ifosfamide or DTIC) supplemented by

Table 22.4 Chemotherapy in melanoma.

Drug	Response rate* (%)
Single agents	
DTIC	22
Alkylating agents	10
Methotrexate	7
Cytosine arabinoside	10
Actinomycin D	13
Vindesine	15
Vincristine	10
Mitomycin C	14
Hydroxyurea	10
Nitrosoureas	14
Combination chemotherapy†	
DTIC + vinca	17
DTIC + nitrosourea	17
DTIC + vinca + nitrosourea	24
Vinca + nitrosourea	24
Vinca + nitrosourea + procarbazine	30

*Complete and partial response together. Most response rates refer to cutaneous lesions. Responses are uncommon in visceral lesions.
† Typical regimens.

autologous marrow transplantation, though this has not as yet proven more beneficial than conventional chemotherapy and should not be used outside controlled clinical trials.

There is also evidence of occasional responses to tamoxifen, though reports are still scanty. Interestingly, there are well-documented historic cases of remission (or, alternatively, sudden unexpected relapse) in melanoma patients who have become pregnant, clearly suggesting a degree of hormone-related tumour behaviour.

An alternative approach, for patients with primary melanoma of an extremity and with locoregional or recurrent disease, is the use of regional *cytotoxic* perfusion. Although this was used in the 1960s and 1970s as an adjuvant to primary surgical treatment, there is no convincing evidence that it reduces the likelihood of metastatic disease. Melphalan and cisplatin are most commonly used, the latter particularly in hepatic metastases. Responses are relatively common (up to 40%) though generally partial and short-lived. Regional perfusion has mostly been used for unresectable limb lesions with recurrent disease, or for widespread skin metastases confined to a single limb.

Immunotherapy

Reports of occasional spontaneous regression of disease in melanoma, coupled with the demonstration of antigen and antimelanoma antibodies in the sera of a few patients with the disease, have led to the use of 'active immunotherapy' in this disease. Non-specific intralesional treatment with bacille Calmette–Guérin (BCG) produces local responses in patients with recurrent cutaneous or nodal disease, and α-interferon has also been used in this way [28]. Unfortunately, most responses are short-lived, and of little or no value for patients with recurrent visceral or bone metastases.

Recently, the identification of peptides associated with melanoma has led to the development of new approaches towards vaccines, either for primary or secondary prevention [29]. The best known peptide (melanoma antigen (gene) family, MAGE), a recombinant peptide epitope, is able to produce an immune response which, it is hoped, will prove to be protective.

Biological response modifiers and hyperthermia

Following the interest in immunotherapy of melanoma in the 1970s, attention has more recently turned to the use of interferon, a biological response modifier of established value in other neoplasms, notably B-cell lymphoid tumours (see Chapter 6). The interferons α, β and γ have all been shown to have activity, in about 10–20% of patients, though most responses are short-lived, generally in patients with a relatively small tumour burden. Alpha-interferon is sometimes used for intralesional therapy and may occasionally result in complete disappearance of the injected lesion. Recent studies have attempted to assess α-interferon in combination with chemotherapy, or as a single agent at high doses, with varying success [30].

Interleukin-2 has also been used over the past 5 years, either as a single agent or with cultured autologous lymphocytes which then become cytolytic for the autologous tumour cells. These lymphokine-activated killer (LAK) cells have a response rate reportedly up to 25% with a few unmaintained long-term responses. Unfortunately, interleukin/LAK cell therapy has numerous dose-related side-effects, making it difficult to use (see Chapter 6).

Hyperthermia, the use of heat treatment for cancer, has also been used with some success in melanoma, especially when combined with limb perfusion using melphalan chemotherapy. Although cell kill appears better at temperatures above 41–45°C, toxic reactions at this level can be severe and milder hyperthermia (39–40°C) is more commonly used. Studies of this approach continue, under the supervision of the European Organization for Research and Treatment of Cancer and WHO.

Palliative radiotherapy

Palliative irradiation is undoubtedly useful in selected patients with troublesome deposits, particularly in brain or bone. Although melanoma is not among the more radiosensitive of malignant diseases, resistance can partly be overcome by the use of large infrequent fractions of treatment. Long-term local control of both primary and metastatic lesions, is achieved in about 25% of cases. Newer approaches, including neutron and charged particle therapy, radiosensitizers and hyperthermia, are all being investigated. A further interesting type of regional treatment using novel irradiation is the concept of boron neutron capture therapy [31], exploiting the uptake of phenylalanine (a molecule important in melanogenesis) into melanin-producing melanoma cells. The phenylalanine is coupled to boron to produce the boron-labelled melanin substrate analogue $^{10}B_1$-p-boronophenylalanine. If these cells are irradiated with non-toxic thermal neutrons, the ^{10}B nuclide 'captures' the neutrons, then disintegrates to produce a high-energy lithium atomic nucleus together with an α-particle. The energy is deposited locally, selectively destroying the melanin-synthesizing melanoma cells. This technique has been used in patients with melanoma, with encouraging early results [31].

Prognosis

Prognosis in melanoma is always difficult to determine, a reflection of the multitude of potentially important features (Table 22.2). The sharp increase in incidence of melanoma in wealthier social groups is reflected in a higher mortality rate in these same social classes. For both sexes, people in more affluent social classes are about 50% more likely to die of melanoma than the most economically deprived group, presumably related to access to foreign holidays and more time spent in the sun. The average length of life lost in patients with melanoma is greater than a decade.

Young patients seem to do better than older age groups. Overall, about 90% with melanoma are alive 5 years after diagnosis, whereas only 74% of young men survive that long. Taking all age groups together, a little over 50% of patients with stage I disease will survive 5 years free of recurrence (Fig. 22.6), though it is important to recognize that late relapses occur, so that 5-year survival figures are not definitive. About one-quarter of patients with clinical stage I disease have lymph node involvement at diagnosis (pathological stage II), 75% of these later develop evidence of dissemination. A further 20% of patients with true stage I disease develop distant metastases without ever having had local lymph node enlargement. About 20% of all patients destined to develop recurrent disease will remain disease-free during the first 5 years from diagnosis. For this reason a 5-year survival rate of 60% for stage I melanoma signifies an overall cure rate of about 50% of all patients with early stage of disease. There is also a difference dependent on the primary site of the lesion. Analysis of over 12 000 cases from the Swedish Cancer Registry [32] demonstrated a worse prognosis for scalp and neck lesions, followed by those on the lower limbs and trunk.

Early detection of recurrence appears to give the best opportunity for effective secondary treatment, so patients who have had resection of thick primary lesions require close follow-up [33], for example 2-monthly for the first year and 3-monthly in the second.

For patients with regional lymphadenopathy at diagnosis, the cure rate is probably no more than 15%, while those with disseminated disease at presentation have a median survival of less than 6 months. These dreadful figures will only improve with increased public and pro-

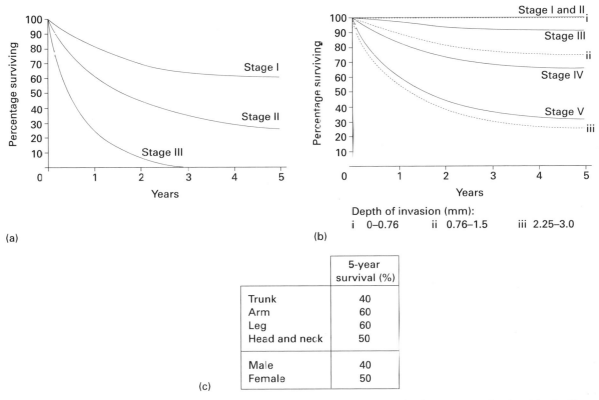

Fig. 22.6 Prognosis in melanoma: (a) prognosis related to stage grouping; (b) prognosis related to microstage (I–V) and depth of invasion (dashed lines); (c) prognosis related to site and sex.

fessional awareness resulting in earlier diagnosis and treatment. Although both chemotherapy and 'immunotherapy' are at present relatively ineffective, it is at least now widely accepted that disseminated melanoma is not totally resistant to treatment.

Skin lymphomas

These are discussed separately in Chapter 26.

Miscellaneous rare tumours

Dermatofibrosarcoma protuberans

This is a soft-tissue sarcoma arising in the skin. It develops as firm nodules which grow slowly and may become large and be locally invasive. In general, it does not metastasize but may recur after simple excision. Wide excision is the

treatment of choice. Radiotherapy may be useful if major surgery (for example, amputation) would otherwise be required.

Kaposi's sarcoma

Originally described by Moritz Kaposi in 1872, this sarcoma was rare in Europe until recently [34]. Kaposi initially described the tumour in elderly Ashkenazi Jewish men, and its incidence in Europe remained low at about 0.3 per million before the acquired immune deficiency syndrome (AIDS) epidemic. In Africa, however, it is common, accounting for 10% of all cancers in Kenya and Uganda. There is a much higher frequency both in renal allograft recipients and in patients with AIDS. The tumour appears to be sustained by immunosuppression which if discontinued, may allow regression of the neoplasm. It is increasingly regarded as a sexually transmitted disease, six times more common, for example, in homosexual or bisexual men than in other AIDS risk groups in the USA [35]. It is clearly linked to infection with human herpes virus 8 (p. 9 and p. 25).

Pathologically there is a proliferation of endothelial vascular channels with numerous interweaving bands of spindle cells, consistent with proliferating endothelium. In the classic form of the disease a pigmented nodule appears on the leg or foot, often growing slowly. It may ulcerate, but lymph node spread is unusual until multiple new lesions have appeared and the disease is more advanced. The disease often results in brawny infiltration with diffuse swelling of the thigh or lower leg. This is a very indolent, unresponsive type of tumour. In children, lymph nodes appear early with a clinical picture similar to lymphoma. In AIDS, the nodular and lymphadenopathic forms convey lesions also appearing on the mucous membranes. Speed of progression varies greatly with the presentation often atypical by contrast to 'classical' Kaposi's sarcoma, with lesions at mucosal or inconspicuous sites. This form of disease seems more prevalent in homosexual males than in other groups with human immunodeficiency virus (HIV) positivity.

Nodular localized disease is treated with radiotherapy. It is a sensitive tumour and single fractions of 8 Gy using electrons are effective, with a complete response rate of 60–90%. In cases of 'classic' non-AIDS-related Kaposi's sarcoma, radiotherapy doses may need to be higher. The tumour is also sensitive to chemotherapy, effective agents (with response rates) including actinomycin D (90%), DTIC (60%), liposomal doxorubicin (70%), bleomycin (60%), paclitax and etoposide (35%) which has the advantage of oral administration. Combination chemotherapy gives a high proportion of complete responders. The usual combinations are actinomycin D and vinblastine, or actinomycin, vincristine and DTIC. α-Interferon produces tumour responses in about 40% of patients who have AIDS, and is increasingly regarded as first-line therapy in selected patients with epidemic cutaneous Kaposi's sarcoma [34].

In the classic form of the disease, patients live for many years. In AIDS-related cases the prognosis is much worse, patients dying of opportunistic infections in addition to the sarcoma.

Merkel cell (primary cutaneous neuroendocrine) tumours

These curious and unusual tumours, often presenting as a discrete nodular mass, have attracted increasing attention in recent years. Histologically they are round cell tumours containing neurosecretory granules, and resemble small-cell carcinoma. They can be surprisingly radiosensitive, and response rates of over 90% have been documented, suggesting that the traditional approach (surgical resection) may be unnecessary. Nevertheless, 40% are locally recurrent and 55% give rise to regional node metastases. The overall 2-year survival rate is 72% (slightly better in women). So far under 1000 cases have been reported in the world literature.

Extramammary Paget's disease

These lesions are located near apocrine sweat glands, in the anogenital region, breast areola and axillae. They are probably a form of carcinoma *in situ*, and present as red, scaly plaques, slowly increasing in size. They are usually removed surgically.

Metastatic carcinoma

Nodules of secondary carcinoma are not infrequently found in the skin, especially with cancer of the breast, penis, vulva and melanoma. If the diagnosis is in doubt, excision biopsy may be necessary. Treatment is generally directed toward the underlying disease if possible. Radiotherapy is often extremely useful for ulcerating or painful deposits.

References

1 Department of Health, *Health Education Authority (UK). Sun Conscious? Fashion and Beauty— the New Testament.* London: Health Education Authority, 1998.

2 Yamagiwa K, Ichikawa K. Experimental study of the pathogenesis of carcinoma. *Cancer Res* 1918; 3: 1–29.

3 Wakefield M, Bonett A. Preventing skin cancer in Australia. *Med J Australia* 1990; 152: 60–1.

4 Zanetti R, Rosso S, Martinez C *et al.* The Multicentre South European Study 'Helios' I. Skin characteristics and sunburns in basal cell and squamous cell carcinoma of the skin. *Br J Cancer* 1996; 73: 1440–6.

5 Rosso S, Zonetti R, Martinez C *et al.* The Multicentre South European Study 'Helios' II. Different sun exposure patterns in aetiology of basal cell and squamous cell carcinoma of the skin. *Br J Cancer* 1996; 73: 1447–54.

6 Rees JL. The melanoma epidemic. reality, and artefact. *Br Med J* 1996; 312: 137–8.

7 Anonymous. Do sunscreens prevent skin cancer? *Drug Therapeutics Bull* 1998; 36: 49–51.

8 Adami J, Frisch M, Yuen J. Evidence of an association between

non-Hodgkin's lymphoma and skin cancer. *Br Med J* 1995; 310: 1491–5.

9 Gorlin RJ. Nevoid basal cell carcinoma syndrome. *Medicine (Baltimore)* 1987; 66: 98–113.

10 Hayward NK. The current situation with regard to human melanoma and genetic inferences. *Curr Opin Oncol* 1996; 8: 136–42.

11 Goldberg LH. Basal cell carcinoma. *Lancet* 1996; 347: 663–7.

12 Lear JT, Harvey I, de Berker D *et al.* Basal cell carcinoma. *J Roy Soc Med* 1998; 91: 585–8.

13 Ashby MA, Smith J, Ainslie J *et al.* Treatment of non-melanoma skin cancer at a large Australian centre. *Cancer* 1989; 63: 1863–71.

14 Mohs FE. *Chemosurgery in Cancer, Gangrene and Infections.* Springfield, Illinois: C. Thomas, 1956.

15 Avril M-F, Auperin A, Margulis A *et al.* Basal cell carcinoma of the face: Surgery or radiotherapy? Results of a randomised study. *Br J Cancer* 1997; 76: 100–8.

16 MacKie RM, Fruedenberger T, Aitchison TC. Personal risk-factor chart for cutaneous melanoma. *Lancet* 1989; ii: 487–90.

17 Elwood JM. Melanoma and sun exposure: contrasts between intermittent and chronic exposure. *World J Surg* 1992; 16: 157–65.

18 Green A, Swerdlow AJ. Epidemiology of melanocytic naevi. *Epidemiol Rev* 1989; 11: 204–21.

19 Anderson DE Smith J, McBride CM. Hereditary aspects of malignant melanoma. *J Am Med Assoc* 1967; 200: 741–6.

20 Bale SJ, Dracopoli NC, Tucker MA *et al.* Mapping the gene for hereditary cutaneous malignant melanoma-dysplastic nevus to chromosome 1p. *N Engl J Med* 1989; 320: 1367–72.

21 Clark WH, From L, Bernadino EA, Mihn NC. The histogenesis and biologic behaviour of primary human malignant melanomas of the skin. *Cancer Res* 1969; 29: 705–27.

22 Breslow A. Tumour thickness level of invasion and node dissection in stage I cutaneous melanoma. *Ann Surg* 1975; 182: 572–5.

23 Rivers JK, Roof MI. Sentinel lymph-node biopsy in melanoma: is less surgery better? *Lancet* 1997; 350: 1336–7.

24 Cascinelli N, Mrabito A, Santinami M *et al.* Immediate or delayed dissection of regional nodes in patients with melanoma of the trunk: a randomised trial. *Lancet* 1998; 351: 793–6.

25 Davis NC, McLeod R, Beardmore G, Little J, Quinn R, Holt J. Melanoma is a word not a sentence. *Australia NZ J Surg* 1976; 46: 138.

26 Piepkorn M, Weinstock MA, Barnhill RL. Theoretical and empirical arguments in relation to elective lymph node dissection for melanoma. *Arch Dermatol* 1997; 133: 995–1002.

27 Barranco SC, Romsdahl MM, Humphrey RM. Radiation response of human melanoma cells grown *in vitro. Cancer Res* 1971; 31: 830–3.

28 Cohen MH, Jessup JM, Felix EL *et al.* Intralesional treatment of recurrent metastatic cutaneous malignant melanoma. *Cancer* 1978; 41: 2456–63.

29 Morton DL, Ravandrath MH. Current concepts concerning melanoma vaccines. In: Dalgleish AG, Browing MJ, eds. *Tumor Immunology.* Cambridge University Press, 1996: 241–68.

30 Marabito A. Effect of long-term adjuvant therapy with interferon alpha-2a in patients with regional node metastases from cutaneous melanoma: a randomised trial. *Lancet* 2001; 358: 866–9.

31 Mishima Y, Honda C, Ichihashi M *et al.* Treatment of malignant melanoma by single thermal neutron capture therapy with melanoma-seeking ^{10}B-compound. *Lancet* 1989; ii: 388–9.

32 Thörn M, Adami HO, Ringborg U *et al.* The association between anatomic site and survival in malignant melanoma: an analysis of 12 353 patients from the Swedish Cancer Registry. *Eur J Cancer* 1989; 25: 483–91.

33 Sylaidis P, Gordon D, Rigby H, Kennedy J. Follow-up requirements for thick cutaneous melanoma. *Br J Plastic Surg* 1997; 50: 349–53.

34 Antman K, Chang Y. Medical progress: Kaposi's sarcoma. *N Engl J Med* 2000; 342: 1027–38.

35 Levine AM. AIDS-related malignancies: the emerging epidemic. *J Natl Cancer Inst* 1993; 85: 1382–97.

23 Bone and soft-tissue sarcomas

Sarcomas are cancers of mesenchymal tissues. Although they are uncommon there is a great variety, and a working classification is given in Tables 23.1 and 23.2. They occur in both children and adults and some types, such as osteosarcoma and Ewing's sarcoma, are most frequent in adolescence. There is a slight male preponderance. The age-specific incidence is shown in Fig. 23.1.

Bone sarcomas

The best understood aetiological factor in bone sarcoma is ionizing irradiation [1]. From 1917 to 1926 many factories were established in the USA and Canada in which there was large-scale production of watches and instruments coated with paint which was made luminous by the action of radium on zinc sulphide. The deplorable factory conditions and the habit of the young female employees of pointing their brushes in their mouths led to osteosarcoma of the jaw and at sites remote from the skull. The cumulative risk of developing osteosarcoma was as high as 70% over the ensuing 40 years.

External beam radiation produces a bone or soft-tissue sarcoma in one in 3000–5000 treated patients. The latent period is 5–30 years (median 10 years). Radiation-induced bone sarcoma is especially likely to occur in children and is one of the commonest second cancers complicating cancer treatment. The major risk of radiation-induced bone cancer is in children with heritable retinoblastoma, and with Ewing's sarcoma, where the relative risk is increased 350-fold. The absolute risk in Ewing's sarcoma is 7%. In other childhood cancers,

the relative risk is 30×. The absolute rate is only 0.1–0.5% [2]. The frequency of osteosarcoma and other bone sarcomas is greatly increased in patients with Paget's disease, the tumour arising in the affected bone. This and prior radiation account for the increased frequency of bone sarcoma in the elderly.

Osteosarcoma occurs with a 500-fold increased incidence in patients who are cured of the familial form of retinoblastoma (see Chapter 24, p. 377). In this disease there is loss of both alleles at 13q14. Allele loss at this site has been found in sporadic cases of osteosarcoma. Loss of heterozygosity and mutation of the *p53* tumour suppressor gene on chromosome 17p is a frequent finding in sporadic osteosarcoma. A cancer familial syndrome, the Li–Fraumeni syndrome, in which sarcomas in childhood are associated with an increased incidence of cancer at an early age in close relatives, is associated with a germline mutation in *p53*. Only 4% of sporadic cases of osteosarcoma, with no suggestive family history, are associated with germline *p53* mutation [3].

In Ewing's sarcoma a characteristic translocation t(11;22) has been found both in cell lines and in primary tumours. The same translocation has been shown in neuroepithelioma and Askin's tumour, suggesting that all three round cell tumours arise from a common lineage. The translocation leads to the expression of an aberrant protein which contains part of either the *FLIa* or *ERG* gene [4]. These transcripts occur in 95% of cases. Three other genes are occasionally partners. The detection of the transcript may be useful diagnostically in distinguishing other small round cell tumours.

Although rare, primary malignant bone tumours are

Table 23.1 Primary malignant bone tumours.

Osteosarcoma
Usually high-grade malignancy, most benign form is parosteal osteosarcoma. Usually metaphyseal. Can be in flat bones. Peak ages 12–24 and 50–80

Ewing's sarcoma
High-grade malignancy. Diaphyseal in long bones, often in flat bones. Age 5–30

Chondrosarcoma
Variable malignancy. Usually metaphyseal. Age 40–60

Other spindle cell tumours
Malignant fibrous histiocytoma ⎫
Fibrosarcoma ⎪ Age 30–50. Long bones. Metaphyseal usually,
Haemangiopericytoma ⎬ similar distribution to osteosarcoma
Haemangioendothelioma ⎭

Other round-cell tumours
Primary lymphoma of bone
Mesenchymal chondrosarcoma
Angiosarcoma

Giant-cell tumour
Occasionally malignant. Epiphyseal. Age 30–40

Table 23.2 Staging system for bone sarcomas.

Stage	Histological grade	Site
IA	Low	Intracompartmental
IB	Low	Extracompartmental
IIA	High	Intracompartmental
IIB	High	Extracompartmental
III	Regional or distant metastases Any grade or local extent	

very important and their management is changing. Until the late 1960s the treatment was usually by amputation or radiotherapy alone, and the results were poor, with osteosarcoma and Ewing's tumour cured in only 10–20% of patients.

In recent years the management of malignant bone tumours has changed considerably. Local control of disease can often now be achieved without amputation by the use of internal prosthetic replacement. The use of intensive chemotherapy pre- and postoperatively has prolonged survival in both Ewing's tumour and osteosarcoma.

These changes have meant that the management of these uncommon tumours has become highly specialized. These tumours are best managed in centres with special experience in the complex surgery and chemotherapy (and sometimes radiotherapy) which is increasingly employed.

Osteosarcoma

This is the commonest malignant tumour of bone (31%) and accounts for 3–4% of all childhood malignancies. In the UK there are approximately 150 new cases each year. The term osteosarcoma is now preferred to osteogenic sarcoma, which is a confusing term because many different bone tumours make bone within their substance.

Pathology

The tumour usually arises in the epiphyseal region and consists of malignant osteoblasts which make osteoid. Within the tumour there may be areas of chondroblastic or fibroblastic differentiation so that small biopsies may not be representative. The tumour cells produce alkaline phosphatase which is a useful cytochemical marker. Typically, the tumour contains mixed fibroblastic, osteoblastic and chondroblastic elements, but other forms are the telangiectatic type, in which there are blood-filled spaces in the tumour, and the small-cell variant, which may be difficult to distinguish from Ewing's sarcoma. The histological differential diagnosis includes other forms of primary malignant bone tumour or soft-tissue sarcoma, especially malignant fibrous histiocytoma of bone. Histological grading of the degree of malignancy gives a rough guide to prognosis and is a prognostic variable which is

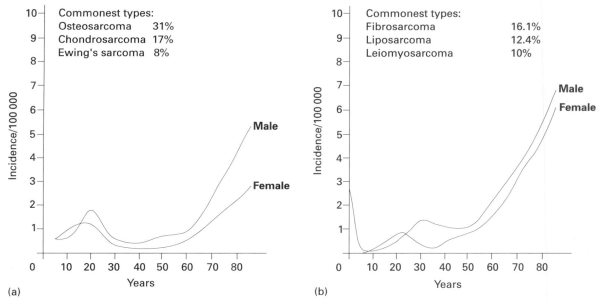

Fig. 23.1 Age-specific incidence of (a) bone, and (b) soft-tissue sarcomas.

taken into account in assessing comparisons between treatments.

Local invasion occurs when the tumour breaks through the bone and the periosteal surroundings (Fig. 23.2) and invades the soft tissue including the nerves and blood vessels around the joint. A staging system has been proposed, based on grade and compartmental extension (Table 23.2).

Juxtacortical (parosteal) osteosarcoma is an unusual variant in which new bone formation is especially dense and which presents as a large exostosis. The pathology and clinical behaviour are less malignant. A further variant, periosteal osteosarcoma, has an intermediate degree of malignancy. Osteosarcoma arising in Paget's disease occurs in an older age group and often develops in flat bones. The tumours are usually aggressive and metastases occur early.

Clinical features

The disease mostly affects adolescents, the peak incidence being in the age range 10–20 years during the adolescent growth spurt. Boys are affected more often than girls (1.5 : 1). Most of the tumours occur around the knee, and the lower femur and upper tibia account for 60% of all cases. The presentation is with pain and swelling, often brought to attention by minor trauma. The pain is typically worse

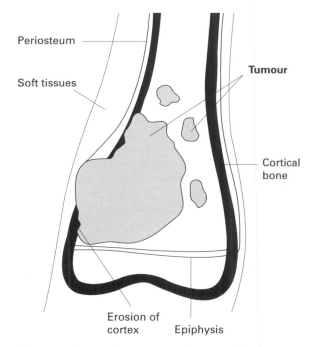

Fig. 23.2 In this central osteosarcoma the tumour has arisen next to the epiphysis. It has eroded the cortical bone, broken through the periosteal barrier and spread into the soft tissues. The 'islands' of the central tumour are actually connected to the main tumour mass when seen in three dimensions.

at night and may be present for many weeks before swelling appears. Nocturnal bone pain is always a serious symptom in oncology. On examination there is usually a firm swelling which may be warm and tender with limitation of movement of the joint.

Radiological appearances

Generally there is a destructive lesion in the metaphyseal region, usually but not always with new bone formation in spicules. There may be a Codman's triangle caused by elevation of the periosteum (Fig. 23.3). The parosteal variety is associated with slow growth, exostosis and dense new bone, and the telangiectatic type with rapidly progressive destruction. The way in which the radiological appearances are produced by the tumour extension is clearly shown in X-rays of thin sections taken through the whole specimen (Fig. 23.4).

Investigation

Routine investigation should include chest X-ray, isotope

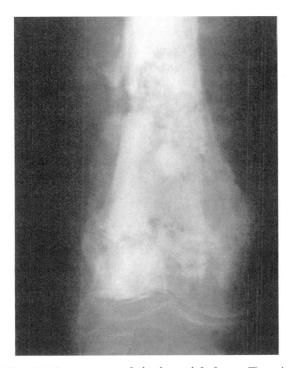

Fig. 23.3 Osteosarcoma of the lower left femur. There is extensive bone destruction, with elevation of the periosteum (Codman's triangle) and new bone formation.

bone scan which may show skeletal metastases, and a computed tomography (CT) scan of the thorax. This should be performed before surgery. Computed tomography scanning is the most sensitive method of detecting pulmonary metastases and these will be present in about 30% of cases. If local resection is contemplated (see below) magnetic resonance imaging (MRI) (or CT if MRI is not available) scan of the affected limb is essential to delineate tumour extent (Figs 23.5 and 23.6) including the extent of the soft-tissue component and the intramedullary extension. In interpreting MRI scans care must be taken not to confuse oedema with soft-tissue infiltration. The serum alkaline phosphatase is frequently elevated.

Treatment

SURGERY

Before 1980, amputation was the main surgical treatment. For tumours around the knee, the amputation is at mid-thigh level. To be of value the stump must extend at least 10 cm from the ischial tuberosity. Higher tumours, or those which extend high up the femoral shaft, are treated by disarticulation.

In recent years conservative surgery has been used wherever possible. A massive internal prosthesis is inserted after removal of the tumour (Fig. 23.7). In some countries a bone allograft is used. The functional results of prostheses are excellent for the lower femur and upper tibia, but somewhat less satisfactory in the upper humerus. Pathological fractures and/or extensive infiltration along the bone shaft or into soft tissue make prosthetic replacement less feasible. Conservative limb-preserving surgery is now increasingly performed for pelvic tumours, either with removal of part of the pelvic ring without reconstruction (for tumours of the pubis and ischium not involving the hip joint) or with insertion of a metallic prosthesis. Local recurrence of the tumour is becoming less common with skilful surgery and with the use of preoperative chemotherapy. Local recurrences can usually still be successfully treated by amputation.

CHEMOTHERAPY

The use of complex and intensive adjuvant chemotherapy has resulted in an increase in survival from 20 to 25% without chemotherapy to 45–80% with treatment.

Modern adjuvant programmes typically use cisplatin, doxorubicin, ifosfamide and high-dose methotrexate. It is still not clear whether the dose of methotrexate is important. Unreliable retrospective analyses suggest that a high

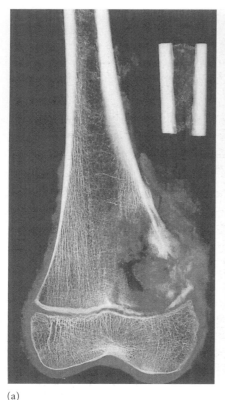

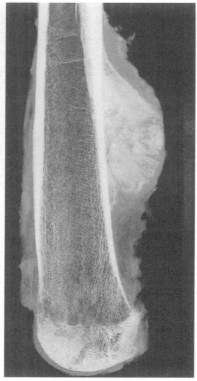

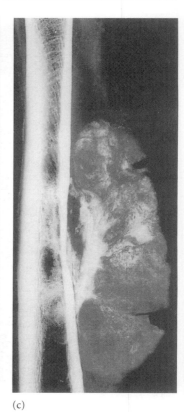

(a)   (b)   (c)

Fig. 23.4 Fine-detail X-rays of sagittal longitudinal slabs of resection specimens of osteosarcoma. (a) Classical osteosarcoma of distal femur in a boy aged 14 years. The lesion stops at the unfused epiphysis. It is destroying the cortex and extends sub-periosteally, lifting the periosteum and forming a Codman's triangle. There are spicules of new bone formation. This is the commonest site for osteosarcoma. The insert shows the normal intramedullary cavity higher in the femur. (b) Parosteal osteosarcoma in an 18-year-old-male, arising from the posterior aspect of the distal femur (the typical site of this tumour). The tumour is confined to the outer aspect of the cortex and contains trabecular bone which is covered with fibrous tissue on the outer surface. The bone cortex is intact and the medulla is not involved. The fused epiphysis is visible. (c) Periosteal osteosarcoma of the mid-femur in a woman aged 50 years. The tumour is made up of radiolucent tumour cartilage and shows patchy calcification. In a few places there is a trabecular pattern with mineralized tumour osteoid. There is involvement of the subadjacent medulla. We are indebted to Dr Jean Pringle of the Royal National Orthopaedic Hospital for these preparations.

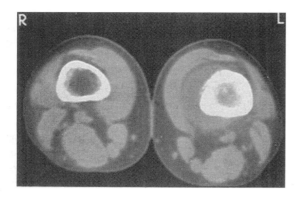

peak serum level (more than 1 mmol) is associated with better survival.

Ifosfamide has been widely used in recent protocols of treatment. There is some evidence that response rates are higher when the drug is given in very high dose (more than $15 \, g/m^2$) but the toxicity is greatly increased and the effect on survival is unknown. Although other agents such

Fig. 23.5 CT scan of osteosarcoma of the left femur. At this level the bone X-ray was only slightly abnormal. The scan shows erosion of the cortex, periosteal reaction and considerable soft-tissue swelling.

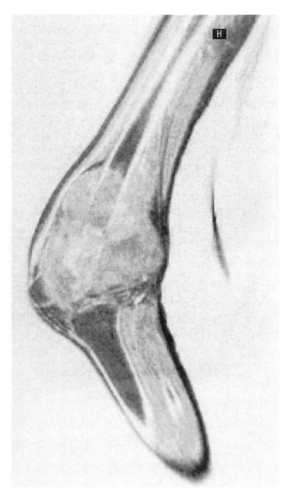

Fig. 23.6 MRI scan of the lower femur in a 16-year-old girl with osteosarcoma. A large soft-tissue mass surrounds the lower femur, extending into the soft tissues.

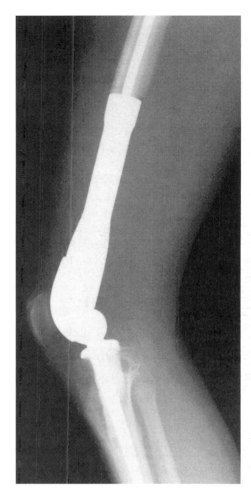

Fig. 23.7 Endoprosthetic replacement of osteosarcoma of the distal femur. Following chemotherapy the tumour was resected and the lower femur and knee replaced by the prosthesis. Chemotherapy was then continued for 3 months. This patient walks normally, can run and climb stairs.

as cyclophosphamide, bleomycin and actinomycin are sometimes used, there is little evidence to suggest they are effective. In large-scale studies about 60% of patients with no detectable metastases at presentation are cured (Fig. 23.8a) [5,6].

It is now usual to employ chemotherapy before surgery (induction or neoadjuvant chemotherapy) as well as post-operatively (Fig. 23.9). This has the advantages of starting systemic treatment early, of allowing time for the manu-facture of an endoprosthesis, of facilitating surgery if the tumour reduces in size, and of allowing histological as-sessment of response when the tumour is resected. The hope that non-responding tumours would have a better prognosis if the chemotherapy was changed postopera-

tively has not been fulfilled. A better strategy appears to be to give all the most active drugs initially. Survival is better in patients whose tumours show a good histological response (Fig. 23.8b).

TREATMENT OF PULMONARY METASTASES [7]
Patients who develop pulmonary metastases may still be curable by surgery. If a patient develops pulmonary metastases, CT scanning should be used to determine if he or she is operable. Adjuvant chemotherapy after amputa-tion may not only delay or prevent pulmonary metastases but also benefits patients by reducing the number of pul-

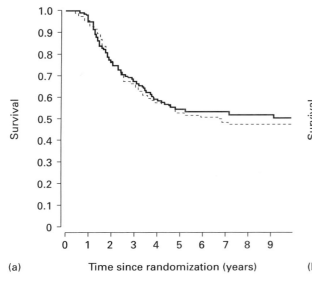

(a) Time since randomization (years)

(b) Time from surgery (years)

Fig. 23.8 (a) A recent randomized trial [6] of two chemotherapy regimens in osteosarcoma. Survival at 5 years is 55% with few recurrences after that time. (b) Survival in the two arms of the trial according to whether there was a good (A) or poor (B) histological response.

monary metastases when they do occur, sometimes allowing a potentially curative resection. The prognosis after metastasectomy is better if the lesions are unilateral, if there are less than six, if they appear late after chemotherapy has stopped, and if they are entirely resected. When a metastasis is detected chemotherapy is often started using agents which have not previously been given, and if no new metastases have appeared within 2–3 months, thoracotomy is undertaken. This approach helps to prevent needless thoracotomies in patients destined to develop further pulmonary metastases early and to die quickly of their disease.

RADIOTHERAPY
Before modern chemotherapy was introduced, high-dose radiotherapy to the primary tumour was used in order to avoid amputation in those destined to die of metastases. If these did not occur within 6–12 months a delayed amputation was performed. Unfortunately, local radiotherapy seldom provides long-lasting control of the primary and local recurrence and fractures often occur. Radiotherapy is still of value in palliation of an advanced tumour and in treatment of painful bone metastases.

Whole-lung irradiation (17.5 Gy in 20 fractions) has been used to prevent pulmonary metastases. Some studies have shown prevention, or delay in onset, of pulmonary metastases, others have not and the value of this treatment remains uncertain. Its use has been superseded by chemotherapy.

Parosteal and periosteal osteosarcoma

Parosteal osteosarcoma is a rare slow-growing variant which arises from the surface of the bone, usually the distal posterior femur (Fig. 23.4b). It metastasizes late and adjuvant chemotherapy is not indicated. Treatment is by

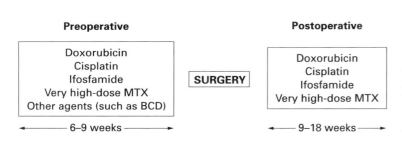

Preoperative

Doxorubicin
Cisplatin
Ifosfamide
Very high-dose MTX
Other agents (such as BCD)

SURGERY

Postoperative

Doxorubicin
Cisplatin
Ifosfamide
Very high-dose MTX

← 6–9 weeks →   ← 9–18 weeks →

Fig. 23.9 Schematic representation of a typical chemotherapy programme for osteosarcoma. BCD is a combination of bleomycin, cisplatin and actinomycin D. MTX is methotrexate. Limb preservation surgery is increasingly employed.

wide local excision. Periosteal osteosarcoma (Fig. 23.4c) is rare and is of a higher grade than parosteal lesions. There are usually areas of chondroblastic differentiation. Although less likely to metastasize than classical central tumours, chemotherapy may be indicated.

High-grade surface osteosarcomas

These are rare variants which can occur at any age. Histologically and clinically they are indistinguishable from central high-grade tumours, and are treated in the same way. They should not be mistaken for periosteal tumours which have a reduced tendency to metastasize.

Small-cell osteosarcoma

A rare variant of osteosarcoma, these tumours resemble Ewing's sarcoma and may contain cytoplasmic glycogen. The tumorous cells produce alkaline phosphatase indicating their osteoblast origins, as does the presence of tumour osteoid. They metastasize rapidly and, although responsive to chemotherapy, the prognosis is less good than for other variants.

Chondrosarcoma

This is the second commonest bone tumour but occurs later in life than osteosarcoma, with a peak incidence at 40–60 years. It may arise *de novo* as a sarcomatous transformation of benign enchondromata, in multiple enchondromatosis (Ollier's disease) and, rarely, in Paget's disease.

Presentation

These tumours are usually slow growing. The commonest site is the pelvis, followed by the femur, humerus, scapula and ribs. The most usual symptom is a painful swelling, but in slow-growing lesions pain may not be a symptom at first. The disease tends to grow more rapidly in younger patients.

The X-ray typically shows a destructive bone lesion with areas of calcification normally as flecks (rather than spicules as in osteosarcoma) (Fig. 23.10).

Pathology [8]

The low-grade tumour resembles cartilage but without tumour osteoid being formed and with a greater degree of cellular pleomorphism. Low-grade tumours tend to be locally invasive and not to metastasize, but pulmonary metastases are frequent in high-grade tumours. Some-

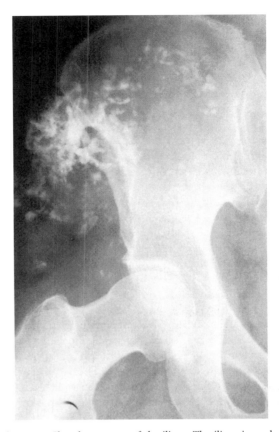

Fig. 23.10 Chondrosarcoma of the ilium. The ilium is eroded by the tumour which shows patchy calcification. The tumour extends into the soft tissues laterally.

times low-grade tumours change to a more malignant variety after repeated local recurrence. At this stage a spindle cell component may dominate the histological appearance.

Treatment and prognosis

The mainstay of treatment is surgery, with complete removal of the tumour with associated soft tissues. In a long bone this can sometimes be accomplished, without amputation, by *en bloc* resection and insertion of an endoprosthesis. In the pelvis a surgical approach is often impossible. It is essential that the initial resection is radical with wide margins. Local recurrence will otherwise occur, requiring much more extensive surgery. Radiotherapy is used as a palliative treatment but the tumour is radioresistant and local control is usually short-lived. From the little evidence available the tumour also appears to be resistant to cytotoxic drugs [9] unless the tumour is dedifferentiated, when responses may occur to drugs such as cisplatin, doxorubicin and ifosfamide.

Prognosis is largely determined by histological grade. Ten-year survival is 80% for grade I tumours and 25% for grade III.

Mesenchymal chondrosarcoma

This rare variant occurs in teenage children and young adults. The axial skeleton and skull bones are often affected. The tumour shows calcification on plain X-ray. The tumour contains small-cell components which may enable distinction from a round-cell sarcoma difficult. It responds to chemotherapy but radical excision is essential for survival. Radiation may be used if the resection margins are not clear at operation. Chemotherapy regimens are usually based on cisplatin, doxorubicin and ifosfamide.

Ewing's sarcoma

This is a malignant round-cell tumour of bone whose aetiology is unknown. The characteristic chromosomal translocation is discussed on p. 344. The peak incidence is 10–20 years and, like osteosarcoma, it is slightly more common in males (1.5 : 1). It is very rare in Africans and African-Americans.

Presentation

Pain and swelling are the usual symptoms and may be present for many months before diagnosis. Pulmonary symptoms, due to metastases, may first bring the patient to the doctor. The flat bones of the pelvis are the commonest site of involvement although the femur is the commonest single bone to be involved, and the tibia and humerus less frequently. The tumour can also arise in the vertebrae, skull and ribs (Fig. 23.11b). Fever and weight loss are not infrequent, especially with large and metastatic tumours.

Pathology

The tumour usually arises in the diaphysis and occasionally in the metaphysis. Epiphyseal involvement is unusual. Histologically it consists of small round cells. It resembles and must be distinguished from non-Hodgkin's lymphoma, metastatic neuroblastoma and some types of rhabdomyosarcoma. On conventional histology it may be impossible to distinguish Ewing's sarcoma from primitive neuroectodermal tumours (PNETs) of other types (such

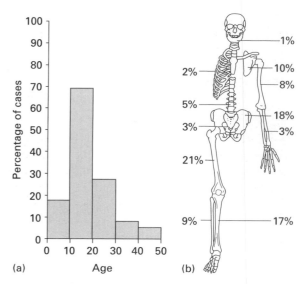

Fig. 23.11 Ewing's sarcoma: (a) age at onset; (b) site of primary tumour.

as Askin's tumour). Indeed, it seems likely that classical Ewing's sarcoma and PNET are part of a spectrum of round-cell tumours showing varying degrees of neural differentiation. Immunohistochemical techniques will show neural markers in PNETs (such as neurone-specific enolase, and the neural cell adhesion molecule). When PNET presents in bone it seems that the prognosis is not substantially different from that for Ewing's sarcoma [10]. Differentiation from lymphoma can be made by use of antibodies to the common leucocyte antigen (which stain lymphoma) and by the lack of surface immunoglobulin in Ewing's sarcoma. Ewing's tumour usually stains with antibodies to MIC2, an antigen almost always present in the tumour cells.

The tumour typically permeates the medullary and cortical bone, and for this reason wide margins are needed in planning radiotherapy or surgery. Glycogen can often be demonstrated in the cytoplasm by the periodic acid–Schiff stain, and the distinction from these other tumours can usually be made on clinical, radiological and biochemical grounds. Metastases to lung and to the bones occur frequently.

Investigation

Diagnosis is by biopsy and expert opinion on the histology. The X-ray usually shows a diffuse erosion in a flat bone (Fig. 23.12) or in the diaphyseal region of a long

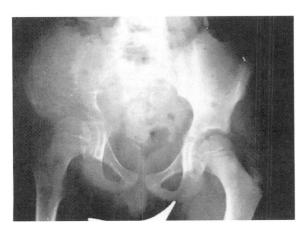

Fig. 23.12 Ewing's sarcoma of the right ilium. The bone is diffusely expanded by a large radiolucent tumour.

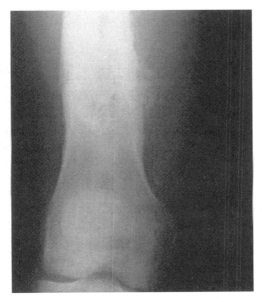

Fig. 23.13 X-ray of Ewing's tumour of the femur. Note the diaphyseal position, the periosteal elevation, and the new bone formation.

bone (Fig. 23.13). There is a marked periosteal reaction, sometimes with an 'onion skin' appearance, usually with evidence of a soft-tissue mass which is often extensive.

Further investigation should include a full blood count which may show anaemia and leucocytosis in advanced or rapidly progressive cases; chest X-ray, CT scan of the primary site and of the thorax which may show single or multiple metastases; isotope bone scan to detect bone metastases which are common; plasma lactate dehydrogenase and liver function tests; and urine vanillyl mandelic acid if there is a possibility that the diagnosis is neuroblastoma. MRI scanning is invaluable in indicating the degree of intramedullary and soft-tissue extension of the tumour. About 20% of patients have radiologically detectable metastases at diagnosis. Sensitive molecular tests can detect Ewing's tumour cells in the bone marrow of an even greater proportion (up to 50% in some series) associated with a somewhat worse prognosis.

Treatment

This must be both local and systemic. Local treatment alone is associated with cure in only 10–20% of cases, and the prognosis has been improved considerably by the addition of adjuvant chemotherapy.

LOCAL TREATMENT

Unlike most primary bone sarcomas, Ewing's sarcoma is radiosensitive. Until recently the mainstay of local treatment was radical megavoltage radiotherapy. Doses of 55–65 Gy are given to the primary site in 2-Gy fractions, over 6–7 weeks. Care must be taken not to irradiate all the soft tissues of a limb to this dose, or troublesome oedema will occur below the irradiated site. In practice this involves careful avoidance of a strip of soft tissue the whole length of the treatment field (Fig. 23.14). Additionally, the last 15–20 Gy are given to a smaller field around the residual tumour, that is, using a 'shrinking field' technique.

In recent years troublesome late local recurrences have been seen in some patients after treatment with radiotherapy and chemotherapy. For this reason there is increasing use of surgical excision and endoprosthetic replacement of bone as an adjuvant to chemotherapy and radiotherapy. Surgery alone may sometimes be sufficient to gain control, but because of the permeating nature of the tumour, a combination of surgery and radiation is sometimes necessary. Another reason for wishing to avoid radiation is the risk of later development of radiation sarcoma. The 20-year risk of induction of a radiation sarcoma after treatment of Ewing's tumour in childhood is 7%. The problem is that surgery for large tumours often proves to be histologically intralesional so that follow-up radiation cannot be avoided. The decision between surgery and radiation is therefore highly complex, especially in pelvic tumours [11]. Malignant round-cell bone tumours should be managed by those who are very familiar with these problems and not in hospitals with limited experience.

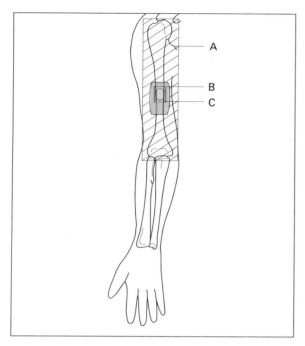

Fig. 23.14 Radiation fields in Ewing's sarcoma. (A) The whole bone is irradiated to a modest diaphyseal humeral dose (30 Gy). (B) The field is shrunk down to the tumour and adjacent bone to 45 Gy. (C) The tumour itself is boosted to 60–70 Gy. If the tumour is well clear of the epiphyses these may not be included in the radiation field.

CHEMOTHERAPY

Adjuvant chemotherapy is an essential part of management and has been responsible for the improved prognosis in recent years [12]. The most useful agents are doxorubicin, cyclophosphamide, vincristine, actinomycin D and ifosfamide. Responses are also seen with etoposide, methotrexate and nitrosoureas. A variety of different combinations is in use, with none showing a clear superiority. It is probable that all first-line agents should be used and that the dose of drugs should be kept as high as possible. In recent years the tendency has been to use chemotherapy very intensively over a period of 9–12 months rather than to use lower doses for 1–2 years. A typical regimen begins with ifosfamide, doxorubicin and vincristine for 12 weeks followed by local treatment (with surgery and radiotherapy). Chemotherapy is continued postoperatively, with actinomycin substituted for doxorubicin when the maximum dose of doxorubicin has been reached. The patient must be kept under regular review during this time with regular blood counts and chest X-rays, with bone scans when clinically indicated.

Prognosis

In localized disease, the use of radical local treatment with the most intensive chemotherapy regimens has now led to 5-year survival rates of 50–60%. Most of these children have probably been cured. Although many factors have contributed to this improved survival there is little doubt that chemotherapy has been the major influence.

Pelvic lesions have a worse prognosis than limb tumours. Very small tumours (for example, in the jaw, and in the small bones of the hand and feet) have an excellent prognosis and it is not clear how much chemotherapy is necessary in these cases. The main determinants of prognosis are tumour volume and the presence of metastases. Large tumours are more likely both to recur locally and to metastasize.

Patients presenting with metastatic disease may frequently obtain a complete response of the tumour followed by later relapse. With conventional chemotherapy the outlook remains poor, although patients with only a few pulmonary metastases have a reasonable chance of cure. For the rest, these very high-risk patients are increasingly considered for very high-dose chemotherapy with autologous bone marrow or peripheral blood stem cell support. Preliminary results suggest that a minority of these patients may be cured by this procedure, depending on their remission status at the time of high-dose therapy.

Giant-cell tumour of bone (osteoclastoma)

This tumour occurs at age 20–40 and typically involves the epiphysis of a long bone. It causes a well-defined lytic lesion which eventually erodes the cortex of the bone, giving rise to soft-tissue extension. The presentation is with pain and swelling typically around the knee, the tumour occurring with equal frequency in the lower femur and upper tibia. X-ray shows a lytic lesion. Similar cystic changes can be caused by aneurysmal bone cysts or the cystic lesion of osteitis fibrosa cystica (primary hyperparathyroidism).

Pathologically the tumour consists of giant cells and spindle cells. Occasionally the appearances are frankly malignant and the tumour is then more locally invasive and metastases may occur. The tumours can be graded (I–III) according to the appearance of the stromal cells. There is some dispute about whether radiation treatment encourages malignant transformation. This is an uncommon development in the tumour and usually it is the more aggressive (grade III) tumours which are irradiated, so the issue is not clear.

The treatment is usually by thorough curettage of the

entire cavity of a localized lesion. The cavity can then be filled by bone chips. More extensive lesions can be treated by excision and endoprosthetic replacement of bone. Some tumours are not amenable to surgery, for example those in vertebrae. In these cases, radiotherapy at modest dose (40–50 Gy) over 4–5 weeks is the mainstay of treatment. There is no known effective chemotherapy, although drugs used in osteosarcoma treatment have been used. Solitary pulmonary metastases can be excised, sometimes without recurrence.

Other malignant spindle cell tumours of bone (malignant fibrous histiocytoma, fibrosarcoma)

These tumours have a similar anatomical distribution to osteosarcoma but occur in the 30–50 year age range, and in the diaphysis a little more commonly. The fibrosarcomas are often of low grade. Many of the tumours are associated with a long history of pain before the diagnosis is established by X-ray followed by biopsy. Malignant fibrous histiocytoma consists of spindle cells with histiocytic-like cells. The radiological features are of bone lysis. The tumour is of high grade. Treatment is by overall excision, but there is clear evidence of chemosensitivity and the tumour is now treated with chemotherapy as well. It is sensitive to high-dose methotrexate, ifosfamide and doxorubicin [12]. The prognosis is poor with surgery alone (30% overall survival at 3–4 years) but it seems that chemotherapy will improve this. Like osteosarcoma, these tumours tend to be resistant to radiotherapy, although radiotherapy may be helpful as an adjuvant to surgery, or for local recurrence. Fibrosarcoma is treated by surgical excision. Although chemotherapy may be considered in high-grade lesions, there is little information on the chemosensitivity of this rare tumour.

Bone tumours of vascular origin

Haemangioendothelioma is a locally invasive tumour which does not usually metastasize. The lesion can occur at any age and is radiologically lytic. It may be multicentric. Treatment is by excision. Haemangiopericytoma is a vascular tumour, taking on a spindle cell appearance and of variable malignancy. Treatment is by surgery. Angiosarcoma is an exceedingly rare undifferentiated tumour. The tumour arises from vascular endothelium (demonstrated by staining for factor VIII). Although usually solitary, multiple contiguous bones may be involved. The tumour is excised if possible. Little is known of its chemosensitivity.

Non-Hodgkin's lymphoma of bone

Non-Hodgkin's lymphoma may occur in bone and be completely localized with no evidence of disease elsewhere. Nevertheless, the risk of spread is great. The tumours are lytic and destructive, typically having ill-defined margins. Both high-grade and low-grade tumours are described. In Europe they are usually B-cell disorders, but T-cell lymphomas are possibly more common in Japan. An associated soft-tissue mass is often present. Full staging is essential (see Chapter 26) to determine if there is systemic spread and to ensure that the bone lesion is not a metastasis from a nodal lymphoma. Radiotherapy (30–40 Gy) controls the local disease, and systemic chemotherapy is now usually given, especially if there is any doubt about whether the tumour is localized, and in all high-grade tumours. In elderly patients with clinically localized disease it is permissible to follow an expectant policy and treat with cytotoxic agents only if metastasis occurs. Very rarely, the tumour may arise at a number of bone sites in a multifocal distribution.

Soft-tissue sarcomas

Progress in the management of adult sarcomas has been hampered by the relative rarity and heterogeneity of these tumours. In addition, they are relatively unresponsive to radiotherapy and chemotherapy, and many of these tumours have a high incidence of local recurrence after surgery. In adults the clinical behaviour of these tumours is becoming clearer, and one or two important points in management have begun to emerge. In childhood sarcomas the picture is different, with some degree of responsiveness to chemotherapy proving the rule, leading in many instances to an improvement in survival rate (see Chapter 24).

Aetiology

The overall incidence in adults is two per 100 000, accounting for 1% of all cancers. Most cases of soft-tissue sarcoma are sporadic. Soft-tissue sarcoma is one of the tumours which occurs in the Li–Fraumeni syndrome (p. 344). Patients with von Recklinghausen's disease have a tendency towards malignant change in fibromatous or neurofibromatous lesions (neurofibrosarcoma is the typical tumour type). Angiosarcoma of the liver occurs more frequently in workers who are chronically exposed to PVC. Patients with gross lymphoedema may rarely

Table 23.3 Soft-tissue sarcoma: a simplified classification.

Tissue of origin	Benign neoplasm	Sarcoma
Fibrous tissue	Fibroma (single or multiple, as in fibromatosis)	Fibrosarcoma (including dermatofibrosarcoma protruberans)
Muscle		

Striated	Rhabdomyoma	Rhabdomyosarcoma
		  Embryonal
		  Alveolar
		  Pleomorphic
		  Botryoidal

Smooth	Leiomyoma (including uterine 'fibroids')	Leiomyosarcoma
Mixed origin		Malignant fibrous histiocytoma (possibly a mixture of other pathologies)
Fat	Lipoma	Liposarcoma
Blood vessels	Angioma, haemangioma	Haemangiosarcoma, Kaposi's sarcoma, lymphangiosarcoma, haemangiopericytoma
Peripheral nerves	Neuroma, neurofibroma neurilemmoma (including Schwannoma)	Neurofibrosarcoma, malignant neurilemmoma (including malignant Schwannoma and neuroepithelioma)
Pleura and peritoneum		Mesothelioma
Unknown		Synovial cell sarcoma Alveolar soft part sarcoma (malignant non-chromaffin paraganglioma)

develop a lymphangiosarcoma of the oedematous limb (Stewart–Treves syndrome), most typically in the upper arm, following radiotherapy for breast carcinoma. Soft-tissue sarcoma may also arise in a previously irradiated area. The latency and frequency are similar to that for bone sarcoma.

Pathology and molecular genetics

Soft-tissue sarcomas can arise wherever mesenchymal tissue is present (Table 23.3). The commonest varieties in adults result from malignant transformation of fibrous tissue (fibrosarcomas); striated muscle (rhabdomyosarcoma); smooth muscle (leiomyosarcoma); fat (liposarcoma); and blood vessels (haemangiopericytoma, angiosarcoma). Tumours of peripheral nerves (schwannoma, neurofibrosarcoma, etc.) are discussed in Chapter 11 and mesothelioma in Chapter 12. Other rarer tumours occur and are discussed below. The characteristic cytogenetic changes which accompany some sarcomas are described in the appropriate sections.

Gene mutations

The discovery that the molecular changes that occur in soft-tissue sarcomas provide potential targets for therapy, and aid classification has led to a dramatic conceptual and practical advance.

Gastrointestinal stromal cell tumours (GIST) are benign but may become malignant. When they do they frequently overexpress a mutant, active, signal transduction receptor tyrosine kinase called c-KIT. Dramatic responses to the tyrosine kinase inhibitor ST1571 (used in chronic granulocytic leukaemia—see p. 450) have shown that the tumour growth is at least partially stimulated by c-KIT [13].

Inflammatory myofibroblastic tumours may become high-grade sarcomas and overexpress the mutant tyrosine kinase ALK.

Desmoplastic round-cell tumours are related to Ewing's sarcoma and express the *EWS–WTI* fusion protein (p. 344). This is a transcriptional regulator that induced platelet derived growth factor (PDGF-α) which is a mitogen. It is not yet known if inhibitors will cause tumour regression.

Other sarcomas overexpressing receptor tyrosine kinases are *congenital fibrosarcoma* and *mesoblastic nephroma* (N-TRK-3 in both) and *dermatofibrosarcoma protuberans* (PDGF-β). The signal transduction protein *Ras* is overexpressed in neurofibrosarcomas.

From the point of view of diagnostics/classification characteristic translocations have been found in myeloid liposarcoma and synovial sarcoma (see below).

Fibrosarcoma

These tumours are composed of fusiform fibroblasts which form collagen strands and reticulin. The histological definition of malignancy may be difficult, and well-differentiated tumours such as dermatofibrosarcoma protuberans seldom metastasize but may be locally invasive. Anaplastic tumours invade locally and also spread rapidly to the lungs.

The tumours usually arise on the limbs or trunk but may occur in any soft tissue. Typically, the patient notices a painless firm lump. In dermatofibrosarcoma protuberans, the history is of a slowly enlarging skin nodule becoming violaceous and later ulcerating.

Malignant fibrous histiocytoma

This term has become more widely used as a pathological entity. It is not a new disease and cases previously diagnosed as poorly differentiated fibrosarcoma or pleomorphic rhabdomyosarcomas are now often included in this category. It is probable that the term does not describe a specific tumour but an appearance which can be found in sarcomas of many types. The typical histological pattern is one of malignant spindle cells often arranged in a 'storiform' or herring-bone fashion. As with fibrosarcomas, the presentation is usually with a painless lump or nodule, though this tumour can also occur as a primary bone tumour (p. 355).

Liposarcoma

These tumours present in middle age and occur in subcutaneous fat and in retroperitoneal tissues. They do not arise from pre-existing lipomas. There are four histological types.
1 Well differentiated (with mature fat).
2 Myxoid which has a characteristic t(12;16) (q13;p11) translocation.
3 Round-cell type.
4 A pleomorphic variant.

The translocation in the myxoid tumour deregulates the *CHOP* gene which is involved in adipocyte differentiation.

Rhabdomyosarcoma

This is a complex group of tumours with several distinct subtypes.

EMBRYONAL RHABDOMYOSARCOMA
These tumours occur in early childhood and young adult life. They consist of malignant spindle and round cells, and often occur in the head and neck and orbit (see Chapter 24).

ALVEOLAR RHABDOMYOSARCOMA
This tumour is composed of large, round and polygonal cells. It occurs in adolescents and young adults and has a wider, anatomical distribution, often presenting in the trunk. These are highly malignant tumours and metastasize early.

PLEOMORPHIC RHABDOMYOSARCOMA
In these tumours the cells vary greatly in size and shape, and giant cells are often present. Many are now classified as malignant fibrous histiocytoma. They occur in adult life (over the age of 30), usually on the limbs, arising from deep muscle groups.

BOTRYOIDAL RHABDOMYOSARCOMA ('SARCOMA BOTRYOIDES')
These tumours consist of polypoid growths in the urinary and genital tracts, usually in young children. Histologically the tumour consists of an area of cells with high mitotic activity surrounded by acellular oedematous tissue.

Leiomyosarcoma

The uterus is the commonest site of origin. The tumours probably occur as a result of malignant change in a uterine fibroid (leiomyoma). The histological diagnosis is usually made after hysterectomy for fibroids. Other leiomyosarcomas arise from smooth muscle at other sites such as subcutaneous tissue, stomach, bowel and retroperitoneum.

Synovial sarcoma [14]

These tumours arise around joints, bursae and tendon sheaths. The cell of origin is not known but may not be the synovial lining cell. Pathologically the monophasic form consists of sheets of spindle cells, and in the biphasic form there are 'glandular' spaces lined by cuboidal epithelial cells. The tumours may contain calcified areas. Tumours with few mitoses and a large 'glandular' component may have a better survival. A consistent chromosomal translocation is present, t(X;18) (p11.2;q11.2). There are two alternative chromosomal breakpoints, one associated with the monophasic appearance, and the other with the biphasic. Synovial sarcomas occur in young adults, especially in the hands, feet and knees, but do not involve the joint lining. They present as hard lumps near a joint. Local spread and metastasis occur and local recurrence after excision is frequent. They are relatively chemosensitive tumours. The prognosis is better for small tumours (>75 cm) and if there is no neural or vascular invasion.

Angiosarcoma, lymphangiosarcoma and haemangiopericytoma

Angiosarcomas are rare, highly malignant neoplasms arising from the vascular endothelium itself. There are rare instances of their occurring in the liver (Chapter 15). They usually arise in the skin, subcutaneous tissues and glandular sites such as breast and thyroid. Lymphangiosarcomas may arise in areas of chronic oedema (for example, in the arm after mastectomy). Haemangiopericytoma (glomus tumour) is thought to arise from the contractile cells (pericytes) in small blood vessels. It usually occurs in the extremities and retroperitoneal spaces but is also found in the head and neck; benign and malignant variants occur.

Kaposi's sarcoma

This important tumour is discussed in Chapter 22. It arises from endothelial cells and presents as pigmented skin lesions which grow slowly. Formerly, the tumour was commonest in Jewish and Italian men, and was much more frequent in West Africa than in Europe or the USA. This has changed with the recognition of acquired immune deficiency syndrome (AIDS), in which Kaposi's sarcoma occurs much more frequently, and with a much more aggressive course. This tumour is associated with a human herpes virus (HHV) type 8 (see p. 9).

Alveolar soft part sarcoma

This rare neoplasm occurs in young adults, usually women. It is usually a slow-growing tumour, occurring typically in the extremities, and typically arising in the thigh in adults and in the head and neck in children.

Although lung metastases usually occur, they grow slowly and may be compatible with long survival.

Epithelioid sarcoma

This is a rare tumour occurring on the extremities and with a tendency to spread to skin, bone and draining nodes. The cell of origin is unknown, but the histological appearances can be similar to a carcinoma or chronic inflammatory lesion. As with other tumours, the presence of an undiagnosed mass on a limb or intra-abdominally should raise the suspicion of a sarcoma. Diagnosis and staging should precede surgical excisions whenever possible, and the operative procedure should be carefully planned.

'Clear cell sarcoma' (soft part melanoma)

This tumour typically arises in the extremity, usually around the knee in a young adult. Ultrastructurally the tumour contains premelanosomes and is a form of undifferentiated melanoma.

Diagnosis, investigation and staging

Clinical staging in soft-tissue sarcoma is important for management and also offers a guide to prognosis. Chest X-ray is important since many of these tumours metastasize to the lungs. Lymph node metastases are frequent, particularly in alveolar rhabdomyosarcoma and Ewing's sarcoma. Other important distant sites include the liver, bone marrow and brain.

Staging investigation should therefore include chest X-ray and CT scan of the thorax, since the latter is the most sensitive means of detecting pulmonary metastases. MRI scanning is essential to determine the extent of the tumour and infiltration into local structures. Operability is better assessed by this means than by any other.

Although there is no generally accepted staging system, the classification of the American Joint Committee is useful prognostically (Table 23.4).

Management of the primary tumour

Biopsy is always required for an accurate diagnosis. The most satisfactory procedure is a needle biopsy followed by a planned approach to local and systemic treatment in collaboration with medical and radiation oncologists and surgeons. Sadly, the patient with a lump on a limb is often operated upon ('shelled out') by an inexperienced sur-

Table 23.4 Stage grouping of soft-tissue sarcomas [15].

Stage I	Low-grade (1) tumour. No nodal or distant spread ($G_1 T_{1-2} N_0 M_0$)
Stage II	Intermediate grade (2) tumour. No nodal or distant spread ($G_2 T_{1-2} N_0 M_0$)
Stage III	High-grade (3) tumour. No nodal or distant spread ($G_3 T_{1-2} N_0 M_0$)
Stage IV	A Tumour of any grade with lymph node metastases only ($G_{1-4} T_{1-2} N_1 M_0$)
	B Distant metastases ($G_{1-4} T_{1-2} N_{0+1} M_1$)

T_1 tumours are less than 5 cm diameter (subgroup A)
T_2 tumours are more than 5 cm diameter (subgroup B)
Grade is based on necrosis, pleomorphism and mitotic activity

geon who has no prior knowledge of the diagnosis. Such operations are often marginal or even intralesional resections which subsequently may pose formidable problems in management. Where a sarcoma is suspected preoperatively and confirmed by frozen section, it is unwise to attempt an excision biopsy at the same procedure since such surgery is inadequate and definitive surgery must be undertaken at a second operation. This problem also arises when excision biopsy of a 'benign' mass has been attempted, and the diagnosis of malignancy was not suspected even at operation. Examples are leiomyosarcoma of the uterus which is usually diagnosed after hysterectomy for fibroids, and soft-tissue sarcomas of the head and neck region, which frequently present with cervical lymphadenopathy rather than with the primary tumour itself.

Traditionally, radical surgery has usually been recommended for soft-tissue sarcomas arising in the extremities, and amputation has been widely used. For high lesions of the thigh, this may require disarticulation or even hemipelvectomy in an attempt to control the tumour. These radical operations were introduced because of the risk of local recurrence.

Removal of the tumour without a wide margin of normal tissue (so-called marginal excision) carries an average local failure rate of 80%. Wide local excisions are accompanied by failure rates of up to 45% with surgery alone. Radical excisions, such as compartmentectomy (see below) or amputation have local failure rates of less than 10%. These figures led to the adoption of radical surgery as the mainstay of treatment.

The common problem of distant metastases, coupled with the realization that radiotherapy can play a useful part in local control, has led over the past 10 years to a modification of this view. Wide surgical excision, coupled with high-dose irradiation, may sometimes be accepted as a satisfactory alternative, with a happier outcome than can be achieved by amputation. The radiation dose must be high (at least 60 Gy in 6 weeks) to minimize the risk of local recurrence. For tumours of the limbs the dose can

often be taken to 70 Gy. The affected compartment should be considered at risk and uniformly irradiated to this high dose. A strip of skin and subcutaneous tissue should be left unirradiated to allow adequate lymphatic drainage from the distal limb. A proportion of these patients develop local recurrence which may well require amputation, but wide local excision combined with radical radiotherapy offers a satisfactory method of local control in the large majority (80–90%) of all patients with soft-tissue sarcomas of the extremities. Surgical removal of the whole of the affected compartment (compartmentectomy) is usually recommended. These are often technically more difficult operations than amputation, in view of the important structures which have to be preserved, as well as the need to resect a large volume of tissue with primary closure wherever possible (Fig. 23.15). Radiotherapy is not always recommended for grade 1 (very low grade) tumours treated with wide local excision since the risk of recurrence is low. It may also not be needed for higher-grade tumours of smaller size where the risk of local recurrence is judged to be low. Each case must be decided on its merits. The dose and timing of radiation and the use of preoperative radiotherapy, are issues requiring further study.

Radiotherapy treatment is particularly valuable in soft-tissue sarcomas with multiple or extensive primary sites, such as soft-tissue angiosarcomas or Kaposi's sarcoma. Recent reports in both of these tumours confirm a high degree of local control using wide-field irradiation, sometimes in combination with surgery, with durable remissions (possibly cures) lasting 10 years and more, even in patients with multifocal sites of primary disease, for example on the scalp.

Hyperthermia has been used as an adjunct to radiation therapy, but there has not yet been a controlled comparison of this technique. Hyperfractionated and accelerated radiotherapy are also being assessed in current trials.

The management of soft-tissue sarcomas of childhood is further discussed in Chapter 24.

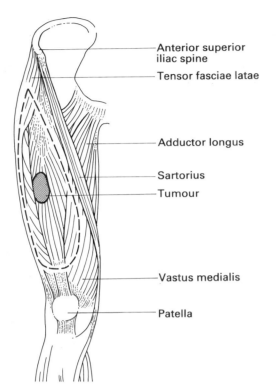

- Anterior superior iliac spine
- Tensor fasciae latae
- Adductor longus
- Sartorius
- Tumour
- Vastus medialis
- Patella

Fig. 23.15 Compartmentectomy. The diagram illustrates the wide surgical excision of soft tissue, situated, in this case, in the rectus femoris.

Chemotherapy [16]

A number of agents are effective in producing partial (or occasionally complete) remissions in patients with local recurrence and/or metastatic disease. A wide variety of agents has been shown to have activity, although in general the response rates to single agents are low and of brief duration. In the occasional patient a complete and durable response to chemotherapy is obtained. Many classes of drug have activity (Table 23.5). Doxorubicin is one of the most active and widely used agents. It has been extensively used alone and in combination with ifosfamide, itself an active drug with a response rate of 25%. In advanced disease the two-drug combination has not appeared superior to doxorubicin alone. Other drugs with activity include methotrexate, actinomycin and vinca alkaloids.

Undoubtedly, the most responsive of these tumours are the embryonal rhabdomyosarcomas, in which the success of combination regimens (particularly employing vincristine, actinomycin D, doxorubicin and cyclophosphamide) for metastatic disease has led to their routine use as adjuvant treatment immediately following local radiotherapy and/or surgery. At least 60% of patients with embryonal rhabdomyosarcomas can be cured with modern adjuvant chemotherapy, and cure is even possible in patients with evidence of residual disease postoperatively and in a proportion of patients with metastatic disease. The majority of these patients will be children or young adults, and these encouraging results have not so far been seen with other forms of soft-tissue sarcoma in adults.

Table 23.5 Chemotherapy in soft-tissue sarcoma.

Drug regimen	Approximate response rate (%)
Single agents	
Ifosfamide	25
Doxorubicin	25
DTIC	15
Cyclophosphamide	10
Vincristine	10
Methotrexate	10
Cisplatin	10
Actinomycin	10
Combination chemotherapy	
Doxorubicin, DTIC, ifosfamide	25–35
Vincristine, actinomycin, cyclosphosphamide (VAC)	20
Vincristine, doxorubicin, DTIC (VADIC)	35
Doxorubicin, cyclophosphamide methotrexate (ACM)	30
Cyclophosphamide, vincristine, doxorubicin, DTIC (CyVADIC)	40
Cyclophosphamide, vincristine, doxorubicin, actinomycin (CyVADACT)	35

A wide variety of single agents and combination regimens has been used in advanced soft-tissue sarcomas (Table 23.5). The higher response rates were reported with doxorubicin and dacarbazine, a careful review of over 350 patients has indicated that the response rate is approximately 25% of patients. A much smaller proportion of patients will achieve complete response but the addition of cyclophosphamide and vincristine to these two drugs has increased the response rate only to about 40%, at the cost of considerable toxicity. A recent patient-data based meta-analysis has shown that doxorubicin-based chemotherapy prolongs progression-free survival in localized soft-tissue sarcoma with a small effect on overall survival (Fig. 23.16).

Newer agents include ifosfamide, with a reported response rate of 30%, making it one of the most active of all single agents yet encountered. Epirubicin is also active with similar response rates. Attempts at improving these figures have centred on the use of these drugs in combination.

The use of chemotherapy as an adjuvant to surgery with or without radiotherapy remains controversial. The trial sizes have been far too small to detect differences of less than 20% in survival, and improvements of this size are clearly implausible with present drugs.

The problem is made more difficult by the heterogeneity of histology, grade, stage and site. At present adjuvant chemotherapy is best offered in the setting of a trial, or in younger adults with high-grade tumours where the risk of metastasis is very high. The role of signal transduction inhibitors remains to be determined but offers exciting opportunities for progress.

For advanced, metastatic disease other studies will be necessary to elucidate small but possibly important differences in chemotherapy effectiveness and also to monitor toxicity. If the initial promising results with ifosfamide can be confirmed, it may be possible to increase the cure rate by including this drug in adjuvant programmes.

Survival

The survival correlates with stage and site: 5-year survival for stage I is 80%; stage II, 60%; stage III, 30%; and stage IV, 10%. The more distal the tumour, the better the prognosis. Lymph node spread is important prognostically and is commoner in rhabdomyosarcoma and synovial sarcoma. The prognosis for retroperitoneal tumours is poor, with 5-year survival of 15–35%. This figure is worse for higher-grade lesions and those where no surgical removal is possible.

References

1 Souhami RL. *The Aetiology of Bone Sarcomas*. In: Souhami RL, ed. *Clinics in Oncology: Bone Tumours*, Vol. 1. London: Baillière Tindall, 1987.

2 Hawkins M, Kinnier-Wilson M, Burton HS *et al*. Radiotherapy, alkylating agents, and risk of bone cancer after childhood cancer. *J Natl Cancer Inst* 1996; 88: 270–3.

3 Brugieres L, Gardes M, Moutou C. Screening for germ line p53 mutations in children with malignant tumors and a family history of cancer. *Cancer Res* 1993; 53: 452–5.

4 Delattre O, Zucman J, Melot T *et al*. The Ewing family of tumors: a sub-group of small round-cell tumours defined by specific chimeric transcripts. *N Engl J Med* 1994; 331: 294–9.

5 Link MP, Goorin AM, Miser AW *et al*. The effect of adjuvant chemotherapy on relapse free survival in patients with osteosarcoma of the extremity. *N Engl J Med* 1986; 314: 1600–6.

6 Souhami RL, Craft AW, Van den Eijken JW *et al*. Randomised trial of two regimens of chemotherapy in operable osteosarcoma: a study of the European Osteosarcoma Intergroup. *Lancet* 1997; 350: 911–17.

7 Saeter G, Hole J, Stenwig AE *et al*. Systemic relapse of patients with osteogenic sarcoma: prognostic factors for long-term survival. *Cancer* 1995; 75: 1084–93.

8 Mankin HJ, Cantlay KD, Lipielo L *et al*. The biology of human chondrosarcoma. 1. Description of the case, grading and biochemical analyses. *J Bone Joint Surg [A]* 1980; 62: 160–76.

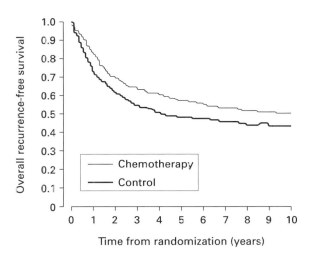

Patients at risk

Chemotherapy	436	366	305	249	173
Control	394	306	262	213	141

Fig. 23.16 Kaplan–Meier curves of local recurrence free interval (RFI), distant RFI, overall recurrence-free survival, and overall survival for adjuvant chemotherapy vs. control. From [16].

9 Earl HM. Chemotherapy of rare malignant bone tumours. *Baillière's Clin Oncol* 1987; 1: 223–41.

10 Terrier P, Henry-Amar M, Tricke TJ *et al*. Is neuroectodermal differentiation of Ewing's sarcoma of bone associated with an unfavourable prognosis? *Eur J Cancer* 1995; 31A: 307–14.

11 Scully SP, Temple HT, O'Keefe RJ *et al*. Role of surgical resection in pelvic Ewing's sarcoma. *J Clin Oncol* 1995; 13: 2336–41.

12 Paulussen M, Ahrens S, Dunst J *et al*. Localized Ewing tumour of bone: final results of the Cooperative Ewing's Sarcoma Study CESS 86. *J Clin Oncol* 2001; 19: 1818–29.

13 Joenssu H, Roberts P, Sarlomo-Rikala M *et al*. Clinical response induced by the tyrosine-kinase inhibitor STI571 in metastatic gastrointestinal stromal tumor expressing a mutant c-kit proto-oncogene. *N Engl J Med* 2001; 344: 1052–6.

14 Cagle LA, Mirra JM, Storm FK *et al*. Histologic features relating to prognosis in synovial sarcoma. *Cancer* 1987; 59: 1810–14.

15 American Joint Committee on Cancer. *Manual for Staging of Cancer*. Philadelphia: JB Lippincott, 1988.

16 Sarcoma Meta-analysis Collaboration SMAC. Adjuvant chemotherapy for localised resectable soft tissue sarcoma of adults: meta-analysis of individual data. *Lancet* 1997; 350: 1647–54.

24 Paediatric malignancies

An approach to cancer in children

The diagnosis of cancer in a child is an exceptional and painful test of the strength of family life. Happy families usually cope better with the shock, grief and disruption. When the diagnosis has been made, the physician must take time to be alone with the parents, explaining the diagnosis, prognosis and approach to investigation and treatment. Over half of all children with cancer are cured, so for many tumours a cautiously optimistic account can be given. The parents will sometimes feel angry about the diagnosis and may direct this towards the doctor. Often the parents themselves feel that they have been responsible in some way, in that there is a genetic factor to which they have contributed, or that the cancer has arisen as a result of avoidable physical or mental trauma or faulty diet. Increasingly, parents are concerned about avoidable delays in diagnosis. They need to express these feelings and must be reassured that they are not to blame. They must feel confident in the hospital and its staff.

Talking to children and their parents requires tact, humanity, patience and a clear head. Every new case will prove an additional test of these qualities, and the doctor will have to deal with the guilt, anguish and anger of the parents as well as the physical and emotional suffering of the child. All children, except for the very youngest, need some account of why they are in hospital and what is likely to happen, and with older children and adolescents these explanations will need to be accurate and complete. It is impossible to make any generalization about how much to tell. Children of 6–8 years will understand that they are ill, and grasp the elements of treatment. At 10–11 years they will know more, and teenagers will know about cancer and leukaemia. The physician must talk to the child and try to gauge his or her feelings and understanding. For children of about 11 years or more, a personal and private relationship with the doctor is important. They often want to ask questions directly and are anxious to avoid upsetting their parents. At other times they may feel that the truth is being filtered by their parents. The doctor should try to encourage the family to be open with each other with respect to the illness. Honesty and frankness are important in gaining the parents' trust and in helping them to participate in treatment.

The complexity of treatment makes it difficult for any doctor to provide detailed answers to all the questions which a parent or the child might ask, but it is essential that a single, experienced clinician should be seen to be in charge of the team, so that both the patient and the parents can identify with an individual.

With most childhood cancers, the disease is brought under control and the child feels and looks well, except for the side-effects of treatment. These side-effects come to dominate the illness, since the acute anxiety about the diagnosis fades with time and with the induction of a remission or disappearance of the tumour. The nausea, vomiting and hair loss, and the disruption of school and family life because of frequent hospital trips, all place a great strain on the child and family, who will need support and reassurance from the medical team. A skilled multidisciplinary team is an essential part of management. Case discussion with nursing staff, counsellors, psychologists and medical staff is a useful way of ensuring that treatment and support are made as effective as possible. In teenagers the disruption to school work, the blow to body image and development, and the possible loss of contact with friends, mean that family and school will need to act in harmony with the hospital staff to try and minimize the stress of the illness and the disruption to the child's education.

After successful treatment the long-term sequelae of treatment may bring problems—intellectual and neurological impairment following brain tumours such as medulloblastoma (see Chapter 11), growth defects after extensive radiation (see Chapter 5) and infertility after chemotherapy.

If the disease recurs, the implications for prognosis are usually grave. If there is still a chance of cure, intensive treatment may be needed again and the depression of morale in the child and family will make extra support necessary. If the chance of cure is slim or non-existent, the parents must be told and the aims of palliative treatment explained. Many parents still hope that a cure will be found, yet they must at the same time begin to accept the likelihood of the child's death. The conflict may be great and there must be an opportunity for the family to express their feelings. Parents should know that freedom from pain or discomfort is usually possible, and that the child's survival will not be uselessly prolonged.

Parents may be angry that relapse has occurred and feel that they had been wrong to allow aggressive treatment with its attendant side-effects, and all to no avail. This anger may be directed at the medical team. At this difficult stage, discussion and explanation are essential. Senior staff

must remember that those who are less experienced may themselves need to be reassured and supported.

Very young children do not have a clear idea of death but may express their fears of separation in play or in conversation. Adolescents will usually have an adult perception of death. In dealing with a dying child the doctors should allow the patient and family to indicate how far and fast they wish to go in discussion and should not force unpalatable facts upon them. Many families need to retain some hope of recovery in dealing with the situation. At the same time the doctor must listen to, and understand, expressions of anger and grief as part of the process of acceptance that the child will die.

Tumours of childhood

Although all childhood tumours are uncommon, cancer is the commonest natural cause of death in childhood—of all causes, second only to accidents. The incidence figures for the UK are shown in Table 24.1. Extraordinary advances have been made in the management of almost all of the common childhood tumours. With a better understanding of the diseases and far more effective treatments, cure is frequently achieved. As treatment policies become more sophisticated, paediatric oncology has become a specialized branch of cancer treatment. There is little doubt that childhood cancer is best treated in a specialized paediatric oncology centre. With some tumours, the chances of survival are possibly improved by 10–15% [1].

Diagnostic group	Cases per year	0–1	1–4	5–9	10–14
Leukaemia					
Acute lymphoblastic	323	16.3	58.6	26.6	14.9
Acute non-lymphocytic	64	9.5	7.3	4.1	5.6
Lymphomas					
Hodgkin's disease	58	–	1.4	4.3	9.8
Non-Hodgkin's lymphoma	70	2.2	5.0	7.1	7.5
Brain and spinal cancer	290	27.3	30.9	27.2	22.7
Neuroblastoma	74	32.1	14.9	2.7	0.4
Retinoblastoma	33	21.9	6.0	0.5	–
Wilms' tumour	70	12.9	16.6	4.0	0.5
Bone					
Osteosarcoma	32	–	0.2	1.7	6.3
Ewing's sarcoma	28	–	0.6	2.7	4.2
Soft-tissue sarcoma	80	11.9	8.9	6.1	6.3
Germ cell and gonadal cancer	39	6.9	4.7	1.4	3.9
All cancers	1240	153.6	161.1	92.8	91.7

Table 24.1 Average annual registrations and incidence rates per million population in the UK, 1978–87.

Conversely, in cancers such as Wilms' tumour, where results may be equal in survival to those in non-specialist centres, this is often at the expense of overtreatment in the non-specialist hospitals [2]. In recent years units for the care of adolescents with cancer have been established in some cancer centres. These units are based on the principles of paediatric cancer units, but with special expertise in managing the cancers found in this age group and the particular emotional consequences of cancer at this age.

Aetiology and incidence (Table 24.1)

Little is known of the aetiology of childhood tumours. Ionizing radiation may be a predisposing cause, either when given during pregnancy or as a result of deliberate irradiation, for example to the thymus for thymic hyperplasia which has been responsible for an increased risk of thyroid carcinoma. Transplacental carcinogens have long been thought to be a possible cause of childhood cancer. The clearest demonstration of the potential importance of this mechanism is shown by the association of adenocarcinoma of the vagina in teenage girls with treatment of the mother 20 years previously with diethylstilboestrol for early threatened abortion.

Genetic factors are frequently involved [3]. Several tumours of childhood are now known to be associated with chromosomal abnormalities. Some of these are acquired and are discussed in the sections on the tumours concerned. Others are heritable (constitutive) abnormalities, and these are listed in Table 3.4 (see p. 29). Some congenital malformations appear to be associated with paediatric tumours. There is an increased risk of tumours (usually neurogenic sarcomas) developing in children with von Recklinghausen's disease. The rare syndrome of hemihypertrophy may be associated both with Wilms' tumour and hepatoblastoma. Wilms' tumour can be associated with aniridia and a wide variety of congenital abnormalities.

In addition to inherited non-malignant diseases in which there is an increased risk of cancer, there are inherited gene mutations which give rise to a high risk of cancer without any other manifestations. One of the best-known examples is retinoblastoma, which has a marked familial incidence particularly in the bilateral form of the disease, where half the offspring of affected children will themselves develop the disease. The Li–Fraumeni syndrome, due to *p53* mutation, is another example of a high risk of cancer in families of children with sarcoma (see p. 344).

Other genetic influences remain to be elucidated. If a child with an identical twin develops acute leukaemia, then the risk of the twin also developing this disease is high. The overall risk of cancer in childhood is 1 : 600, but in siblings 1 : 300.

Geographical and racial variations also exist, which may eventually throw further light on aetiology. Liver cancer is commoner in the Far East, retinoblastoma in India, intestinal lymphoma in Israel and Burkitt's lymphoma in Uganda. In the UK and the USA the proportion of various groups of tumours is reasonably constant; 20–25% consist of tumours of the central nervous system (CNS) and eye, 33% are leukaemias, and 35% are solid tumours (chiefly Wilms' tumour and neuroblastoma). Most of these tumours have their maximal incidence at ages 0–4 years, although some, such as bone tumours and lymphomas have a later peak, between 6 and 14 years. In general, younger children appear to have a better survival than older groups, particularly with neuroblastoma and retinoblastoma. With the relative improvement in treatments of other paediatric illnesses, cancer has assumed an increased importance as a cause of death despite the many advances in management.

Childhood tumours of the CNS are common, and are discussed with adult brain tumours in Chapter 11; leukaemia is discussed in Chapter 28 and paediatric lymphomas in Chapter 26.

Neuroblastoma

After brain tumours, leukaemia and lymphoma, neuroblastoma is the commonest of paediatric tumours, accounting for some 7% of the total. Over 80% of cases occur below 4 years of age. Most cases are sporadic but there are reports of twins with both affected, as well as families with two or more affected siblings.

Pathology

Neuroblastomas are embryonal tumours which arise from neural crest tissue, which itself normally develops into the adrenal medulla and sympathetic ganglia [4]. The common primary sites are therefore the adrenal medulla and the sympathetic nervous tissue in the retroperitoneum.

However, tumours may also arise in the posterior mediastinum and spine, predominantly extradurally from paravertebral ganglia (Fig. 24.1). Because of their derivation from the adrenal medulla, elaboration and secretion of adrenal medullary hormones or metabolites are characteristic of these tumours (see below).

Neuroblastomas undergo spontaneous regression and differentiation. Small neuroblastomas are not infre-

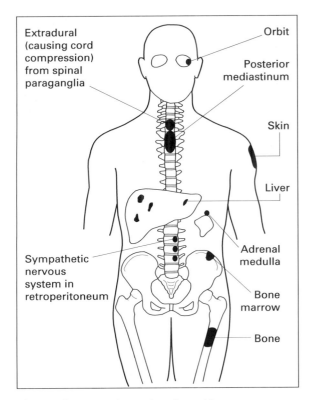

Fig. 24.1 Common primary sites of neuroblastoma.

Table 24.2 Presenting symptoms of neuroblastoma.

Constitutional
Fever, malaise, weight loss, anaemia

Primary site
Adrenal: pain and abdominal mass
Presacral: loss of bladder control, frequency of micturition
Paravertebral: spinal cord compression
Cervical sympathetic: Horner's syndrome
Olfactory bulb: unilateral nasal block and epistaxis

Metastases
Liver: pain, weight loss, fever
Bone: pain (preceding X-ray change), anaemia, pathological
    fractures
Orbit: proptosis
CNS: malignant meningitis

Remote effects
Diarrhoea: ?due to secretion of vasoactive intestinal polypeptide
Myoclonus or opsoclonus
Hypertension

Neuroblastomas tend to spread very widely, by local, lymphatic and haematogenous routes, and important sites of blood-borne dissemination include bone marrow (often forming clusters of large, poorly differentiated cells), the liver (sometimes resulting in enormous hepatomegaly) and bone (often with a single destructive lesion as the typical neuroblastoma deposit). Unlike other paediatric soft-tissue tumours, the lungs are seldom the site of metastases. Skin and periorbital metastases are common.

Clinical features

Clinical presentation is unusually varied, due to the variety of primary sites, the early wide dissemination and the secretion of pharmacologically active metabolites (Table 24.2). The commonest presentation is of an abdominal mass, sometimes painless but often accompanied by mild or recurrent abdominal pain. Other common syndromes include irritability, fever, lethargy, anaemia or bone pain from a metastasis. Occasionally, lymph node or skin metastases, hepatomegaly or proptosis are the first clinical signs. Subcutaneous metastases often have a blue/black colour. Liver metastases may be painful. Other primary sites of presentation include presacral neuroblastoma causing urinary frequency or obstruction; posterior mediastinal tumours causing dyspnoea; intraspinal tumours causing spinal cord compression; cervical sympathetic

quently found in the adrenals in foetal autopsies. In infancy there is a widely disseminated form of the disease (stage 4S) that undergoes spontaneous regression. In other cases the tumour shows pathological features indicating varying degrees of differentiation from small round undifferentiated cells to ganglion cells and Schwann-cell like stroma. The degree of neural differentiation is related to improved prognosis as is lower mitotic rate and absence of necrosis. Neuroblastomas are often positive on periodic acid–Schiff (PAS) staining, and express a variety of neuroendocrine markers (chromogranin-A, synaptophysin, neurone-specific enolase). Electron microsocopy may show dense neurosecretory granules.

The N-*myc* gene, found on chromosome 2p24, is frequently amplified. More than 10 copies per cell is a strong indicator of poor prognosis. Assessment of amplication is now a routine part of pathological examination. Deletion of chromosome 1p is present in 40%. This region of chromosome 1 may contain a tumour suppressor gene and loss of heterozygosity at this site may predict early relapse. Gain of genetic material at 17q is frequent and is associated with poor prognosis.

tumours causing Horner's syndrome; and olfactory bulb tumours (aesthesioneuroblastoma) causing nasal obstruction and epistaxis. There is an association between neuroblastoma and myoclonic or opsoclonic movements, though the mechanism is unclear. Rarely, secretion of large amounts of catecholamines and intestinal peptides can cause sweating, pallor and diarrhoea.

Diagnosis and investigation

The definitive diagnosis is by biopsy of the affected site but a confident diagnosis may already have been made biochemically. Catecholamine metabolites are produced in about 90% of all children with neuroblastomas, and screening for urinary metabolites should be undertaken if the diagnosis is suspected. Homovanillic acid (HVA) or vanillyl mandelic acid (VMA) are the most reliable and widely used measurements. The diagnosis can often be made on a random urine sample. Both HVA and VMA should be measured since either metabolite may be increased.

Plain X-ray of the abdomen will frequently demonstrate calcification in the primary tumour, typically with a diffuse pattern. Liver metastases may also calcify. The chest X-ray is often normal, though abnormal mediastinal shadowing often occurs with primary intrathoracic tumours (typically in the posterior mediastinum). Parenchymal lung metastases are very unusual. Skeletal survey and isotope bone scanning are useful in detecting osseous metastases. Bone marrow aspiration is mandatory in all cases of neuroblastoma. Over 40% of children have marrow involvement even when bone X-rays are normal. Computed tomography (CT) and/or magnetic resonance imaging (MRI) and abdominal ultrasonography give excellent delineation of tumour as well as providing accurate imaging of the liver.

Meta-iodobenzylguanidine is taken up by adrenergic nervous tissue and can be used to identify both primary and metastatic neuroblastoma: 10% of cases show no uptake. Early diagnosis by screening urine of all 6-month-old-babies has been attempted in Japan. The effectiveness in saving life has not been proved and trials in Europe have not confirmed its value. Some small tumours may be detected early but these may regress spontaneously.

Differential diagnosis

The clinical diagnosis of neuroblastoma is not always straightforward, particularly if the child presents with failure to thrive and without other obvious abnormalities to suggest a diagnosis of malignancy. The most important distinction in children presenting with an obvious abdominal mass lies between neuroblastoma and Wilms' tumour. Other abdominal tumours which may cause diagnostic difficulty include hepatoblastoma and intestinal lymphoma. If the child presents with bone metastases, these may be difficult to distinguish radiologically from a primary Ewing's tumour, bone lymphoma or even a nonmalignant cause such as osteomyelitis or tuberculosis.

Difficulty may also occur when the child presents with spinal cord compression, when a variety of malignant and non-malignant causes must be considered. These include intraspinal cysts, neurofibroma, spinal tuberculosis, primary intraspinal tumours, medulloblastoma and other tumours which seed within the CNS (see Chapter 11), or other rare causes of extradural compression, such as Hodgkin's disease.

Clinical staging

Clinical staging of neuroblastoma is important both prognostically and also as a means of selecting the most appropriate treatment. Although several classification schemes have been suggested, all are based on an accurate assessment of the detailed extent of spread. Although it is known that the degree of histological differentiation (that is, tumour grade) may influence prognosis, this information, though potentially useful, is difficult to fit into a simple staging classification. The same can be said for catecholamine excretion and age, though age at diagnosis is probably the single most important prognostic factor [5]. The most widely used classification [6] is based on extent of disease so as to produce a system that is practical for clinical use (Table 24.3).

Up to 70% of children have disseminated tumour at diagnosis, often in the bone marrow. The prognosis worsens with increasing stage. However, the IV-S category has been defined because these children have a surprisingly good prognosis, with a survival rate similar to patients with stage I tumours. Most IV-S patients are under the age of 1 year. Children below the age of 1 year have a much better prognosis even with stage IV disease. Within this group those with stage IV and without tumour N-*myc* amplification have a very good outcome.

In addition to age and disease extent, the primary site is also prognostically important. Tumours arising in the mediastinum and the neck have a better prognosis than those in the abdomen, probably since more are localized at the time of diagnosis. This is particularly true with thoracospinal lesions which produce early spinal cord

Table 24.3 International staging system for neuroblastoma [6].

Stage I	Localized tumour confined to the area of origin; complete gross excision, with or without microscopic residual disease; identifiable ipsilateral and contralateral lymph nodes negative microscopically
Stage IIA	Unilateral tumour with incomplete gross excision; identifiable ipsilateral and contralateral lymph nodes negative microscopically
Stage IIB	Unilateral tumour with complete or incomplete gross excision; with positive ipsilateral regional lymph nodes; identifiable contralateral lymph nodes negative microscopically
Stage III	Tumour infiltrating across the midline with or without regional lymph node involvement; or unilateral tumour with contralateral regional lymph node involvement; or midline tumour with bilateral regional lymph node involvement
Stage IV	Dissemination of tumour to distant lymph nodes, bone marrow, liver and/or other organs (except as defined in stage IV-S)
Stage IV-S	Localized primary tumour as defined for stage I or II with dissemination limited to liver, skin and/or bone marrow

Table 24.4 Guidelines for treatment of neuroblastoma.

Stage I	Surgery alone
Stage II	Surgery with postoperative irradiation is considered if surgery incomplete
	Chemotherapy sometimes used for stage IIB after incomplete excision unless the child is less than 6 months old
Stage III	Chemotherapy followed by 'debulking' surgery with local irradiation and further chemotherapy
Stage IV	As for stage III, but intensive chemotherapy is the mainstay of treatment
Stage IV-S	If possible no treatment is given. If the child has symptoms because of tumour size, surgery ± minimal chemotherapy is justified

compression. Curiously, pelvic tumours also appear to have a better prognosis, and more frequently undergo differentiation to ganglioneuroma or even a spontaneous remission; again this may relate to the fact that most of these children are under the age of 15 months.

Other, biological, factors correlate with prognosis. These include N-*myc* amplification, high mitotic rate, hypodiploidy and karyotypic abnormalities of chromosome 1 which are all associated with a poor prognosis. Hyperdiploidy and normal N-*myc* are associated with better outcome. Serum neurone-specific enolase and serum ferritin, if elevated, have also been reported as associated with a worse prognosis.

Clinical management

Current clinical management of neuroblastoma is unsatisfactory and refinements in treatment are continuously being suggested. Unlike many of the paediatric malignancies, chemotherapy has not yet made a significant improvement in the survival of these children, though the chemosensitivity of this tumour is not in doubt.

Local treatments with surgery and/or radiation therapy are therefore critically important, and may be curative in children with localized disease. In one surgical series, a 2-year survival rate of 84% was achieved by the use of surgery alone in apparently localized cases. Radiotherapy is usually recommended after incomplete excision, but probably best avoided where surgery appears complete. Long-term survivors have certainly been documented where surgery was incomplete, but supplemented by postoperative radiotherapy, though the contribution of radiotherapy is difficult to quantify since almost all patients will have had at least a partial or subtotal surgical excision. Most children with clinical stage II and III disease will be in this category. Even in children with stage IV disease, in whom chemotherapy may be the most important part of treatment, attention must be paid to controlling the primary disease.

In stage IV cases chemotherapy is usually the first treatment, but radiotherapy and surgery will often be required at a later stage in order to achieve control of the bulky primary tumour. Some surgeons feel that in this situation preoperative irradiation makes surgery technically easier. In these more advanced cases, the local treatment is usually withheld until at least two cycles of chemotherapy have been given.

Guidelines for treatment of neuroblastoma are given in Table 24.4. Combinations of vincristine, cyclophosphamide, actinomycin D and doxorubicin are usually

Table 24.5 Chemotherapy for neuroblastoma.

Single agents
Vincristine
Actinomycin D
Doxorubicin
Cyclophosphamide
Ifosfamide
Cisplatin/carboplatin
Etoposide/teniposide
High-dose melphalan

Combination chemotherapy

VAC I	Vincristine, actinomycin and cyclophosphamide
VAC II	Vincristine, doxorubicin and cyclophosphamide
OPEC	Vincristine
	Cisplatin
	Etoposide
	Cyclophosphamide
VECI	Vincristine
	Carboplatin
	Teniposide
	Ifosfamide

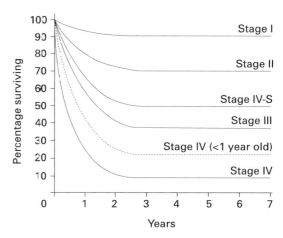

Fig. 24.2 Survival related to stage in neuroblastoma.

used. Agents such as cisplatin, etoposide and ifosfamide are increasingly used in combination therapy. All of these drugs have been shown to be active as single agents in neuroblastoma (Table 24.5). With these more intensive regimens (such as OPEC, Table 24.5) the response rates are 60–70% but only 25–30% of advanced disease is cured. The use of high-dose chemotherapy and autologous bone marrow transplantation may improve survival in high-risk cases [7]. Patients who receive high-dose therapy after complete or partial chemotherapy response are more likely to be long survivors: the toxicity of these treatments is diminishing and further trials are in progress. Targeted radiotherapy also appears to hold some promise, using ^{131}I meta-iodobenzylguanidine either as primary therapy or at relapse.

Although overall results remain disappointing, survival has improved in recent years as a result of better diagnosis, treatment strategy, biochemical monitoring and possibly chemotherapy. Survival is clearly related to age and stage (Fig. 24.2), and children living beyond 3 years from diagnosis are usually considered cured.

Wilms' tumour

Incidence and aetiology

Wilms' tumour (nephroblastoma) accounts for about 8%

of all paediatric tumours, with a peak incidence below the age of 4 years. Inherited cases are less than 1%. With neuroblastoma it forms much the largest group of intra-abdominal malignancies of childhood. However, there are pronounced behavioural differences between these two tumours, particularly in their response to treatment.

Although most cases are sporadic, there is a familial form. Aniridia, gonadal dysplasia and mental retardation may be associated with Wilms' tumour, as may musculoskeletal deformity. Chromosomal analysis shows deletion at the level of band 13 of the short arm of chromosome 11p13 (Fig. 24.3). Cases with small deletions do not show mental retardation. The *Wt1* gene [8] is a transcription factor. Other described germline abnormalities are XX/XY mosaicism and trisomy 8 or 18. The peak age of incidence is 3–5 years, though it has on rare occasions been discovered at birth. There is a slight male preponderance.

Pathology

Almost the whole kidney can be replaced either by a centrally or peripherally placed tumour, often exhibiting areas of patchy haemorrhage or degeneration, and sometimes with a lobulated appearance. Necrosis and cystic change are both common, and although a very large size may be attained without obvious extrarenal involvement, extension of solid cores of tumour cells along the renal vein and inferior vena cava are common. Other direct sites of spread may include the perinephric fat, colon, adrenal gland or liver as well as the renal pelvis itself, and the local draining lymph nodes. Occasionally, the tumour may be extrarenal in origin, presumably arising in ectopic cell rests from mesonephric crest migration.

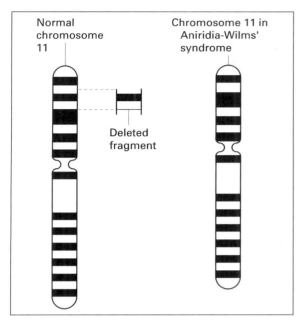

Fig. 24.3 Deletion of part of the short arm of chromosome 11 in aniridia–Wilms' syndrome.

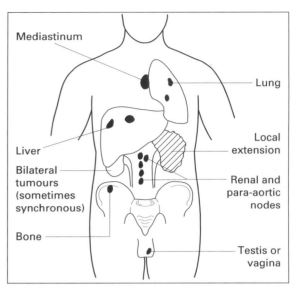

Fig. 24.4 Common sites of metastasis in Wilms' tumour.

Histologically, Wilms' tumour contains both mesenchymal and epithelial elements, often admixed and with differing stages of maturity [9]. Within the epithelial element, there is usually evidence of a renal origin with embryonic tubular or glomerular structures sometimes lined by recognizable epithelium and occasionally arranged in rosettes. The most favourable histological group usually contains all three elements. A monomorphic epitheliae form is particularly favourable. Undifferentiated stroma may form a large proportion of the tumour, though this too may show areas of differentiation to form smooth muscle, bone or cartilage. A variety of histological types have been described, which probably represent differing degrees of differentiation. Some tumours are so undifferentiated as to defy unequivocal histological diagnosis. About 5% of tumours are anaplastic. Nuclear enlargement and hyperploidy are associated adverse features. Typically, such tumours have a great propensity to metastasis. There is a particular form of bone-metastasizing tumour which is probably a distinct entity. More highly differentiated forms also occur, and a specific group of 'mesoblastic nephromas', with only minimal nuclear pleomorphism and mitotic activity, a very low metastatic potential, and often surgically curable. Loss of heterozygosity on the short arm of chromosome 11 has been widely reported as the most consistent karyotypic abnormality in the tumour.

Clinical features

The common presentation is with a symptomless, painless abdominal mass more commonly on the left and often discovered by the parent or during a routine examination. There may be recurrent abdominal pain of moderate severity. Abdominal distension is common, though unlike neuroblastoma these tumours tend not to cross the midline. Haematuria occurs in 30% of cases. Hypertension is unusual but is occasionally severe and sometimes accompanied by complications such as retinopathy or encephalopathy. It is thought to be due to excess renin production by the tumour or to renal ischaemia from renal artery stenosis. Fever, anorexia and lethargy may also be presenting symptoms.

About one-fifth of children with Wilms' tumour have evidence of distant metastases at presentation, though figures from central referral hospitals suggest a much higher incidence (up to 60–70%), representing a preponderance of advanced and complicated cases. Direct spread to extrarenal fat and other local organs is common, and local nodal spread occurs predominantly to the para-aortic and other intra-abdominal lymph node groups. Haematogenous spread occurs typically to the lung parenchyma, brain and bone, though liver, mediastinum, vagina and testis are well-known secondary sites (Fig. 24.4). Bilateral presentation occurs in 5% of cases which are usually regarded as being bilateral primary tumours rather than secondary spread. Bilateral Wilms' tumour can also be metachronous. Children with bilateral tumours are younger and have 10 times the incidence of associated congenital anomalies.

Investigation and staging

Plain chest and abdominal X-rays will help to define the extent of the primary tumour and demonstrate obvious pulmonary metastases. Computed tomography scanning of the chest is more sensitive but may not alter management since small metastases (not visible on chest X-ray) respond to chemotherapy. Abdominopelvic ultrasonography will give accurate preoperative information as to the size and extent of disease. Visualization of the inferior vena cava is important prior to surgery and can be achieved with ultrasound or contrast venography. The most precise definition of tumour size is achieved with CT or MRI scanning of the abdomen.

Routine urine examination often reveals microscopic haematuria, and measurement of catecholamine excretion will be necessary in cases which are difficult to distinguish clinically from neuroblastoma especially if there is hypertension. Isotope bone scanning is usually recommended since symptomless bone secondaries may be present. These investigations should help distinguish the true Wilms' tumour from a variety of malignant and non-malignant conditions which it may clinically resemble.

Although neuroblastoma is the most important differential diagnosis, other intra-abdominal childhood tumours may cause difficulty, such as retroperitoneal sarcoma and hepatoblastoma. Important non-malignant causes of childhood abdominal masses include renal haematomas, hydronephrosis, multilocular cystic kidney, horseshoe kidney, perirenal haematoma and splenomegaly.

Staging systems have become more logical with increased understanding of the natural history of these tumours and of the importance of complete surgical removal. At present, the National Wilms' Tumour Study Staging System (Table 24.6) is most widely used.

This staging system has now been successfully used for 10 years, and data are accumulating to suggest that extent of disease at operation and the presence of lymph node involvement are the most influential prognostic factors. Large referral centres have better results than smaller hospitals where the occasional case is treated, a finding with the unavoidable implication that non-specialist clinicians should be strongly dissuaded from treating a child with a curable cancer.

Management

There should be close co-operation between paediatric surgeon, radiotherapist, paediatric oncologist and pathologist to ensure that all clinicians will have the opportunity to assess each child before surgery is performed. There has been some controversy over the use of preoperative biopsy because of the risk of intra-abdominal dissemination of tumour. If this is done it should be a fine-needle biopsy to

Table 24.6 Staging and guidelines for the management of Wilms' tumour.

Stage I	Tumour limited to the kidney, and completely resected. Renal capsule intact, tumour removed without rupture, no residual disease	Surgery and vincristine
Stage II	Tumour extends beyond kidney but is completely resected. Penetration is into the perirenal soft tissue or fat; infiltration of renal vessels outside the kidney, or para-ortic lymph node involvement. No residual tumour	Surgery; adjuvant combination chemotherapy using vincristine and actinomycin D
Stage III	Residual tumour confined to the abdomen, or tumour biopsied or ruptured before or during surgery. Involved lymph nodes beyond para-aortic chains; tumour not completely resected	As for stage II but whole-abdominal irradiation for diffuse spread, and chemotherapy includes doxorubicin
Stage IV	Distant blood-borne metastases (usually to lung, liver, bone and/or brain). Lymph node metastases beyond the abdomen	Surgery and more intensive combination chemotherapy
Stage V	Bilateral tumours at presentation	Individual treatment often including bilateral renal surgery with low-dose postoperative radiotherapy and adjuvant combination chemotherapy

minimize the risk of intra-abdominal dissemination. Even in the presence of obvious metastatic disease, careful assessment of operability should be made since control of the primary tumour without surgery is always difficult. The advent of effective irradiation and chemotherapy has allowed surgeons to reconsider operating on children whose tumours were inoperable at first presentation.

Guidelines for the management of Wilms' tumour are set out in Table 24.6. Surgical removal should be performed in order both to remove the tumour in its entirety, without biopsy or other disturbance of the capsule, and to assess the extent of intra-abdominal disease with careful delineation of any area of residual tumour. Before resection it must be confirmed that the contralateral kidney is intact. Enlarged lymph nodes should generally be resected or at least biopsied. There is no substitute for surgical experience and the planning of the surgery must be meticulous. Surgery should not be attempted if the tumour is fixed and if there is hepatic infiltration. Under these circumstances chemotherapy is usually given first as well, as if there are metastases.

Postoperative chemotherapy with combinations of vincristine, actinomycin D and/or doxorubicin should be used (Table 24.7). However, the possible roles of preoperative chemotherapy and routine postoperative irradiation of the tumour bed remain controversial. There is a growing evidence that preoperative chemotherapy is valuable in the management of doubtfully resectable tumours.

Although postoperative radiotherapy has been employed routinely for 30 years or more as an adjuvant to surgery, the development of effective chemotherapeutic regimens has led to a reappraisal of the role of radiotherapy [10].

In stage I disease, postoperative radiotherapy confers no benefit and 10 weeks' treatment with doxorubicin and vincristine are as effective as longer periods.

Children with stage II disease should be treated postoperatively with combination chemotherapy. Combination chemotherapy using vincristine and actinomycin D, if intensive, gives as good a result as regimens using doxorubicin (with its attendant cardiotoxicity).

Stage III disease has presented a bigger challenge. Evidence from European trials has indicated that preoperative chemotherapy reduces the stage of tumour at surgery and may allow radiotherapy to be omitted from the programme. If radiotherapy is omitted it is probable that three-drug regimens are necessary.

Stage IV disease should be treated with intensive combination chemotherapy. The successful treatment of disseminated Wilms' tumour demands an aggressive approach, often requiring surgical resection of residual pulmonary and hepatic metastases with additional use of both radiotherapy and chemotherapy.

In patients with bilateral (stage V) disease, surgery is attempted only after initial chemotherapy has reduced the tumour mass as far as possible. The aim of surgery is then to preserve as much of both kidneys as possible. Chemotherapy is usually continued postoperatively. If surgical clearance is impossible, and the disease cannot be eradicated, bilateral nephrectomy and transplantation is a last resort.

Table 24.7 Chemotherapy in Wilms' tumour.

	Response rate (complete and partial)(%)
Single agents	
Vincristine	70
Doxorubicin	60
Actinomycin D	40
Cyclophosphamide	35
Etoposide	30
Cisplatin	30
*Combination therapy**	
Actinomycin D and vincristine	95
Vincristine and doxorubicin	90
Vincristine, doxorubicin, cyclophosphamide	90

*Response rates are approximate as these combinations have not been thoroughly tested in metastatic disease, and different combinations are used in different stages of the disease.

Unlike neuroblastoma the routine use of chemotherapy has radically altered the outlook in this disease, which was the first of the solid tumours in which adjuvant chemotherapy was established as an important part of the initial management. Most patients tolerate this treatment without too much difficulty. Avoidance of radiotherapy wherever possible has undoubtedly reduced the long-term complications such as growth retardation within the irradiated area, scoliosis and radiation-induced second tumours—often an unresectable and rapidly fatal sarcoma. Trials are in progress to clarify further the details of postoperative treatment. At present, important chemotherapy-induced complications include nausea and vomiting, peripheral neuropathy, alopecia and skin reactions (including recall phenomena in previously irradiated areas following actinomycin D treatment).

Treatment of recurrent disease is always difficult because of the previous administration of chemotherapy and radiotherapy. The same agents may again be effective, particularly in cases where recurrence is late, well after discontinuation of the initial adjuvant chemotherapy. Other drugs such as cisplatin, vinblastine, bleomycin and etoposide may be of value in children resistant to first-line treatment. Palliative irradiation (sometimes in combination with surgery) may also be useful for brain, lung, extradural, bony and hepatic metastases.

Prognosis

The prognosis in Wilms' tumour has improved greatly as a result of routine adjuvant chemotherapy, though a better understanding of the role of surgery, radiotherapy and supportive care has also contributed. At present, the prognosis in this disease is better than for any other childhood malignancy and the overall survival rate is now 80–90% (Fig. 24.5). Several prognostic factors are known to be important including age at diagnosis (the younger the better), histological findings such as degree of differentiation (with a better prognosis in well-differentiated tumours) and tumour stage. Prognosis for stage I disease is excellent with 5-year survival rates of at least 90%; with stage IV disease this falls to 54%.

Malignant mesenchymal tumours (soft-tissue sarcoma)

Incidence, aetiology and classification

This very heterogeneous group of tumours account for 7% of childhood tumours, with an incidence of 0.8 per

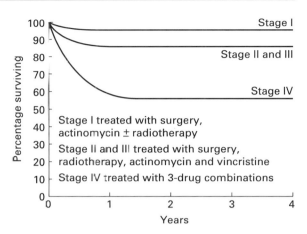

Fig. 24.5 Survival related to stage in Wilms' tumour.

Table 24.8 Childhood soft-tissue sarcoma.

	Relative frequency (%)
Rhabdomyosarcoma	52
Fibrosarcoma (including histiocytoma)	10
Mesenchymoma	6
Synovial sarcoma	6
Liposarcoma	4
Leiomyosarcoma	2
Vascular sarcomas	5
Others	15

100 000 children. The tumours become much less common after 14 years of age. Little is known of their cause, although genetic factors are important in the Li–Fraumeni syndrome (see Chapter 23, p. 344). In alveolar rhabdomyosarcoma a 12;13 translocation occurs.

The histological types of soft-tissue sarcoma in children are similar to those found in adults (see Chapter 23), but the relative frequency is different, with rhabdomyosarcoma and fibrosarcoma predominating (Table 24.8). Histological diagnosis may be difficult. Advances in molecular genetics may help in classification.

Rhabdomyosarcoma

This tumour is the commonest soft-tissue sarcoma of childhood. *Embryonal rhabdomyosarcoma* is the most frequent histological type, with a peak incidence at 2–5 years. *Alveolar rhabdomyosarcoma* is commoner in adolescence.

The tumours can arise at a variety of sites: in the head and neck (chiefly the orbit, nasopharynx, oropharynx or palate), the pelvis (particularly bladder, uterus and vagina) or, less commonly, the extremities or trunk.

PATHOLOGY [11]

There are four main histological subtypes of rhabdomyosarcoma: embryonal, alveolar, pleomorphic and mixed types. The first two account for more than 90% of all cases. Macroscopically, the tumours are usually nodular, often with a surrounding inflammatory and oedematous reaction. Although they may appear to be circumscribed, true encapsulation is very uncommon. Sarcoma botryoides has a characteristic macroscopic appearance, described as resembling bunches of grapes, which consist of mucinous polyps of tumour.

Microscopically, these tumours are highly malignant. Pathological diagnosis can be difficult, particularly if cross-striation is regarded as an essential part of the histological diagnosis (Fig. 24.6). Differentiation from other small round-cell tumours can be made by showing positivity for desmin and vimentin, and lack of staining with markers for Ewing's tumour or lymphoma. *Embryonal rhabdomyosarcoma* is often poorly differentiated, with long slender spindle-shaped cells with a single central nucleolus and eosinophilic cytoplasm, often without obvious cross-striations. The cells usually have an irregular pattern without the cellular arrangements which are characteristic of alveolar rhabdomyosarcoma. *Sarcoma botryoides* is a polypoid form of embryonal rhabdomyosarcoma. The embryonal group is the commonest form of paediatric rhabdomyosarcoma and accounts for the majority of head, neck and genitourinary cases.

Alveolar rhabdomyosarcoma arises more commonly on the limbs and trunk. Microscopically, these tumours have a more organized pattern and the cells tend to be separated by connective tissue bands. The typical cell is round with scanty eosinophilic cytoplasm which is sometimes vacuolated and may contain glycogen. Cross-striations are often seen, and giant multinucleate cells are common. Pleomorphic rhabdomyosarcomas are rare in childhood, and almost always arise in skeletal muscle.

All varieties are *highly* malignant and exhibit rapid growth with early dissemination. Early lymph node involvement is common, producing obvious lymphadenopathy which may be the initial presenting feature, particularly in head and neck tumours. Blood-borne metastases are also frequent, particularly to lung and marrow, though other sites such as brain, liver and other

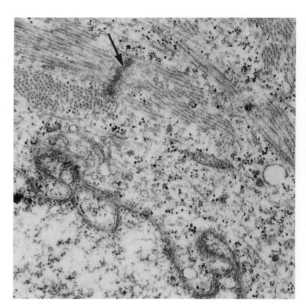

Fig. 24.6 Electron micrograph of a portion of rhabdomyoblast. Thick and thin filaments are shown, and there is formation of Z bands (arrowed) ($\times 26\,600$).

Table 24.9 Pathology and prognosis in rhabdomyosarcoma [11].

Prognosis	Pathology
Good	Botryoid, spindle cell
Intermediate	Embryonal
Poor	Alveolar undifferentiated
Uncertain	Rhabdoid

soft-tissue sites may also be involved. However there are prognostic implications of the pathology as shown by the International Classification (Tables 24.9 and 24.10).

CLINICAL FEATURES

Clinically, the commonest presentation is with a painless mass either clearly visible in the case of extremity and trunk lesions, or causing displacement as with the characteristic proptosis of orbital rhabdomyosarcoma which accounts for 30% of all head and neck cases. A grouping of major sites has been summarized by an international workshop as shown in Table 24.11.

In the pelvis, the commonest primary sites are the genitourinary tract and perianal area. Bladder tumours are more common in boys and present with urinary symptoms. There may be hydronephrosis. Vaginal tumours present with a vaginal mass or bleeding. Deep-seated

Table 24.10 Preclinical staging of childhood rhabdomyosarcoma.

T	T_1	Confined to organ of origin (subgroup according to size < or > 5 cm)
	T_2	Spread to adjacent structures (subgroup according to size < or > 5 cm)
N	N_0	No involved nodes
	N_1	Regional nodes involved
	N_X	Uncertain
M	M_0	No distant metastases
	M_1	Distant metastases

Stage grouping (and 5-year survival rates)

Stage				5-year survival (%)
I	T_1	N_0 or N_X	M_0	78
II	T_2	N_0 or N_X	M_0	65
III	Any T	N_1	M_0	67
IV	Any T	Any N	M_1	26

parameningeal tumours may cause indirect symptoms such as facial and other cranial nerve palsies and discharge from the ear with tumours in the middle ear; airway obstruction and nasal discharge from nasopharyngeal primaries. Dysphagia may occur with tumours in the oropharynx. Lymph node metastasis is common with testicular and genitourinary sites and may be the presenting sign, but is very unusual with head and neck (particularly orbital) primaries.

INVESTIGATION AND STAGING

Important investigations include a chest X-ray and thoracic CT scan; bone scan; ultrasonography of the liver; and CT and/or MRI scanning of the abdomen (in patients with abdominopelvic primary tumours). In head, neck and orbital cases, detailed plain radiographs, CT and/or MRI scanning are essential to determine the local extent of the primary site. In the orbit, scanning may show extension into the nasal or maxillary sinus when it is then considered as parameningeal. Intracranial extension is uncommon. For parameningeal sites, MRI scans will frequently reveal invasion of the skull base and intracranial extension. An ear, nose and throat examination is necessary. In other head and neck sites an examination under

anaesthesia may be necessary to delineate the tumour. In genitourinary sites CT has largely rendered urography unnecessary. Computed tomography of the abdomen is also necessary in paratesticular tumours to identify enlarged para-aortic lymph nodes. Numerous staging systems have been proposed, but these have now been pulled together to form a widely accepted system of pretreatment staging based on the tumour node metastasis (TNM) system (Table 24.10).

MANAGEMENT [12,13]

As with most paediatric tumours, current management is complex and, for the majority of patients, includes surgery, radiotherapy and chemotherapy since none of these modalities alone gives satisfactory results. This integrated multimodal approach to treatment has led to a substantial improvement in prognosis. Until recently, radical surgical removal of the primary was always felt to be mandatory, a view which has undergone revision in recent years. Combination chemotherapy should now be used as the initial treatment, followed by local treatment with surgery and radiotherapy. Although surgery should be as complete as possible, careful judgement is required in order to avoid the risk of long-term mutilation. This has led, for example, to an increasing preference for wide excision (including compartmentectomy) rather than amputation for children with tumours of the extremities. When coupled with radical postoperative irradiation and early (adjuvant) chemotherapy this approach gives acceptably low local recurrence rates and allows for later amputation in the small number of cases where local recurrence occurs in the absence of more generalized disease.

With more deeply situated primary tumours such as nasopharynx, primary surgery plays no part other than to

Table 24.11 Major sites of rhabdomyosarcoma.

1 Orbit (non-parameningeal)
2 Head and neck (non-parameningeal)
3 Head and neck (parameningeal), nasopharynx, nasal cavity, paranasal sinuses, middle ear, pterygoid fossa
4 Genitourinary
5 Limbs
6 Other

establish the histological diagnosis. In some of the deeply situated but more accessible abdominopelvic primaries, the role of surgery is more uncertain, though it is increasingly accepted that major procedures such as total cystectomy or exenteration should not be performed in the first instance since effective irradiation and chemotherapy may result in cure with far less long-term damage. Combinations of chemotherapy and irradiation are increasingly used to achieve local control in orbital rhabdomyosarcoma, and it is sometimes possible to save the eye. Embryonal and alveolar rhabdomyosarcoma are relatively sensitive to irradiation (particularly embryonal rhabdomyosarcoma), though high doses are required for effective control (50–60 Gy over 5–6 weeks).

Chemotherapy has now been established as an important part of treatment in both metastatic and recurrent cases, and also as an adjuvant to local treatment. Many agents are known to produce objective responses in significant numbers of patients, including vinca alkaloids, alkylating agents, actinomycin D, doxorubicin, methotrexate, ifosfamide, cisplatin, carboplatin and etoposide (Table 24.12). Chemotherapy of metastatic disease usually produces only temporary remission. Treatment with combination chemotherapy is preferable using, for example, vincristine, actinomycin D and cyclophosphamide, though actinomycin D should not be given synchronously with radiation because of dangerous recall phenomena, and cyclophosphamide is usually deferred until after radiotherapy because of the danger of myelosuppression. Adjuvant chemotherapy is usually continued for 9 months. Localized tumours require only 6 months' therapy. Tumours in special sites may require particular treatment strategies; for example, in parameningeal tumours prophylactic treatment with intrathecal chemotherapy and cranial irradiation may be needed.

Table 24.12 Chemotherapy in rhabdomyosarcoma in childhood.

Single agents	
Vincristine	Mitomycin C
Actinomycin D	Cisplatin
Doxorubicin	Ifosfamide
Cyclophosphamide	Etoposide

Combination chemotherapy regimens
Vincristine, actinomycin D, cyclophosphamide
Vincristine, actinomycin D, cyclophosphamide, doxorubicin
Other regimens including cisplatin, ifosfamide and etoposide as part of study protocols especially in poor-prognosis disease

At present, multicentre studies in both Europe and the USA are attempting to provide answers to several unresolved issues such as the need for radiotherapy, the most acceptable and effective form of adjuvant chemotherapy, and the duration of adjuvant treatment.

PROGNOSIS

The stage of disease is the most important prognostic factor; both the extensiveness of the primary lesion (which will govern the likelihood of resectability) and the presence of metastases affect survival. Overall 5-year survival rates according to pretreatment stage are given in Table 24.10. As with other paediatric tumours, age at presentation also affects prognosis. The median survival is better for children under 7 years. Younger children have less extensive disease at the time of diagnosis, and in general a more favourable tumour type (predominantly embryonal rhabdomyosarcoma) than older children. Site may also be important, and orbital tumours in general have a better prognosis although other head and neck tumours, particularly nasopharynx, have a poor prognosis presumably due to their inaccessibility, late presentation and unsuitability for surgical resection as well as propensity for spread to the CNS.

Recurrence tends to occur early, usually (90%) within the first 2 years.

Retinoblastoma

Incidence and inheritance

Retinoblastoma is a rare but important tumour with a familial incidence. The rate appears to have doubled over the past 40 years and it now has a frequency of one case per 15 000 live births, accounting for about 3% of all childhood malignancies. Its increasing incidence is due in part to the fact that it is an inherited disease in which survival is increasing, which in turn leads to an increase in the number of children born to previously affected parents.

Most children with retinoblastoma have a normal karyotype. In those with associated mental retardation (see below) a deletion on the long arm of chromosome 13 is present (13q14). Chromosome loss, and loss of heterozygosity at this site can be shown in all patients. Tumour formation only occurs when both genes are lost.

The *Rb* gene codes for a nuclear phosphoprotein which is DNA-binding. The introduction of the normal *Rb* gene product suppresses tumorogenicity. The *Rb* gene may be inactivated in other tumours, for example small-cell carcinoma of the lung and breast cancer. The gene product appears to have a general cell cycle suppressor function.

Patients with retinoblastoma have a greatly increased likelihood of developing a second tumour. Those with bilateral (inherited) disease have a 20% risk of a monocular cancer of which the commonest is osteosarcoma, and occasionally Ewing's sarcoma, Wilms' tumour and soft-tissue sarcoma.

Most cases of retinoblastoma are sporadic (non-familial). When familial, it is inherited by an autosomal dominant gene, though some individuals can apparently carry this defective gene without developing the tumour. Sporadic non-familial cases are mostly unilateral, with only a small risk that the offspring of these patients will subsequently develop the disease (Fig. 24.7). However, in sporadic bilateral cases, there is a 50% chance of the offspring developing the disease. In retinoblastoma families, most affected children will themselves develop bilateral disease so that in apparently unilateral familial cases, a close watch must be kept on the contralateral eye. In genetic counselling (Table 24.13) it is also important to recognize that about 4% of normal parents of an affected child produce more than one child with the disease. Retinoblastoma can on rare occasions be associated with mental retardation, microcephaly and skeletal deformity; a deletion at 13q14 may be observed. A group of patients has been reported in which bilateral retinoblastoma was associated with pinealoblastoma.

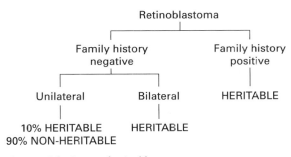

Fig. 24.7 Inheritance of retinoblastoma.

Pathology

Retinoblastoma is thought to arise from a retinal neuroepithelial progenitor. Microscopically, the tumour typically consists of an admixture of undifferentiated and small cells with deeply staining nuclei and scant cytoplasm, though larger cells are often found, sometimes with a tendency to rosette formation around the central cavity.

Retinoblastoma is typically multifocal. This is presumably due to spread of tumour within the retinal layers, as well as to synchronous tumour development within different parts of the retina in cases of bilateral disease, since spread via the optic nerves and chiasm does not generally occur. The commonest route of spread, the so-called 'endophytic type' of tumour, is forward into the vitreous humour, and this growth within the globe tends to occur before other involvement of periglobal structures. The 'exophytic' growth pattern is when the tumour arises from the outer retinal layers and grows outwards. Retinal detachment may occur during this process, but extension of growth into the choroid does not usually occur other than with very large tumours. Seeds of tumour may break off and implant themselves in the eye. Invasion of the choroid increases the risk of haematogenous spread. Invasion of the sclera may also occur, carrying a poor prognosis; the optic nerve itself may be directly invaded by the tumour via the lamina cribrosa, and the tumour may thence spread to the subarachnoid space with dissemination of tumour cells into the cerebrospinal fluid, with consequent seeding along the base of the brain.

Blood-borne metastases occur, most commonly to the bone marrow, liver, lymph nodes and lungs.

Clinical features

Most children present under the age of 2 years, usually with a white pupil (leucocoria), or, less commonly, with strabismus, glaucoma, defects in visual fixation, or inflammatory changes within the eye. Any family history of

Table 24.13 Genetic counselling in retinoblastoma.

Bilateral disease is almost always familial

Offspring of survivors of hereditary retinoblastoma, or of bilateral sporadic cases, will have a 50% chance of developing the tumour

Unaffected parents with a child with unilateral disease have a 1–4% chance of having another affected child

Survivors of unilateral sporadic disease have a 7–10% chance of having an affected child, and are therefore presumed to be silent carriers

If two or more siblings are affected there is a 50% chance that subsequent siblings will have the tumour

Unaffected children from retinoblastoma families may occasionally (5%) carry the gene, but if they have an affected child the risk in subsequent children is 50% since the parent is then identified as a silent carrier

retinoblastoma should immediately raise suspicion, and the most important investigation is a careful ophthalmological examination by an experienced ophthalmic surgeon. This gives an assessment of tumour site, extent, involvement of the contralateral eye and evidence of multicentricity. Only the ophthalmologist can reliably exclude important non-malignant diseases such as *Toxocara* infection or retinal dysplasia; biopsy is accepted as unwise since this may provide a pathway for tumour dissemination.

Investigation

Tumour calcification may also be present radiologically. Chest X-ray, full blood count and isotope bone scanning should be performed in all cases, with cerebrospinal fluid examination whenever there is a suspicion of CNS involvement. CT and MRI scanning are now used to assess disease extent.

Staging

Size, site and multicentricity of tumour have led to the widely accepted clinical staging system which has now been in clinical use for over 25 years (Table 24.14). This simple system depends on ophthalmoscopic examination with accurate diagrammatic representation of the retinal lesion in relation to standard reference landmarks such as the optic nerve head, ora serrata (junction of the retina and ciliary body) and so on.

Treatment [14]

Treatment depends on the presenting stage. In recent years, treatment philosophy has altered sharply away from immediate or early enucleation of the more severely affected eye, to a more conservative policy with a much greater reliance on chemotherapy and radiotherapy as the preferred local technique. The excellent results of this approach (see below) are highly dependent on careful ophthalmological assessment in every case. Eradication of tumour with preservation of vision has in most cases become a realistic aim.

With very small tumours (less than 7 mm diameter) cryosurgery and photocoagulation are both effective, though with tumours near the optic disc or macula, external beam irradiation is preferable because light coagulation close to these critical parts of the eye carries a risk of permanent visual damage. For these tumours, external irradiation using a single lateral field is both simple and effective.

For larger tumours (3–10 mm) brachytherapy (see Chapter 5) with radioactive cobalt plaques is frequently used, but smaller tumours near the optic disc or macula are better treated with external beam irradiation. With single tumours above 10 mm, external beam irradiation of the whole eye is frequently used and usually requires multifield treatment to ensure homogeneous irradiation of the whole globe, particularly where there is vitreous seeding. Use of an anterior field allows for more adequate sparing of the contralateral eye even though the lens and cornea are unavoidably treated. This technique is also suitable where there are multiple tumours confined to one eye. A dose of 35 Gy in 3–4 weeks is sufficient to control most intraocular retinoblastomas. With posteriorly situated tumours, a lens-sparing approach is preferable, using contact lenses to locate the cornea.

With obvious infiltration of the optic nerve, enucleation is preferable.

Chemotherapy has become the preferred initial treatment for bilateral tumours in infants and in older children with extensive bilateral disease (when it is frequently combined with external beam radiation). This approach has avoided some of the bony deformity that is the inevitable consequence of radiation on the growing skull. With bilateral tumours, preservation of sight is more difficult, and it is best to treat each eye individually on its own merits rather than assuming that enucleation of the worse eye will invariably be required. Where there is residual tumour in the orbit, postoperative irradiation should certainly be given to include the whole orbit and optic foramen. A dose of 50 Gy in 5 weeks is both effective and well tolerated in children requiring postoperative irradiation of the orbit, in whom the radiation tolerance of the eye is no longer a consideration. Particular care is required to ensure immobilization either by means of a head cast or with sand bags.

In all cases of retinoblastoma, treatment planning must be precise, aiming to cover all areas of disease without unnecessarily jeopardizing the lens of both the affected and the contralateral eye. Unfortunately, with the radiation dose required to control most retinoblastomas (35–40 Gy in 3.5–4 weeks), significant complications are still common. The commonest complication, cataract formation, is unavoidable when anterior beams are used, though not all cataracts are clinically significant and, if necessary, lens extraction is fairly simple and effective. Vascular injury from irradiation, though easily visible to the ophthalmologist, rarely impairs vision, though occasionally retinal haemorrhage may result in secondary glaucoma which can be troublesome. Irreversible damage to the orbital bones is a frequent complication preventing normal growth. Following radiation there is a greatly increased risk of second cancer, especially bone sarcoma. The tumours are most likely to occur in the irradiated site, although the risk of tumour elsewhere is also greatly increased. Over a 20-year period the relative risk is increased 350-fold with 12% of patients developing a second malignant neoplasm. The use of anthracyclines and alkylating agents may add to this risk. Enucleation of the affected eye is often necessary.

Cytotoxic chemotherapy is increasingly used. It has a clear role in bilateral disease, in poor-risk tumours with optic nerve invasions (detected following enucleation) or choroidal invasion, in relapsed disease (in the orbit or metastatic) and when disease recurs in a sole remaining eye. Vincristine, carboplatin and etoposide are the drugs most usually employed in combination chemotherapy. The results of treatment for advanced and extraocular retinoblastoma are poor. Adjuvant chemotherapy for these high-risk tumours has improved the chances of cure. Surgical or radiation cure is rare in patients with massive orbital disease or extensive optic nerve involvement at presentation. In these very advanced cases, death is as likely to result from intracranial involvement as from distant metastases, and although combination chemotherapy, whole-brain irradiation and intrathecal chemotherapy have undoubtedly produced worthwhile responses, no cures have yet been reported.

Prognosis [15]

The results of treatment are very good (Table 24.14), particularly in early cases and where specialized facilities and experienced clinicians are available. Cure rates of 90% have been achieved in the UK as a whole; in one large series, children with stage I and II disease had a cure rate of 100%, and even those with stage IV and V disease had a cure rate of 75%. When conservative measures have failed, enucleation of the eye can be curative, though there is still

a 10–15% overall mortality rate due to intracranial spread or distant metastases. A few children, successfully treated, will later die from a second radiation-induced tumour (usually osteosarcoma).

Histiocytoses

This is a group of disorders comprising 3–4% of paediatric tumours, whose origin is from the macrophage/monocyte series of cells. These cells arise in the bone marrow, circulate briefly as blood monocytes and then migrate to tissues where they form fixed macrophages in the liver, spleen, lung, bone marrow and tissues (histiocytes) or are antigen-presenting (dendritic cells). The disorders in class 1 are often multifocal, sensitive to cytotoxic agents and irradiation, and can be fatal.

The classification of histiocytoses has recently been altered and is now based on the nature of the histiocytic infiltrate.

1 Class 1 histiocytosis is characterized by the presence of the Langerhans' cell. These cells may not be genuinely malignant and may respond to immunological mediators. Under electron microscopy the cells show typical Birbeck granules. Opinion is still divided as to whether this is a malignant disease. In some cases, however, monoclonality of cells has been demonstrated [16].

2 Class 2 lesions are characterized by a reactive macrophage infiltrate. The two disorders in this category are the rare and rapidly fatal disease familial erythrophagocyte lymphohistiocytosis, and infection-associated haemophagocyte syndrome.

3 Class 3 are malignant histiocytic tumours, including monocytic leukaemia (see Chapter 28).

Langerhans' cell histiocytosis (LCH, class 1 histiocytosis) [16]

This used to be called histiocytosis X, which included the spectrum of syndromes of Letterer–Siwe disease,

Table 24.14 Staging and prognosis (percentage 3-year survival) in retinoblastoma.

Stage I	Single or multiple tumours of size less than 4 disc diameters at or behind the equator (90–100%)
Stage II	Single or multiple tumours of size 4–10 disc diameters at or behind the equator (90–100%)
Stage III	Tumours anterior to the equator or a single tumour larger than 10 disc diameters at or behind the equator (70–85%)
Stage IV	Multiple lesions, some greater than 10 disc diameters. This group includes any lesion extending anteriorly to the ora serrata (70–75%)
Stage V	Massive tumours involving over half the retina, or tumours with vitreous seeding (33–70%)
Stage VI	Residual orbital disease. Extension into the optic nerve and through the sclera (30%)

eosinophilic granuloma and Hand–Schüller–Christian disease. Letterer–Siwe disease, an acute disease with onset in infancy, is characterized by hepatosplenomegaly, lymph node enlargement, thrombocytopenia and skin rash. A greasy, scaly scalp or nappy (diaper) rash is usually the presenting feature. Widespread infiltration of the skin, liver, lungs, spleen and bone marrow gives rise to hepatic dysfunction, dyspnoea and marrow failure. Lytic lesions in bone are common. The form of the disease, previously called eosinophilic granuloma, forms a spectrum ranging from a single, isolated bone lesion, typically in older children, to multiple punched-out bone lesions. The prognosis is worse below the age of 3 years. Presentation is usually with bone pain or lymphadenopathy. The disease may regress spontaneously. Other patients present with multiple eosinophilic granulomas. Occasionally, diabetes insipidus may occur, due to pituitary involvement as well as exophthalmos from orbital deposits (Hand–Schüller–Christian disease). Enlargement of liver and spleen occurs, as does skin infiltration, but the disease is less aggressive than Letterer–Siwe disease. As with eosinophilic granuloma, the disease may become quiescent and does not usually relapse if the activity ceases for 3–4 years. Diabetes insipidus is permanent, and chronic neurological disability may occur as cirrhosis with portal hypertension.

Prognosis and treatment

Mortality is highest in infants and in children with organ infiltration (lung, liver, bone marrow). Single bone lesions can be treated by curettage and local steroid injection. Radiation in low dosage is often dramatically effective but carries the risk of bone sarcoma in later life. More generalized disease can be treated with cytotoxic drugs of which the most useful are prednisolone, vinblastine, etoposide, chlorambucil and methotrexate. However, the disease may follow a very indolent course and may even remit completely even without treatment, and it is important to avoid toxicity. In many cases (especially those where the disease is confined to the bone or skin) treatment can be withheld for long periods of time.

Rare paediatric tumours

The tumours described above, the intracranial tumours of childhood, and the leukaemias and lymphomas, constitute 92% of all childhood malignancies; the remaining 8% are made up of a variety of uncommon diseases seen only sporadically even in large paediatric centres. Some, such as hepatoblastoma and orchioblastoma, are true paediatric tumours whereas others, such as adenocarcinoma of the kidney or transitional cell carcinoma of the bladder, are essentially adult tumours seen very rarely in the paediatric age group. The principles of management of some of these rare paediatric malignancies are not yet clearly established. The importance of a joint approach with full pretreatment assessment by paediatric surgeon, radiotherapist and paediatric oncologist (working closely with a histopathologist with special experience in these tumours), cannot be emphasized too strongly.

Hepatoblastoma

This rare tumour occurs in children below the age of 5 years. It is occasionally associated with Wilms' tumour. It can be associated with anomalies such as hemihypertrophy as well as with familial ademomatous polyposis coli (FAPC) and the Fanconi syndrome. In cases associated with FAPC there is germline mutation of the *APC* gene on chromosome 5q. Cytogenetic abnormalities in tumours are deletions in 1p, 1q and 11p (a site commonly involved in the Beckwith–Wiedemann sydrome in which hepatoblastoma may occur).

The pathological features are immature hepatic epithelial cells or a mixture of these cells with mesenchymal elements [17]. It usually arises in the right lobe and presents with a visible asymptomatic mass which later causes pain and weight loss. Like hepatocellular carcinoma (which occurs in children over the age of 5 years), the tumour produces α-fetoprotein (AFP) which may be elevated above the normal infantile range. The tumour can be delineated by ultrasound and CT scanning. Arteriography is essential if an unusual resection is to be attempted. Occasionally the tumour is associated with thrombocytosis (thrombocytopenia is more likely to indicate a vascular tumour).

The tissue diagnosis is usually made by biopsy to exclude other liver tumours. It does not appear possible to cure these children without complete surgical excision. Up to 75% of the liver can be removed but haemorrhage can be severe and great skill is necessary. Preoperative chemotherapy is now given to most cases of hepatoblastoma. The tumour shrinks and surgical excision is facilitated.

Cisplatin and doxorubicin are the most effective agents. Responses are also reported to alkylating agents such as ifosfamide. Serum AFP can be used to assess response to treatment. Prognosis is worse the more sections of the liver that are involved, if there is diffuse invasion, and if there are metastases. A very high AFP and node involvement are adverse indicators.

Germ cell tumours

All of the adult germ cell tumours (see Chapters 17 and 19) are occasionally seen in childhood. In addition, specific childhood forms occur though none is common.

SACROCOCCYGEAL GERM CELL TUMOURS

These are the most common germ cell tumours of childhood and the commonest tumour of the newborn. The female:male ratio is 4:1. The tumour arises on the inner margin of the distal part of the coccyx. The tumour is often external with variable internal components between the coccyx and the rectum. Approximately 10% of tumours in the newborn are malignant, but above 3 months of age 50% are malignant. Where possible tumour should be surgically excised. When this is not possible, and if there are malignant elements (embryonal carcinoma, choriocarcinoma), chemotherapy should be given. If a good response is obtained surgical excision may then be possible.

HEAD AND NECK GERM CELL TUMOURS

Ten per cent of childhood teratomas arise in the head and neck. The sites are very variable (orbit, soft tissue, nasopharynx), and they may cause respiratory obstruction. Treatment is with surgery and chemotherapy (if malignant). Pineal teratomas are discussed in Chapter 11.

TESTICULAR GERM CELL TUMOURS

The main histological variants are the yolk sac tumour (endodermal sinus tumour, Teilum tumour, orchioblastoma), embryonal carcinoma and differentiated tumour. Below the age of 2 years, yolk sac tumours are probably less likely to metastasize than in older children. The differentiated tumours are benign. Before effective chemotherapy was available, 9% of children under 2 years old were alive 2 years after treatment, while only 25% of older children survived. This difference may be less marked since the advent of platinum-based chemotherapy. The management follows the guidelines outlined for adult testicular tumours (see Chapter 19).

SEX CORD AND STROMAL TUMOURS OF THE TESTIS

Leydig cell tumours and Sertoli cell tumours occur rarely, the Leydig cell tumour at age 4–5 years and the Sertoli cell tumour below the age of 2 years. Leydig cell tumours, which may be accompanied by testicular virilization, are slow growing and cured by orchidectomy. Sertoli cell tumours may cause feminization, and orchidectomy is adequate treatment.

Gonadoblastomas are very rare tumours, chiefly found in patients with testicular feminization (XY or XY/XO karyotype with dysgenetic gonads and feminine phenotypes). The tumour develops in an abnormal gonad which is frequently indeterminate or no more than a rudimentary streak. The testes may be maldescended, in which case they are present in the inguinal canals or abdomen.

OVARIAN GERM CELL TUMOURS

The classification of these tumours is discussed in Chapter 17. Dysgerminomas, embryonal carcinoma and teratoma are managed as outlined in that chapter; as in adults, surgery and combination chemotherapy are the major modalities.

Late sequelae of treatment of cancer in childhood

As more children and adolescents survive cancer, we are becoming increasingly aware of late effects of treatment. The importance of these problems has, in turn, led to a re-examination of the primary treatment in some stages of some tumours, if the same survival can be achieved at less long-term cost. There are three areas of particular concern: effects on growth, gonadal function and the occurrence of second cancers.

Growth [18]

Studies in acute lymphoblastic leukaemia where both chemotherapy and prophylactic cranial irradiation were administered have shown significant decreases in height during treatment, which is regained to a varying degree when treatment stops. The site of damage is not definitely known but growth hormone deficiency and a lack of responsiveness of the epiphysis to growth hormone, induced by chemotherapy, certainly play a part. In children treated with radiation for brain tumours, growth retardation is greater in those who are also given chemotherapy. It is not known which cytotoxic agents are most likely to produce growth impairment.

Radiation of a growing epiphysis results in an arrest of bone growth at that site. The dose required to produce a permanent closure of the epiphysis is not known with certainty, but most schedules of treatment for cancer will do so. In a young child this may lead to a gross disparity in limb length, failure of development of the spine (after mantle treatment for Hodgkin's disease, for example) or asymmetry of the chest wall.

Gonadal function [19]

Children treated with nitrosoureas and procarbazine for brain tumours have a high incidence of gonadal dysfunction[19,20]. Although puberty progresses normally, follicle-stimulating hormone levels are high (and luteinizing hormone to a lesser degree). In later life the boys have small testes and severe oligospermia. In girls, ovarian function appears to return to normal and prospects for fertility are good. It is not known if their menopause will be premature. In some acute lymphoblastic leukaemia protocols, spinal irradiation may affect either the ovaries or the testes.

In boys who do not receive alkylating agents there is much less germinal epithelial damage. If mustine, vincristine (oncovin), prednisone and procarbazine therapy has been given for Hodgkin's disease severe oligospermia and high follicle-stimulating hormone levels are the rule. Damage appears to be less long lasting if treatment is given prepubertally.

Second cancers

The possibility of inducing a second cancer by treatment is particularly important in childhood cancers because of the long period of risk. One of the commonest types of second cancer is bone sarcoma [21], and the relative risk depends on the primary diagnosis (Table 24.15). The secondary cancer is usually osteosarcoma and it typically develops in the radiation field (though this is often not the case in the inherited form of retinoblastoma (Fig. 24.7)).

Acute non-lymphoblastic leukaemia may develop after treatment with chemotherapy-alkylating agents and nitrosoureas appear to be the drugs most likely to be associated. The risk seems higher after treatment for Hodgkin's disease (where radiation is often also given). Leukaemia is also more common after brain tumour treatment. Overall, the relative risk of leukaemia determined by the Late Effects Study Group was 14 [22]. A recent re-

Table 24.15 Relative risk of bone cancer according to primary diagnosis.

Diagnosis	Relative risk
Retinoblastoma	350
Ewing's sarcoma	250
Rhabdomyosarcoma	30
Wilms' tumour	30
Hodgkin's disease	30

port from the same group has confirmed an even higher incidence of solid tumours, particularly breast cancer—two-thirds occurring in patients who received both chemotherapy and radiation, and with an overall incidence in women [23].

Cancer in children of survivors

Apart from an increased risk of cancer in children of survivors of hereditary cancer such as retinoblastoma, there does not appear to be an excess incidence of cancer in offspring of survivors of paediatric cancer [24].

References

1 Stiller CA. Centralisation of treatment and survival rates for cancer. *Arch Dis Childhood* 1988; 6: 3–23.
2 Pritchard F, Stiller CA, Lennox EL. Overtreatment of children with Wilms' tumour outside paediatric oncology centres. *Br Med J* 1989; 299: 835–6.
3 Mott MG. The molecular genetic basis of childhood neoplasia. *Clin Oncol* 1995; 7: 279–86.
4 Ambros IM, Zellner A, Roald B *et al*. Role of ploidy, chromosome 1p and Schwann cells in the maturation of neuroblastoma. *N Engl J Med* 1996; 334: 1505–11.
5 Evans AE, D'Angio GH. Prognostic factors in neuroblastoma. *Cancer* 1987; 59: 1853–9.
6 Brodeur GM, Pritchard J, Berthold F *et al*. Revisions of the International Criteria for neuroblastoma diagnosis, staging, and response to treatment. *J Clin Oncol* 1993; 11: 1466–77.
7 Matthay KK, Villablanca JG, Seeger RC *et al*. Treatment of high-risk neuroblastoma with intensive chemotherapy, radiotherapy autologous bone marrow transplantation and 13-*cis*-retinoic acid. *N Engl J Med* 1999; 341: 1165–73.
8 Gessler M, Poustk AA, Cavenee W *et al*. Homologous deletion in Wilms' tumours of a zinc-finger gene identified by chromosome jumping. *Nature* 1990; 343: 774–8.
9 Beckwith JB. Wilms' tumour and other renal tumours of childhood. In: Finegold M, ed. *Pathology of Neoplasia in Children and Adolescents*. Philadelphia: W.B. Saunders, 1986: 313–32.
10 D'Angio GJ, Breslow N, Beckwith JB *et al*. Treatment of Wilms' tumour: Results of the third National Wilms' Tumour Study. *Cancer* 1989; 64: 349–60.
11 Newton WA, Geham EA, Webber BL *et al*. Classification of rhabdomyosarcomas and related sarcomas. Pathological aspects and proposal for a new classification—an Intergroup Rhabdomyosarcoma Study. *Cancer* 1995; 76: 1073–85.
12 Maurer HM, Beltangady M, Gehan EA *et al*. The Intergroup Rhabdomyosarcoma Study 1. A final report. *Cancer* 1988; 61: 209–20.
13 Flamant F, Rodary C, Voute PA, Otten J. Primary chemo-

therapy in the treatment of rhabdomyosarcoma in children: trial of the International Society of Paediatric Oncology preliminary results. *Radiotherapy Oncol* 1985; 3: 227–36.

14 Harnett AN, Hungerford J, Lambert G *et al.* Modern lateral external beam (less sparing) radiotherapy for retinoblastoma. *Ophthal Paediatr Genet* 1987; 8: 53–61.

15 Sanders B, Draper GJ, Kingston JE. Retinoblastoma in Great Britain 1969–80, incidence, treatment and survival. *Br J Ophthalmol* 1988; 72: 576–83.

16 Willman CL, Busque L, Griffith BB *et al.* Langerhans cell histiocytosis (histiocytosis X): a clonal proliferative disease. *N Engl J Med* 1994; 331: 154.

17 Haas JE, Muczynski KA, Krailo M *et al.* Histopathology and prognosis in childhood hepatoblastoma and hepatocarcinoma. *Cancer* 1989; 64: 1082.

18 Clayton PE, Shalet SM, Morris-Jones P *et al.* Growth in children treated for acute lymphoblastic leukaemia. *Lancet* 1988; i: 460–2.

19 Livesey EA, Brook CGD. Gonadal dysfunction after treatment of intracranial tumours. *Arch Dis Childhood* 1988; 63: 495–500.

20 Jenney ME, Levitt GA. The quality of survival after childhood cancer. *Eur J Cancer* 2002; 38: 1241–50.

21 Hawkins MM, Kinnier-Wilson M, Burton HS *et al.* Radiotherapy, alkylating agents and the risk of bone cancer after childhood cancer. *J Natl Cancer Inst* 1996; 88: 270–8.

22 Meadows AT, Baum E, Bellani-Fossati F *et al.* Second malignant neoplasms in children: an update from the Late Effects Study Group. *J Clin Oncol* 1985; 3: 532–8.

23 Bhatia S, Robinson LL, Oberlin O *et al.* Breast cancer and other second neoplasms after childhood Hodgkin's disease. *N Engl J Med* 1996; 334: 745–51.

24 Sankila R, Olsen JH, Anderson H *et al.* Risk of cancer among offspring of childhood-cancer survivors. *N Engl J Med* 1998; 338: 1339–44.

25 Hodgkin's disease

The prognosis of Hodgkin's disease has greatly improved, both for patients with localized disease who are often curable by radiotherapy, and for those with disseminated disease treated with cytotoxic drugs. Success has been achieved not only because of the introduction of new methods of treatment, but also because it has become apparent how radiotherapy and chemotherapy can be employed to best advantage. There have also been improvements in staging techniques and a better understanding of the patterns of spread which have led to more rational treatment.

Incidence and epidemiology

The incidence of Hodgkin's disease rises steeply from the age of 10–20 years. There is a slight fall in middle-age, followed by a rise after 50 years to reach a maximum at age 70 years and over (Fig. 25.1). The male : female ratio in Western countries is about 1.5 : 1. Although the relative age incidence varies in different parts of the world, the male predominance usually holds (Table 25.1).

The reported variation in incidence appears to reflect genuine differences in the frequency of the disease rather than in the accuracy of diagnosis.

In some countries such as Colombia and Nigeria the incidence in childhood (age 5–14) is five times that in the UK, but in adult life it is four times less common. In these countries the history also tends to be less favourable compared with western Europe and North America. In Japan and possibly other Far Eastern countries, the incidence appears to be substantially lower than in the West.

Aetiology

Genetic, family and social factors

There is a significant excess of human histocompatibility antigen identity in affected siblings. In the family of a patient the risk of siblings having the disease is greater than normal, possibly about six times that of the normal population, with siblings of the same sex most likely to be affected. The disease is slightly more frequent in higher socioeconomic groups. The meaning of rare, but dramatic, clusters of cases is unknown but suggests an environmental rather than a genetic cause [1].

Infections

The infectious agent which has the strongest claim to an

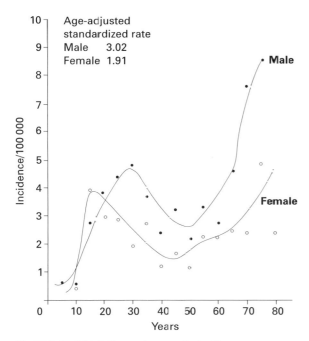

Fig. 25.1 Hodgkin's disease. Age-specific incidence.

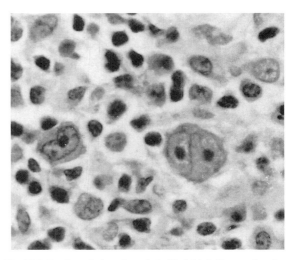

Fig. 25.2 Section of a lymph node in Hodgkin's disease, showing typical binucleate RS cell and mononuclear Hodgkin's cell (×400).

Table 25.1 Hodgkin's disease. Annual incidence rates (per 100 000) in various countries.

	Male	Female
England	2.2	1.3
USA		
Whites	2.3	1.4
African-Americans	1.3	0.7
Japan	0.6	0.3
Sri Lanka	0.1	0.1

genome and latent membrane protein does not prove that it is a cause of transformation—the same findings are present in non-neoplastic proliferation.

Pathology

The Hodgkin Reed–Sternberg (HRS) cell

Lymph nodes from patients with Hodgkin's disease contain two categories of cells. The first is the cell which is the hallmark of the disease and which is thought to be the malignant component—the RS cell or its mononuclear counterpart (Fig. 25.2). The second consists of a pleomorphic cellular infiltrate, the composition of which varies considerably in different patients.

The malignant cells are large, often with slightly basophilic cytoplasm. The nuclei are usually lobulated and there may be two or more in a single cell. The classical RS cell has two or more nuclei, usually with large nucleoli which are acidophilic. The mononuclear variety of cell is sometimes seen in reactive inflammatory nodes, and cells with a similar appearance to RS cells may occasionally be found in infective lesions (infectious mononucleosis) and other lymphoproliferative disorders such as phenytoin-induced lymph node enlargement and non-Hodgkin's lymphoma. The HRS cell is a B lymphocyte derived from the germinal centre of lymph nodes [3]. The mechanism provoking the infiltrate of normal cells that make up the

association with Hodgkin's disease is the Epstein–Barr virus (EBV) [2]. This virus infects B cells, the acute infection being controlled by a cytotoxic T-cell response. A history of infectious mononucleosis (which is caused by EBV) in the previous 3 years is associated with a four-fold risk of Hodgkin's disease. Cells similar to Reed–Sternberg (RS) cells have been found in lymph node biopsies from patients with infectious mononucleosis. The EBV genome can be detected in RS cells in 75% of cases of mixed cellularity histology, 40% of nodular sclerosing variety, but not in lymphocyte predominant disease.

The role of EBV remains open, since the finding of viral

bulk of the nodal enlargement in the disorder is unclear. Their function is known.

The techniques of immunohistochemistry and molecular genetics have been used in Hodgkin's disease to characterize the RS cell. Immunophenotyping shows B-cell characteristics in RS cells. CD20 and CD15 are usually expressed. CD30, an activation antigen on lymphoid cells, is strongly expressed on RS cells (and on other lymphomas and so-called Ki-1 positive lymphomas). Soluble CD30 is found in the serum of untreated patients.

To date, no consistent karyotypic abnormality has been found in Hodgkin's disease although a variety of chromosomal translocations have been detected.

Classification

The histological classification which is now widely used is based on the revised American–European classification [4] which divides the microscopic appearance into five categories.
1 *Lymphocyte rich.* The appearances are of small lymphocytes with scarce RS cells and mononuclear variants. These are sparse within B-lymphocyte rich node.
2 *Nodular lymphocyte predominant.* The tumour has a nodular appearance with mononuclear Hodgkin's cells that have a B-cell phenotype that differs from typical RS cells. The disease usually presents as stage 1 disease. There is a risk of development of a B-cell non-Hodgkin's lymphoma, usually after an interval of 10 years.
3 *Nodular sclerosis.* There are broad bands of collagen separating cellular nodules of Hodgkin's disease. The tumour contains mononuclear 'lacunar' cells which are typical of this form. Nodular sclerosing disease has been subcategorized into two groups where group 1 has a lymphocyte-predominant infiltrate in the nodules and group 2 has a more pleomorphic appearance with numerous RS cells. Patients in group 1 have been reported to have a better prognosis [5].
4 *Mixed cellularity.* The infiltrate is pleomorphic with lymphocytes, macrophages, eosinophils and polymorphs.
5 *Lymphocyte depleted.* There is either diffuse fibrosis with fewer RS cells, or a reticular type with numerous RS cells or their mononuclear variant.

The nodular sclerosing and mixed cellularity categories make up 80–90% of all cases. Prognostically, lymphocyte-predominant histology is most favourable and lymphocyte-depleted histology least so. Most of the relationship between prognosis and histology relates to disease stage. In patients of similar tumour stage, histology has little influence on outcome.

Sometimes the pathologist has great difficulty in deciding if the patient has Hodgkin's disease or not, and mistakes can occur. The clinician should be very careful in cases which have atypical histology obtained from nonnodal sites, and with clinically odd presentations such as isolated disease presenting in the gut or skin. The differential histological diagnosis includes the following.
1 Reactive nodes with immunoblasts which may be seen in infectious mononucleosis, other herpes virus infections or toxoplasmosis.
2 Hypersensitivity to drugs such as phenytoin.
3 Angioimmunoblastic lymphadenopathy (see Chapter 26).
4 T-cell lymphoma (see Chapter 26).
5 Metastatic melanoma.
6 Non-Hodgkin's lymphoma, particularly the distinction from sclerosing B-cell mediastinal lymphoma and Ki-1 lymphoma (Chapter 26).

In patients with proven Hodgkin's disease, other histological abnormalities may be found. The spleen or liver may show granulomatous infiltration of unknown cause. After intensive chemotherapy the lymph nodes may show an unusual appearance, with vascular invasion and atypical, lymphocyte-depleted histology with few inflammatory elements—appearances similar to a non-Hodgkin's lymphoma.

Abnormal immunity in Hodgkin's disease

Host defence against infection is abnormal in advanced Hodgkin's disease even before treatment. Radiotherapy and chemotherapy can impair these defence mechanisms still further. In advanced disease there are depressed delayed-hypersensitivity reactions to a variety of antigens including tuberculin *Candida*, mumps and histoplasmin.

There is little doubt that patients with Hodgkin's disease are especially susceptible to opportunistic infections. These include infections with bacteria such as *Pseudomonas* and tuberculosis, fungi such as *Candida* and *Aspergillus*, and viruses such as herpes zoster and herpes simplex. In all of these diseases, susceptibility is probably due to depressed cell-mediated immunity (CMI).

The more advanced the disease, the greater the likelihood of anergy, but there is little clinical value in tests of immune competence as part of the routine investigation of a newly diagnosed case. The degree of spread of the disease is better assessed by more straightforward investigations.

The treatment of patients with advanced disease with cytotoxic drugs is hazardous for many reasons; one of the most important is the profound additional depression of immunity which may lead to fatal infection.

Clinical features

In the vast majority of cases the clinical presentation is straightforward [6]. The patient has accidentally noticed an enlarged, painless lymph node in the neck or elsewhere, and a biopsy gives the diagnosis. The initial site of presentation (Fig. 25.3) includes cervical nodes (70% of all cases), axilla (25%) and inguinal area (10%). The lymph nodes usually grow slowly and are sometimes visible on photographs months or years before being noticed by a patient. Occasionally the nodes are described as growing very rapidly and sometimes they are tender if there has been a recent upper respiratory infection. The nodes may fluctuate in size with such infections and may mislead the physician into believing that the node enlargement is only inflammatory.

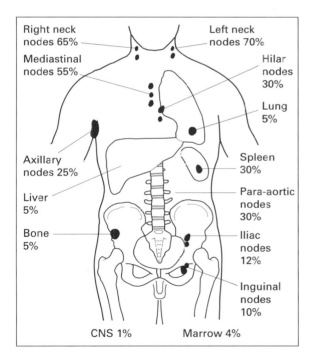

Fig. 25.3 Frequency of sites of involvement at presentation in patients with Hodgkin's disease.

Twenty-five per cent of all patients have constitutional symptoms at presentation. Fever is the commonest of these and is generally of low grade but may occasionally be hectic, up to 40°C, which usually occurs in the evening and falls to normal in the morning. In advanced disease, bouts of fever lasting 1 or 2 weeks may occur (Pel–Ebstein fever) but this is unusual and not specific for Hodgkin's disease. Drenching sweats may occur at night, waking the patient from sleep. Lesser degrees of sweating occur in many normal individuals and are hard to evaluate. Weight loss occurs and is especially associated with advanced or bulky disease. The triad of constitutional symptoms (fever, sweats and more than 10% loss of body weight) is of great importance since cases with one or more of these have a poorer prognosis.

Generalized pruritus occurs in 5–10% of patients at the time of presentation, but many patients will develop this symptom during the course of the disease when it relapses. If severe, it can be a most disabling symptom, the skin becoming excoriated from scratching, especially at night. The cause is unclear. The symptom abates with successful treatment. Alcohol-induced pain is felt in involved lymph nodes in a very small number of patients (2–5%). It is aching or stabbing in nature, comes on within minutes of drinking and lasts from a few minutes to an hour. It is chiefly associated with mediastinal disease of nodular sclerosing histology.

Other rare systemic features of Hodgkin's disease include autoimmune haemolytic anaemia (although a positive antiglobulin test in the absence of haemolysis is more common) and immune thrombocytopenia. A variety of erythematous skin rashes may occur, including erythroderma, erythema multiforme, psoriasiform lesions and bullous eruptions.

Enlarged nodes may produce symptoms due to compression. Examples include limb oedema and pain due to nerve entrapment; cough, stridor or superior vena caval obstruction from mediastinal disease; obstruction of the inferior vena cava or the ureters by para-aortic nodes; and obstructive jaundice due to nodes in the porta hepatis. Internal mammary node enlargement may give rise to a chest wall mass in the parasternal region. In contrast to non-Hodgkin's lymphoma, the tonsil and Waldeyer's ring are rarely involved, and when this does occur it is usually associated with upper cervical node involvement.

Hodgkin's disease occasionally presents as a pulmonary lesion and then must be distinguished from infection or other bronchial neoplasms by sputum cytology, culture and biopsy. Endobronchial Hodgkin's disease is very rare—the clinical features being wheezing and haemoptysis. Much more commonly, pulmonary infiltration occurs from direct spread from enlarged hilar or mediastinal nodes. Pulmonary nodules of Hodgkin's disease are easily missed on conventional chest X-rays, and CT scans are very useful when the diagnosis is in doubt. Pleural infiltration usually presents as an effusion, and is nearly always associated with mediastinal and pulmonary disease. If the mediastinal disease is massive, the pleural effusion may be due to lymphatic obstruction rather than direct invasion by tumour. The same is true for chylous effusions. A diagnosis of pleural infiltration can only be made reliably by biopsy or by a computed tomography (CT) scan showing nodules of tumour in the pleura or subpleural lung. Cytological examination is usually unrewarding since RS cells are rarely found.

Bone marrow involvement occurs at presentation in approximately 5% of patients and is nearly always associated with widespread disease elsewhere, and with constitutional symptoms. The diagnosis is by marrow trephine biopsy. The number of positive routine marrow biopsies in patients with early stage disease is very small, but a normal blood count does not preclude involvement in those with advanced disease. Marrow involvement is, however, more likely if there is anaemia, thrombocytopenia or leucopenia. The disease is focal within the marrow, so false negative biopsies are frequent.

Occasionally the bones are involved in a more localized way by Hodgkin's disease, either by direct spread from adjacent nodes, or by metastatic spread (in which case there is usually widespread disease elsewhere). The commonest histology is nodular sclerosis. The presentation is with pain, the serum alkaline phosphatase is elevated, X-rays may show either osteoblastic or osteolytic lesions, and an isotope bone scan is positive. A solitary bone deposit does not necessarily indicate stage IV disease (that is, diffuse involvement of an extranodal tissue; see Table 25.2) and may respond to local treatment, with a good prognosis.

Skin and subcutaneous infiltration are uncommon as presenting features but may occur in the context of aggressive disease over lymph node masses or in their drainage areas. The nodules of tumour are often painless but may ulcerate. Subcutaneous lesions may occur in the breasts. Primary cutaneous Hodgkin's disease is a great rarity.

When Hodgkin's disease involves the central nervous system (CNS) it is usually spinal rather than cerebral. This is a rare presentation and usually occurs by extension through the intervertebral foramina from adjacent lymph nodes to cause epidural compression. The clinical features are of root pain, paraesthesiae or spinal cord compression. All are medical emergencies because there is a serious risk of paraplegia (see Chapter 8). Laminectomy and radiotherapy are the usual methods of diagnosis and treatment.

Table 25.2 Staging classification for Hodgkin's disease.

Staging classification	
Stage I	Involvement of a single lymph node region or of a single extralymphatic site or organ
Stage II	Involvement of two or more node regions on the same side of the diaphragm, or of a localized extranodal involvement and one or more lymph node regions on the same side of the diaphragm (IIE)
Stage III	Involvement of lymph nodes on both sides of the diaphragm which may include the spleen (IIIS) or a localized extranodal site (IIIE) or both (IIISE)
Stage IV	Diffuse involvement of one or more extralymphatic organs

Notes

1 Suffix A: no constitutional symptoms. Suffix B: constitutional symptoms present. These are fevers, night sweats and/or loss of 10% or more of body weight over 6 months. Pruritus is not included

2 Localized extranodal involvement can at times be difficult to distinguish from stage IV disease. A good working rule is that localized spread means that the lesion in question could still be treated with radiotherapy

3 Stage III disease can be usefully subdivided according to the extent of intra-abdominal node involvement. Stage III means involvement of spleen, splenic, coeliac or portal nodes or any combination of these. Stage III2 means involvement of para-aortic, iliac or mesenteric nodes with or without upper abdominal disease

4 In the case of the marrow or liver, diffuse involvement means the demonstration of any amount of unequivocal Hodgkin's disease since localized spread at these sites is not recognized and radiotherapy not regarded as a treatment option

If the diagnosis is known, prompt treatment with radiotherapy and steroids is usually adequate. Compression of the spinal cord may be localized and does not necessarily constitute an indication for chemotherapy. Hodgkin's disease may on rare occasions present with leptomeningeal spread, with a clinical syndrome of basal malignant meningitis causing cranial nerve palsies, or symptoms and signs of raised intracranial pressure.

The gut is rarely the primary site of Hodgkin's disease and the diagnosis should be viewed with suspicion, since gastrointestinal non-Hodgkin's lymphomas are so much more common. Nevertheless, there are isolated cases of the disease arising in the oesophagus, stomach, small and large bowel. The presentation is usually indistinguishable from other tumours at these sites. When the disease occurs in the small bowel it usually affects the terminal ileum and may cause malabsorption syndrome.

The urinary tract is seldom clinically involved, and the commonest manifestation is ureteric compression with hydronephrosis. It is very unusual for direct renal infiltration to be clinically apparent. Rarely, cases of nephrotic syndrome occur which are due to immune complex glomerulonephritis or to compression of the renal veins by tumour masses.

Hodgkin's disease may be accompanied by paraneoplastic syndromes (see Chapter 9). In the CNS, patients may rarely develop progressive multifocal leucoencephalopathy. This is a relentless, fatal, demyelinating disorder, now known to be caused by a papovavirus and characterized by dementia, disorientation and focal signs leading to coma and death. Subacute cerebellar degeneration may occur with progressive ataxia, especially truncal ataxia, due to degeneration of Purkinje cells in the vermis. It usually does not improve with treatment of the disease. The Guillain–Barré syndrome occurs in the disease more commonly than would be expected by chance. Segmental, granulomatous, angiitis may occur in the brain, which may respond to treatment of Hodgkin's disease and which is possibly related to varicella-zoster infection.

Patterns of spread

In early Hodgkin's disease some lymph node groups are much more commonly involved than others (Fig. 25.3). By far the commonest site of presentation is the neck, while involvement of mesenteric nodes is rare. Following localized treatment, adjacent lymph nodes are the most frequent sites of relapse, a finding which led to the introduction of extended-field radiotherapy. In more detailed analyses, certain patterns of spread have been found. Bilateral cervical node enlargement is unusual unless there is also mediastinal disease; mediastinal disease is itself frequently associated with involved neck nodes. Unilateral upper cervical nodes involved with nodular sclerosing disease are seldom associated with disease at other sites. Nodular sclerosing Hodgkin's disease in the mediastinum is more frequently found in women and is not usually associated with subdiaphragmatic disease. Splenic involvement is uncommon when the presentation is with isolated inguinal node enlargement. Splenic disease, as the sole intra-abdominal site, recurs in only 10% of patients. In the abdomen the coeliac plexus is the commonest site of node involvement.

When the disease involves the liver or bone marrow, splenic disease is nearly always present. Involvement of the liver with sparing of the spleen is so unusual that the pathological findings should be questioned. It is not clear if splenic involvement is a source of dissemination, although vascular invasion in splenic Hodgkin's disease may signify a worse prognosis.

Staging classification [7,8]

The Ann Arbor classification is widely used as a description of clinical or pathological stage and is outlined in Table 25.2. This staging notation (with explanatory notes) is used throughout this chapter. The original Ann Arbor scheme did not take account of bulk of disease, number of sites of involvement or laboratory findings—such as erythrocyte sedimentation rate (ESR) and lactate dehydrogenase—which influence prognosis. The scheme has been revised to take account of these changes and modern imaging methods.

Clinical stage refers to the anatomical description of the extent of the disease on the basis of clinical examination, chest X-ray, CT and isotope scans is based on information obtained by biopsy and other surgical procedures.

Pathological stage refers to staging based on histological identification of additional sites of spread.

When comparison was made between the results of clinical and pathological staging (based on laparotomy) it was found that for each clinical stage there was a 25–30% chance of error as judged by pathological stage. Although modern scanning techniques have reduced the false negative rate of clinical staging, occult intra-abdominal disease in normal size para-aortic nodes and spleen is impossible to detect reliably.

Investigation

Clinical examination

The presence of constitutional symptoms should be noted. The sites of disease should be carefully documented, and a diagram or measurement made of the major nodal masses.

Haematology and biochemistry

Full blood counts are normal in most patients with localized nodal disease without constitutional symptoms (stages IA and IIA). Mild anaemia, polymorphonuclear leucocytosis and a high ESR are more common with advanced disease. The anaemia is usually normochromic or slightly hypochromic and is typical of the anaemia of chronic disease. Autoimmune haemolytic anaemia may rarely occur at presentation. Lymphopenia usually signifies advanced disease but eosinophilia, which occurs in a few patients, has no prognostic significance. The ESR is a somewhat unreliable guide to extent and activity of disease but a high ESR (above 40) is usually associated with more widespread disease.

Liver enzymes and plasma bilirubin are often abnormal with hepatic involvement, but isolated, modest elevation in aspartate transaminase or glutamyl transpeptidase sometimes occurs in the absence of proven involvement. The plasma alkaline phosphatase is often elevated, particularly in patients with advanced disease. Usually it is the liver isoenzyme which is responsible, but bone phosphatase may sometimes be contributory. An elevated alkaline phosphatase is not conclusive evidence of extensive disease if it is an isolated finding.

Routine X-rays

Chest X-ray

The chest X-ray is an essential examination. Enlargement of mediastinal and bronchopulmonary lymph nodes is very common, and the anatomical distribution of the lymph node groups is shown in Fig. 25.4. Mediastinal adenopathy is particularly common in women with nodular sclerosing disease. Massive mediastinal node enlargement may occur, leading to superior vena caval obstruction (Fig. 25.5). The thymus may be involved and often the mass projects laterally to the right and is seen anteriorly on lateral films. The bronchopulmonary lymph nodes may be enlarged with more subtle radiological

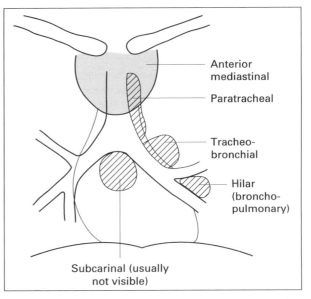

Fig. 25.4 Anatomical distribution of the major lymph node groups which may be involved in Hodgkin's disease.

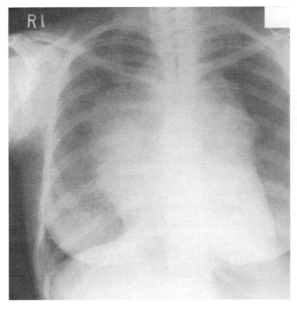

Fig. 25.5 Chest X-ray showing a very large, well-defined mediastinal mass. The patient was a woman of 22, with nodular sclerosing Hodgkin's disease.

changes. Usually there is associated mediastinal node enlargement.

The pulmonary changes may be due to compression of a bronchus, to direct intrapulmonary extension from a lymph node mass or, less commonly, to localized intrapulmonary Hodgkin's disease. Bronchial compression may cause atelectasis of a whole lobe with associated consolidation within the collapsed area. Direct extension from lymph nodes (Fig. 25.6) is not infrequent. In patients who have been previously treated with radiation to mediastinal nodes, extension of the disease into the lung may be very difficult to distinguish radiologically from radiation pneumonitis and fibrosis. Tuberculosis and other infections may produce similar radiological appearances. A chest X-ray may also show enlargement of the cardiac shadow due to a pericardial effusion, or erosion of a rib or the sternum due to local extension from lymph nodes.

Other imaging techniques

Ultrasound examination may demonstrate enlarged nodes and may be of value in the upper abdomen (see Chapter 4). The technique depends critically on the experience of the radiologist, so that assessment of its accuracy and value in routine use is difficult. In experienced hands the technique is useful to monitor response, since it is entirely non-invasive and can be easily repeated.

Thoracic CT scan will determine whether there is intrapulmonary spread of disease and will demonstrate small pulmonary and subpleural nodules of tumour. Involvement of mediastinal nodes is demonstrated by the technique. The additional information may lead to a change in treatment policy and the scans are of value in the planning of involved field radiotherapy.

In the abdomen, CT scanning is less sensitive than lymphography (see below) in demonstrating abnormal pelvic, iliac and lower para-aortic nodes if these are not enlarged, but it is useful in the upper abdomen, where lymphography is of limited value. Small foci of hepatic or splenic disease cannot be demonstrated. Computed tomography scanning of the abdomen is especially valuable if it shows widespread disease in asymptomatic patients, because the management will be altered.

Both ultrasound and CT scanning may alter treatment policy, but are not as accurate as laparotomy and give no information about microscopic splenic involvement.

Bone scanning may be useful in demonstrating isolated areas of involvement. The information obtained from routine use is limited; but if there is bone pain, it is an essential investigation, since a positive scan may change

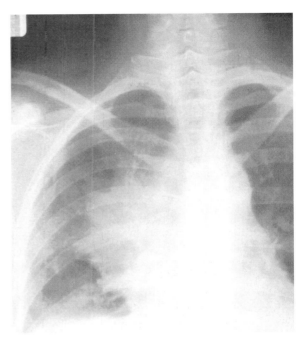

Fig. 25.6 Involvement of hilar nodes with extension into the lung on the right.

treatment policy if the cause of the abnormality is Hodgkin's disease. The areas shown up on scan must be examined radiologically since increased uptake on a bone scan has many causes.

The distinction between fibrosis and active disease can sometimes be made by gallium scanning. This technique is of value if the patient is being investigated for relapse after previous treatment. Higher-dose gallium scanning is now usually used. Another indication is in determining whether a residual mediastinal abnormality, after chemotherapy, contains active tumour. In lymphography lymphatic channels are cannulated, and low-viscosity contrast material is injected slowly. X-rays of the pelvis and abdomen are taken at the time of injection and the next day. Although the technique provides information about the involvement of lymph nodes that may not be enlarged on CT scan, it has largely been abandoned because it is difficult, technically uncomfortable and hypersensitivity reactions can occur.

Barium studies of the stomach and bowel are unnecessary unless there are clear symptoms requiring investigation. In the stomach the usual radiological appearance of Hodgkin's disease is of a mass indenting the barium, occasionally with appearances suggesting ulceration (Fig. 25.7). In the small and large bowel the typical appearance is of a long segment of infiltration with a coarse and distorted mucosal pattern and thickening of the bowel wall. The involvement may be patchy and discontinuous.

Percutaneous biopsy

Some of the indications for percutaneous biopsy have already been discussed. Marrow trephine is a worthwhile investigation in patients for whom treatment may be with radiotherapy alone, since an involved marrow will indicate the need for chemotherapy. However, in localized Hodgkin's disease without constitutional symptoms only 5% of patients will have a positive trephine biopsy. Diagnosis may be difficult because typical RS cells may not be present. The mononuclear Hodgkin's cell may be found and may be sufficient for diagnosis. The involvement is usually focal so there are considerable sampling errors.

Percutaneous liver biopsy is not a reliable investigation since Hodgkin's disease may sometimes be focal within the liver. It can be useful in selected cases with abnormal liver function tests, constitutional symptoms or hepatomegaly, and if positive may remove the need for further staging procedures. There may be a considerable problem in interpreting liver biopsy material even if obtained at laparotomy. Focal mononuclear infiltrates are frequently found, and pathologists are usually reluctant to diagnose the disease on the basis of occasional malignant-looking mononuclear cells. In both liver and marrow, non-caseating granulomata may be found, the cause of which is unknown, and these should not be confused with Hodgkin's disease.

Staging laparotomy and splenectomy

The introduction of laparotomy and splenectomy in the 1960s showed that even in patients with clinical, localized (stage I or II) supradiaphragmatic disease there was a significant chance of finding disease below the diaphragm. Although this led to a greater understanding of the mode of spread of Hodgkin's disease the advent of modern imaging techniques and the increased efficacy of chemotherapy have meant that the procedure has now a greatly diminished role in preoperative staging.

There is no purpose to be served by a staging laparotomy and splenectomy if no change in the proposed treatment will follow. There is no known therapeutic benefit from removing a diseased spleen. In clinically and radiologically localized disease above the diaphragm, a laparotomy will disclose subdiaphragmatic disease in 40% of patients. However a policy of limited assessment followed by radiotherapy, with chemotherapy if relapse occurs, does not lead to reduced survival. Patients who are known beyond doubt to have stage IIIB, IVA or IVB disease, on the basis of clinical evidence and preliminary investigations, should not be subjected to laparotomy since drug treatment will be used (see below). In centres where it is routine practice to use chemotherapy for massive mediastinal disease and stage IIIA disease (Table 25.2), a laparotomy is also unnecessary.

Treatment policy is therefore seldom changed by laparotomy. Furthermore splenectomy carries additional roles in patients who are already immunosuppressed by the disease and its treatment. Splenectomy adds to this susceptibility with increased risk of infection with *Haemophilus influenzae* and *Pneumococcus*. Staging laparotomy is now used only in specific circumstances where a fundamental change in policy would result. This means that patients who have been treated for supradiaphragmatic disease with radiotherapy alone must be carefully watched for early symptoms of subdiaphragmatic relapse which will occur in a substantial minority.

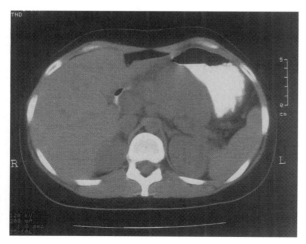

Fig. 25.7 CT scan of the abdomen in a patient with stage III Hodgkin's disease. A large mass of lymph nodes is displacing the barium-filled stomach to the left.

Treatment

There is now a good chance of cure for all patients, even when they present with extensive disease. The mainstay of treatment of localized disease is radiotherapy, with chemotherapy for advanced disease, and combined modality treatment in particular clinical situations. The best chance of cure is when the patient first presents. Careful assessment of the best treatment strategy is critical at this stage. While many patients can still be cured after relapse, recurrence of disease usually worsens the outlook.

The methods of using radiotherapy and drugs are changing. An understanding of the principles of these treatments in the disease is important in planning the correct approach in each patient.

Principles of radiotherapy

Like all lymphomas, Hodgkin's disease is highly sensitive to radiotherapy. The probability of long-term control (Fig. 25.8) at the irradiated site is dependent on dose. The dose which is needed to eradicate clinically inapparent disease in adjacent nodes, or in nodal areas in remission after chemotherapy, is less than that required for enlarged nodes and bulky tumour masses. The usual practice has been to treat both the involved and adjacent fields to the same dose level—usually in the region of 40 Gy in 25 daily fractions.

There has been considerable debate over many years as to whether it is preferable to treat only the sites of clinical involvement (involved field, IF) or whether to extend the field to adjacent nodes (extended field, EF). Now that chemotherapy for relapse after radiation failure is so much more successful than it was at the time when EF radiation was first introduced, the long-term survival advantage for EF rather than IF is not apparent (see below). Radiation fields commonly employed are the mantle field for treating disease in the neck, mediastinum and axillae, and the inverted Y field for nodes in the para-aortic and iliac regions (Fig. 25.9). The lungs, larynx and humeral heads are shielded. When large mediastinal masses are irradiated the field is often progressively contracted as resolution occurs, to avoid irradiating large volumes of lung (see Chapter 5). Recently there has been an increasing tendency to reducing the size of the radiation fields in localized disease especially when chemotherapy is given additionally (see below). The long-term effects of radiation are of increasing concern particularly secondary fibrosis and cardiac toxicity.

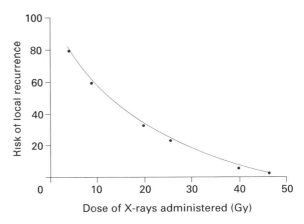

Fig. 25.8 The relationship between local recurrence rate and dose of radiation administered.

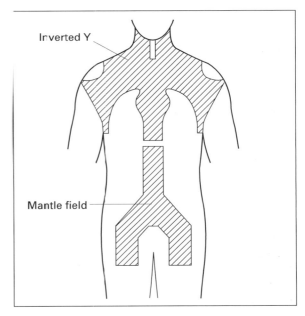

Fig. 25.9 Mantle and inverted Y fields. These are commonly employed fields.

Principles of chemotherapy [9]

Many classes of cytotoxic agents show activity against Hodgkin's disease. The approximate response rates obtained with the different drugs, when used as single agents in advanced disease, are shown in Table 25.3.

When cytotoxic drugs are used as single agents the likelihood of a complete response is small and, if obtained, the response is not usually sustained for more than a few months.

The major step forward was the development of combination chemotherapy. The drug regimen which has been most widely employed is MOPP (mustine, vincristine, prednisone and procarbazine) schedule. The details of this and other commonly employed regimens are given in Table 25.4. A total of six cycles of chemotherapy produces responses in a far higher proportion of cases than with single-agent treatment. Equally important, most of the responses are complete and are sustained when chemotherapy is stopped. Current policies typically use either six cycles in total or two further cycles after achieving complete remission. Regimens have been developed in which seven or eight drugs have been combined into a single cycle usually over 10–14 days. Response rates are high but the regimens have not yet been shown to be more effective than standard combination. An example is the BEACOPP regimen. Previously untreated patients have a 40–50% chance of long-term relapse-free survival with these regimens and may be cured. The likelihood of achieving sustained complete response seems to be somewhat less in men, in patients over the age of 40 years, in those with marked constitutional symptoms and in patients with multiple sites of disease, especially if bulky. In these patients, alternating regimens of different drugs (for example, MOPP and ABVD (doxorubicin, bleomycin, vinblastine and dacarbazine)) may improve response and survival. There are several other alternating combinations in common use such as LOPP (chlorambucil, vincristine, procarbazine and prednisolone)/EVAP (etoposide, vinblastine, doxorubicin and prednisolone). Response rate, duration and survival are much worse if the patient has previously been treated with single- or multiple-drug therapy. Previous radiotherapy does not seem to jeopardize response, although the toxicity may be greater (see below). The general principles of administration of the drugs are discussed in Chapter 6.

The response to chemotherapy is usually rapid, with disappearance of fever and reduction in tumour masses. Following treatment there appears to be no advantage in maintenance chemotherapy although the use of a different regimen such as ABVD may increase the length of remission.

Risk-adapted treatment

Some patients with apparently localized disease, treated with radiotherapy may relapse at distant sites. This is

Table 25.3 Approximate response rates to cytotoxic drugs (%).

	Complete response	Partial response	Total
Alkylating agents			
Nitrogen mustard	10	50	60
Cyclophosphamide	10	45	55
Chlorambucil	15	45	60
Vinca alkaloids			
Vincristine	30	30	60
Vinblastine	30	30	60
Other agents			
Prednisolone	0	60	60
Procarbazine	20	35	55
Doxorubicin	10	45	55
Bleomycin	5	40	45
DTIC	5	40	45

Table 25.4 Combination chemotherapy regimens and approximate response rates (%).

ChlVPP (28-day cycle; for LOPP substitute vincristine for vinblastine)
Chlorambucil (6 mg/m^2 days 1–14 p.o.)
Vinblastine (6 mg/m^2 days 1, 8 i.v.)
Procarbazine (100 mg/m^2 days 1–14 p.o.)
Prednisolone (40 mg days 1–14 p.o.)

ABVD (28-day cycle)
Doxorubicin (25 mg/m^2 days 1, 15 i.v.)
Bleomycin (10 mg/m^2 days 1, 15 i.v.)
Vinblastine (10 mg/m^2 days 1, 15 i.v.)
DTIC (375 mg/m^2 days 1, 15 i.v.)

EVAP (alternates with LOPP every 28 days)
Etoposide (150 mg/m^2 days 1, 2, 3; max. 200 mg)
Vinblastine (6 mg/m^2 days 1, 8; max. 10 mg)
Doxorubicin (25 mg/m^2 days 1, 8)
Prednisolone (25 mg/m^2 days 1–14; max. 200 mg)

MOPP (28-day cycle)
Mustine (6 mg/m^2 days 1, 8 i.v.)
Vincristine (2 mg (max) or 1.4 mg/m^2 days 1, 8 i.v.)
Procarbazine (100 mg/m^2 days 1–19 p.o.)
Prednisolone (40 mg/m^2 days 1–14 p.o.)

i.v., intravenously; p.o., by mouth.

because there is more widespread microscopic disease than is detected at diagnosis (a fact confirmed by past experience with staging laparotomy). Most of these patients can receive chemotherapy on relapse and some may be cured.

Other patients have clinical and biochemical features indicating a bad prognosis even if the disease appears localized.

These considerations, and the increasing evidence that radiation therapy is an important cause of later second cancer, has led to attempts to define patients who should receive chemotherapy as part of initial treatment, and to reduce the extent of radiation by adding chemotherapy as an adjuvant or associated initial treatment.

A simple prognostic score (Table 25.5) has been devised by an International Collaborative group [8] based on biochemical and clinical factors for patients with advanced disease treated with chemotherapy allowing identification of patients in whom more intensive treatments might be considered as initial treatment.

Management as determined by stage

In the following discussion, guidelines are given as to the management of Hodgkin's disease at presentation according to clinical and pathological stage. Clinical practice varies, so a consensus view is presented.

Clinical stage IA, IIA

In this category patients have one or more groups of nodes involved on one side of the diaphragm, and investigation (occasionally including laparotomy and splenectomy) has failed to show disease elsewhere. For this group of patients

Table 25.5 Prognostic score for patients with advanced Hodgkin's disease*.

Factor
Serum albumin < 4 g/dl
Haemoglobin < 10.5 g/dl
Male
Stage IV disease
Age > 45
WBC > 15 × 10^9/l
Lymphocyte < 0.6 × 10^9/l

*Each factor scores 1. Taken from [9].

radiotherapy produces good results. The usual practice for patients with cervical and mediastinal disease is to irradiate the mantle field (Fig. 25.9) to a dose of 40–44 Gy in 20–25 fractions. For those presenting with inguinal node disease the inverted Y field is generally used. The use of chemotherapy in localized disease and the treatment of massive mediastinal disease are discussed separately. The best method of management when laparotomy has not been performed is a matter of considerable controversy. The overall likelihood of undiagnosed intra-abdominal disease (usually high para-aortic or splenic) is 35%. Three treatment strategies have been advocated.

1 To treat with either mantle field or IF irradiation only, and to rely on salvage irradiation or chemotherapy on relapse. The advantage of this approach is that it avoids overtreatment of a large number of patients, especially those with good histology, low risk scores and below 40 years of age in whom the risk of occult intra-abdominal disease is low (20%). About 70% of all patients will be cured by this approach. However, the question of whether treatment on relapse is as effective as early treatment is still somewhat controversial. More recent trials have shown that, in those patients with 'poor' prognostic factors, combined radiation and chemotherapy offers better survival than radiation alone. In the 'good' prognosis group survival is not worse if chemotherapy treatment is delayed, although relapse is, as expected, more frequent in those treated with radiotherapy alone.

2 To treat with total nodal irradiation (TNI) including the spleen. This is associated with results which are the equivalent of relying on staging laparotomy, but many patients will be overtreated by this approach, and if systemic relapse occurs soon after TNI, the toxicity of chemotherapy may be very considerable. The late effects of radiation are of increasing concern. This approach using very extensive radiation has therefore largely been abandoned.

3 To treat with mantle radiotherapy followed by six cycles of ChlVPP (chlorambucil, vinblastine, procarbazine and prednisone) or MOPP, or with chemotherapy followed by irradiation. Again many patients will be overtreated and long-term sequelae of radiotherapy and chemotherapy are worrying (see below). Excellent long-term disease-free survival is usually obtained and this approach may be safest if the histology and other prognostic factors (such as ESR) are adverse. A meta-analysis using individual patient data has shown that the 10-year risk of disease relapse is greater (by 12%) in patients receiving reduced radiation fields, but survival is unchanged because of the efficacy of chemotherapy on relapse [10]. Similarly the use of

Acute toxicity of chemotherapy

Bone marrow suppression

This is a common accompaniment of all standard chemotherapeutic regimens in Hodgkin's disease. Most centres make dosage reductions in response to depressed blood counts, rather than delay the cycle, although delay may be necessary on occasions. The toxicity tends to be cumulative and particular care should be taken as treatment progresses, especially in the elderly, in those who have received EF radiotherapy in the past and in ill patients with extensive disease. After TNI the problem is particularly severe since over 50% of the adult haemopoietic marrow is within the irradiation field. Recovery of the marrow after TNI takes years and is often incomplete, so chemotherapy should be introduced with caution in these patients.

Immunosuppression

Treatment adds to the depression of CMI which is commonly present in advanced disease. Lymphopenia is an invariable consequence of EF irradiation and persists for several months after treatment. Depression of CMI is induced by most cytotoxic agents, especially alkylating agents and steroids. For this reason, herpes zoster and herpes simplex are very common in heavily treated patients and may be life-threatening. Less common nowadays is reactivation of tuberculosis, but other opportunistic infections such as *Pneumocystis*, cytomegalovirus and aspergillosis are occasionally seen.

Long-term complications of radiation

Radiation pneumonitis, leading to fibrosis, is a relatively common complication if the radiation dose is above 40 Gy. For this reason very large mediastinal masses require special consideration. Chemotherapy is often used to produce tumour shrinkage before irradiation, though it is not clear whether it is sufficient to irradiate the residual volume only. For smaller nodal areas complications are exceptionally rare.

With earlier radiation techniques there was an increased risk of myocardial infarction and cardiac death which was greater with higher total dose and larger mediastinal radiation fields. The relative risk has fallen from about six-fold to two-fold using modern techniques. Occasionally, mediastinal irradiation may cause pericarditis with a pericardial effusion which usually resolves. This may cause pain but is usually asymptomatic. Constrictive pericarditis is an extremely uncommon complication of mediastinal irradiation using modern techniques.

Clinical hypothyroidism is an infrequent (5%) complication of mantle field irradiation, although transiently elevated thyroid-stimulating hormone levels are more frequent (30%). Radiation damage to the bowel following infradiaphragmatic irradiation may uncommonly occur giving rise to diarrhoea (sometimes bloody), steatorrhoea and intestinal obstruction. It is related to both the volume and the total dose administered, and it is more likely to occur if the bowel has been tethered in one site by previous inflammation or surgery.

In the CNS the commonest symptom of radiation damage is Lhermitte's syndrome of tingling and paraesthesiae in the legs, often provoked by neck flexion. This usually passes off with no sequelae. Transverse myelitis should not occur with modern planning techniques. Very high repeated doses over peripheral nerves can rarely lead to peripheral neuropathy, usually within 1–5 years.

Impaired spermatogenesis occurs with doses of irradiation to the testes as low as 50 cGy and is more rapid, complete and long-lasting with higher doses, being invariable and often permanent above 5 Gy (see Chapter 5). During pelvic irradiation, with effective shielding, the dose should be below 100 cGy. The dose which causes permanent cessation of ovarian function is higher than for the testis. Oophoropexy is sometimes carried out to take the ovaries outside a possible pelvic irradiation field (see above).

Long-term complications of chemotherapy
(see Chapter 6)

Female fertility may be depressed after MOPP, but the effect is inconsistent. Persistent amenorrhoea and the onset of the menopause are more likely to occur in older premenopausal women. Amenorrhoea frequently occurs during treatment but normal menstruation usually returns and many patients have had normal children after treatment. The hazard of teratogenicity during chemotherapy, on the other hand, is usually regarded as an indication for termination.

Azoospermia is almost inevitable after MOPP or its variants. Procarbazine and the alkylating agents appear to be responsible. Recovery from sterility is rare. Sperm storage before chemotherapy is strongly advised for men who are concerned about the effects on fertility. In advanced Hodgkin's disease oligospermia is common before treatment begins.

During the first 5 years after MOPP chemotherapy the

cumulative risk of herpes zoster is approximately 15%, and after MOPP with TNI is 50%. Disseminated zoster (9%) is more common in those receiving combined modality treatment than with chemotherapy or radiation alone (2%). Bacterial infections, especially pneumococcal, also occur more often, particularly in children, in patients over 50 years and probably in those who have undergone splenectomy.

Second malignancies [15,17,18]

In recent years it has become apparent that, following chemotherapy for Hodgkin's disease, there is an increased risk of the patient developing a second malignancy. The association was first documented for acute non-lymphocytic leukaemia (ANL). At present, the risk of developing ANL in the 7 years after chemotherapy alone, or after combined modality treatment, is approximately 2%. However, in patients over the age of 40 years, the risk of ANL may be higher. It is now apparent that the risk of solid tumours is greater than that of leukaemia and occurs with a relative risk of 4 for lung cancer, 17 for non-Hodgkin's lymphoma and 2 for all other tumours. Lung cancers and breast cancer are especially likely to occur in the radiation field, as are bone sarcomas. However, the relative risk is greatest for combined modality treatment. The cumulative probability is shown in Fig. 25.10.

Both alkylating agents and procarbazine are potential carcinogens, but the cause of the increased incidence of ANL is not known. It may be less common after ABVD; however, this regimen has been introduced into clinical practice more recently than MOPP, and since the leukaemia risk is highest more than 5 years after chemotherapy, it is too soon to assume that ABVD is not as leukaemogenic. The risk of leukaemia relates to survivors rather than to those treated. It is important to appreciate that the risk of Hodgkin's disease is far greater than the hazard from a second malignancy.

References

1 Glaser ST, Jarrett RF. The epidemiology of Hodgkin's disease. *Baillière's Clin Haematol* 1996; 9: 401–16.
2 Chapman ALN, Rickinson AB. Epstein–Barr virus in Hodgkin's disease. *Ann Oncol* 1998; 9 (55): 550–16.
3 Küppers R, Rajewsky K. The origin of Hodgkin and Reed–Sternberg cells in Hodgkin's disease. *Ann Rev Immunol* 1998; 16: 471–93.

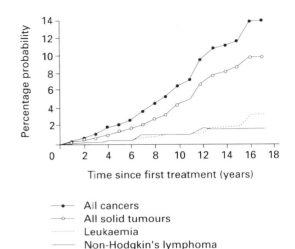

Fig. 25.10 Second malignancies after treatment for Hodgkin's disease. From [17] with permission.

4 Harris NL. A revised European–American classification of lymphoid neoplasms: a proposal from the International Lymphoma Study Group. *Blood* 1994; 84: 1361–92.
5 MacLennan KA, Bennett MH, Tu A *et al*. Relationship of histopathological features to survival and relapse in nodular sclerosing Hodgkin's disease: a study of 1659 patients. *Cancer* 1989; 64: 1686–93.
6 Urba WJ, Longo DL. Hodgkin's disease: review article. *N Engl J Med* 1992; 326: 678–87.
7 Lister TA, Crowther D, Sutcliffe SB *et al*. Report of a committee convened to discuss the evaluation and staging of patients with Hodgkin's disease: Cotswolds Meeting. *J Clin Oncol* 1989; 7: 1630–6.
8 Hasenclever D, Diehl V. A prognostic score for advanced Hodgkin's disease. *N Engl J Med* 1998; 339: 1506–14.
9 Canellos GP, Anderson JP, Propert KJ *et al*. Chemotherapy of advanced Hodgkin's disease with MOPP, ABVD and MOPP alternating with ABVD. *N Engl J Med* 1992; 327: 1478–84.
10 Specht L, Gray RG, Clarke MJ, Peto R. Influence of more extensive radiotherapy and adjuvant chemotherapy on long-term outcome of early-stage Hodgkin's disease: a meta-analysis of 23 randomised trials involving 3888 patients. *J Clin Oncol* 1998; 16: 830–40.
11 Loeffler M, Bronsteanu O, Hasenclever D *et al*. Meta-analysis of chemotherapy versus combined modality treatment trials in Hodgkin's disease. *J Clin Oncol* 1998; 16: 818–29.
12 Hoppe RT. Development of effective salvage treatment programs for Hodgkin's disease: an ongoing clinical challenge. *Blood* 1991; 77: 2093–5.
13 Schellong G. Paediatric Hodgkin's disease: treatment in the late 1990s. *Ann Oncol* 1998; 9 (Suppl. 5): 115–19.
14 Shafford EA, Kingston JE, Malpas JS *et al*. Testicular function

following the treatment of Hodgkin's disease in childhood. *Br J Cancer* 1993; 68: 1199–204.

15 Batia S, Robison LL, Oberlin O *et al.* Breast cancer and other second neoplasms after childhood Hodgkin's disease. *N Engl J Med* 1996; 334: 745–51.

16 Hancock S, Hope R. Long-term complications of treatment and causes of mortality after Hodgkin's disease. *Semin Radiat Oncol* 1996; 6: 225–42.

17 Swerdlow AJ, Douglas AJ, Vaughan-Hudson G *et al.* Risk of second primary cancers after Hodgkin's disease by type of treatment: analysis of 2846 patients in the British National Lymphoma Investigation. *Br Med J* 1992; 304: 1137–43.

18 Tucker MA, Coleman CN, Varghese A, Rosenberg SA. Risk of second cancers after treatment for Hodgkin's disease. *N Engl J Med* 1988; 318: 76–81.

Incidence and aetiology [1]

Recent years have seen a considerable growth in our knowledge of the aetiology of non-Hodgkin's lymphomas (NHLs). They are a heterogeneous group of neoplasms which, in Western countries, occur predominantly in the elderly. The overall age-specific incidence is shown in Fig. 26.1, but this obscures markedly different age incidences with some rarer forms of NHL (which occur in childhood or early adult life). It seems clear that the incidence of NHL is rising quite rapidly but the causes are not fully known. The acquired immune deficiency syndrome (AIDS) epidemic has contributed to the rising incidence of B-cell lymphomas.

Geographical distribution

In 1958, Burkitt reported cases of a lymphoma occurring in the jaw and abdomen of Ugandan children. The jaw tumours occurred maximally at 3 years of age. Burkitt showed that the tumour appeared in regions of high humidity—the wet tropical areas. The tumour was then reported in Papua New Guinea in the same climatic regions. Cases are now reported in the Western countries, but with an incidence of only 1% of that in Africa. Western cases have few jaw tumours and in Middle-Eastern cases the ileocaecal region is more usually involved. The Epstein–Barr virus (EBV) was identified in cultured tumour cells from African cases, and almost all African cases have high serum titres of anti-EBV. Since almost all the normal

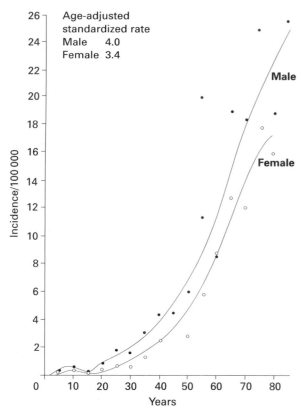

Fig. 26.1 Age-specific incidence of NHL.

population has been infected a cofactor has been postulated—possibly falciparum malaria. This is also suggested by the lower incidence of the tumour in cities and in regions where malaria has been controlled. The age of onset is higher in children who have migrated to areas of high malaria endemicity.

Lymphomas are a common Middle-Eastern cancer (10% of all cancer cases), but they differ from European cases in that many are intestinal, often arising in a background of diffuse small-intestinal thickening generally termed immunoproliferative small-intestine disease. Current hypotheses favour the view that this is an early stage of lymphoma.

A lymphoma characterized by skin rash, hepatosplenomegaly and hypercalcaemia was reported in 1977 in patients from the southern Japanese island of Kyushu. Later, cases were described in the UK in patients from the Caribbean and in the USA. T-lymphotrophic viruses isolated in Japan and in the USA were shown to be identical. This virus is designated human T-cell lymphotropic

retrovirus-1 (HTLV-1). The virus is transmitted in breast milk and possibly in semen. It seems that HTLV-1 lymphoma may also be endemic in eastern China. It is not clear what environmental stimulus causes activation of an infection acquired in infancy—the age of onset of the overt disease is 40–60 years. The overall incidence in Japan is five per 100 000 and three per 100 000 in the Caribbean. HTLV-1 also causes spastic paraplegia in Jamaica.

Viral causes

There is compelling evidence that *HTLV-1 retrovirus* is the cause of adult acute T-cell leukaemia/lymphoma. The virus appears to act early in oncogenesis causing transformation that leads to further genetic alteration. This results in malignant, clonal, change no longer dependent on the virus. Transformation depends on a protein (*Tax*) that interacts with other cellular activators leading to activation of factors causing lymphoid proliferation (such as interleukin-2, IL-2) and deregulating cell cycle control.

Epstein–Barr virus is implicated in the pathogenesis of endemic Burkitt's lymphoma, AIDS-related lymphomas, angiocentric T/natural killer (NK) lymphoma and possibly Hodgkin's disease. EBV can transform lymphoid cells, but it is not clear how it might maintain this state. The full expression of transforming proteins is only possible in conditions of profound immune suppression, such as after bone marrow transplantation, and this is probably the way in which post-transplant lymphoid proliferations are caused. In chronic latent infection other transforming events must occur such as c-*myc* mutation, and overexpression of *BCL*-6.

Kaposi's sarcoma herpes virus (human herpes virus type 8, HHV8) has been found in a rare lymphoid malignancy known as primary effusion lymphoma (PEL) often in patients with AIDS. Infection with HHV8 is far more common in AIDS than PEL. A cofactor is presumably needed for transformation—possibly EBV infection. HHV8 codes for a variety of proteins that might interfere with B-lymphoid and endothelial cell function including a viral cyclin, a viral IL-6 and a viral G protein-coupled receptor.

Lymphomas in other immunodeficiency states

Table 26.1 indicates the wide range of disorders predisposing to NHL, with the majority clearly suggesting states of immune deficiency. Patients with AIDS are at high risk of developing NHL [2]. The clinical features of these lymphomas are discussed on p. 414. Almost all are B-cell

Table 26.1 Disorders predisposing to development of lymphoma.

Congenital
Chediak–Higashi syndrome
Ataxia telangiectasia
Wiskott–Aldrich syndrome
Swiss-type agammaglobulinaemia
Klinefelter's syndrome
Coeliac disease
Bloom's syndrome
X-linked lymphoproliferative disease

Acquired
Acquired immune deficiency syndrome (AIDS)
Chronic immune suppression (e.g. renal allograft recipients)
Sjögren's syndrome
Rheumatoid arthritis
Common variable hypogammaglobulinaemia

tumours. In organ transplant recipients, lymphomas account for one-third of all the associated malignancies. The tumours are usually immunoblastic and often intracranial. If the immunosuppression has included cyclosporin A in high dose, the lymphomas are more frequent and often nodal or intestinal. With other immunosuppressive treatment, intracerebral lymphoma is more common. In ataxia telangiectasia and Wiskott–Aldrich syndrome there is a high incidence of lymphoma. In these cases, and in transplant recipients, there are well-documented associations with EBV infections.

In the X-linked lymphoproliferative syndrome (discussed above) immune deficiency in young boys is associated with overwhelming EBV infection.

Coeliac disease

Patients with this disease have a 200-fold increase in incidence of lymphoma of the intestine. The tumours are T cell in origin and have distinct clinical features (p. 419).

Molecular genetics of lymphoma [3]

A reciprocal translocation of chromosomal material between chromosome 8 and 14 t(8;14) (q24;q32) occurs in tumour cells in Burkitt's lymphoma. More than 80% of tumours have this translocation. Translocations between 8 and 22 t(8;22) and from 2 to 8 t(2;8) occur in the remaining 20%. The immunoglobulin (Ig) heavy chain locus is located at 14q32 and the light chain was found at 2p11 and at 22q11. Each of these sites is the site of gene rearrangement in the normal B lymphocyte. The break on the 8 chromosome is always at band 8q24 which is the c-*myc* proto-oncogene site.

There is now known to be heterogeneity at the site of the Ig locus break. The c-*myc* is abnormally expressed for B cells, although it is at a level appropriate for proliferating cells. The endemic cases do not show c-*myc* rearrangement, but the sporadic cases do.

Follicle-centre cell lymphomas of the follicular type and some diffuse large cell lymphomas show a characteristic chromosomal translocation in 85% of cases. This is between 14q32 (the heavy chain locus) and 18q21. The breakpoint on chromosome 18 is rearranged in the majority of follicular lymphomas. The gene is *bcl*-2 (B-cell leukaemia and lymphoma 2) which codes for a mitochondrial protein that inhibits apoptosis. The expression of *bcl*-2 is associated with worse prognosis in large-cell lymphomas.

T-cell malignancies also show non-random chromosomal abnormalities. The most common site is at 14q11 which is the site of the T-cell receptor gene (α and β chains).

It is still not clear what role these lympho-specific translocations play in oncogenesis. They sometimes appear to develop earlier in the cell lineage than the phenotype of corresponding tumour would suggest and to be related to control of proliferation appropriate to that cell lineage. A recently defined abnormality has been a t(2;5) translocation in anaplastic large cell lymphoma producing a tyrosine kinase (ALK) that may be a drug target. In mucosa-associated lymphoid tissue lymphomas a t(1;14) translocation activates *bcl*-10 which may protect the cell from apoptosis. In small lymphocyte lymphomas a t(9;14) is often present which activates *PAX*-5, a transcription factor that may stimulate B-cell proliferation in some lymphomas.

An important clinical application of molecular techniques has been the detection of rearrangement of antigen–receptor genes as a manifestation of clonality. These genes (T-cell receptor genes and Ig genes) rearrange during normal development of the cells, producing an antigen-specific clone. Neoplastic expansion of a clone is accompanied by a specific rearrangement which can be detected at low levels using molecular and immunological techniques.

Pathology [2,4]

The classification of lymphomas has been in a state of constant change for many years. The problem has been that lymphomas that can be shown to be derived from different cells, or at different stages of lymphoid differentiation, may nonetheless have very similar prognoses and require similar treatments. A purely clinical description, ignoring biology, lacks a rational scientific basis; while a classification based on biology alone becomes a list of entities providing little help to the clinician. Gradually a consensus has emerged in which modern methods of determining the cell of origin and the characteristic genetic abnormalities have been linked to practical clinical considerations concerning treatment and prognosis. This is summarized in the World Health Organization (WHO) classification which is closely aligned to others (such as revised European–American lymphoma, REAL) that have had wide acceptance (Table 26.2). The Kiel classification (Table 26.3) is similar but also groups according to clinical behaviour.

During fetal life precursors of T lymphocytes are formed and migrate to the thymus, and thence to the developing lymph nodes and spleen. Maturation into mature T cells takes place at various stages, especially in the thymus. The sequence of maturation can be defined by their surface antigen structure. Monoclonal antibodies to T-cell surface antigens have been especially helpful in this respect. The sequence of maturation is shown in Fig. 26.2. By the time the T cell leaves the thymus its function as a helper cell or cytotoxic/suppressor cell is established.

In the lymph nodes the T cells lodge in the paracortical region (Fig. 26.3) and around the central arterioles in the spleen. Some T cells recirculate from the lymphatic system to the blood and thence back to the lymph nodes where

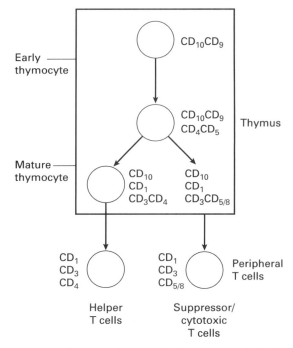

Fig. 26.2 T-cell surface phenotype during maturation in the thymus. The T-cell antigens are identified by monoclonal antibodies and are helpful in categorizing the various forms of T-cell lymphoma and leukaemia.

Table 26.2 The WHO classification of NHL.

B-cell neoplasms	T and putative natural killer cell neoplasms
B-cell chronic lymphocytic leukaemia/lymphocytic lymphoma	T-cell prolymphocytic leukaemia
B-cell prolymphocytic leukaemia	T-cell large granular lymphocyte leukaemia
Mantle cell lymphoma	Natural killer cell leukaemia
Follicular lymphoma	Natural killer cell lymphoma, nasal and nasal-type
Splenic marginal zone lymphoma	Mycosis fungoides
Marginal zone B-cell lymphoma (MALT type)	Sézary syndrome
Nodal marginal zone lymphoma ± monocytoid cells	Angioimmunoblastic T-cell lymphoma
Hairy cell leukamia	Peripheral T-cell lymphoma unspecified
Diffuse large cell lymphoma subtypes: medistinal (thymic), intravascular, primary effusion	Subcutaneous panniculitis T-cell lymphoma
Burkitt's lymphoma	Adult T-cell leukaemia/lymphoma (HTLV-1 positive)
Plasmacytoma	Anaplastic large cell lymphoma (T- and null cell types)
Plasma cell myeloma	Primary cutaneous anaplastic large-cell lymphoma
	Subcutaneous panniculitis-like T-cell lymphoma
	Enteropathy-type T-cell lymphoma
	Hepatosplenic γδ T-cell lymphoma

Table 26.3 Kiel classification of NHL

B cell	T cell
Low grade	Low grade
Lymphocytic (chronic lymphocytic and prolymphocytic leukaemia)	Lymphocytic (chronic lymphocytic and prolymphocytic leukaemia)
Lymphoplasmacytic	Cutaneous (cerebriform cell-Sézary's mycosis fungoides)
Plasmacytic	Lymphoepithelioid (Lennert's lymphoma)
Centroblastic/centrocytic	Angioimmunoblastic
Follicular ± diffuse	T zone
Centrocytic (now known as mantle zone)	Pleomorphic small cell (HTLV-1)
High grade	*High grade*
Centroblastic	Pleomorphic larger cell (HTLV-1)
Immunoblastic	Immunoblastic
Large-cell anaplastic (Ki-1)	Lymphoblastic
Burkitt's lymphoma	Large-cell anaplastic (Ki-1)
	Lymphoblastic

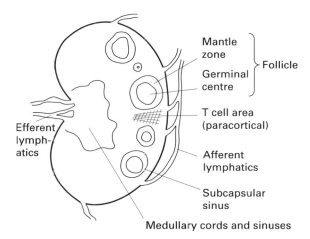

Fig. 26.3 Lymph node structure.

they enter the paracortical region through postcapillary venules.

Early B lymphocytes are formed in the fetal liver and subsequently in the bone marrow. From there they migrate to the lymph nodes. They are found in the follicles which consist of an outer mantle zone of small lymphocytes and a germinal centre composed of cells where the nucleus is either irregular in shape or large and round. In lymphoma the cells with a nucleus of irregular outline are called cleaved cells or *centrocytes* and those with a large round non-cleaved nucleus are *centroblasts*. Some B lymphocytes recirculate between nodes and blood. After contact with antigen, B cells transform into antibody-secreting plasma cells.

As B cells terminally differentiate, the genes which code for the enormous variety of potential Ig molecules rearrange to code for one Ig molecule only. At this point the 'clonal' nature of the cell is established. Similarly, rearrangement of the genes which code for the four components of the T-cell antigen–receptor occurs during T-cell clonal development in the thymus. This rearrangement can be detected relatively simply using molecular biological techniques. In a cell suspension which may contain lymphoma cells (which are clonal), clonal rearrangement can be detected if as few as 5% of the cells constituting the tumour population. Gene rearrangement is therefore a useful technique for determining, for example, marrow contamination. Detection of a chromosomal abnormality (such as the t(14;18) translocation in follicular lymphoma) by polymerase chain reaction (PCR) is even more sensitive but is not possible in tumours which do not have such abnormality.

Macrophages, or mononuclear phagocytes, are formed from pluripotent haemopoietic stem cells in the marrow. They are liberated into the bloodstream as monocytes and lodge in tissues at sites of inflammation (histiocytes). They also play a part in repopulating the 'fixed' tissue phagocytic cells — Kupffer cells, splenic, alveolar and peritoneal macrophages. The antigen-presenting cells (dendritic cells) in lymph nodes and spleen may also be part of the mononuclear phagocyte system.

A simplified guide to the stage in differentiation of lymphocytes to which various NHLs and leukaemias correspond is shown in Fig. 26.4 and a synopsis of the immunological classification of lymphoreticular neoplasms is shown in Table 26.2.

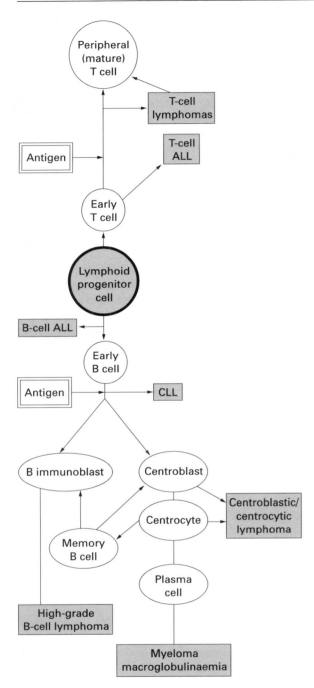

Fig. 26.4 Simplified scheme of cell origin of NHLs: origin of B-cell and T-cell lymphomas, and origin of macrophage tumours.

The following cell types have been identified: small lymphocytes (B and T), lymphoplasmacytic cells, plasma cells, centrocytes (small and large), centroblasts (small and large), immunoblasts (B and T) and lymphoblasts (B and T).

B-cell neoplasms make up the majority of NHLs (Table 26.2). The most common are all the follicular lymphomas which are derived from the B cell of the follicle centre. However, these cells do not always form follicles and may also give rise to a diffuse lymphoma.

T-cell lymphomas probably constitute about 10% of NHLs (Table 26.2). The T-cell lymphomas can be divided into three broad categories: cutaneous lymphomas, thymic lymphomas and peripheral T-cell lymphomas. Morphologically they are diffuse, with a wide variety of cellular morphology.

It is not yet clear how many lymphomas are neoplasms of malignant macrophages or NK cells. Those which are should not, strictly speaking, be called lymphomas. Histochemical evidence has suggested that they may account for 5% of diffuse large-cell lymphomas. The situation is uncertain because of the lack of a clonal marker for macrophages.

Although the immunological classification of lymphoma is logical and in many respects superior, the pathological diagnosis in most departments rests on conventional light microscopical appearances (Fig. 26.5).

Clinical features

Non-Hodgkin's lymphomas usually arise in peripheral lymph nodes, but may also develop at a wide variety of extranodal sites. The clinical features of extranodal lymphomas are described later (see pp. 417–24).

Nodal lymphomas

Presentation

Painless enlargement of a lymph node is the most frequent presentation of NHL, and the commonest site is the neck. Sometimes the nodes fluctuate in size, which can lead to delay in diagnosis. Non-Hodgkin's lymphomas tend to be more widespread at presentation than Hodgkin's disease and to be present at more unusual lymph node sites, for example Waldeyer's ring. Although the presentation is usually straightforward, the enlarging lymph node mass may cause initial symptoms due to compression, for ex-

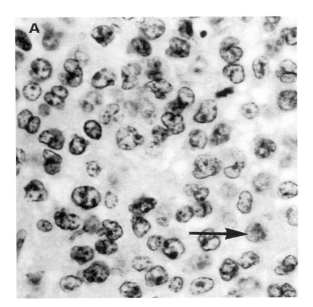

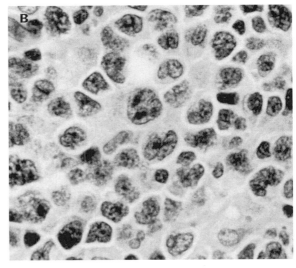

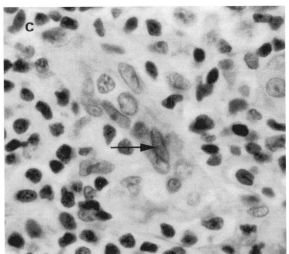

Fig. 26.5 Histological appearance in NHL (original magnification × 400). (A) Follicle centre cell lymphoma predominantly containing centrocytes but with scattered centroblasts (arrowed). (B) Follicle centre cell lymphoma composed principally of centroblasts. (C) Peripheral T-cell lymphoma showing proliferating high endothelial venules (arrowed) and a mixture of small and large lymphocytes, some with clear cytoplasm, others showing an irregular nuclear outline.

ample swelling of the arm or leg, simulating deep venous thrombosis or superior vena caval obstruction (SVCO).

Retroperitoneal lymph node enlargement can result in backache and obstructive renal failure, and nodes in the aorta hepatis may cause obstructive jaundice.

Widespread infiltration of the liver is usually accompanied by weight loss, anorexia and fever.

Even without liver involvement, constitutional symptoms are not infrequent, with weight loss, night sweats and fever. Intra-abdominal lymphoma may present with fever of unknown origin, especially if there is hepatic or bone marrow involvement.

Clinical examination must be meticulous. The neck

should be carefully examined, and it is often easier to determine the extent of disease in the neck if the examination is carried out from behind the patient. Node enlargement should be sought in the pre- and postauricular regions, in the occipital, supra- and infraclavicular areas, and deep behind the sternomastoid. The axilla should be carefully examined in both the apex and the walls. Epitrochlear nodes are often missed. In the abdomen the size of the liver and spleen should be noted and an attempt made to examine abdominal and retroperitoneal nodes by deep palpation. The inguinal nodes are often slightly enlarged in normal individuals, but pathological inguinofemoral nodes may extend

Table 26.4 Lymph node enlargement simulating lymphoma.

Follicular histology
Reactive hyperplasia
Rheumatoid arthritis and related arthritides
Angiofollicular hyperplasia
Toxoplasmosis

Diffuse histology
Phenytoin sensitivity
Dermatopathic lymphadenopathy
Metastatic carcinoma and melanoma

Other histologies
Sinus histiocytosis with massive lymph node enlargement
Infectious mononucleosis
Cat scratch fever
Metastatic carcinoma (especially melanoma)

downwards into the medial aspect of the thigh. Examination of the oro- and nasopharynx should be routine, as should rectal examination which may lead to detection of large masses of pelvic nodes.

Diagnosis and investigation

The diagnosis is by node or tissue biopsy. Although there is usually little difficulty about the diagnosis, other conditions may simulate lymphoma (see Table 26.4) especially at extranodal sites, and precise immunological classification is becoming increasingly important in management. For these reasons, a lymph node biopsy should be regarded as an important clinical investigation and not as a trivial affair.

Inexperienced surgeons sometimes biopsy a superficial node, which shows reactive hyperplasia, or a node in the neck or groin which may not be obviously abnormal. If there is a deeper, clearly pathological node this should be removed. Immunohistochemistry helps a great deal in diagnosis, particularly in distinguishing large-cell lymphomas from anaplastic carcinoma, and in the diagnosis of T-cell tumours. Some of these investigations can only be done on fresh or frozen tissue, so the biopsy should not all be placed in formaldehyde and the pathologist will advise as required. If the node shows reactive hyperplasia, or an equivocal result, one should not hesitate to biopsy another node if the clinical suspicion is high. If the nodes are in an inaccessible site it may be necessary to proceed to laparotomy or mediastinotomy. It is often better to do this than repeatedly to biopsy equivocally enlarged peripheral nodes.

Staging notation

The staging notation is the same as that employed for Hodgkin's disease (see Table 25.2). Unlike Hodgkin's disease the great majority of patients will have stage III or IV disease at presentation.

In the investigation of NHL there are certain routine tests which are inexpensive, harmless, and sometimes rewarding, and these should be performed. A chest X-ray may show hilar, mediastinal or paratracheal node enlargement. Parenchymal lung lesions are less common as are pleural effusions, but the latter occur not infrequently when there is massive mediastinal disease. Occasionally the effusion is chylous due to rupture of lymphatics in the mediastinum. Lung infiltrates and effusions which contain lymphoma cells usually occur when there is associated mediastinal or hilar disease.

The blood count may show anaemia, which is usually normochromic and typical of the anaemia of chronic disease (with a low serum iron and iron-binding capacity).

Occasionally it is due to autoimmune haemolysis, and a Coombs' test and reticulocyte count should be performed if this is suspected. The blood film may show circulating lymphoma cells. However, immunological methods may detect a malignant population which is not apparent on the blood smear, and the proportion of patients with blood involvement will certainly prove to be higher than the present 10% of cases identified by the blood film. Recent methods of demonstrating monoclonality in B cells have been applied to bone marrow and have suggested a high level (30–50%) of involvement in both follicular and diffuse lymphomas. An abnormal blood film implies marrow disease, but this may not always be detected on aspiration and biopsy. Conversely, marrow involvement on biopsy is not always associated with an abnormal peripheral blood picture. The blood urea and electrolytes should be measured to exclude renal failure. The liver enzymes should also be measured since a rise in alkaline phosphatase and transaminases may indicate liver infiltration, and the alkaline phosphatase and bilirubin may be elevated if there are nodes in the aorta hepatis causing compression.

Other investigations include computed tomography (CT) scanning of the abdomen or pelvis to demonstrate intra-abdominal or pelvic disease, an intravenous urogram if there is evidence of renal impairment, and X-rays and bone scan if there is bone pain or tenderness at a particular site. Before the advent of CT, lymphography was widely used to demonstrate pelvic and para-aortic nodes. Most patients (80%) with nodular lymphoma have abnormal lymphograms, and approximately 60% of those with diffuse lymphoma. Computed tomography scanning is a less troublesome alternative to lymphography and has about the same sensitivity. It has the advantage of being able to demonstrate nodal masses in the mesentery and in the upper abdomen—sites poorly demonstrated by lymphography.

How far should these tests be done as a routine and combined with more invasive tests such as liver or marrow biopsy? This depends on what the treatment strategy is to be. If there is a prospect that the disease is localized and the patient might be cured by radiotherapy, extensive investigation is needed to define the true extent of the disease. But if the treatment is to be with palliative local radiotherapy—for example, in an elderly patient with clinically localized disease—then invasive investigations are meddlesome. If the histology and clinical features indicate widespread poor-prognosis disease then intensive chemotherapy will be used and it becomes irrelevant to persist with unpleasant investigations such as liver biopsy.

Most cases of NHL presenting as a nodal disease should be regarded as widespread, irrespective of histology [5]. In both nodular and diffuse lymphomas it is likely that there will be evidence on mediastinal and abdominal CT, and a not inconsiderable chance of detecting disease in the marrow or liver. While 30% of patients have clinically localized disease (stages I and II) at presentation, after sequential investigation the proportion falls to about 15%. Laparotomy makes little contribution to assessment of spread.

Follicular lymphoma [6]

Centroblastic and centrocytic follicular lymphomas constitute 30–40% of all cases. They are tumours of the follicle centre (B cell) and are a mixture of small cleaved centrocytes and large centroblasts. Depending on the proportion of these cells they are referred to as follicular small cleaved (centrocytic) mixed or large-cell (centroblastic) lymphoma. The distinction from diffuse lymphomas of the follicular centre cell is occasionally arbitrary since a single node may show follicular and diffuse changes, especially in the large-cell (centroblastic) types. Spontaneous fluctuations in lymph node size and even regressions occur.

An unusual form of lymphoma with a nodular appearance is the lymphoma derived from small B cells surrounding the follicle. This has a different phenotype from the follicular centre cell.

The tumours always express CD19, CD20, CD22 and frequently express CD19. The translocation from 18q21 to 14q32 at the site of the heavy chain enhancer has been previously discussed (p. 403). The resulting overexpression of *bcl*-2 may block programmed cell death, contributing to expansion of the tumour. The large-cell variants appear to have the highest growth fraction and small-cell the lowest, and this may account for the greatest likelihood of cure of the large-cell variant by chemotherapy.

The tumours occur in middle or old age with painless (often prolonged) enlargement of nodes. Involvement of marrow and blood is frequent, especially in the centrocytic types. Clinical stage I and II disease occurs in 40% of cases, but only 20% have stage I and II after investigation.

Stage I and II

Studies have suggested that a watch-and-wait policy confers no disadvantage, and may be the preferred option. In practice, patients may find this hard to accept, especially if the nodes are highly visible.

In this group localized or extended-field irradiation produces impressive results, with 60–80% of patients free of the disease at 10 years. Recurrence is frequent at adjacent lymph node sites, but further radiation can be given. The current data suggest that about 50% of patients will be cured by treatment of involved and adjacent lymph nodes [7]. Additional chemotherapy has not yet been shown to be unequivocally beneficial when radiation is used. However, in stage II disease in the elderly population, excellent symptomatic control can be obtained with the use of intermittent oral chlorambucil, sometimes combined with prednisolone.

Stage III and IV

Some of these patients with low-grade follicular lymphomas will live for several years without symptoms from their disease (Fig. 26.6). There has been considerable debate about how soon treatment (with chemotherapy) should begin. The median period before symptoms develop is 4 years. It seems that no advantage in survival is obtained with an immediate treatment policy over a watch-and-wait approach [6].

With low-dose oral chemotherapy, symptoms can usually be brought under control. However, with this approach, relapse will occur relatively quickly and the interval between treatments will shorten.

A promising new agent is the purine analogue fludarabine [8]. It is relatively free of immediate side-effects, and 50% of patients relapsing after chlorambucil have a remission. Myelosuppression and immunosuppression are

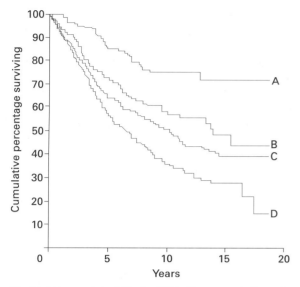

Fig. 26.6 Prognosis in follicular NHL. The curves indicate the death rate from lymphoma according to stage at presentation. A, stage I/IE (*n*=2441); B, stage II/IIE (*n*=186); C, stage III/IIIE (*n*=397); D, stage IV/IVE (*n*=423). The relationship between prognosis and clinical stage is clearly shown. Fifteen-year overall cause-specific survival is 37%. Data from the British National Lymphoma Investigation.

cumulative and limit dose and duration. Interferon-α has been shown to prolong progression-free survival in some trials, and there is some suggestion of improved overall survival. It is used after or with chemotherapy and may justify the increased toxicity. Rituximab (an anti-CD20 monoclonal antibody) produces responses in drug-insensitive relapse [9]. Its role in early treatment is being defined as well as exploration of the schedule of administration.

Poor prognosis is indicated by systemic symptoms, high serum lactate dehydrogenase and poor performance status. A high response rate can be achieved with more intensive chemotherapy. Early studies with cyclophosphamide, vincristine and prednisolone did not, however, show any advantage to this approach. Subsequently, even more intensive doxorubicin-containing therapy has been shown to produce a high rate of complete response. Longer-term follow-up, however, has failed to show a convincing benefit for more intensive therapy [10]. The role of high-dose chemotherapy (with bone marrow or blood stem cell support) is under evaluation in young and high-risk patients. Prolonged remissions can be obtained. There may be an

advantage to 'purging' the stem cells (used for reinfusion) of contaminating B cells. A survival value of the high-dose procedure has still not been conclusively demonstrated. Myelodysplasia is a frequent complication. The role of allongenic transplantation is still to be determined.

Mantle cell lymphoma [11]

This is a relatively infrequent lymphoma (5–10% of cases).

This is the term used in the REAL classification. Previous terms were *centrocytic, intermediate lymphocytic* or *diffuse small cleaved cell lymphoma*. It affects men more than women, usually aged about 60 years. It presents as widespread nodal disease often with marrow and spleen involvement. It may present as a primary disorder in the spleen, or as a generalized nodular infiltrate in the gastrointestinal tract [12]. The malignant B cells appear as small cleaved cells occasionally admixed with larger blastic cells. They express CD20, CD19 and CD22 and surface Ig and IgD. There is a t(11;14) translocation which moves *BCL*-1 to be next to the Ig heavy chain enhancer. This results in overexpression of cyclin D. This overexpression is associated with worse prognosis but probably plays a role in pathogenesis and is a target for new agents. The presence of blastic cells is adverse prognostically.

Treatment is unsatisfactory. The tumour responds to COP (cyclophosphamide, vincristine, prednisolone), CHOP (cyclophosphamide, H-doxorubicin, O-vincristine and prednisolone) and other regimens, but only for a short time. Responses to fludarabine are short-lived. Rituximab is an anti-CD20 monoclonal antibody that can induce remissions although these do not last long usually. Overall, 25% of patients are alive at 5 years. High-dose chemotherapy is being evaluated. The bowel disease is difficult to treat. It is diffuse, unresectable and responds poorly.

Stage I and II follicular large-cell (centroblastic) lymphoma

This is a much less common form and has a more rapid course. In true stage I disease radiation therapy may cure some patients. Relapse-free survival is prolonged if chemotherapy (such as CHOP) is added. Chemotherapy alone with CHOP or ProMACE (prednisone, methotrexate, A-doxorubicin, cyclophosphamide and etoposide)–MOPP (mustine, vincristine, prednisone and procarbazine) produces excellent results. At present the weight of evidence favours intensive chemotherapy as the mainstay of treatment, and the role of radiation is less clear.

Adult diffuse intermediate- and high-grade lymphoma

Included in this category are follicular large-cell lymphoma (see below) and the diffuse tumours called centrocytic/centroblastic, large-cell, immunoblastic, undifferentiated and pleomorphic peripheral T-cell lymphomas. The largest group is the diffuse large-cell type. Diffuse large-cell lymphoma is the commonest form of NHL. Most of the tumours are B cell in origin, many of them having the immunophenotype and genetic abnormalities associated with follicular cell lymphoma (CD+, bcl-2 rearrangement, bcl-6 expression). T-cell tumours can appear identical clinically and it is not clear if there is any prognostic significance to the cell type. Immunoblastic tumours are usually of B-cell origin, and lymphoblastic may be B or T cell. The justification for grouping them all therapeutically is that there is no clear reason for adopting different treatment strategies in each type.

The patients are usually middle-aged or older. Most cases are stage III or IV but large-cell types are localized (stage I or II) in 25% of cases. Routine investigation includes chest and abdominal CT scanning and bone marrow aspiration and biopsy. An international prognostic index [12] used age performance status serum, lactate dehydrogenase (LDH), stage and extranodal spread to define four risk groups depending on age (Table 26.5 and Fig. 26.7).

Radiotherapy alone is not adequate treatment for stage II disease, and the relapse rate in stage I disease is 40%. Treatment for stage I and II cases therefore now includes combination chemotherapy. Radiotherapy to the involved field with three cycles of CHOP has been shown to be superior to eight cycles of CHOP without radiation both with respect to progression-free survival and overall survival [13]. For stage III and IV disease, treatment is with intensive combination chemotherapy. The CHOP regimen has been widely used (Table 26.6) but several more intensive combinations have been used. These regimens have incorporated the following features: additional agents such as methotrexate, cytosine arabinoside and etoposide, treatment at closer intervals to avoid the problem of relapse between cycles, and the use of multidrug combinations (such as ProMACE–CytaBOM (cytarabine, bleomycin, O-vincristine and methotrexate); Table 26.6) to overcome drug resistance. Typically, treatment durations of 6–8 months are used, but the MACOP-B (methotrexate, A-doxorubicin, cyclophosphamide, O-vincristine, prednisolone and bleomycin) regimen lasts only 12 weeks, with chemotherapy cycles being given weekly. The regimens are very myelosuppressive, and mucositis is common especially with MACOP-B. A randomized comparison of three of these regimens with CHOP has, however, failed to show any survival advantage and CHOP remains the standard chemotherapy approach [14]. The best results require the maximum dosage and the risks of toxicity are constantly present. The more intensive programmes are not suitable for elderly or infirm patients, and considerable care is needed in all patients regardless of age.

Table 26.5 International Diagnostic Index for NHL*.

Factor†	Score	
	0	1
Age	<60	≥60
P.S.	0,1	2 3 4
Stage	1, II	III, IV
Extranodal disease	<2 sites	>2 sites
LDH	Normal	High

Low risk score 0, 1
Low intermediate risk score 2
Higher intermediate risk score 3
High risk score 4, 5

P.S., performance status.
*Originally defined for diffuse lymphomas it applied to follicular lymphomas as well.
†To these factors may be added β_2-microglobulin in plasma (lower score when normal) and obesity (higher score).

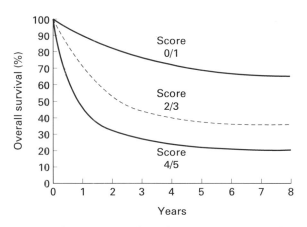

Fig. 26.7 The 5-year survival rates for aggressive NHL according to the International Prognostic Index Score (see Table 26.5).

Table 26.6 Combination chemotherapy regimens in advanced diffuse nodal NHL.

CHOP (21 days)
Cyclophosphamide (1 g/m^2 day 1)
H-doxorubicin (70 mg/m^2 day 1)
O-vincristine (2 mg i.v. day 1)
Prednisolone (100 mg p.o. days 1–5)

M-BACOD (21 days)
Methotrexate (200 mg/m^2 days 1, 8, 15; with folinic acid)
Bleomycin (15 mg/m^2 day 1)
A-doxorubicin (45 mg/m^2 day 1)
Cyclophosphamide (600 mg/m^2 day 1)
O-vincristine (2 mg/m^2 day 1)
Dexamethasone (6 mg/m^2 p.o. days 1–5)

Pro(M)ACE-CytaBOM (21 days)
Prednisolone (60 mg/m^2 days 1–14)
A-doxorubicin (25 mg/m^2 day 1)
Cyclophosphamide (650 mg/m^2 day 1)
Etoposide (120 mg/m^2 day 1)
Cytarabine (300 mg/m^2 day 1)
Bleomycin (15 mg/m^2 day 8)
O-vincristine (2 mg/m^2 day 8)
Methotrexate (120 mg/m^2 day 8; with folinic acid)

MACOP-B
Methotrexate (400 mg/m^2 days 8, 36, 64)
A-doxorubicin (50 mg/m^2 days 1, 15, 29, 43, 57, 17)
Cyclophosphamide (350 mg/m^2 days 1, 15, 29, 43, 57, 71)
O-vincristine (2 mg/m^2 days 8, 22, 36, 50, 64, 78)
Prednisolone (75 mg/m^2 p.o. days 1–84, reducing)
Bleomycin (20 mg/m^2 days 22, 50, 78)

---

i.v., intravenously; p.o., by mouth.

With many of these regimens complete response rates (in single-institution selected series) are 80% or greater. Relapse is uncommon after 3 years, and cure rates of 60% are achieved depending on the composition of the patient groups included, with respect to the prognostic index. If complete response is not attained the outlook is poor—most patients die within 2 years. Failure to attain early complete response may be an indication for autologous or allogeneic stem cell transplantation (see below).

Adult lymphoblastic lymphoma [15]

These are diffuse high-grade lymphomas characterized by cells with scant cytoplasm, small nucleoli and nuclei which may be of a convoluted or non-convoluted form. The mitotic rate is high. There is often strong phosphatase activity. The immunophenotype is variable but many are T-cell tumours. Both T-cell and B-cell forms express terminal deoxyribonucleotidyl transferase. The cells may show a variety of T-cell markers (Fig. 26.2) and some have a clearly 'thymic' pattern of antigen expression. B-cell types may show common acute lymphoblastic leukaemia antigen (CALLA). Chromosomal breaks at the location of the T-cell receptor α and δ chains are frequent (14q11).

The disease is most frequent in adolescence and in young adults, and in males more than in females. A mediastinal mass and SVCO are frequent. There is widespread nodal involvement. Bone marrow involvement is frequent and the distinction between this and lymphoblastic leukaemia is sometimes a matter of definition. Many haematologists will call this leukaemia if there are more than 25% of lymphoblasts in the marrow. Although involvement of the central nervous system (CNS) at diagnosis is unusual, it may occur during the course of the disease especially if there is marrow involvement.

Treatment has depended to some degree on whether these patients have been regarded as having leukaemia or lymphoma and on whether they are children or adults. There is no clear clinical basis for this. In children, haematology units have used either acute lymphoblastic leukaemia (ALL) protocols or those based on the LSA2L2 regimen (p. 416). Both these regimens are relatively successful but the LSA2L2 probably cures only half of the patients; other regimens such as cyclophosphamide, vincristine, methotrexate and prednisolone (COMP) or A-COP (A-doxorubicin, cyclophosphamide, O-vincristine and prednisolone) appear to be at least as effective. All employ intrathecal treatment as prophylaxis for CNS disease. Established CNS disease is treated as described on p. 421. With the introduction of intensive chemotherapy regimens the prognosis has improved, with a 3-year relapse-free survival rate of 60%. Poor prognostic features are age greater than 30, high initial white blood count and a failure to obtain complete response. The role of high-dose chemotherapy (and autologous marrow or blood stem cell support) is under investigation for these patients.

Small non-cleaved cell lymphomas (SNCC lymphomas, Burkitt's lymphoma, lymphoblastic lymphoma—Burkitt's type)

These tumours are characterized by diffuse infiltration of lymph nodes with cells with a round nucleus with multiple nucleoli, scanty cytoplasm containing lipid and macrophages. The distinction between Burkitt's and non-Burkitt's type is somewhat arbitrary. The cells are B cells with surface IgM. They express HLA-DR, CALLA, CD19,

CD20 and CD21—all B-cell markers. The chromosomal translocations are described on p. 403.

In Western countries about 30% of childhood NHL and 1–2% of adult cases are of Burkitt type. In so-called 'endemic' areas (equatorial Africa, New Guinea) the incidence is 40 times higher than in the West, where the incidence is 2 per million below the age of 20.

The presentation and management of Burkitt's lymphoma in childhood is discussed below (p. 415). Adult patients have traditionally been treated with one of the regimens outlined in Table 26.6. This may not be the correct policy, and in recent years there has been increasing evidence of improved results if protocols based on the childhood regimens are adopted. Recent results are comparable with those obtained in children. The regimen consisted of CHOP with intermediate-dose methotrexate, and cytosine arabinoside and methotrexate given intrathecally.

Primary mediastinal B-cell lymphoma (PMBL) [16]

This is a recently defined entity. It occurs in young adults with a female preponderance. It presents with the typical symptoms of an anterior mediastinal mass: cough, dysphagia, hoarse voice, chest pain and SVCO. The tumour remains localized to the mediastinum where it may invade locally into adjacent lung and pleura. It consists of medium to large B cells often with marked fibrosis. The tumour expresses CD20 and other B-cell markers. It is not distinguishable histologically from other diffuse large-cell B-cell tumours. The likely origin is in thymic B cells. Various chromosomal abnormalities have been described. Mutation of the *bcl*-6 gene, common in other large-cell lymphomas, is absent in PMBL.

The differential diagnosis includes other mediastinal lymphomas and tumours. PMBL is the commonest mediastinal lymphoma in adults. Immediate chemotherapy is the first step in management. SVCO responds rapidly and emergency radiation is not usually needed. The regimens are anthracycline-containing and there is no clear superiority for any. Mediastinal radiation is often given after chemotherapy especially if response is incomplete (although the presence of fibrosis makes this difficult to assess). There is no certain evidence that it is necessary. Extensive masses and invasion are associated with worse outcomes. In these patients, and those with a poor response to initial therapy, high-dose chemotherapy with stem cell support has been used. Approximately 60% of patients appear to be cured with current approaches.

Ki-positive lymphomas [17]

This is a rather distinctive lymphoma which expresses CD30 (Ki-1) from the outset (other lymphomas may express CD30 later in their clinical course). The cells are large and may contain phagocytosed red cells. Breaks in chromosome 5 are often present. Seventy per cent are of T-cell origin.

The tumours often occur in children or young adults. Skin rash may be present at presentation. The treatment is as for high-grade lymphoma. Approximately 50% of patients will be long-term survivors.

Lymphoplasmocytic lymphoma and Waldenström's macroglobulinaemia [18]

These lymphomas occur in the elderly. They are tumours of small lymphocytes mixed with plasma cells which often produce IgM in large quantities. Typically they present with lymph node enlargement, anaemia and symptoms of hyperviscosity: bleeding, retinal haemorrhages, mental confusion, renal impairment. On examination there may be hepatomegaly, splenomegaly (which may be massive but is often not present) and lymph node enlargement. Patients may have distal sensorimotor peripheral neuropathy and cranial nerve palsies (in these patients the IgM is often directed to a myelin-associated protein). Rarely these may be urticarial red skin lesions due to dermal infiltration (Schnitzler's syndrome).

Investigation reveals anaemia, high erythrocyte sedimentation rate (ESR), monoclonal Ig which may be a cryoglobulin, and abnormal platelet function. The bone marrow shows focal infiltration with small lymphocytes with occasional plasma cells. There is involvement of spleen, liver and lymph nodes. Pulmonary infiltration may be due to tumour of opportunistic infection.

Treatment is with plasmapheresis if hyperviscosity is life threatening. Alkylating agents fludarabine and 2-deoxychloroadenosine are both effective treatments, but relapse occurs. The therapeutic role of anti-CD20 antibody is being assessed.

Angioimmunoblastic T-cell lymphoma

This disease, which for several years was not thought to be malignant, is a T-cell lymphoma characterized by proliferating vascular endothelium replacing the paracortical region, interspersed with T cells and plasma cells. It presents with lymph node enlargement, rash, hepatosplenomegaly, fever and dysproteinaemia with polyclonal hyperglobulinaemia. Initial response to treatment is not sustained and a progressive lymphoma supervenes.

Bone marrow transplantation in non-Hodgkin's lymphomas [19]

Although modern combination regimens will cure 50–60% of patients with high-grade NHL, those who relapse are seldom, if ever, curable by conventional chemotherapy. High-dose chemotherapy with autologous bone marrow transplantation or peripheral blood stem cell support can achieve a five- to seven-fold increase in drug dosage. Whether this is adequate to cure a patient with a tumour resistant to lower doses is the essential question which surrounds the procedure. Above these doses non-haematological toxicity is likely to be fatal. Major improvements in supportive care, the use of autologous peripheral blood stem cell support and haemopoietic growth factors have all reduced the morbidity and mortality from the procedure.

Evidence from uncontrolled trials [10] shows that in relapsed patients about 30–40% of cases will live beyond 3 years after high-dose treatment and 60–75% of patients will have a major response. Prognostic factors include general health, tumour mass, the responsiveness of the tumour to previous chemotherapy and the number and variety of previous regimens. These encouraging results have led to the use of the procedure in first remission in high-risk patients, or in patients failing to achieve complete response (CR) with the first treatment. The problem here is that in those patients who have a CR the cure rate may be as high as 60%, and in the others a wide variety of prognostic factors means that randomized comparison of the new treatment is essential.

The first randomized trial has now been reported [19] in which patients who had relapsed after chemotherapy, but who still had chemosensitive disease, were treated either with chemotherapy and irradiation alone or with the addition of high-dose therapy. A clear relapse-free survival and overall survival advantage was found in those receiving the high-dose treatment although the numbers of patients randomized was small (109 patients). High-dose therapy should be considered in patients who fail to achieve CR with initial treatment, in selected patients with poor-prognosis tumours (such as high-grade T-cell lymphomas, adult lymphoblastic lymphoma, poor-prognosis high-grade nodal lymphoma of follicular centre cells) even in first CR, and patients who, after first relapse, achieve a second CR.

One problem with autologous stem cell or marrow transplantation is the potential contamination of the transfused cells by tumour. A wide variety of 'purging' procedures has been adopted to eliminate residual tumour cells, but, as yet, there is no convincing evidence that these are necessary or effective. The problem therapeutically is mainly the residual disease in the patient rather than in the transfused cells.

HIV- and AIDS-related non-Hodgkin's lymphomas [20,21]

The occurrence of NHL in patients infected with human immunodeficiency virus (HIV) is now regarded as part of the definition of AIDS. These lymphomas are usually diffuse large-cell immunoblastic or SNCC lymphomas (Burkitt's-like) and other diffuse large-cell types. Ki-1 anaplastic large-cell lymphoma may occur, of B-cell type.

Typically, the NHL occurs in a patient who has had AIDS for 1–2 years and whose CD4 cell count is very low. Most patients present with widespread disease, and extranodal sites are often involved (CNS 40%, bone marrow 35%, gastrointestinal 25% and numerous other sites less frequently). Some patients have a previous history of progressive lymphadenopathy. It is estimated that as more patients with AIDS live longer (due to antibiotic therapy) one-third or more will develop NHL. Coincident infection with HTLV-1 is increasingly recognized, especially in intravenous drug abusers. The EBV may be a factor in pathogenesis.

Chemotherapy appears to improve survival. Haematological toxicity may be ameliorated by granulocyte colony-stimulating factor but immunosuppression is a serious problem. The CR rates are relatively low and median survival is about 6 months. Poor prognostic features are AIDS present before diagnosis of NHL, poor performance status, low CD4 count and extranodal disease. Treatment of CNS disease is discussed on p. 421.

Non-Hodgkin's lymphoma in childhood

Incidence and aetiology

Non-Hodgkin's lymphomas are rather more common in children than Hodgkin's disease (1.5 : 1) and are the third most frequent childhood cancer. Approximately 0.6 per 100 000 children below 15 years of age develop the disease each year, with a peak onset age of 6–10 years (Fig. 26.1). A variety of inherited diseases predispose to childhood NHL

(Table 26.1). The other aetiological factors are discussed on p. 402.

Pathology

The distinction between childhood NHL and leukaemia is to some extent a semantic one. Many childhood lymphomas spread to the bone marrow and the frequency of diagnosis of marrow involvement is increasing as techniques for the demonstration of monoclonality of B cells (for example, light chain restriction) improve. A convention is to regard more than 25% infiltration as compatible with lymphoma. The lymph nodes almost always show diffuse involvement, and follicular patterns are very rare. The main types are shown in Table 26.7. Diffuse lymphoblastic lymphoma is the commonest type. Some of these tumours show a convoluted nuclear morphology, and react with anti-T-cell reagents—these are T-cell tumours. Others show surface Ig—these are B-cell tumours. Other tumours have neither T nor B markers.

Approximately 20% of cases are large-cell lymphomas which are of diverse lineage. Some appear to be tumours of the follicle centre cell, others are B-cell immunoblastic tumours, while yet others express T-cell histiocytic markers. Many of these tumours express the CD30 antigen (Ki-1, *Ber*-h2) which characterizes activated B and T cells. The majority of these appear to be peripheral T-cell tumours.

Table 26.7 Pathology of childhood NHL.

Diffuse lymphoblastic lymphoma: B cell, T cell
Diffuse large-cell lymphoma
Burkitt's lymphoma

Childhood NHL has a greater tendency to involve extranodal sites such as the gut, bone marrow and CNS. The lymph nodes of Waldeyer's ring and the mediastinum are frequently involved. The distribution of the main mass of disease at presentation is shown in Table 26.8, and a staging system in Table 26.9. About 50% of the tumours arising in the mediastinum are of T-cell origin.

Childhood B-cell lymphomas

The majority of NHLs in childhood are B-cell tumours. These diffuse lymphomas are either of large-cell type or consist of small non-cleaved cells (SNCCs). The large-cell lymphomas are usually found in boys and are often extranodal, occurring in the nasopharynx, lung, mediastinum, bone, soft tissues and tonsils.

The SNCC lymphomas are either Burkitt's lymphoma, or a form in which the cells are more pleomorphic. Burkitt's lymphoma occurs predominantly in Africa but is occasionally seen in Western countries. In Africa, the presentation is usually with jaw or orbital tumours which

Table 26.8 Distribution of main primary site of disease in children with NHL (%).

Intra-abdominal	30
Peripheral nodes	25
Mediastinal	22
Skeleton	7
Nasopharynx	10
Subcutaneous and skin	3.5
Epidural	1
Thyroid	0.5
Testis	0.5
Breast	0.5

Table 26.9 A simple staging system for childhood NHL and SNCC (Burkitt's) lymphoma.

Stage	Description
IA	Single nodal area, or single extranodal site excluding the mediastinum
IIA	Single extranodal tumour with involved regional nodes. Two or more nodal areas on one side of the diaphragm. Primary gut lymphoma and mesenteric nodes
III	Two or more nodal sites above and below the diaphragm. All primary intrathoracic tumours. Extensive primary intra-abdominal disease. All paraspinal or epidural tumours
IV	Involvement of CNS or marrow
Burkitt's lymphoma	
I	Single extra-abdominal site
II	Multiple extra-abdominal sites
III	Intra-abdominal tumour
V	Intra-abdominal tumour with extra-abdominal sites

grow rapidly. Other sites of involvement include the ovaries, retroperitoneal tissues, kidneys and glandular tissues such as breast and thyroid. Invasion of the lymph node and marrow is infrequent.

Spread to the CNS is common and occurs early, often with paraplegia and cranial nerve palsy. A staging system which relates to prognosis is shown in Table 26.9. In Western countries SNCC lymphoma is more likely to present with an abdominal mass, or with enlarged cervical nodes. Marrow involvement is more frequent than in African cases.

Many childhood B-cell lymphomas are generalized diseases with a risk of marrow and CNS involvement. However, some cases have a lower risk of meningeal spread. These cases include localized tumours of the gut, and patients with localized nodal disease. With localized gut lymphoma it is not clear if any treatment should be given after a complete resection, but it is the usual practice to treat with chemotherapy. Central nervous system prophylaxis does not appear to be necessary in these cases.

Childhood T-cell lymphomas

These tumours often present with anterior mediastinal or cervical node enlargement. They disseminate rapidly to the bone marrow, the CNS and the testes. The cells may have convoluted nuclei and focal acid phosphatase activity in the cytoplasm. They usually exhibit T-cell markers, reacting with T-cell monoclonal antibodies, and also express CD30 (see above). In childhood, Ki-1 (CD30-positive) lymphomas may be accompanied by a skin rash (lymphomatoid papulosis) which may be the presenting feature on which a rapidly evolving lymphoma develops.

Histologically, the mediastinal tumours are described as lymphoblastic. The distinction between the childhood and adult forms of lymphoblastic lymphoma is arbitrary, and this and the treatment are more based on historical patterns of care rather than on clear evidence that such distinctions are important.

The patients are usually males and there may be SVCO at presentation which may need urgent treatment (usually with steroids and vincristine) before the diagnostic biopsy can be taken. This therapy can make subsequent diagnosis difficult, but the situation may be life-threatening and aggravated by biopsy under anaesthetic. Marrow failure from infiltration, or CNS symptoms, may be the presenting feature.

In many large treatment series these childhood tumours have not been characterized by modern methods. It now appears that many pleomorphic large-cell lymphomas of childhood are T-cell tumours even when there is no mediastinal mass present.

Diagnosis and investigation

Diagnosis is by lymph node or tissue biopsy. Initial staging investigations should be performed quickly since progress of the disease may be rapid. A marrow aspiration and biopsy should be performed and the cerebrospinal fluid (CSF) examined for cells. Biochemical tests of liver and kidney function are necessary with measurement of plasma calcium and urate since tumour lysis syndrome (see Chapter 8) may occur when treatment starts.

Precise immunohistochemical definition of the tumour is now often possible. Although at present the relationship to prognosis is not clear, in the next few years the application of these techniques may allow a more precise definition of risk and therefore lead to greater precision in selecting treatment.

Treatment

Large-cell non-Hodgkin's lymphoma

During the 1960s the prognosis of acute lymphoblastic leukaemia in childhood was improving rapidly with the use of more intensive drug regimens and prophylactic treatment of the CNS. Childhood lymphomas were, however, still rapidly fatal, 85% of children dying within 1 year and only 10–15% surviving 5 years.

Many modern protocols of treatment are derived from the LSA2L2 programme introduced by Wollner in 1971. 5-year survival of 70–80% is now obtained, with few children relapsing beyond this time. The protocols have the following components.
1 An intensive induction regimen using cyclophosphamide, vincristine, doxorubicin, prednisolone and intrathecal methotrexate.
2 A consolidation phase using antimetabolites—cytosine arabinoside, thioguanine, asparaginase.
3 A maintenance phase lasting 1 year, using sequential alternating pairs of drugs.
The results of protocols of this type are shown in Fig. 26.8. Survival is better in stage I and II disease.

In a randomized study [22] in paediatric NHL of all stages comparing the LSA2L2 protocol with the slightly less aggressive regimen COMP—cyclophosphamide, vincristine, methotrexate and prednisolone—the Children's Cancer Study Group in the USA found the COMP regimen to be slightly less effective. Other regimens have been

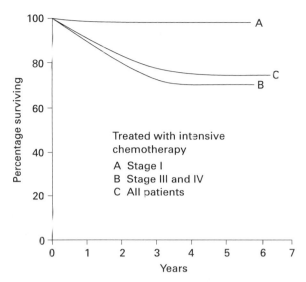

Fig. 26.8 Results of intensive chemotherapy of large-cell NHL in childhood.

based on German protocols for acute leukaemia, and on high-dose cyclophosphamide [23], which are as successful as LSA2L2. There is better disease-free survival at 2 years for localized disease (81%) than for generalized disease (46%). In non-localized disease the LSA2L2 protocol proved better than the COMP regimen for patients with lymphoblastic disease.

Lymphoblastic lymphoma in childhood tends to present with mediastinal disease and includes many cases of T-cell lymphoma. Non-lymphoblastic disease tends to be more localized and have an intra-abdominal presentation. In cases with a better prognosis (stage I and II disease, Table 26.9) a recent trial has shown that radiotherapy can be omitted from the treatment and that treatment of moderate intensity combined with intrathecal methotrexate is associated with a 4-year survival of nearly 90% [22]. There are considerable potential long-term advantages in reducing the amount of chemotherapy and radiation which these children receive. Failure of bone growth, bone cancers, leukaemia and sterility are sequelae of childhood treatment which may be avoided if less intensive treatment can be given without diminished survival.

The optimum treatment for the tumours expressing CD30 has not yet been defined, but regimens based on COMP or the LSA2L2 programme have generally been employed.

Other regimens have been used, some of which include cranial irradiation as prophylactic CNS treatment. With

the LSA2L2 protocol, using intrathecal methotrexate only, the incidence of CNS relapse is about 16%. The incidence is probably lower when cranial irradiation is used in addition. The risk of CNS disease appears to be low for those with stage I nodal disease, and those whose intra-abdominal lymphoma has been resected.

Small non-cleaved cell lymphoma (including Burkitt's lymphoma) [24,25]

The chemotherapy approach is rather different from lymphoblastic lymphoma, with greater emphasis on high doses of alkylating agents. Treatment does not need to be prolonged beyond 10 weeks, but should be very intensive during this time. Radiation therapy has no part to play in initial treatment. Almost all children will have a complete remission but 50% will relapse. Cure is still possible if CNS relapse occurs, but many regimens now include some form of CNS prophylaxis.

Children who survive 2 years are cured. The 2-year disease-free survival figures for each stage (Table 26.9) are: I and II, 80%; III, 65%; and IV, 40%. In stage III it is advisable to remove as much bulk as possible before treatment. With 90% removed the results approach those for stage I. More aggressive regimens are being developed for stage IV cases. Very high-dose chemotherapy with autologous peripheral stem cell support is being assessed, and newer agents such as ifosfamide and etoposide are being introduced into protocols.

Extranodal presentation of non-Hodgkin's lymphoma

Non-Hodgkin's lymphomas may present at a variety of extranodal sites, and when they do there are particular problems in diagnosis and management. In addition to presentation at an extranodal site, there may be involvement of these sites at a time when the nodal lymphoma relapses and disseminates. In this latter circumstance, this is usually part of a generalized spread of the disease. Treatment will be palliative if there has been intensive previous chemotherapy.

The account which follows concerns the management of NHLs presenting at an extranodal site, in the absence of clinically overt disease elsewhere.

Gastrointestinal lymphoma [26]

Lymphomas may occur at any site in the gastrointestinal

tract, but the stomach and the small intestine are most frequently involved. The aetiology and pathogenesis are not well understood. The gut-associated lymphoid tissue in a normal individual shows a well-defined pattern of lymphocyte traffic. Immunoglobulin-bearing cells in the follicle centre of small-intestinal lymphoid nodules (Peyer's patches) migrate into the bloodstream and return to the lamina propria of the small bowel, where they differentiate to plasma cells. A similar 'homing' mechanism may take place with gastric and large-bowel lymphocytes and with lymphocytes bearing Ig of other classes.

Non-Hodgkin's lymphoma of the stomach

Pathology and clinical features

Lymphoma of the stomach is an uncommon tumour, comprising less than 0.5% of all gastric neoplasms. The patient is usually middle-aged or elderly, but the disease can affect young adults. In many cases the tumour begins as a low-grade lesion in the mucosa with destruction of the glandular tissue — 'lymphoepithelial lesions'. This low-grade tumour may occur diffusely in the stomach and remain localized to the stomach wall for several years. Some tumours are of large-cell type and spread early to adjacent lymph nodes.

The two most widely used staging systems are given in Table 26.10.

The presentation of gastric lymphoma is similar to that of adenocarcinoma of the stomach, with nausea, anorexia and upper abdominal discomfort as the chief symptoms and occasionally haematemesis, or chronic iron-deficiency anaemia, being associated. Barium meal shows a large gastric ulcer or appearances similar to adenocarcinoma of the stomach. On endoscopy, a malignant ulcer is usually seen, but occasionally the appearances can simulate a benign gastric ulcer. Biopsy evidence can be misleading since the specimen may show small lymphocytes

which are hard to distinguish from an inflammatory infiltrate. There is a close association between the low-grade gastric lymphoma of mucosa-associated lymphoid tissue and infection with *Helicobacter pylori* [27].

Treatment

In the past, treatment of gastric lymphoma has usually been by surgical resection if possible. The lack of randomized trials means that clear-cut guidance concerning non-surgical treatment is difficult.

If the diagnosis of a low-grade lymphoma has been made on biopsy and *H. pylori* infection is present, it is usual to treat the infection with antibiotics and a proton-pump inhibitor. About 60% of patients will show a complete histological response of the tumour which will be at the molecular level in half of these. The remission may last several years. If relapse occurs or there is a failure to achieve CR many physicians would use chemotherapy as the next step keeping surgery in reserve. The 'correct' chemotherapy is not known, but it seems reasonable to use combination therapy (for example, CHOP or equivalent) in younger patients and chlorambucil in the elderly.

For higher grade stage I tumours and those not associated with *H. pylori*, surgery is often the first treatment, but a formal comparison with chemotherapy has not been made [28]. For localized high-grade tumours and all tumours of stage II or worse there is a higher risk of relapse. These relapses may be outside the abdomen (in 50% of cases of stage II$_1$ or III disease). Stage II$_2$ low-grade tumours may be treated by gastric and upper abdominal radiotherapy but increasingly the preference is to use chemotherapy. Stage III high-grade tumours are usually treated with combination chemotherapy. For stage II$_2$ or III, chemotherapy seems the most appropriate treatment, and it is clearly indicated for stage IV disease.

Small-bowel lymphoma [29]

Pathology

Lymphoma of the small intestine represents the most common gut tumour of children below the age of 10 years and there is a rise in incidence in adults above the age of 50 years. There is a male preponderance (with a male : female ratio of 5 : 1) and there are two predisposing conditions. In long-standing untreated coeliac disease there is an increased incidence of intestinal lymphoma, and in this situation the lymphoma has now been shown to be of T-

Table 26.10 Staging systems for gastric lymphoma.

	TNM	Ann Arbor
Limited to stomach wall	I	I
Mucosa alone	IA	
Submucosa	IB	
Serosal	IC	
Adjacent (perigastric) nodes	II	II$_1$
Non-adjacent intra-abdominal	III	II$_2$
Nodes outside abdomen	III	III
Disseminated, non-nodal disease	IV	IV

cell type and the bowel is usually widely involved. In the Middle East, there is a high incidence of intestinal lymphoma which is usually preceded by a diffuse plasma cell and lymphocytic proliferation in the small bowel, known as immunoproliferative disease of the small intestine. In this early phase there is an excess production of the heavy chain of IgA (α-chain disease). At this early stage, the disease may respond to treatment with antibiotics, but it subsequently progresses and a B-cell lymphoma develops which may be rapidly evolving. The secretion of heavy chains in the blood may disappear with the onset of lymphoma.

In the typical case of intestinal lymphoma in Europeans, no predisposing cause can be detected. The neoplasm arises in the lymphoid tissues of the mucosa of the bowel, invades and ulcerates the mucosa, and penetrates through the bowel wall to the serosal surface. Histologically, many small-bowel lymphomas are of the diffuse large-cell type, but in adults some of the lymphomas are of lower grade [29].

Clinical features

The presentation is usually with subacute or acute intestinal obstruction with colicky abdominal pain, vomiting and constipation. There may be diarrhoea or even malabsorption, but this is unusual. Gastrointestinal haemorrhage occurs, usually of a chronic type leading to iron-deficiency anaemia. When perforation occurs the clinical picture is typical of perforation of the bowel at any site. Occasionally, patients may present with ascites, usually chylous in nature, but sometimes due to widespread dissemination of intraperitoneal lymphoma. With more extensive abdominal disease there may be fever and anaemia.

The diagnosis is usually made at laparotomy or by a barium follow-through examination which may show infiltration of the bowel wall with ulceration and segments of narrowing, above which are areas of bowel dilatation.

The management of NHL of the small intestine is often difficult. This is in part due to the fact that the disease often presents as an acute surgical emergency. The prognosis is dependent on an adequate surgical excision of the tumour. A simple system of staging related to prognosis is shown in Table 26.11.

All cases should be further staged with chest X-ray and bone marrow aspiration. A liver biopsy should be performed during the laparotomy. Complete local excision of the tumour with the cut ends free of disease, and without involvement of mesenteric nodes, will frequently result in

Table 26.11 Staging of intestinal lymphoma.

IA	Single tumour confined to gut
IB	Two or more tumours confined to gut
IIA	Local node involvement
IIB	Local extension to adjacent structures
IIC	Local tumour with perforation and peritonitis
III	Widespread lymph node enlargement
IV	Disseminated tumour (to liver, spleen and elsewhere)

a cure, and the role of radiation therapy and adjuvant chemotherapy is still to be determined in this type of case. If the lymphoma is of low-grade histology and complete excision has been carried out, then it is probable that no further treatment is needed. If, as is more likely, there is local node involvement and the histology is of a diffuse large-cell type, most oncologists would treat the patient further, and in recent years the tendency has been to use combination chemotherapy. There is a particular danger in the use of combination chemotherapy in patients in whom the tumour has not been resected completely, with perforation of the bowel wall a result of tumour lysis. This has a high mortality. In unresectable tumours it is therefore prudent to begin chemotherapy in lower doses both to allow healing of the bowel wall as the tumour regresses more slowly, and to avoid neutropenia which will add to mortality if perforation occurs. Without combination chemotherapy the 5-year survival of diffuse lymphomas of the gut is about 20%, and of follicular lymphomas about 50%, but this clearly depends on the stage.

The combination of drugs usually employed will include cyclophosphamide, vincristine, doxorubicin and prednisolone in various regimens as for diffuse NHLs at other sites (Table 26.6). In children, the likelihood of CNS involvement is small and it does not appear that prophylactic treatment of the CNS is an essential part of management.

The lymphoma complicating coeliac disease presents particular problems. The preferred designation is 'enteropathy-associated T-cell lymphoma'. The mean time of onset is 7 years after the diagnosis of coeliac disease but may be many years later. The lymphoma does not regress on a gluten-free diet and, typically, patients do not show antigliadin antibody in the blood. Cutaneous and pulmonary spread of the lymphoma is characteristic. The small bowel is frequently involved with an ulcerative lesion which may be the harbinger of the malignant change. Resection of the lymphoma is carried out where possible. Although chemotherapy is usually given postoperatively, the prognosis is poor due to the poor nutritional state of the patient and the risks of perforation and haemorrhage.

Alpha-chain disease [30]

The lymphoma which follows immune proliferative small-intestine disease (IPSID) is characterized by a transformation of the nodular mucosal infiltrate into a high-grade B-cell lymphoma where there is secretion of α-heavy chain (subclass 1). Recent studies have suggested that IPSID is a neoplasm from the beginning. Although in the early stage IPSID may regress with antibiotics, when it transforms to a high-grade tumour treatment with chemotherapy is difficult and usually unsuccessful.

Lymphomatous polyposis [12]

This is a rare disease in which polyps occur in the ileocae-cal region in patients over 50 years of age. The polyps consist of a centrocytic tumour and the mesenteric nodes are usually involved. The tumour disseminates widely early on. Treatment with chemotherapy produces regression but the prognosis is poor. (See also mantle zone lymphoma, p. 410.)

Non-Hodgkin's lymphoma of bone
(see also Chapter 23, p. 355) [31]

Non-Hodgkin's lymphoma frequently invades the marrow and may sometimes cause localized bone lesions with pain, vertebral collapse and pathological fractures. Occasionally, NHL presents as a bone lesion and most of these cases are of large-cell lymphoma formerly called 'reticulum cell sarcoma of bone'. Sometimes the lesion is localized with no evidence of NHL at other sites, even after extensive investigations. In children, isolated lymphoma of bone may be mistaken for Ewing's sarcoma. Immuno-histochemical studies will usually resolve any diagnostic difficulty. In most cases of NHL of bone the lesion is confined to one bone, and a long bone is usually affected. The antecedent history is often very long and the lesions are often very large with extensive soft-tissue infiltration.

The diagnosis is based on the finding of a bone lesion in the absence of widespread lymphoma at other sites including the bone marrow. Pretreatment staging therefore includes CT scanning of the abdomen and mediastinum and a bone marrow examination.

Although radiotherapy (40–45 Gy) produces local con-

trol in over 90% of cases, and should encompass a generous margin of normal bone and soft tissue, dissemination to lymph nodes occurs in approximately 50% of cases. It is usual practice therefore to give combination chemotherapy before radiotherapy. It is not known whether, in the era of intensive chemotherapy, radiation treatment can be dropped, and at present local treatment is given even if the chemotherapy response is excellent. In the very elderly it is reasonable to treat with radiation alone in the first instance.

Central nervous system involvement with lymphoma

Primary lymphomas of the brain and spinal cord occur but are rare. Usually the CNS is involved as part of the pattern of spread of generalized disease and there is a particular tendency for the CNS to be involved in diffuse lymphomas, especially of childhood, of T-cell type and when there is marrow involvement.

Primary lymphoma of the brain [32,33]

These uncommon tumours occur more frequently in AIDS, in renal allograft recipients and in those on long-term immunosuppressive therapy. The histological appearances are usually of a high-grade lymphoma with centrocytic, centroblastic and lymphoplasmacytic forms. They arise in the cerebrum in 70% of cases, cerebellum and brainstem (25% of cases) and rarely in the spinal cord. They tend to be multicentric, and perivascular infiltration is common. Presentation is with the signs and symptoms of a brain tumour (see Chapter 11). Although rare in the spinal cord, seeding into the CSF occasionally occurs late in the disease. An unusual complication is migration of lymphoma cells into the vitreous of the eyes causing visual loss. Patients do not usually show lymphoma elsewhere at presentation or later in the disease. Bone marrow and CSF examination are essential staging investigations.

In non-AIDS-related cases, treatment was traditionally with radiotherapy but the disease was difficult to control, local relapse being common even after doses as high as 45–50 Gy. Chemotherapy is now usually given either alone or before irradiation. Combinations are based on high-dose methotrexate and cytosine arabinoside. Response rates of 60–80% (depending on criteria) are achieved. Relapse is frequent with a 2-year survival of 60%.

If CSF seeding has occurred, it is very difficult to cure

the disease even with chemotherapy, neuraxis radiation and intrathecal treatment.

At the start of the AIDS epidemic CNS lymphoma was recognized as an associated tumour. The tumour is a high-grade B-cell neoplasm, typically occurring in patients already gravely ill with AIDS (many cases being diagnosed at autopsy). The presentation is with focal neurological signs, cranial nerve palsies, fits and mental confusion. On CT scan the tumour mass may be difficult to delineate and ring-enhancing lesions may make distinction from toxoplasmosis difficult. Treatment is difficult and unsuccessful. The patients are ill and immunocompromised. Radiation may help localized disease. Chemotherapy is associated with a great likelihood of opportunistic infection.

Secondary lymphoma of the central nervous system

Involvement of the CNS occurs in about 9% of all cases of NHL. The clinical presentation is either with lymphomatous meningitis (55%) or with extradural compression (45%) (see Fig. 26.9). The great majority of patients have diffuse large-cell (centroblastic) lymphoma or diffuse centrocytic lymphoma as the primary disease. Light

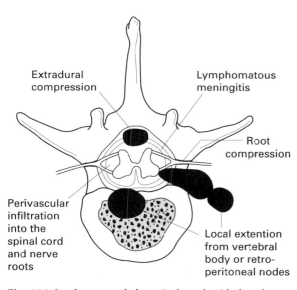

Extradural compression

Lymphomatous meningitis

Root compression

Perivascular infiltration into the spinal cord and nerve roots

Local extention from vertebral body or retroperitoneal nodes

Fig. 26.9 Involvement of the spinal cord with lymphoma. Extradural compression may result from lymphomatous involvement of the vertebral body or by extension from para-aortic nodes. Leptomeningeal infiltration is probably haematogenous and is particularly common when bone marrow is involved.

microscopical evidence of involvement of the bone marrow at diagnosis is present in 70% of cases, probably an underestimate if more sensitive tests of involvement are undertaken. Patients usually have advanced nodal spread at diagnosis, and involvement of retroperitoneal nodes is common. Lymphomatous involvement of the CNS is particularly frequent in childhood lymphomas and in lymphomas of T-cell type.

The clinical presentation of lymphomatous meningitis is with cranial nerve palsies, mental confusion and raised intracranial pressure. Root lesions frequently occur due to compression and perivascular infiltration. The CSF is examined cytologically and, if possible, surface markers (light chain restriction, T-cell markers) should be identified in an attempt to distinguish the cells from reactive lymphocytes which might be found in tuberculous or fungal meningitis and which may be part of the differential diagnosis.

Epidural compression usually occurs in the thoracic spine, but nerve roots may be compressed, including the cauda equina. These patients usually have retroperitoneal lymphoma and sometimes intravertebral deposits. The clinical syndrome is with a paraparesis and is a medical emergency whose management is discussed in Chapter 8.

Lymphomatous meningitis is a serious complication and very few patients in whom it has developed will be cured. The management is with intrathecal chemotherapy using methotrexate in combination with cytosine arabinoside and craniospinal irradiation. Patients at high risk (many childhood lymphomas and T-cell lymphomas in childhood and adolescence) should receive prophylactic treatment of the CNS with intrathecal methotrexate and cranial irradiation in an attempt to avoid this complication. The complication is less frequent in adults. Regimens for systemic treatment often include drugs which penetrate the CSF and these may confer adequate protection. Alternatively, the risk of CNS disease in adults may be lower than had been predicted.

Non-Hodgkin's lymphoma of the nasopharynx and Waldeyer's ring

Non-Hodgkin's lymphoma may present in the lymphoid tissue of the oropharynx and nasopharynx, in the absence of clinical evidence of disease elsewhere. The nose and nasopharyngeal tumours are much more common in China and South America. These tumours may have the phenotype of NK cells and show a distinct pathology of vascular destruction. Others are T-cell or B-cell tumours. The tumours in Waldeyer's ring are usually B-cell tumours and histology may be follicular or diffuse, centroblastic or centrocytic. The presentation is with difficulty in swallowing and nasal congestion. There may be enlargement of cervical lymph nodes, or evidence of disease elsewhere.

Approximately 20% of patients have localized disease (stage I) and 40% have involvement of cervical nodes (stage II). Lymphangiography will demonstrate that half of the patients with stage III disease have involved abdominal nodes (stage III). Approximately 50% of patients have stage III disease at presentation, and 10% of patients stage IV disease (in bone marrow or liver). Patients who present with stage I disease do not usually prove to have more extensive disease on investigation.

The gastrointestinal tract may be involved, and a barium meal and follow-through should be performed as part of the initial investigations.

For patients with disease localized to Waldeyer's ring and cervical nodes, treatment is usually with radiotherapy. Many patients (possibly 60%) will be free of disease at 5–10 years. For patients with stage III and IV disease, treatment is with chemotherapy, but it is not clear if the prognosis has been greatly improved by modern regimens. Survival depends on stage and cell type, NK cell tumours having a good prognosis. For all groups 2-year survival is only 60%.

Ocular non-Hodgkin's lymphoma

Uncommonly the conjunctiva, the orbit and the globe of the eye can be the site of NHL. Orbital lymphomas present with unilateral proptosis, external ocular palsy and intraocular lymphoma with visual disturbance. Conjunctival lymphoma presents with swelling of the lid and visible tumour.

These tumours are uncommon, and their prognosis is not known with certainty. They must be distinguished from the more frequent benign lymphoid proliferations which affect the eye, especially pseudolymphoma of the orbit. They are usually treated with local radiotherapy, but systemic spread probably occurs in about half the cases.

Non-Hodgkin's lymphoma of the lung

Non-Hodgkin's lymphoma may spread to the lung either directly from mediastinal nodes or as part of a more widespread dissemination (usually in advanced and drug-resistant cases). Both Hodgkin's and NHL may involve the lung and cause considerable diagnostic difficulty.

Lymphomatoid granulomatosis

This disease usually arises in the lung. It consists of a pleomorphic infiltrate, often involving vessel walls with areas of necrosis and atypical lymphoid cells. The disease is indolent often over many years. Malignant invasive lymphoma occurs in up to 50% of cases, even if the disease is not considered malignant at the onset. In some cases T-cell monoclonal proliferation has been demonstrated (by T-cell receptor gene rearrangement). Cases have been described in AIDS. Spread to the skin and CNS occurs. Local resection may be curative. More widespread disease has a worse prognosis but long-term remissions may be obtained by steroids and chemotherapy. The EBV genome has been demonstrated in one case.

Cutaneous non-Hodgkin's lymphoma

The skin is a frequent site of *secondary spread* of NHL of all types. It is usually involved in the context of disseminated and often drug-resistant disease. Clinically, there are subcutaneous lumps or papular infiltrates in the dermis. The treatment is of the underlying disease where possible. Superficial X-rays are very helpful in controlling troublesome lesions, and electron therapy is useful for widespread cutaneous infiltrates.

The skin may also be the site of a *primary lymphoma*. These tumours are of many types and are often indolent. They can be broadly classified into those of T-cell and B-cell origin, of which the T-cell variants (primary cutaneous T-cell lymphomas) are the commonest.

Primary cutaneous T-cell lymphoma (PTCL) [34,35]

The two major syndromes are *mycosis fungoides* and *Sézary's syndrome*.

This disease is uncommon. It seldom occurs in black people and has an equal sex incidence. The onset is usually at 50–70 years of age, though many cases may have a long history with an origin much earlier in life. There are stages in the clinical evolution, although in individual cases they are often not easily separable.

The lesions typically occur on the trunk and buttocks and may be very itchy. In the *erythematous* or *pretumour* stage there is a rash which may resemble psoriasis with fine red scaly patches. There are often poikilodermatous changes which suggest the diagnosis. This phase may last for many years with numerous diagnoses offered. The diagnosis can only be substantiated by biopsy and by showing monoclonality of T cells by molecular methods.

There is acanthosis, parakeratosis and clusters of histiocytes (Darier–Pautrier abscesses).

In the *infiltrative* or *plaque* stage there are indurated plaques. Microscopically, there is infiltration of the upper dermis and epidermis with lymphoma cells which are helper T cells. There is usually no significant lymph node enlargement. If the nodes do enlarge, they may show 'dermatopathic lymphadenopathy' and, later, clear evidence of tumour infiltration. In the *tumour* stage the lesions enlarge and ulcerate. Involvement of internal organs may occur.

In the erythrodermic phase (Sézary's syndrome). The skin shows infiltration with T cells. Lymph node enlargement and hepatomegaly may be present. The patient complains of intense itching, the skin becomes red and thickened and may be swollen. Hair is lost and palmar hyperkeratosis occurs with dystrophy and loss of nails. The circulating cells were called *cellules monstreuses* by Sézary. They do not infiltrate the marrow until late in the disease. Hepatosplenomegaly may occur and there may be lymph node enlargement.

The most important prognostic factor is extent of disease. A staging system is shown in Table 26.12.

Treatment in the first stage is with steroid creams and topical nitrogen mustard or nitrosoureas. Cutaneous hypersensitivity to nitrogen mustard can be troublesome. Local radiation can be used for unsightly lesions. More widespread disease responds to psoralens and ultraviolet light A (PUVA) and whole-body election beam therapy; PUVA is complicated by secondary skin cancers in a few patients. Whole-body electrons cause depilation and loss of sweating. Neither appear to change prognosis. Wide-field irradiation is the treatment usually, used in the mycotic stage.

Chemotherapy responses occur. There is no benefit from aggressive early treatment using combination chemotherapy of the type used for other lymphomas. Responses to alkylating agents and anthracyclines is variable and usually short-lived. Responses have been reported to fludarabine and 2-chlorodeoxyadenosine. Interferon also produces responses, some of which are long lasting. New approaches that have shown some clinical effectiveness are the retinoid bexarotene, anti-CD5 and 6 monoclonal antibodies and the use of toxin-coupled antibodies to the IL-2 receptor.

Prognosis is related to stage. Patients with stage IA disease probably have a normal lifespan with few of them progressing to tumour stage. For stage 2 disease, survival is 85% at 5 years and 70% at 10 years. More extensive skin disease, nodal involvement, tumour stage and visceral involvement are all poor prognostic factors (Table 26.12).

Primary cutaneous B-cell cutaneous lymphoma (PCBCL) [36]

This is a group of disorders of which the commonest form is probably derived from germinal centre B cells. It presents as a single red patch or nodule, without ulceration, occurring at any site. The diagnosis may present difficulty both clinically and pathologically. Radiation is used for localized lesions, but the disease responds to chemotherapy using a conventional combination of drugs. The localized disease is associated with an excellent prognosis — greater than 90% survival at 10 years. There is a large-cell variant affecting the leg in women that has a worse outcome (50% at 5 years).

Malignant angioendotheliomatosis

This disorder is characterized by widespread skin lesions, fever, dementia, neurological signs and organ failure. There is intravascular proliferation of atypical mononuclear cells within small blood vessels. Recent studies have shown this to be a lymphoid tumour with positive B-cell markers and numerous karyotypic abnormalities.

Table 26.12 Staging system for primary cutaneous T-cell lymphoma.

T_1	Plaques occupying less than 10% of body surface
T_2	Plaques over more than 10%
T_3	Tumours
T_4	Generalized erythroderma (Sézary's syndrome)
N_0	No clinically or pathologically involved nodes
N_1	Nodes enlarged, pathology negative
N_2	Pathologically involved
N_3	Clinically and pathologically involved
M_0	No visceral involvement
M_1	Visceral involvement

Stage group

1A	$T_1 N_0 M_0$
1B	$T_2 N_0 M_0$
2A	$T_{1-2} N_1 M_0$
2B	$T_3 N_{0,1} M_0$
3	$T_4 N_{0,1} M_0$
4A	$T_{1-4} N_{2,3} M_0$
4B	$T_{1-4} N_{0-3} M_1$

Non-Hodgkin's lymphoma of the thyroid

These tumours usually present as a rapidly enlarging thyroid mass in middle-aged or elderly women. They are associated with Hashimoto's thyroiditis, and areas of thyroiditis may be found in the gland on biopsy. Histologically, they are usually diffuse large-cell tumours which are generally of B-cell type. Follicular and plasmacytoid forms are unusual, and T-cell tumours are rare. The evolution of the disease in a gland affected by autoimmune disease is reminiscent of the development of lymphomas in Sjögren's syndrome. The mass does not take up radioactive iodine and cannot be distinguished clinically from other thyroid cancers. Diagnosis is made by biopsy or thyroidectomy. Radical surgery has little role in management, however, since the tumours are sensitive to radiotherapy.

Staging investigations are necessary since the prognosis is excellent with local treatment if the disease is confined to the gland. These investigations should include chest X-ray, abdominal CT scan and/or lymphogram, and marrow aspiration and biopsy. Relapse in the gut is relatively frequent and a small-bowel barium examination may be useful.

If there is no local extension of the tumour from the gland and no evidence of involvement of adjacent nodes, radiotherapy (40 Gy in 4 weeks) to the gland and adjacent nodes will cure 90% of patients. Only 50% of patients with local and nodal extension will be cured, and the prognosis is also worse over the age of 65 years. Adjuvant chemotherapy should therefore be considered in these cases, and is clearly necessary for patients with more widespread disease. It seems likely that T-cell tumours will also require chemotherapy. There are, as yet, few data to show whether chemotherapy will improve the prognosis.

Non-Hodgkin's lymphoma of the testis

Non-Hodgkin's lymphoma of the testis is usually a diffuse large-cell (centroblastic) lymphoma. The patients are generally over the age of 50 years—an age when seminoma and teratoma are uncommon. The tumours are mostly unilateral but there is a considerable risk of contralateral involvement. Presentation is with a painless enlargement of the testis. After investigation most patients are found to have stage I or II disease (Ann Arbor system, Table 25.2). The disease has a tendency to spread to abdominal nodes and to Waldeyer's ring. Occasionally, CNS relapse occurs.

Staging investigations should include lymphangiogram and/or CT scan of the abdomen, and bone marrow exam-

ination. Localized disease (IE and IIE) can be treated with radiotherapy to the pelvic and para-aortic lymph nodes. Bilateral or advanced (stage III and IV) disease carries a poor prognosis and systemic chemotherapy is required. The prognosis is not good. Overall 60% of patients have died at 3 years.

Tumour lysis syndrome

This syndrome of hyperuricaemia and renal failure is particularly likely to occur in patients with Burkitt's lymphoma, those with large intra-abdominal tumours, and with T-cell tumours with a large mediastinal mass. The cause, prevention and treatment of tumour lysis syndrome are discussed in Chapter 8.

References

1 The emerging epidemic of non-Hodgkin's lymphoma. Current knowledge regarding aetiological factors. *Cancer Res* 1992: 52. (Suppl).

2 Isaacson PG. Pathology of malignant lymphomas. *Curr Opin Oncol* 1992; 4: 811–20.

3 Sarris A, Ford R. Recent advances in the molecular pathogenesis of lymphomas. *Curr Opin Oncol* 1999; 11: 351–63.

4 Harris NL, Jaffe ES, Stein H *et al*. A revised European-American classification of lymphoid neoplasms: a proposal from the International Lymphoma Study Group. *Blood* 1994; 84: 1361–92.

5 Aisenberg AC. Coherent view of non-Hodgkin's lymphomas. *J Clin Oncol* 1995; 13: 2656–75.

6 Gupta RK, Lister TA. Management of follicular lymphoma. *Curr Opin Oncol* 1996; 8: 360–5.

7 MacManus MP, Hoppe RT. Is radiotherapy curative for stage I and II low grade follicular lymphoma? Results of long-term follow-up study of patients treated at Stanford University. *J Clin Oncol* 1996; 14: 128–290.

8 Tallman MS, Hakimian D. Purine nucleoside analogs: emerging roles in indolent proliferative disorders. *Blood* 1995; 86: 2463–74.

9 McLaughlin P, Grillo-Lopez AJ, Link BK *et al*. Rituximal chimeric anti-CD20 monoclonal antibody therapy for relapsed incident lymphoma: half of patients respond to a four dose treatment program. *J Clin Oncol* 1998; 16: 2825–33.

10 Dana BW, Bahlberg S, Nathwani BN *et al*. Long-term follow-up of patients with low-grade malignant lymphomas treated with doxorubicin based chemotherapy or chemoimmune therapy. *J Clin Oncol* 1993; 11: 644–51.

11 Leonard JP, Schattner EJ, Coleman M. Biology and management of mantle cell lymphoma. *Curr Opin Oncol* 2001; 13: 342–7.

12 International NHL Prognostic Factors Project. A predictive

model for aggressive Non-Hodgkin's lymphoma. *N Engl J Med* 1993; 329: 987–94.

13 Miller TP, Dahlberg MS, Cassady JR *et al*. Chemotherapy alone compared with chemotherapy for localised intermediate and high-grade non Hodgkin's lymphoma. *N Engl J Med* 1998; 339: 21–6.

14 Fisher RI, Gaynor ER, Dahlberg S *et al*. Comparison of a standard regimen (CHOP) with three intensive chemotherapy regimens for advanced non-Hodgkin's lymphoma. *N Engl J Med* 1993; 328: 1002–6.

15 Piccozi VJ, Coleman CN. Lymphoblastic lymphoma. *Semin Oncol* 1990; 17: 950–1104.

16 van Besien K, Kelta M, Bahaguna P. Primary mediastinal B-cell lymphoma. a review of the pathology and management. *J Clin Oncol* 2001; 19: 1855–64.

17 Kadin ME, Sakko K, Berliner N *et al*. Childhood Ki-1 lymphoma presenting with skin lesions and peripheral lymphadenopathy. *Blood* 1986; 68: 1042–9.

18 Dimopoulous MA, Galan IE, Matsouka C. Waldenstrom's macroglobinaemia. *Hematology/Oncol Clin N Am* 1999; 13: 1351–66.

19 Philip T, Guglielmi C, Hagenbeek A *et al*. Autologous bone marrow transplantation as compared with salvage chemotherapy in relapses of chemotherapy-sensitive non-Hodgkin's lymphoma. *N Engl J Med* 1995; 333: 1540–5.

20 Levine AM, Sullivan-Halley J, Pike MC *et al*. HIV related lymphoma: prognostic factors predictive of survival. *Cancer* 1991; 68: 2466–72.

21 Sander AS, Kaplan L. AIDS lymphoma. *Curr Opin Oncol* 1996; 8: 377–85.

22 Anderson JR, Wilson JF, Jenkin DT *et al*. Childhood non-Hodgkin's lymphoma. The results of a randomized therapeutic trial comparing a 4-drug regimen (COMP) with a 10-drug regimen (LSA2-L2). *N Engl J Med* 1983; 308: 559–65.

23 Hvizdala EV, Berard C, Callihan T *et al*. Lymphoblastic lymphoma in children — a randomized trial comparing LSA2L2 with the A-COP therapeutic regimen: a Paediatric Oncology Group Study *J Clin Oncol* 1988; 6: 26–33.

24 Philip T, Pinkerton R, Biron P *et al*. Effective multiagent chemotherapy in children with advanced B-cell lymphoma: who remains the high-risk patient? *Br J Haematol* 1987; 65: 159–64.

25 Murphy SB, Magrath IT. Workshop on paediatric lymphomas: current results and prospects. *Ann Oncol* 1991; 2 (Suppl. 2): 219–23.

26 Isaacson PG, Spencer J. Malignant lymphoma of mucosa associated lymphoid tissue. *Histopathology* 1987; 11: 445–62.

27 Wotherspoon AC, Doglioni C, Diss TC *et al*. Regression of primary low grade B-cell gastric lymphoma of the mucosa-associated lymphoid tissue type after eradication of *Helicobacter pylori*. *Lancet* 1993; 342: 575–7.

28 Liu HT, Hsu C, Chen CL *et al*. Chemotherapy alone versus surgery followed by chemotherapy for stage I/IIE large cell lymphoma of the stomach. *Am J Hematol* 2000; 64: 175–9.

29 List AF, Greer JP, Cousa JC *et al*. Non-Hodgkin's lymphoma of the gastrointestinal tract. An analysis of clinical and pathological features affecting outcome. *J Clin Oncol* 1988; 6: 1125–33.

30 Ben-Ayed F, Halphen M, Najjar T *et al*. Treatment of alpha chain disease-results of a prospective study in 21 Tunisian patients by the Tunisian-French Intestinal Lymphoma Study Group. *Cancer* 1989; 63: 1251–6.

31 Bacci G, Jaffe N, Emilani E *et al*. Therapy for primary non-Hodgkin's lymphoma of bone and a comparison of results with Ewing's sarcoma. *Cancer* 1986; 57: 1468–72.

32 Pollock IF, Lunsford LD, Flickinger JC, Dameshek HL. Prognostic factors in the diagnosis and treatment of primary central nervous system lymphoma. *Cancer* 1989; 63: 939–46.

33 De Angelis LM, Yahaloin J, Thales AT, Khan U. Combined modality treatment for primary CNS lymphoma. *J Clin Oncol* 1992; 10: 635–43.

34 Willemze R, Meijer CJLM. EORTC classification for primary cutaneous lymphoma. a comparison and the REAL classification and the proposed WHO classification. *Ann Oncol* 2000; II (Suppl. I): 11–15.

35 Koh HK, Foss FM, eds. *Cutaneous T Cell Lymphoma*. (Haematology/Oncology Clinics in North America Series). Philadelphia: W.B. Saunders, 1995, 2000.

36 Pandolfino TL, Siegel RS, Kuzel TM. *et al*. Primary cutaneous B-cell lymphoma: Review and current concepts. *J Clin Oncol* 18: 2151–68.

Myeloma and other paraproteinaemias

Myeloma

Incidence and aetiology

Myeloma (multiple myeloma, myelomatosis, plasma cell myeloma) is chiefly a disease of the elderly (Fig. 27.1), and is almost twice as common in males as in females. Annual incidence is approximately four per 100 000 and is twice as frequent in American black as in white people. The incidence has increased over the past 40 years [1]. Family clusters have been reported, with an increased incidence in first-degree relatives. Use of serum electrophoresis in screening programmes reveals a far higher incidence of paraproteinaemia—a monoclonal immunoglobulin (Ig) band—and up to 3% of an asymptomatic population over the age of 70 years have a monoclonal gammopathy. Most of these have a form of 'benign' paraproteinaemia (see p. 428) but a minority subsequently develop symptomatic myeloma. As with other B-cell neoplasms, there appears to be an unequivocal relationship between radiation exposure and subsequent development of myeloma [2]. An increased incidence has been reported in a group of American radiologists, presumably due to life-long radiation exposure, and also in survivors of Nagasaki and Hiroshima with a delay of 20 years.

Pathogenesis

Immunoglobulin abnormalities

Multiple myeloma is a B-lymphocyte neoplasm character-ized by continued synthesis and release of Igs (Table 27.1), with neoplastic proliferation of a clone of B lymphocytes resulting in large numbers of immature plasma cells which infiltrate the bone marrow and which can occasionally be found in the blood. The oncogenic event may occur earlier in the B-cell differentiation pathway but clonal expansion occurs at the plasma cell stage (Fig. 27.2). Production of large amounts of a monoclonal Ig is therefore characteristic of multiple myeloma.

The basic structure of normal Igs consists of two polypeptide light chains (with molecular weights of 22 kDa) and two heavy chains (molecular weights of 55–70 kDa), held together by covalent (disulphide) and noncovalent bonds (Fig. 27.3). There is variability in heavy chain structure, with five separate types of heavy chain γ, α, μ, δ and ε, these differences forming the basis of the five classes of immunoglobulin, IgG, IgA, IgM, IgD and IgE. Furthermore, there are altogether 10 different heavy chain sequences, four γ, two α, two μ and only one each of δ and ε. Of the γ immunoglobulins, IgG_3 is particularly prone to polymerize, as are IgA and IgM. There are, however, only two types of light chain—kappa (κ) and lambda (λ). IgG, IgD and IgE are found in the plasma as single molecules with a molecular weight of 160–200 kDa. IgM is a macroglobulin (molecular weight 900 kDa) synthesized as a pentamer of IgG structure. IgA is formed by plasma cells in the gut and respiratory tract, and is therefore found in external secretions such as saliva, tears, bronchial and gastrointestinal mucosa, as well as in the blood. It has an important role in primary defence against invading pathogens.

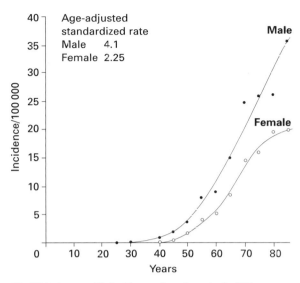

Fig. 27.1 Age-specific incidence of myeloma in the UK.

Table 27.1 Immunoglobulin-producing neoplasms.

Benign (but see text)
Monoclonal gammapathy of unknown significance
Cold agglutinin disease

Malignant
Myeloma
Waldenström's macroglobulinaemia
Primary amyloidosis
Non-Hodgkin's lymphomas
Heavy chain diseases (γ, α or μ)

Normal Igs are diverse in their detailed structure, synthesized in response to a variety of antigenic stimuli. Each Ig molecule recognizes one antigenic structure only, and the portion of the molecule which confers this specificity is known as the idiotypic determinant. By contrast, in myeloma the product of the neoplastic plasma cell clone is an Ig of a single homogeneous structure (that is, a single idiotype), the myeloma or M protein (not to be confused with IgM), or paraprotein. There is always light-chain restriction, that is, to either κ or λ type.

In most patients, whole Ig molecules are often synthesized, but in about one-quarter there may be a disproportionate production of one component so that free light chains are produced. In approximately 1% of patients (often termed non-secretors), no monoclonal protein can be detected in the plasma or urine.

When free light chains are secreted into the blood, they cross the glomerular membrane and are detectable in the

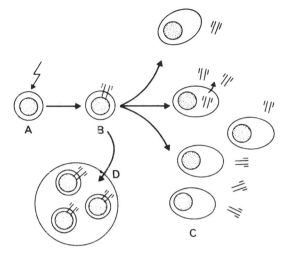

Fig. 27.2 Pathogenesis of myeloma: (A) oncogenic event in a B cell; (B) expansion of a clone of malignant B cells; (C) proliferation of plasma cells leading to bone lesions and production of paraprotein; (D) suppression of normal B cells leads to hypogammaglobulinaemia.

urine. They have the unusual property of producing a cloudy precipitate (Bence-Jones protein) when the urine is heated to 50–60°C, with dissociation of the precipitate as the temperature is raised near boiling point. Excretion of free light chains occurs in 40–50% of all cases of myeloma, and is detected nowadays by immunoelectrophoresis of the urine.

The major classes of Ig have differing physical properties, which may be clinically relevant since many aspects of the disease are attributable to the physical characteristics or deposition of the Ig itself. For example, IgM has a high molecular weight, and hyperviscosity syndrome is not uncommon (see below). Immunoglobulin A molecules polymerize in the plasma and will also cause hyperviscosity. Excess light chains may be deposited in the renal tubule and contribute to renal failure (see p. 430). Polymerization of light chains is one component of amyloid which also contributes to renal disease. The incidence of the different types of myeloma roughly parallels the concentrations of normal serum Igs and reflects the number of plasma cells normally found in each group. IgG myeloma is the commonest type, followed by IgA. Immunoglobulin M production is rarely due to a true myeloma but is usually part of Waldenström's macroglobulinaemia or non-Hodgkin's lymphoma (see p. 413). Immunoglobulin D myeloma is very uncommon, and IgE exceedingly rare. More than 5×10^9 plasma cells must be

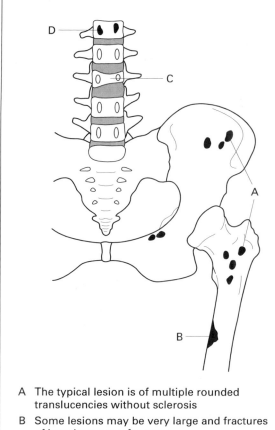

A The typical lesion is of multiple rounded translucencies without sclerosis

B Some lesions may be very large and fractures of long bones are frequent

C Vertebral osteoporosis and collapse is very common

D Loss of the vertebral pedicle is an easily missed sign of infiltration

Fig. 27.3 Diagrammatic representation of bone lesions in myeloma.

Table 27.2 Prognostic features in myeloma.

Good	Poor
Low serum β_2 microglobulin level < 2 mg/l	High serum β_2 microglobulin level > 2 mg/l
Haemoglobin > 10 g/dl	Haemoglobin < 8.5 g/dl
Serum calcium normal	Serum calcium > 2.9 mmol/l
No lytic bone lesions	More than three bone lesions
Low paraprotein level	High paraprotein level
IgG < 50 g/l	IgG > 70 g/l
IgA < 30 g/l	IgA > 50 g/l
Urine light chains < 2 g/day	Light chains > 5 g/day
Plasma urea < 8 mmol/l	Urea > 8 mmol/l

ues and initial haemoglobin (Hb) level. In this formula, larger values imply a worse prognosis [3].

Depression of production of normal Ig is a characteristic feature of the disease and one which helps to differentiate it from benign varieties of a monoclonal gammopathy, though the mechanism of suppression of normal Ig production is not clear. This depression affects all classes of normal Ig and contributes greatly to susceptibility to bacterial infection.

Other causes of monoclonal Ig production (Table 27.2) include monoclonal gammopathy of unknown significance (MGUS), previously erroneously termed 'benign monoclonal gammopathy'. This is common in the elderly and may cause diagnostic difficulty, particularly as it may later progress to myeloma. The current understanding of the MGUS–myeloma relationship is that a spectrum exists from the relatively benign disorder to the frankly malignant. Although MGUS shares certain features with myeloma (excess Ig synthesis and occasional Bence-Jones proteinuria), the marrow plasma cell infiltrate is modest (<10%) and there are no bone lesions. Progression of MGUS to myeloma is well described and may occur slowly, with a period of 'smouldering' disease which can cause difficulty for the clinician.

It is not yet clear which oncogenes or other DNA sequences are the most critical for myeloma development, either *de novo* or within an existing background of MGUS. Initial studies suggest that both the *myc* and *ras* oncogene series may be implicated. It is also known that of the cytokines, interleukin-6 (IL-6) is an important agent capable of stimulating plasma cell growth and differentiation, and lymphotoxin (tumour necrosis factor-β, TNF-β) is a known mediator of osteoclast activation and therefore of myeloma bone destruction [4]. It is now clear that

present for the paraprotein to be detectable as a discrete Ig band.

In myeloma an assessment of tumour mass can be made using a formula which includes haemoglobin, calcium, presence of multiple bone lesions, paraprotein concentration and blood urea. Patients with a large tumour mass (in excess of 0.5×10^{12} cells) have a worse prognosis and respond less frequently to chemotherapy. Some of the important prognostic features are shown in Table 27.2. One of the more successful attempts to determine likely prognosis has used only serum β_2 microglobulin (s-β_2m) val-

myeloma develops as a 'multistep transformation process', with cellular proliferation regulated through several different pathways [5].

Pathological features

Both the bone and the bone marrow are infiltrated by malignant plasma cells, typically round or oval, often with an eccentrically placed nucleus like their normal counterpart. The cytoplasm is densely basophilic due to the RNA-producing paraprotein, with a clear perinuclear zone where the Golgi apparatus is situated. Abnormal forms are often present, sometimes large and bi- or trinucleate, with the nucleus eccentrically placed. The marrow infiltration is often patchy, unlike leukaemia—hence the name multiple myeloma—but the histological diagnosis is highly probable when the level of infiltration exceeds 20% of all nucleated marrow cells, though the diagnosis is not excluded by lesser degrees of involvement. The bone becomes destroyed by the tumour.

Typically the lesions are lytic and fractures are common (Fig. 27.3). The mechanism of lysis is not fully understood but osteoclastic-activating factors produced by the myeloma or mature B cells have been described. Any bone can be affected and common sites include vertebrae, pelvis, skull, ribs and proximal long bones.

The kidney is affected in several ways (Fig. 27.4). First, light chains are taken up by distal renal tubular cells, a major site of catabolism of normal light chains. The massive load of light chains results in tubular damage and large casts of light chains and albumin fill and obstruct the tubule, imposing a further load on the remaining nephrons. Specific defects in tubular reabsorption occur, due to protein aggregation in renal tubule cells, and leading to tubular reabsorptive defects with leakage of amino acids, glucose, potassium and phosphate (acquired Fanconi syndrome).

Second, amyloid deposition in glomerular blood vessels occurs in 10% of patients, particularly in cases where light chains alone are produced. In myeloma this protein consists in part of polymerized light chain fragments. λ light chains are much more likely to lead to amyloid formation. Other features contributing to renal impairment include recurrent hypercalcaemia with dehydration, hypercalciuria and nephrocalcinosis, urate deposition and renal tubular leakage. Urinary tract infection is common and pyelonephritis may develop. Together, these processes constitute 'myeloma kidney'. There may even be renal deposition of malignant plasma cells, typically late in the disease when there is a large tumour mass.

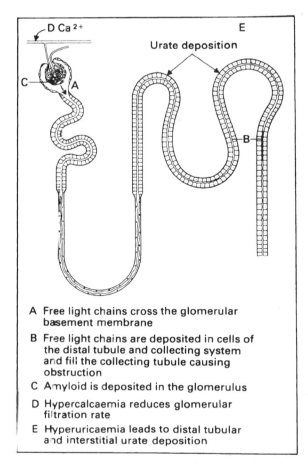

A Free light chains cross the glomerular basement membrane

B Free light chains are deposited in cells of the distal tubule and collecting system and fill the collecting tubule causing obstruction

C Amyloid is deposited in the glomerulus

D Hypercalcaemia reduces glomerular filtration rate

E Hyperuricaemia leads to distal tubular and interstitial urate deposition

Fig. 27.4 Renal damage in myeloma.

Clinical features

Patients with myeloma may be asymptomatic for many years before presenting with weakness, bone pain, anorexia and other symptoms due either to abnormal proliferation of the malignant plasma cells, to direct effects of the abnormal Ig, or to hypercalcaemia.

Diffuse bone pain is often the major complaint, with skeletal abnormalities present in about two-thirds of patients. The pain is typically dull or aching, often felt in the spine, ribs or pelvis. Pathological fractures are common, and acute back pain from a vertebral crush fracture is a frequent first presentation of myeloma. This may lead to acute cord compression (see Chapter 8). In its later stages, multiple myeloma may be among the most painful of all cancers, with multiple sites of vertebral and long bone fracture from widespread malignant infiltration.

Typical radiological appearances include generalized

osteopenia or osteoporosis (particularly evident in the dorsal and lumbar spine and sacroiliac area), and punched-out osteolytic lesions, with little or no sclerosis. Full radiological skeletal survey often reveals unsuspected bone lesions and should always be performed at diagnosis. In addition to the ribs, vertebrae and hips, these lesions are characteristically found in the skull, usually remaining asymptomatic until they reach a large size. Biopsy of any of these sites reveals heavy infiltration with abnormal plasma cells.

Many patients present with fatigue and lassitude due to anaemia, and recurrent bacterial infection due to immunoparesis. Nausea, anorexia and dehydration may be due to hypercalcaemia and lead to deteriorating renal function.

Hyperviscosity syndrome may develop in patients in whom the type and level of abnormal Ig contributes to an increase in plasma viscosity. This is most commonly seen in patients with Waldenström's macroglobulinaemia (see below) but also occurs in patients with myeloma, especially with IgA, IgM and IgG$_3$ paraproteins. Clinically, this syndrome consists of neurological symptoms, chiefly vertigo, confusion and transient ischaemic episodes; retinopathy with distended retinal veins, haemorrhages and papilloedema; and hypervolaemia with increased vascular resistance. A bleeding tendency is frequently due to both thrombocytopenia and clotting disturbances due to interference of the coagulation system by paraprotein, leading to reduced platelet aggregation. Clinically this may cause purpura, epistaxis, mucosal bleeding and retinal haemorrhage. A positive Hess test, reduced thromboplastin generation time and defective clot retraction may all occur.

In addition to cord compression from direct involvement of the vertebrae by myeloma, patients often suffer other neurological complications. Direct extradural involvement may occur through involvement of nerve roots via the intervertebral foramina. Soft-tissue deposits may occur in the orbit or base of skull, leading to proptosis or cranial nerve palsies. Carpal tunnel syndrome may develop, due to amyloid infiltration. Megaloblastic anaemia can occur, possibly due to defective folate metabolism, although many patients have some degree of macrocytosis with no megaloblastic change and of uncertain cause. Recurrent infection is also a common feature of the disease and is frequently one of the presenting complaints. Leucopenia predisposes to infection, as does the generalized depression of normal Igs. This Ig abnormality usually fails to become normal even with 'successful' treatment which may supress the monoclonal Ig band. Some patients also have impairment of phagocytosis and cellular immune responses.

The plasma volume may be high as a result of the increase in total plasma protein, contributing to the anaemia even when the total red cell mass is near normal. The M band is also responsible, by direct coating of erythrocytes, for the raised erythrocyte sedimentation rate (ESR) and erythrocyte rouleaux formation which are so characteristic of myeloma. Typically, the ESR is more than 80 mm/h. Bone marrow involvement is almost invariable, though for diagnostic purposes, direct biopsy of a tender area is more likely to be positive. Abnormal plasma cells can account for up to 95% of the nucleated cell population. A practical point: many haematologists advise against sternal marrow puncture in patients with myeloma, in view of the extreme fragility of bone and the danger of inadvertently entering the mediastinum.

Hypercalcaemia is common, chiefly attributable to bone destruction from abnormal plasma cell proliferation, although other factors which activate osteoclasts have been described [6]. In many patients, a highly potent osteoclast-activating factor has been identified [4,7]. Approximately one-third of patients have an abnormally elevated plasma calcium at diagnosis, and the majority develop hypercalcaemia during the course of the illness. Indeed, myeloma is the diagnosis par excellence which may result in profound and treatment-resistant hypercalcaemia, often of sufficient severity to require emergency treatment (see Chapter 8). The symptoms include polyuria, polydipsia, constipation, nausea, vomiting, dehydration and mental confusion. Hypercalciuria is even more frequent.

Impaired renal function is extremely common. Once hypercalcaemia and renal impairment have developed, a vicious circle becomes established in which there is worsening renal function, increasing hypercalcaemia, further dehydration with falling glomerular filtration rate, and increasing tubular obstruction and dysfunction from light chain deposition. This is a medical emergency and its management is described below.

Diagnosis

In a typical case when there are bone lesions, anaemia, paraproteinaemia, hypercalcaemia, Bence-Jones proteinuria and marrow involvement, there is no diagnostic difficulty. In less florid cases, the differential diagnosis can be extensive and may include the following.

1 Other causes of anaemia, bone pain and hypercalcaemia such as metastatic cancer.

2 Other causes of paraproteinaemia such as MGUS, occult primary tumours (Table 27.3), Waldenström's macroglobulinaemia or lymphomas (Table 27.4).

3 Other causes of lytic lesions in bone such as breast, renal, thyroid or bronchial carcinoma.

4 Other causes of spinal cord compression such as metastatic cancer.

5 Other causes of anaemia and raised ESR such as connective tissue diseases, malignancy and infection especially where cold agglutinins are formed as in *Mycoplasma* infections and infectious mononucleosis, although these patients are generally younger.

6 Solitary plasmacytomas (see below).

7 Primary amyloidosis, which may be accompanied by plasmacytosis in the marrow and also by a proteinuria.

The diagnosis may be difficult if there is minimal marrow involvement, no detectable paraprotein, or a solitary bone lesion on skeletal X-rays. In doubtful cases the marrow examination may have to be repeated. However, if there is no pressing indication for treatment, a period of observation may allow the diagnosis to be established more easily (Table 27.4). Occasionally, immunological testing using light and heavy chain antibodies to establish

Table 27.3 Causes of monoclonal gammaglobulinaemia other than myeloma.

Monoclonal gammopathy of unknown significance

Non-lymphoid and lymphoid malignancy
Carcinoma of breast, gastrointestinal tract, ovary, bladder, prostate and others
Soft-tissue sarcomas
Melanoma
Non-Hodgkin's lymphoma
Waldenström's macroglobulinaemia

Autoimmune diseases
Rheumatoid arthritis
Polyarteritis nodosa

Table 27.4 Causes of macroglobulinaemia.

Benign
Benign macroglobulinaemia
Cold agglutinin disease

Neoplasms
Waldenström's macroglobulinaemia
IgM myeloma
Non-Hodgkin's lymphomas
Chronic lymphatic leukaemia

monoclonality may be necessary to exclude a 'reactive' plasmacytosis.

Treatment

When patients with myeloma present with dangerous manifestations such as dehydration, hypercalcaemia or spinal cord compression, the first treatment should be to correct the metabolic disturbance or serious local problem (see Chapter 8). Intravenous fluid replacement, correction of hypercalcaemia, local irradiation and occasionally decompressive laminectomy should, in these circumstances, take precedence. In the majority of patients, however, the presenting clinical syndrome is more slowly evolving and, in contrast to these clinical emergencies, there will be time to confirm the diagnosis before instituting treatment.

Chemotherapy

Despite recent advances in chemotherapy for myeloma (see below), the traditional approach, using oral melphalan, is still widely used. This form of medication has improved survival from a median of 6–12 months (untreated) to 2–3 years [7,8]. Usually given by mouth, doses vary from 6 to 10 mg/m^2 over 4–7 days every 46 weeks. The addition of oral prednisolone has slightly improved the remission rate. Typical doses range from 60 to 80 mg/m^2 (with melphalan) in divided doses and accompanied by an H$_2$ antagonist such as ranitidine 150 mg twice daily. Despite the introduction of more complex induction chemotherapy regimens, it is not entirely clear whether they provide a higher survival rate [9].

Combined melphalan–prednisolone oral therapy is generally well tolerated, although in long survivors, there is undoubtedly a small risk of development of acute myeloblastic leukaemia related to chronic melphalan therapy [10].

Most patients with myeloma (approximately 75%) will respond to oral chemotherapy, with prompt improvement in symptoms, particularly pain, tenderness and hypercalcaemia. The paraprotein level generally falls within the first three cycles, although the immune paresis of the unaffected Igs usually takes longer to recover, and may never do so. Other parameters such as haemoglobin, albumin and blood urea may return to normal limits and can be useful for monitoring progress. In patients who respond to chemotherapy, it is rarely necessary to continue the initial treatment beyond between six and nine courses, since little further is to be gained. By this time many will have entered a 'plateau' phase, in which no further reduction of the paraprotein occurs, and treatment can reasonably be discontinued; or, disease will be progressing and further strategies will be necessary.

In the past 15 years many more complex regimens have been tested, generally employing intravenous agents, in an attempt to raise remission rates and duration, and ultimately to improve survival [7,11]. The newer regimens generally include a vinca alkaloid, multiple alkylating agents and doxorubicin together with high-dose prednisolone or dexamethasone. Immune modulators such as levamisole have sometimes been used (notably in the USA) and also α-interferon which clearly has activity in this disease, though its use still remains controversial [11]. Although many have reported improved results with complex regimens, intensive (monthly) treatment with conventional melphalan and prednisolone may offer equally good results with fewer side-effects. In the UK, however, a prospectively randomized Medical Research Council myeloma study suggested that the ABCM (doxorubicin, *bis*-chloroethyl nitrosourea, cyclophosphamide and melphalan) regimen may be superior, although the melphalan in this trial was given without a steroid and at relatively modest dose [12]. Intensive regimens are clearly more toxic and may be difficult to apply in an elderly population. One well-known combination of vincristine, infused doxorubicin and high-dose dexamethasone (VAD) requires insertion of a Hickman line, and considerable periods of inpatient care, also making it less widely acceptable.

However, it seems reasonable to offer more intensive regimens such as ABCM (doxorubicin, BCNU, cyclophosphamide and melphalan), VAD or VMCP–VBAP (vincristine, cyclophosphamide, melphalan, and prednisolone alternating with vincristine, BCNU, doxorubicin and prednisolone) to younger, fitter patients. It is also in this group that the initial results of high-dose melphalan therapy—with or without autologous bone marrow transplantation (BMT) —have been promising [13]. With this intensive but single-exposure treatment, complete remission is seen in about one-third of patients, with elimination of malignant plasma cells in the marrow, reduction of paraprotein to undetectable levels and return of normal marrow function. In many cases, the immune paresis has resolved as well, an impressive feature and unusual with conventional treatment. An important study from France, comparing results of conventional with high-dose treatment (including autologous BMT), confirmed response rates of 81% with high-dose therapy (including complete responses in 22%) compared with 57% (complete responders 5%) in the conventionally treated arm [14]. Event-free 5-year survival was 52% compared with 12%. These

are substantial differences which will alter current treatment recommendations in myeloma, particularly since stem cell autotransplantation is widely applicable to reasonably fit patients up to age 65 years. A further group, limited to highly selected younger patients, may possibly derive real benefit from allogeneic BMT if a donor is available [15]. Use of erythropoietin (EPO) has become more widespread as a means of avoiding anaemia without frequent transfusion.

After discontinuation of first-line chemotherapy, patients should be carefully monitored since further treatment will always be required, although sometimes only after many months or years. If treatment is discontinued following a well-documented response, it may be worth reinstituting the same therapy at the point of relapse since a second response is often seen. Relapse is usually detectable by a rise in the monoclonal Ig band, although some patients become symptomatic again without such a rise. Further supportive therapy with blood transfusion, antibiotics or palliative radiotherapy is often required if the patient becomes anaemic, or develops infections or painful bony lesions.

Second-line chemotherapy in myeloma remains unsatisfactory, although successes have been claimed with combinations of doxorubicin, vincristine, nitrosoureas and other agents [7]. This also applies in the 25% of patients who are unresponsive when first treated ('primary chemoresistance'). Responses to secondary chemotherapy are usually of short duration, at the cost of inflicting more undesirable side-effects than are seen with melphalan–prednisolone. In an elderly population, careful judgement is always required before considering such treatment and it is important to establish that no further response can be obtained with first-line chemotherapy. The recent use of thalidomide as a second-line treatment in relapsed myeloma has given this controversial agent a new role [16]. It is capable of reducing serum and urine paraprotein levels, and can be taken orally at a daily dose of 200 mg but increasing to 800 mg in tolerant patients. Toxicity is mostly mild, at least at lower doses (below 600 mg). This antiangiogenic agent may well have a place as maintenance oral therapy in myeloma: studies are currently in progress.

Radiotherapy

Radiotherapy is of great value in multiple myeloma and is often required as part of the initial treatment, particularly for patients who present with painful bone deposits in the vertebrae or long bones, especially if there is a likelihood of pathological fracture or cord compression [9]. Radiotherapy is the most important modality in myelomatous spinal cord compression, either alone or in combination with surgical decompression. Magnetic resonance imaging (MRI) scanning should be performed to define the extent of the compression, and treatment should be started early at the onset of radicular pain. Radiotherapy is often combined with internal fixation, particularly where a weight-bearing long bone is affected by lytic deposits. Since myeloma deposits are relatively radiosensitive, large doses are rarely required [9].

Success has been claimed with systemic or hemi-body irradiation (HBI) in myeloma [17], particularly in patients with symptomatic relapses unresponsive to standard chemotherapy. With HBI, pulmonary complications are unusual if the dose to the upper half of the body is kept below 8 Gy. Overall median survival with this technique is 12 months in drug-resistant cases (with many surviving beyond 2 years), comparable with second-line chemotherapy regimens but generally more acceptable. However, HBI cannot be recommended as first-line therapy to consolidate a chemotherapy remission.

A further recent advance has been the use of pamidronate, clodronate and other bisphosphonate agents to protect against skeletal complications and improve the quality of life in patients with advanced stages of disease [18]. In an MRC study of over 500 patients assessing the potential of oral clodronate as part of primary management, several benefits were noted [19]. Fewer patients receiving clodronate developed vertebral or other pathological fractures, height loss was reduced and hypercalcaemia was also less frequent. The authors recommended that treatment with clodronate should be instigated early in the course of the disease.

Prognosis

Patients with myeloma experience remissions and relapses requiring careful judgement for optimal choice and timing of therapy. Some survive over 5 years, requiring little in the way of chemotherapy, but repeated courses of radiotherapy and general support measures. Such patients usually have a low tumour burden based on simple criteria (Table 27.2). Retrospective analyses have shown that tumour burden is a good predictor of response and survival [9,10]. Median survival in the best groups is approximately 5 years, compared with only 6 months in the worst (Fig. 27.5). Since patients with myeloma often develop renal failure, it is not surprising that simple renal function is generally regarded as the most important prognostic criterion at diagnosis, although in recent years more weight has been given to total tumour mass, initial β_2 mi-

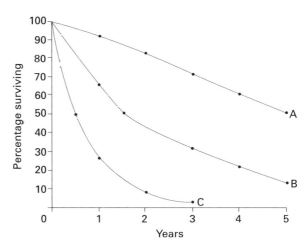

Fig. 27.5 Prognosis in myeloma related to tumour mass.

croglobulin level and number of bone lesions. Apart from disease recurrence and renal dysfunction, other myeloma complications result from progressive pancytopenia both from crowding of normal elements by abnormal plasma cells, and from therapy. Anaemia (often requiring repeated transfusion), infection and thrombocytopenia with bleeding are all common. Occasionally, infection, renal failure and hypercalcaemia may become totally resistant to treatment.

Solitary plasmacytoma [20]

This single-site plasma cell lesion occurs in either bone (common sites including vertebrae, clavicles, sternum or skull) or soft tissue (particularly nasal or oral cavity, bowel or bronchus). The typical histological picture is of malignant plasma cell infiltration, as in myeloma. In many patients, no other evidence of myeloma develops provided adequate local treatment with radiotherapy is given. However, solitary plasmacytoma can be the initial manifestation of myeloma; these patients should be carefully investigated since a proportion with apparently solitary lesions actually have multiple myeloma at the outset. A proportion of patients with solitary plasmacytomas will undoubtedly develop myeloma later, although latent periods of several years are not unusual. Progression is more common in those who present with a plasmacytoma in bone than in those where the site is extramedullary. There is no proven benefit in aggressive chemotherapy for solitary plasmacytomas to prevent the development of generalized myeloma. One-third of patients remain disease-free for 10 years or more, the remainder developing myeloma within a median time period of 2–3 years. Non-secretory disease and persistence of myeloma-specific protein after local treatment are both important adverse prognostic features [21].

Monoclonal gammopathy of unknown significance [22]

There are many diseases in which a monoclonal Ig band is found but without evidence of a plasma cell neoplasm (Table 27.4). The commonest cause, and the one which creates greatest diagnostic confusion, is MGUS, which is a disease of the elderly. It is common, with a prevalence of 0.5% in adults over 40 years and 3% over 70 years of age; it accounts for 40% of all paraproteinaemias. The monoclonal Ig concentration is usually less than 30 g/l. A large majority (85%) have an IgG paraprotein. Without other abnormalities in plasma proteins or symptoms of the kind found in patients with multiple myeloma. Bence-Jones protein is occasionally found. The ESR is usually raised. MGUS requires no treatment, although it clearly predisposes to myeloma. In one series, for example, 22 patients with MGUS went on to develop multiple myeloma at a median time interval of just under 10 years after initial recognition of the M protein. Long-term (30-year) follow-up has confirmed that myeloma develops in up to 16% of those with MGUS, with an annual actuarial rate of 0.8% [7].

Macroglobulinaemia

This group of conditions is characterized by the production of monoclonal IgM (Table 27.4). The correct diagnosis may prove elusive and require months or years of careful assessment as the disease process gradually develops and becomes more clear-cut, particularly in patients with slowly-evolving IgM-producing non-Hodgkin's lymphoma, in whom the paraprotein elevation may precede lymphadenopathy or other lymphoma-related symptoms, or may even masquerade as a genuine case of myeloma.

Benign macroglobulinaemia follows a similar course to other forms of MGUS (see above).

Cold agglutinin disease is a disease of the elderly in which patients suffer vascular disturbances in the extremities due to intracapillary red-cell agglutination in parts of the body exposed to cold. A deep blue–violet discoloration may occur (acrocyanosis) which may lead to gangrene. A moderate haemolysis is usually present, but physical examination is usually normal. The disease is due to a monoclonal IgM which has the property of being a cold agglutinin. If simple measures—gloves or mittens and warm boots—are inadequate, treatment with alkylating agents can be helpful.

Waldenström's macroglobulinaemia (see also p. 413)

This condition, typically occurring in the elderly, is characterized by marrow infiltration with lymphoid cells which have the appearance of an intermediate form between lymphocytes and plasma cells (lymphoplasmacytoid). Monoclonal lymphocytes are present in both blood and marrow, and the morphology is suggestive of a differentiating B-cell neoplasm. There is often an enlargement of lymph nodes, liver and spleen. Unlike IgM myeloma, bone lesions are very uncommon, although diffuse osteoporosis may occur. Monoclonal IgM, is often produced in very large amounts, sometimes producing hyperviscosity.

The patient typically presents with ill-health and weakness, often with night sweats. Symptoms of hyperviscosity may predominate, with headache, mental confusion, retinal haemorrhages and renal impairment. The macroglobulin may produce haemolytic anaemia or act as a cold agglutinin, producing haemorrhage by interaction with platelets and clotting factors. Purpura and bleeding are not infrequent. Investigations reveal anaemia, variable thrombocytopenia, a raised serum IgM and occasionally immune paresis.

The disease is usually only slowly progressive and, in the absence of symptoms, treatment can be withheld. Chlorambucil or cyclophosphamide, usually produce regression of lymphadenopathy and a fall in IgM levels. Fludarabine is also effective but immunosuppressive. Steroids are of little value, but plasmapheresis will produce reduction of viscosity and may be essential if clinical hyperviscosity is present, until chemotherapy has reduced IgM production. Prognosis is variable, but average survival is 3–4 years. In aggressive cases, combination chemotherapy as for myeloma may be valuable.

Heavy chain diseases

These diseases are lymphocyte neoplasms in which there is production of incomplete heavy chains of Ig, without light chains. The first patient was described by Franklin and coworkers in 1964 [23]. So far, only γ, α and μ heavy chain diseases have been described. Interestingly, each has distinct clinical features.

γ Heavy chain disease

γ Heavy chain disease usually affects elderly patients, producing lymphadenopathy, tonsillar enlargement, palatal oedema and hepatosplenomegaly. Bone lesions are unusual. Occasionally there are associated autoimmune diseases such as systemic lupus erythematosus or Sjögren's syndrome. Anaemia is common but marrow biopsy is not always diagnostic. The lymph nodes are sometimes replaced with lymphoplasmacytoid cells; the γ heavy chain fragment is found in serum or urine, and there may also be an immune paresis. Chemotherapy is usually minimally effective. Although this disease may occasionally regress without treatment, survival is usually less than 3 years.

α Heavy chain disease (see also Chapter 26, p. 419)

This is the commonest of the heavy chain diseases, chiefly found in young Mediterranean adults aged 20–30 years, predominantly in the Middle East and South America. It is a disease of the small bowel although occasionally the stomach, large bowel and postnasal space are affected. There is often a lengthy history of gastrointestinal disturbance, and some patients have been previously diagnosed as having immune proliferative disease of the small intestine. Because of massive lymphoid infiltration of the bowel, severe malabsorption and diarrhoea occur and although the histological appearances may initially not appear to be malignant, a true lymphoma usually develops.

α Heavy chains are present in the blood but their detection is difficult. The marrow is not involved and liver, spleen and lymph nodes are not enlarged. The diagnosis is made by small-bowel biopsy. Treatment with chemotherapy at the stage of frank lymphoma is only temporarily effective, and whole-abdominal irradiation has sometimes been used. Before this stage, treatment with oral tetracycline may produce lengthy remissions.

μ Heavy chain disease

In this very rare disease, μ heavy chains are found in the plasma. The clinical disease mimics long-standing chronic lymphatic leukaemia, or a non-Hodgkin's lymphoma, usually with marked visceral organomegaly, and treatment is similar to that used for these diseases.

References

1 Velez R, Beral V, Cuzick J. Increasing trends of multiple myeloma mortality in England and Wales 1950–79: are the changes real? *J Natl Cancer Inst* 1982; 69: 387–92.

2 Cuzick J. Radiation-induced myelomatosis. *N Engl J Med* 1981; 304: 204–10.

3 Cuzick J, Cooper EH, MacLennan ICM. The prognostic value of serum β_2 microglobulin compared with other presentation features in myelomatosis. *Br J Cancer* 1985; 52: 1–6.

4 Tricot G. New insights into the role of microenvironment in multiple myeloma. *Lancet* 2000; 355: 248–50.

5 Hallek M, Bergsagel DL, Anderson KC. Multiple myeloma: increasing evidence for a multistep transformation process. *Blood* 1998; 91: 3–21.

6 Mundy GR, Raisz LG, Cooper RA, Schechter GP, Salmon SE. Evidence for the secretion of an osteoclast stimulating factor in myeloma. *N Engl J Med* 1974; 291: 1041–6.

7 Gahrton G. Treatment of multiple myeloma. *Lancet* 1999; 353: 85–6.

8 Niesvisky R, Siegel D, Michaeli J. Biology and treatment of multiple myeloma. *Blood Rev* 1993; 7: 24–33.

9 Williams CD, Tobias JS. Current management of multiple myeloma. In: Tobias JS, Thomas PRM, eds. *Current Radiation Oncology*, Vol. 2. London: Edward Arnold, 1996: 294–319.

10 Alexanian R, Dimopoulos M. Drug therapy. the treatment of multiple myeloma. *N Engl J Med* 1994; 330: 484–9.

11 Bataille R, Hanousseau J-L. Medical progress: multiple myeloma. *N Engl J Med* 1997; 336: 1657–64.

12 MacLennan ICM, Drayson M, Dunn J. Current issues in cancer: Multiple myeloma. *Br Med J* 1994; 308: 1033–6.

13 Selby PJ, McElwain TJ, Nandi AC *et al.* Multiple myeloma treated with high dose intravenous melphalan. *Br J Haematol* 1987; 66: 55–62.

14 Attal M, Harousseau J-L, Stoppa A-M *et al.* A prospective randomized trial of autologous bone marrow transplantation and chemotherapy in multiple myeloma. *N Engl J Med* 1996; 335: 91–7.

15 Gahrton G, Tura S, Ljungman P *et al.* Allogeneic bone marrow transplantation in multiple myeloma. *N Engl J Med* 1991; 325: 1267–73.

16 Singhal S, Mehta J, Desikan R *et al.* Antitumour activity of thalidomide in refractory multiple myeloma. *N Engl J Med* 1999; 341: 156–7.

17 McSweeny EN, Tobias JS, Blackman G *et al.* Double hemibody irradiation in the management of relapsed and primary chemoresistant myeloma. *Clin Oncol* 1993; 5: 378–83.

18 Bloomfield DJ. Should bisphosphonates be part of the standard therapy of patients with multiple myeloma or bone metastases from other cancers? An evidence-based review. *J Clin Oncol* 1998; 16: 1218–25.

19 McCloskey EV, MacLennan ICM, Drayson MT *et al.* For the

MRC Working Party for Leukaemia in Adults. A randomized trial of the effect of clodronate on skeletal morbidity in multiple myeloma. *Br J Haematol* 1998; 100: 317–25.

20 Frassica DA, Frassica FJ, Schray MF *et al.* Solitary plasmacytoma of bone: the Mayo Clinic experience. *Int J Radiation Oncol Biol Physics* 1989; 16: 43–8.

21 Dimopoulos MA, Goldstein J, Fuller L *et al.* Curability of solitary bone plasmacytoma. *J Clin Oncol* 1992; 10: 587–90.

22 Kyle RA. Monoclonal gammopathy of undetermined significance and smouldering multiple myeloma. *Eur J Haematol* 1989; 51 (Suppl.): 70–5.

23 Franklin EC, Lowenstein J, Bigelow B, Meltzer M. Heavy chain disease. A new disorder of serum gammaglobulin. *Am J Med* 1964; 37: 332–50.

Leukaemias are neoplastic proliferations of white blood cells. Although uncommon, they have been the subject of detailed investigation because of the insights they give into aetiology and pathogenesis of the malignant process. The intensive chemotherapy which has been responsible for the increasing cure rate in acute leukaemia has served as an example for the treatment of other malignancies. Allogeneic bone marrow transplantation (BMT) was developed as a treatment for acute leukaemia. Autologous BMT has also been widely used in treatment of acute leukaemia and some of the findings have been of great importance in designing studies of autologous BMT in solid tumours. For these reasons, the principles of management are described in this chapter, but more detailed discussion and guidance is given in the references listed at the end of the chapter.

Incidence and aetiology [1]

In childhood (below 15 years of age), acute lymphoblastic leukaemia (ALL) accounts for 80% of all cases, acute myeloblastic leukaemia (AML) and its variants accounting for 17%, and chronic granulocytic leukaemia (CGL) approximately 3%. The death rate from acute leukaemia in the population is approximately seven per 100 000. The disease is slightly more common in males (with a male : female ratio of 3 : 2), and its incidence over the last decade appears to have been constant. Acute leukaemia is most common in the elderly (Figs 28.1a.b), and over 15 years of age 85% of cases are AML. In adults, AML and ALL have a very similar prognosis, but childhood ALL has different clinical features and a much better prognosis than adult ALL, or AML at any age.

A variety of aetiological factors have been implicated. Ionizing irradiation is leukaemogenic. Survivors of the Hiroshima and Nagasaki atom bombs have an increased risk of leukaemia, and the risk is greater for those who were near the centre of the explosions. The most frequent types are AML and CGL. The increased incidence began 2 years after the explosion and then declined after 6 years (Fig. 28.1c). Exposure to ionizing irradiation in pregnancy doubles the risk of childhood leukaemia as does irradiation for the treatment of ankylosing spondylitis.

Viral causes are not well established except for the role of the human T-cell leukaemia group of viruses (HTLV) prevalent in Japan and other Asian countries.

Benzene and some of its derivatives predispose to the development of both leukaemia and aplastic anaemia. An excess of leukaemia (predominantly AML) has been reported in refinery workers. Other occupations with increased risk appear to be welders and workers in industries using DDT.

An important cause of leukaemia is anticancer treatment itself. There is an increase in risk of leukaemia after treatment for Hodgkin's disease (see also Chapter 25, p. 399) and ovarian cancer[2]. The risk increases with time from treatment. There is a higher relative risk for young patients. In treatment-related leukaemia, typical chromosomal abnormalities occur of which the most consistent is translocation involving chromosome 11. This also occurs following benzene exposure. The region 11 band 23–32 appears to be consistently involved. The functional effect is to alter cell signalling and growth.

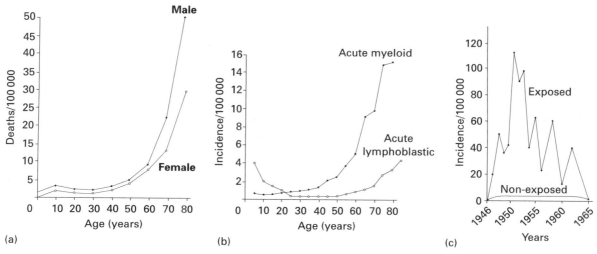

Fig. 28.1 Incidence of leukaemia: (a) age-specific death rates from leukaemia of all types in England (1979); (b) age-specific incidence rates of acute lymphoblastic and myeloblastic leukaemia (Third National Cancer Survey USA, 1969–71); (c) leukaemia incidence in Hiroshima from 1946 onwards, in exposed and non-exposed individuals. From [3] with permission.

Smoking increases the risk of leukaemia by 50%. The risk is mainly for AML and acute myelomonocytic leukaemia (AMML) (see below). The risk of childhood leukaemia is also probably increased in children whose mothers smoked marijuana or who were exposed to benzene and other solvents in pregnancy.

Certain constitutive abnormalities predispose to leukaemia. In Down's syndrome (trisomy 21) there is an increased risk of acute leukaemia—usually ALL in younger patients. Bloom's syndrome, Fanconi's anaemia and ataxia telangiectasia are all autosomal recessive diseases characterized by chromosome breakage and an increased risk of leukaemia. A defective DNA repair mechanism may be responsible; AML is the usual leukaemia in Fanconi's anaemia, and ALL in ataxia telangiectasia.

Pathogenesis

The clonal nature of leukaemia proliferation has been elegantly established by studies on patients who are heterozygous for glucose-6-phosphate dehydrogenase (G6PD). Leukaemic cells have been shown to express only one isozyme in heterozygotes for G6PD with chronic myeloblastic leukaemia (CML). Similar clonality has been shown in acute myeloid leukaemia [4].

The oncogenic event endows the clone with a proliferative advantage, because it is not subject to growth regula-

tion. The leukaemic mass increases, but this does not appear to be the sole reason for the suppression of normal haemopoiesis. In the process of clonal expansion somatic genetic instability gives rise to subclones with diverse features within the tumour.

These genetic changes *consequent* to the leukaemic process may themselves confer a growth stimulus. In CML there is a translocation between chromosomes 9 and 22 (t9;22) (q34;q11). This juxtaposes the *BCR* gene and the *ABL* gene: the fusion protein results is a tyrosine kinase that gives rise to phosphorylation of substrates involved in growth regulation. Several of the translocations in acute leukaemia result in expression of transcription factors which themselves regulate expression of other genes (see below).

The acute leukaemias

Pathology and classification [5]

Acute leukaemias often retain many of the cytoplasmic and membrane characteristics of their normal counterparts, so it is possible to relate the various types of acute leukaemia to a particular stage of myeloid or lymphoid maturation. A simplified scheme is shown in Fig. 28.2.

The diagnosis is made from blood and marrow films. In the typical case there are leukaemic blasts in the blood and the marrow is packed with uniform-looking blast cells.

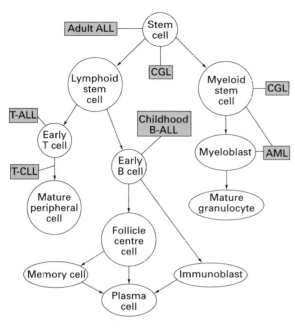

Fig. 28.2 Maturation of haemopoietic and lymphoid cells in relation to types of leukaemia.

Cases of ALL almost always show these appearances but in adult AML the leukaemic process may be much more subtle, with few blasts in the blood. The marrow must show over 30% of blasts for the diagnosis to be made with confidence. When there are less than 20% blasts the diagnosis of myelodysplastic state is usually made (see p. 446).

The acute leukaemias have been subdivided on morphological grounds using a scheme devised by a French–American–British study group [5]. An outline is given in Table 28.1.

In AML, the myeloblasts may contain Auer rods which are pink-staining rod-like inclusions which are probably aberrant forms of the cytoplasmic granules found in normal granulocyte precursors. These granules are often prominent in the cytoplasm in AML and are particularly frequent and often large in the M_3 variety (hypergranular promyelocytic leukaemia). In monocytic leukaemia (M_5) the blasts are large with abundant cytoplasm and in erythroleukaemia (M_6) there are erythroblasts and myeloblasts in the marrow.

The commonest form of ALL (L_1) is characterized by scanty cytoplasm and fewer nucleoli. In the less common form (L_2) the blasts are larger, with a larger nucleolus. This

Table 28.1 A morphological classification of acute leukaemia. (%) Indicates the proportions of the subtypes of acute leukaemia of myeloid and monocytic origins.

Myeloblastic leukaemia (55%)

M_0	Almost no differentiation. Antimyeloperoxidase staining (5% of cases) ?Worse prognosis
M_1	Poorly differentiated. Stains for myeloperoxidase. Auer rods (20% of cases)
M_2	Differentiated beyond promyelocyte. May show t(8;21) and B-cell antigens (30% of cases)

Promyelocytic leukaemia (10%)

M_3	Hypergranular, Auer rods, t(15;17)
M_3 (variant)	Granules absent but myeloperoxidase present

Myelomonocytic leukaemia (20%)

M_4	Granulocyte features but monocyte esterase present, urine lysozyme present. Monocytosis. E_0 variant shows eosinophilia

Monocytic leukaemia (15%)

M_5	Monocytic features (less in children), esterase positive, high white blood count, gum hypertrophy. Urine lysozyme present

Erythroleukaemia

M_6	Rare

Megakaryoblastic

M_7	Rare

Acute lymphoblastic leukaemia

L_1	Small monomorphic cells
L_2	Large heterogeneous cells
L_3	Burkitt-like

Table 28.2 Cytochemistry and lineage characteristics of acute leukaemia.

Phenotypic feature	Leukaemia
Sudan black	+AML −ALL
Myeloperoxidase	+AML −ALL
α-Naphthyl-butyrate esterase	+AML −ALL
Tdt expression	ALL (T and B)
Ig gene heavy chain rearrangement	(B) ALL
TCR gene arrangement	(T) ALL
Cytoplasmic or surface Ig	(B) ALL
TCR expression	(T) ALL

TCR, T-cell receptor; Tdt, a DNA polymerase measured by fluorescence or biochemically.

Table 28.3 Useful cellular markers in acute leukaemia.

Stem cells: tdt, HLA-DR, CD34
Myeloid: CD11, CD13, CD14, CD33
Monocytic: CD11, CD14
Megakaryocytic: CD17, AN51, J15
B cell: C10, CD19, CD20, CD24, tdt, SIg
T cell: CD2, cyCD3, CDS, CD7

Note. Several other markers may be used, and the panel of markers shown is an indication of those in wide use. The markers are, in any case, used in conjunction with morphological and clinical features.
cy, cytoplasmic; SIg, surface immunoglobulin; tdt, terminal deoxyribonucleotide transferase.

form, which is more common in adults, is more easily mistaken for AML and may account for some cases designated as undifferentiated leukaemia. The L_3 form is of large homogeneous cells with prominent nucleoli and basophilic cytoplasm resembling Burkitt's lymphoma cells.

Cytochemical stains help to determine the type of leukaemia if there is doubt. The commonly used stains are shown in Table 28.2. These stains may help to confirm the diagnosis in doubtful cases. In occasional instances of undifferentiated acute leukaemia, the cytochemical stains are unhelpful. In ALL in particular, these markers may help to distinguish common ALL from T-cell ALL and Burkitt's lymphoma (Table 28.3).

Immunological phenotype in leukaemia [6]

The normal maturation sequence of lymphoid and myeloid cells is accompanied by expression of cell surface and cytoplasmic proteins which can be detected by antibodies. In leukaemia this antigen expression can be used to 'phenotype' tumours which reflect different stages of maturation. Some of the subdivisions have little prognostic or therapeutic importance but they help in understanding the pathogenesis of leukaemia. An abbreviated summary is given in Table 28.3.

Chromosomal abnormalities in leukaemia
(Table 28.4)

A wide range of acquired karyotypic abnormalities have now been found in leukaemia and in recent years a more precise definition of the genes involved has become possible. Progress is being made in understanding how these genetic changes lead to the development of leukaemia. It seems likely that, as in other cancers, several sequential changes are necessary for the development of the full malignant characteristics.

In *CML* the Philadelphia (Ph′) chromosome is usually present. This is at chromosome 22q which has a reciprocal translocation from chromosome 9q. This moves the C-*abl* (tyrosine kinase) proto-oncogene from 9 to 22 and fuses it to a gene at the breakpoint cluster region (*bcr*). Production of fusion protein results in a 210-kDa protein in CML (and another, 185 kDa, in ALL). When CML undergoes blastic transformation (see below) further chromosomal abnormalities occur. Cases of CML which are Ph′-negative sometimes have a more restricted *abl–bcr* translocation which is not detected cytogenetically.

In AML and AMML there are specific chromosomal abnormalities associated with the different categories (M_1–M_7) described in Table 28.1. These are outlined in Table 28.4. This represents a very simplified summary of many different abnormalities in a rapidly changing field. In these leukaemias the leukaemic event occurs at the stem cell level and is followed by defective maturation.

In T-cell ALL breakpoints occur at 14q11 which is the site of the T-cell receptor genes (α) and (β) and 7q 33–36 (β T-cell receptor). Translocation of oncogenes such as C-*myc* (t(8;14) (q24;q11)) to this site, similar to that found for immunoglobulin (Ig) genes in Burkitt's lymphoma, may result in disordered cell growth. Another T-cell specific translocation is t(11;14). Chromosome 9p is frequently deleted or translocated in ALL and is especially associated with lymphomatous clinical features. Five per cent of children and 25% of adults with ALL are Ph′-positive, associated with a poor prognosis.

In leukaemia some of the gene translocations and deletions described above involve oncogenes, which may thereby be inappropriately activated or mutated leading to disordered growth. Thus, the receptor for colony-

Table 28.4 Common chromosomal abnormalities in leukaemia.

Leukaemia	Abnormality
CML	t(9;22)(q34.1;q11.2) Demonstrable karyotypically in 80% of cases. More restricted translocation in many of the remainder. In ALL this translocation has a very poor prognosis
AML	
M_2 (M_1 less frequently)	t(8;21)(q22;q211). Good prognosis
M_3	t(15;17)(q22;q11). Good prognosis
M_4	Various translocations involving 11q23, inversion of 16 (good prognosis)
M_5	t(9;11), other translocations of 11q23. Poor prognosis
T-cell ALL	t(11;14) (p13;q11). Poor prognosis t(8;14)(q24;q11). Poor prognosis
B-cell ALL	t(8;14)(q24;q321). Poor prognosis t(1;19)(q23;p13) in pre-B-cell ALL 12p12 breakpoint, 6q–. Common findings
Undifferentiated or AUL	t(4;11)(q21;q23). Very poor prognosis
CLL	Trisomy 12. Worst prognosis Deletion 13q14. Worst prognosis

stimulating factor (CSF-1) is the product of the C-*fms* gene and is expressed in acute non-lymphocyte leukaemia. The intracytoplasmic domain has protein tyrosine kinase activity. CD20 (Table 28.3) is a B-cell protein with signal transduction properties. Both of the fusion proteins resulting from the *abl–bcr* translocation in CML and ALL (above) have tyrosine kinase activity and are leukaemogenic in mice. *p53* is frequently mutated in CML and the resultant protein has defective function, being unable to serve as a check to entry into cell cycle. The AML associated t(8;21) translocation blocks the action of a protein complex (*CBFB–AML1*) that activates several genes. This repression is also achieved by the Inv (16) mutation found in AML. Both are associated with a better prognosis. These examples indicate that the result of the genetic instability is to give rise to proteins which may alter growth and differentiation in the cell.

Clinical features and management

Acute leukaemia in childhood

The disease usually presents at the age of 4–5 years. The symptoms are due to marrow infiltration causing anaemia, thrombocytopenia, infection and bone pain, especially in long bones. As with other forms of acute leukaemia, the history is of a few weeks of malaise, sometimes with fever even in the absence of obvious infection. Oral and pharyngeal ulceration may occur. Although petechiae are often found on examination, presentation with other haemorrhagic phenomena is less common.

On examination the child is usually pale. There may be lymph node enlargement, splenomegaly and slight hepatic enlargement. The bones may be tender on pressure, particularly over the sternum. Skin petechiae are common (and may also be seen on the palate) as are haemorrhages in the eye, either in the retina or as larger subhyaloid haemorrhages. Skin infiltration with leukaemia is uncommon and takes the form of plaques of tumour of purple colour. In the mouth there may be mucosal ulceration and gingivitis.

Occasionally the patient has symptoms of meningeal involvement at presentation. This usually manifests itself as headache, vomiting and neck stiffness. Papilloedema may be present. Cranial nerve palsies may occur as in other forms of malignant meningitis.

Investigation usually reveals anaemia, thrombocytopenia and an elevated total white blood count (WBC) with numerous lymphoblasts. In 40% of cases, the total WBC is not elevated but blasts are usually present. 'Aleukaemic leukaemia' is a term used to describe those cases where blasts are not present in the blood film (approximately 5% of cases). In all cases a bone marrow examination is essential, with cytochemical and immunological studies when possible (as outlined above). A chest X-ray is usually normal, but in T-cell ALL may show a mediastinal mass due to thymic enlargement. This form of ALL is common in adolescent boys. Bone X-rays are not infrequently abnormal and the typical abnormality is of radiolucent bands in the metaphyseal region. Diffuse demineralization also occurs, and discrete osteolytic lesions.

Biochemical investigation may show a raised uric acid

due to rapid proliferation and death of leukaemic cells. A lumbar puncture may show leukaemic cells even though there may be no clinical evidence of disease in the central nervous system (CNS).

REMISSION INDUCTION AND CONSOLIDATION (Fig. 28.3)
There is a risk of death in the first few weeks during induction therapy. This risk can be minimized by supportive measures at, or before, the start of chemotherapy. Anaemia must be corrected. If the kidneys are enlarged or the creatinine raised, the risk of tumour lysis syndrome is greatly increased and steps must be taken to prevent and treat this complication (see Chapter 8, p. 120). With more intensive regimens, such as those used for B-cell ALL and AML, platelet support will be necessary. Infections must be detected early and treated vigorously (see also adult acute leukaemia—supportive measures). In common ALL haematological and clinical remission is induced with vincristine, prednisolone and 1-asparaginase. Vigorous hydration, allopurinol and urinary alkalinization are necessary in the induction period. With this regimen 95% of patients remit within 3 weeks. Children with B-cell ALL do not do well with this standard therapy and more inten-

sive protocols are needed using cyclophosphamide, cytosine arabinoside, anthracyclines and methotrexate.

In AML, remission is induced with cytosine and daunorubicin. Recent trials are assessing the value of using additional drugs such as thioguanine and etoposide. Myelosuppression is much more severe with these regimens and skilled supportive care is needed.

In ALL, following the induction of complete or partial remission, the treatment is intensified by using drugs such as asparaginase, an anthracycline (daunorubicin or doxorubicin), cytosine arabinoside and cyclophosphamide [7]. Methotrexate in high dose may add to the durability of remission. These drugs are myelosuppressive, but at this stage the bone marrow has recovered following the elimination of most of the leukaemic population. Intensification for AML has posed great problems in management. The results for intensive conventional chemotherapy have improved at the time when allogeneic transplantation has been introduced with impressive current results. Many children will not have a donor, which leaves only the alternatives of a matched unrelated donor for patients at high risk of relapse after obtaining remission such as those with monosomy 7, or autologous BMT (usually given after several cycles of intensive consolidation therapy). Trials of these different approaches are in progress.

MAINTENANCE THERAPY IN CHILDHOOD ACUTE LYMPHOBLASTIC LEUKAEMIA
The duration of 'maintenance' chemotherapy has not been defined. With more intensive induction and consolidation regimens, it seems probable that prolonged maintenance therapy will be less necessary. 6-Mercaptopurine and methotrexate are the most widely used drugs, often in conjunction with vincristine and prednisolone. In cases with poor prognostic features (Table 28.5), more aggressive regimens have been used as intermittent pulsed therapy. At the end of treatment a testicular biopsy is sometimes performed, if prophylactic irradiation has not been given, to detect occult disease. Relapse at any site is unusual beyond 1 year after treatment has stopped.

PROPHYLAXIS OF CENTRAL NERVOUS SYSTEM DISEASE
The importance of CNS prophylaxis was demonstrated in the early 1970s. Before that time, infiltration of the meninges by leukaemic cells was responsible for relapse in half of all cases. The lymphoblasts infiltrate the meninges diffusely and extend to the spinal meninges and sheaths of cranial nerves. Clinical presentation is with symptoms of raised intracranial pressure: headache, nausea and vomit-

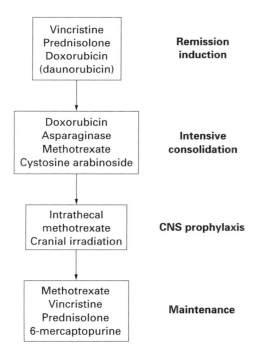

Fig. 28.3 Outline of management of acute lymphoblastic leukaemia in childhood.

ing, with a stiff neck and papilloedema. Convulsions may occur and cranial nerve palsies (particularly VII, VI and III) often develop, and may be the first sign. The diagnosis is made on lumbar puncture when leukaemic blasts are found. The risk of coning from the lumbar puncture is small.

Prophylactic treatment greatly diminishes the frequency of CNS relapse. Nowadays the usual regimen is cranial irradiation (18 Gy in 8–10 fractions over 2 weeks) together with intrathecal methotrexate ($10 \, mg/m^2 \times 4$ over the same period). However, the long-term consequences of CNS radiation have been of sufficient concern to lead to attempts to dispense with prophylactic irradiation [8]. The results are not easy to interpret. It seems that for 'standard risk' ALL (WBC below $50 \times 10^9/l$) intrathecal methotrexate is adequate prophylaxis but that CNS radiation is necessary for all the higher-risk cases. It is not clear if additional drugs (such as cytosine arabinoside) confer additional advantage. Established CNS disease (which now occurs in 5–10% of cases) is treated by intrathecal methotrexate twice weekly with cranial irradiation to a higher dose (often 24 Gy over 2–3 weeks), together with, or followed by, spinal irradiation. Lasting control of CNS disease is, however, unusual. Intrathecal cytosine arabinoside is also used in patients who are thought to be resistant to methotrexate.

TREATMENT AND PROPHYLAXIS OF TESTICULAR DISEASE

Relapse in the testis is common and is one reason for the worse prognosis of ALL in boys. Testicular relapse may be less frequent in regimens including high-dose methotrexate. It occurs in about 25% of prepubertal boys but is less common in older children. Relapse may not be clinically apparent at first — swelling and hardness being late signs. It is usually bilateral, and testicular biopsy shows peritubular leukaemic infiltration. Treatment is by testicular irradiation, generally to a dose of the order of 24 Gy in 2–3 weeks. The role of prophylactic testicular irradiation is still undecided.

TREATMENT ON RELAPSE

If children relapse during initial or maintenance treatment or up to 1 year after cessation of therapy, the outlook is poor and BMT is considered (see below). Following later relapses, remission can usually be reinduced by intensive therapy and may be durable. This may not be the case with modern more intensive regimens, which would then imply that BMT will need to be considered for this group as well [9].

Allogeneic BMT has been used in an attempt to im-

prove results in childhood ALL when the prognosis is poor. The procedure does not have a proven survival advantage over chemotherapy in standard-risk ALL.

The following clinical situations have been regarded as indications for consideration of allogeneic BMT in childhood ALL: second or third remission, especially if relapse occurred while on maintenance therapy; and poor-prognosis cases such as those with t(4;11) acute undifferentiated leukaemia (AUL), t(8;14) B-cell ALL, and Ph'-positive ALL. These children may benefit from BMT in first remission.

Results of BMT in first remission in high-risk cases have been promising, with 55% 3-year relapse-free survival. In standard-risk cases in second remission, 65% 5-year relapse-free survival is reported. The results depend greatly on the factors used to select patients. Autologous BMT or stem cell transplantation has, in general, been rather less impressive than allogeneic, possibly because of marrow contamination but also because some high-dose regimens have not included total-body irradiation (TBI). Newer treatment regimens of combined chemotherapy and TBI may improve results of autologous BMT. Allogeneic BMT has a greater mortality than autologous, partly because of graft-versus-host disease. Conversely, graft-versus-leukaemia may improve results.

If relapse occurs in the CNS despite prophylaxis, a further remission may be obtained with more intrathecal methotrexate or craniospinal irradiation. Methotrexate can also be given through an Ommaya or Rickham reservoir which allows direct delivery of the drug into the cerebral ventricular system. Systemic relapse is inevitable, and further systemic treatment is usually given.

PROGNOSIS

The important prognostic features are given in Table 28.5. Survival is better in girls than in boys and is shown in Fig. 28.4.

Acute lymphoblastic leukaemia in adults

The clinical features are similar to those in children except for the greater percentage of patients with a mediastinal mass. Above the age of 12 years, ALL has a significantly worse prognosis. More cases (20%) are Ph'-positive and at least some cases represent CGL presenting in the acute phase. Only 30% are common ALL, 12% are B-cell ALL, 8% T-cell ALL and 30% of cases are unclassifiable (null cell ALL). Although the long-term prognosis appears to be as poor as in adult AML, adult ALL is usually regarded separately because CNS relapse is common.

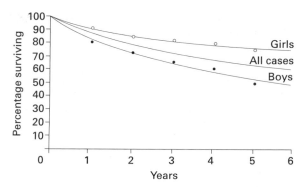

Fig. 28.4 Survival in acute lymphoblastic leukaemia in children.

Table 28.5 Adverse prognostic features in childhood ALL.

1 Cytogenetics
2 CNS disease at presentation
3 Early marrow relapse
4 Testicular relapse
5 T-cell phenotype

The treatment of adult ALL is similar to the childhood disease with the following modifications.

1 Induction treatment is more intense, with regimens which include anthracyclines and asparaginase.

2 More intensive 'consolidation' therapy with cytosine arabinoside and anthracyclines, and recently teniposide.

3 Testicular relapse is less frequent and prophylactic treatment is not given.

Currently, intensive induction regimens in unselected cases produce complete remission in 70–80% of cases with 40% in remission at 3 years [10]. Poor prognostic factors include: age over 60, WBC > 30 000, late achievement of complete response, Ph'-positivity, mature or precursor B-cell phenotype, and abnormal cytogenetics. Prophylaxis of the CNS may, in the future, be avoided for some patients since the high risk of CNS relapse is in patients with B-cell ALL, elevated lactate dehydrogenase or alkaline phosphatase and a high proliferative fraction [11]. Treatment strategies adapted to the prognostic category are being introduced, for example very intensive induction regimens for mature B-cell ALL.

Allogeneic BMT is the preferred treatment in first remission in the high-risk groups defined above. Some centres would consider all first remission ALL over the age of 21 as an indication for BMT on the grounds that the prognosis is worse in adults than in children. Ph'-positive leukaemias show a high rate of remission in first relapse with the use of the signal transduction inhibitor ST1571 (see p. 450).

Following second remission the results of allogeneic BMT are clearly superior since survival rates of 30–40% are obtained. Results with autologous BMT are also clearly superior to chemotherapy alone in second relapse, but not proven to be so in first relapse. Peripheral blood stem cell supported transplant may, however, prove to be the preferred treatment in this situation.

Acute myeloid leukaemia in adults [12]

In most cases the history and physical findings are similar to those in ALL (see above). Bone pain and radiological evidence of bone infiltration are less common in AML, and CNS disease is very unusual at presentation. Lymph node enlargement is also less frequently found than in ALL.

In myelomonocytic (M_4, Table 28.1) and monocytic (M_5) leukaemia, gum infiltration is common, leading to gum 'hypertrophy'. Skin infiltrates are common in these forms and associated features are a high total WBC and high serum and urinary lysozyme which is liberated from the tumour.

Pallor, hepatosplenomegaly, purpura and bone tenderness are the most common physical signs. The WBC is often elevated, with myeloblasts usually demonstrable. Confirmation of the diagnosis is made by bone marrow examination and the use of special stains when appropriate (Table 28.2).

TREATMENT

Remission induction The aim is to induce a complete marrow and clinical remission. To do this, intensive therapy is normally needed with blood, platelet and antibiotic support during the period of hypoplasia which is the inevitable accompaniment of the chemotherapy (see Chapter 8). Combinations of high-dose cytosine arabinoside and daunorubicin are used (Fig. 28.5). Idarubicin and mitoxantrone are possibly more effective than daunorubicin. The blast count usually falls rapidly in the blood and bone marrow with suppression of normal haematopoiesis. The mortality of this stage is now about 10% when skilled support is available. During the hypoplastic period further cytotoxic therapy is often needed if the marrow still shows disease, and this intensifies the hypoplasia and increases the risk.

The induction of remission is therefore a highly skilled

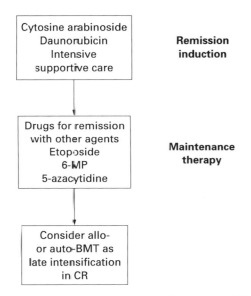

Cytosine arabinoside Daunorubicin Intensive supportive care	**Remission induction**
↓	
Drugs for remission with other agents Etoposide 6-MP 5-azacytidine	**Maintenance therapy**
↓	
Consider allo- or auto-BMT as late intensification in CR	

Fig. 28.5 Outline of management of acute myeloblastic leukaemia.

procedure, best carried out in a unit where the nursing and medical staff are experienced in the problems of bone marrow failure. Careful attention to fluid and electrolyte problems is essential, as is prompt diagnosis and treatment of infection (see Chapter 8). Prophylactic treatment of the CNS is not usually given.

Supportive care Blood product support is essential during the intensive phase of remission induction. As discussed in Chapter 8, platelet transfusion has been a major advance in prevention of death from haemorrhage. The indications for platelet transfusion are discussed on p. 113.

Blood transfusions are essential for anaemia but should be avoided if possible if the WBC is very high (over $100 \times 10^9/l$) because leucostasis in cerebral vessels may occur. Chemotherapy and, if necessary, leucopheresis, should be used to reduce the WBC before transfusion. The use of haemopoietic growth factors is described in Chapter 8. During intensive treatment an indwelling subcutaneously tunnelled intravenous line (Hickman line) is of great help.

To prevent infection patients should be instructed to wash carefully, with particular attention to the perineal region. Dental and oral sepsis should be treated promptly. Food should be cooked and clean — fresh salads are best avoided. Regular examination of the mouth, skin and perineum are essential and cultures should be taken

regularly to detect pathogens such as *Klebsiella* or *Pseudomonas*. Cotrimoxazole is given prophylactically in some units, and it gives protection against the opportunistic pathogen *Pneumocystis carinii*.

Most patients will develop fever at some stage during the period of neutropenia. The management of infection in the neutropenic patient is discussed in Chapter 8. Often no bacteriological diagnosis is made. Most fatal infections are from Gram-negative organisms. Infections occur around Hickman lines, particularly with skin commensals such as *Staphylococcus epidermidis* or *S. aureus*. Vancomycin and teicoplanin are very useful antibiotics for treatment of this complication.

Opportunistic infections cause considerable diagnostic difficulty in a patient with fever and pulmonary infiltration (see Chapter 8). Fungal infection, *Pneumocystis carinii* and, less commonly, cytomegalovirus and other viral infections must be considered.

After blood cultures have been taken at the onset of fever, broad-spectrum intravenous antibiotic therapy is begun. Such regimens usually include an aminoglycoside and a cephalosporin, and metronidazole is often added, particularly if there is clinical deterioration after 24 h. If there are pulmonary infiltrates, treatment with high-dose cotrimoxazole for *Pneumocystis*, amphotericin B for fungal infection and aciclovir for herpes simplex, should be considered.

Results of treatment and new approaches Complete remission occurs in 75% of patients below the age of 60 and 50% above that age. Mitozantrone, etoposide and higher-dose cytosine arabinoside appear to improve remission rates and are incorporated into most recent protocols. More intensive maintenance regimens are also under investigation and may prolong remission duration [13]. Toxicity is increased and intensification is difficult in the elderly. Worse outcome occurs in patients over 60 years, those with a high WBC and poor performance status and patients who have developed AML after a myelodysplastic (9:11) syndrome. Cytogenetic changes are prognostically important: t(q;11), 5q, inv3, are adverse and t(8;21) is favourable (Table 28.4). Overall, 10-year disease-free survival is about 30%.

Although the results of intensive conventional chemotherapy in AML have improved the long-term outlook is still poor for most patients. Approaches using BMT (especially allogeneic) are not appropriate for many patients as AML is mainly a disease of the elderly. Allogeneic BMT is usually carried out in first complete response and, in historical comparisons with conventional treatment, seems to reduce leukaemic relapse by 20%. Some of this benefit may be due to graft-versus-leukaemia effect. Recent studies have indicated a benefit for allogeneic BMT with long-term disease-free survival in about 50% of patients [14]. Against this must be set the acute mortality especially from allogeneic BMT. Autologous BMT has been shown to reduce the risk of relapse [15]. The procedure is more widely applicable than allogeneic BMT, since matched donors are not needed. In allogeneic BMT, high-dose cyclophosphamide and TBI are usually used. In autologous BMT, regimens may be based on chemotherapy alone. Haemopoietic growth factors appear to allow increased treatment intensity without stimulating leukaemic proliferation.

Treatment of relapse Although induction of a second remission is possible in patients who have relapsed after treatment has been discontinued, these remissions are usually short-lived. For young adults and those with favourable prognostic indicators there is a chance of cure by allogenic or autologous BMT usually preceded by re-induction chemotherapy.

Central nervous system relapse is treated in a similar fashion to ALL (see above).

Treatment of acute promyelocytic leukaemia (M_3) Acute promyelocytic leukaemia (APL) accounts for 10% of AML. Induction of remission is complicated by disseminated intravascular coagulation when cytotoxic chemotherapy is given. This seems to be due to release of a procoagulant (cysteine proteinase). The cells differentiate *in vitro* in response to all-*trans*-retinoic acid (ATRA). When patients with APL are treated with ATRA the bone marrow slowly (over 2 months) returns to normal (with loss of the typical t(15;17) karyotype), and disseminated intravascular coagulation does not occur [16]. Side-effects include dry skin, headache and potentially fatal hyperleucocytosis (which may cause pulmonary oedema). Patients relapse after 6 months. New trials suggest that chemotherapy in addition to ATRA will improve results. The breakpoint of t(15;17) is near the gene for the retinoic acid α receptor on chromosome 17 and the use of ATRA is only successful when this translocation is present.

Myelodysplastic syndromes and secondary leukaemia [17]

These include a range of disorders, usually of unknown aetiology, characterized by one or more peripheral cytopenias, with a cellular marrow showing morphological evidence of disordered haematopoiesis. This may include ring sideroblasts, hypogranular polymorphs with abnormally segmented nuclei, and increased numbers of early myeloid cells. Myelodysplastic syndromes (MDS) have an inherent tendency to progress to acute leukaemia.

Myelodysplastic syndromes are classified according to the major abnormality present, but there is often more than one abnormality and precise categorization may be difficult and arbitrary. When ring sideroblasts are the prominent abnormality a diagnosis of sideroblastic anaemia is usually made, and when blast cells are present in modest numbers the disease is labelled as refractory anaemia with an excess of blasts. This has a particular propensity to develop into acute leukaemia. Increasing numbers of patients with ALL secondary to MDS are now being seen. Some are the late effects of chemotherapy for a previous cancer. These leukaemias are characteristically difficult to treat. In younger patients, remission may be obtained with cytosine arabinoside and doxorubicin in 60% of cases, but the relapse rate is high and the toxicity of treatment is considerable. The role of allogenic BMT is not yet fully evaluated.

The chronic leukaemias

There are two main forms of chronic leukaemia: chronic lymphocytic (lymphatic) leukaemia (CLL) and CGL. The former is exceptionally rare below 40 years of age, while the latter can occur at any age, although it is commoner in middle and old age.

Chronic lymphocytic leukaemia [18]

This disease is nearly always a chronic neoplastic proliferation of small B lymphocytes. These B cells are probably early in the B-cell differentiation pathway [19]. The immunoglobulin classes IgM and IgD are present in small amounts on the cell membrane, but no cytoplasmic Ig can be detected. Free light chains can be found in the urine in many patients. Since the tumour is a clonal proliferation, each cell bears the same Ig molecule with the same type of light chain. The phenotype of the B cell is similar to B cells of the mantle zone of lymph nodes. Chromosomal abnormalities (Table 28.4) include trisomy 12 and deletion of 13q14 (the retinoblastoma gene). Both are adverse prognostically. The *bcl*-2 gene is overexpressed resulting in an inhibition of apoptosis.

Clinical features

Over 25% of patients have no symptoms at the time of diagnosis. The disease is discovered because of lymphocytosis noted on an incidental blood count or because enlargement of lymph nodes or spleen is detected on physical examination. In other patients the symptoms are due to noticeably enlarged lymph nodes in the neck or elsewhere, fatigue and malaise due to mild anaemia, infection due to immunosuppression, pain from an enlarged spleen or bruising and bleeding due to thrombocytopenia.

Physical examination reveals painless enlarged lymph nodes which are rubbery and mobile. Many node groups are affected (unlike most lymphomas) and the spleen is often palpable. Massive splenomegaly is unusual at presentation and splenic infarction is less frequent than in CGL.

The diagnosis is made on the blood count. This shows a raised total WBC which may even be as high as 500–1000 $\times 10^9/l$ but is more usually below $100 \times 10^9/l$. The diagnosis must be considered when the lymphocyte count is above $10 \times 10^9/l$. The differential count shows a great excess of small lymphocytes which usually have a normal morphology but which are sometimes larger with less mature-looking nuclei. Cleaved nuclei suggest the diagnosis of follicular-centre cell lymphoma rather than CLL (see Chapter 26). Prolymphocytic leukaemia cells (see p. 448) are larger with more cytoplasm and a distinct prominent nucleolus. Hairy cells (see p. 449) are usually easily distinguished. Occasionally it may be necessary to undertake a lymph node biopsy. In CLL, this shows diffuse infiltration with small well-differentiated lymphocytes. A marrow aspiration and biopsy shows a marked diffuse increase in small well-differentiated lymphocytes in CLL. A blood film is all that is necessary for diagnosis in the great majority of cases.

Occasionally, the lymphocytosis is slight and it is then not clear if the patient has a reactive lymphocytosis or CLL. This problem can now often be solved by examining the cell surface for light chain restriction, and the presence of CD5. In CLL, all the cells are identical and are restricted to one light chain type (κ or λ), while both light chain types are represented in a reactive lymphocytosis.

Anaemia is variable and, when present, indicates extensive marrow infiltration. Autoimmune haemolytic anaemia sometimes occurs. The platelet count may be low as a result of marrow infiltration, hypersplenism, chemotherapy and, occasionally, autoimmune thrombocytopenia. There is suppression of Ig synthesis in many patients, with marked hypogammaglobulinaemia which leads to increased susceptibility to infection.

Staging

It may seem contradictory to stage a leukaemia (see Chapter 4). However, it has been shown that a simple staging classification, based on clinical findings and blood count, has prognostic value. This staging notation is shown in Table 28.6. The worse prognostic categories (III–IV) have greater degrees of marrow failure at presentation.

Treatment [18]

There is no cure for CLL. Treatment undoubtedly produces symptomatic benefit and may prolong survival. This comes from reduction of the leukaemia mass and consequent improvement in marrow function. Clear indications for treatment include troublesome symptoms of fatigue, night sweats and fever, greatly enlarged nodes especially if causing pressure, splenic discomfort and marrow failure causing anaemia and thrombocytopenia. Most patients requiring treatment will have stage II–IV disease.

DRUG TREATMENT

Alkylating agents (especially chlorambucil) are the mainstay of treatment. Steroids (usually prednisolone) are

Table 28.6 Staging of CLL.

Stage		Definition	Median survival (months)
0	A	No enlarged nodes or spleen, Hb > 11 g/dl, platelets > $100 \times 10^9/l$, lymphocytes < $15 \times 10^9/l$	150
I	B	As stage 0 with enlarged nodes	100
II		As stage 0 with enlargement of spleen or liver	70
III	C	As 0, I or II; Hb < 11 g/dl	20
IV		As 0, II, or III; platelets < $100 \times 10^9/l$	20

The staging notation 0–IV was introduced by Rai *et al.* in 1975, and A–C by Binet *et al.* in 1981.

useful in patients developing marrow failure (anaemia, thrombocytopenia) since they do not suppress haemopoiesis. In a patient with anaemia, prednisolone 30–40 mg can be given daily by mouth for 2–3 weeks followed by an alkylating agent. Chlorambucil is given intermittently, 2 weeks on, 2 weeks off, at a dose of about 0.1–0.2 mg/kg. An alternative is to give 2.5 mg/kg over 2–4 days each month. The treatment is continued until the symptoms and signs of the disease have regressed to a considerable extent, and then discontinued. A prolonged period of stable disease may then follow before progression which will then require further treatment. Repeated chemotherapy will ultimately contribute to bone marrow failure. Trials have shown no benefit for treatment with cyclophosphamide, vinblastine and prednisolone (CVP), or the combination of cyclophosphamide, doxorubicin, vincristine and prednisolone (CHOP) compared with chlorambucil.

Some newer agents have been found to be effective. Fludarabine, a nucleoside analogue, produces responses in 60% of patients with 40% complete responses. The response rates are higher when the drug is combined with prednisolone. The drug adds greatly to the immunosuppression which is already present but has a promising role in treatment. 2-Chlorodeoxyadenosine produces responses (but is myelosuppressive), and so does pentostatin. Further exploration of the use of these drugs, alone and in combination, is in progress. Exploration of the use of autologous and allogeneic BMT has just begun in young patients in whom complete remission has been obtained.

RADIOTHERAPY

Splenic irradiation is sometimes used palliatively for painful splenomegaly, often to a dose of 10 Gy in six to eight fractions over 2 weeks. The lymphocyte count falls and the spleen shrinks. Peripheral nodes may diminish in size. Myelosuppression can be troublesome particularly if the spleen (and therefore the treatment field) is very large. Splenectomy is then preferable if the patient is fit enough. If there are painful enlarged lymph nodes these can also be treated effectively by irradiation.

TREATMENT OF INFECTION

The hypogammaglobulinaemia renders patients highly susceptible to bacterial infection. Febrile illnesses such as upper respiratory infections should be treated promptly with antibiotics and patients warned of their susceptibility. Immunoglobulin is sometimes given prophylactically to patients who have recurrent infections. Penicillin is usually given prophylactically to patients who have been splenectomized or who have had an episode of pneumococcal infection.

Prognosis

In this elderly population, death frequently occurs from other causes. Infection contributes to mortality, and as the disease progresses, marrow failure develops, increasing the likelihood of infection and bleeding. Survival is closely related to initial stage of disease (Table 28.6).

Second cancers are possibly more common in CLL than in the general population. A small proportion of patients die from an aggressive malignant transformation with fever, weight loss and rapidly increasing tumour containing large undifferentiated cells. This syndrome (Richter's syndrome) is unusual.

T-cell chronic lymphocytic leukaemia

One of the neoplasms of peripheral (post-thymic) T cells is T-cell CLL. It accounts for 2% of all CLL and the cells are larger and more granular than B-cell CLL. Splenomegaly is commoner and lymph node enlargement is unusual. The cells are CD8+ (suppressor) and CD3+. There is often neutropenia and hypergammaglobulinaemia. Treatment is as for B-cell CLL.

Prolymphocytic leukaemia

This uncommon disease occurs in the elderly. The presentation is like CLL but without much lymph node enlargement and with marked splenomegaly. The WBC is high (in excess of 100×10^9/l). The white cells are larger than CLL cells, with more cytoplasm and a single prominent nucleolus. The cells are B cells with bright staining for surface Ig, although occasional T-cell variants have been described.

Treatment is with chemotherapy and splenic irradiation. Combination chemotherapy is usually used with regimens similar to those used in high-grade non-Hodgkin's lymphoma (see Chapter 26).

Hairy cell leukaemia [20]

The disease occurs more commonly in men (male:female ratio 4:1) aged 50–70 years and is characterized by anaemia, thrombocytopenia and neutropenia, splenomegaly and the presence of cells in the blood which have unusual cytoplasmic villi—so-called hairy cells.

There is little enlargement of lymph nodes and constitutional symptoms (fever, night sweats) are very unusual unless there is an intercurrent infection due to the neutropenia. Pyrexia may be caused by intercurrent mycobacterial infection which is related to neutropenia.

There has been considerable debate as to the nature of the hairy cell. B-cell markers (surface Ig) are usually present and the current view is that the cell is an activated clonal B lymphocyte. The cells contain tartrate-resistant acid phosphatase.

Treatment of hairy cell leukaemia is changing [20]. Interferon (IFN) is effective. Both recombinant α-2a and α-2b have been used. The schedules have varied in frequency (daily or twice weekly), duration (6–18 months) and dose. The complete response rate is about 8% and the partial response rate 75%. Interferon should be given for about 1 year. Deoxycoformycin (Pentostatin) and 2-chlorodeoxyadenosine have been shown to be effective. Deoxycoformycin is well tolerated, with myelosuppression the main side-effect. The complete response rate is 70% with a further 25% showing a partial response. Furthermore, these responses are durable for several years. The drug can be given with IFN, but it is not clear if this improves results. Similar results are obtained with 2-chlorodeoxyadenosine. Myelosuppression and fever are the main toxicities. The advent of these drugs has led to a reappraisal of the role of splenectomy which is now mainly performed in cases where there is no bone marrow infiltration. Four-year survival is now 80%. The prognosis is worse in patients with massive splenomegaly or abdominal lymphadenopathy.

Chronic myeloid leukaemia

Chronic myeloid leukaemia is, in the majority of patients, associated with a specific acquired chromosomal defect. After a period of slow progression the disease transforms into a more malignant variety of leukaemia. It occurs in 1.5 per 100 000 per year.

The chromosomal characteristics of CML have been outlined on p. 438.

Clinical features

These are shown in Table 28.7. The patient may be asymptomatic and the diagnosis made on a routine blood count, but fatigue, anaemia, weight loss and splenic pain eventually occur. Bruising and bleeding may develop. Abdominal pain may be due to stretching of the splenic capsule or may be acute and pleuritic if there has been splenic infarction.

Table 28.7 Clinical and laboratory findings in CML.

	Frequency (%)	
Symptoms and signs		
Malaise and fatigue	80	
Weight loss	60	
Bruising and bleeding	40	
Abdominal discomfort	40	
Splenomegaly	95	
Bone tenderness	70	
Hepatomegaly	50	
Purpura	25	
Typical laboratory findings		
Anaemia	9–12 g/dl	
WBC	$25–1000 \times 10^9/l$	
Granulocytes	40%	
Metamyelocytes	10%	
Myelocytes	30%	
Promyelocytes	5%	
Myeloblasts	3%	
Platelets		
$<150 \times 10^9/l$	10	
$150–400 \times 10^9/l$	40	Cases (%)
$>400 \times 10^9/l$	50	

Peptic ulceration is 10 times more common than in the general population.

On examination there is usually splenomegaly and often sternal tenderness. The spleen is often considerably enlarged. Hepatomegaly and purpura may be present and retinal haemorrhages are not infrequent.

Investigation

The WBC is grossly elevated with an increase in all stages of the granulocyte series, particularly myelocytes. Promyelocytes and myeloblasts are present in smaller numbers than myelocytes unless the presentation of the disease is with acute transformation ('blast crisis'). There is a variable degree of anaemia and the platelet count may be high, because of excess production of abnormal platelets, or low, because of hypersplenism or marrow failure. Thrombocytopenia is an indication that blastic transformation may have occurred. The diagnosis can usually be made from the blood film, and the bone marrow examination (although usually performed) does not contribute to diagnosis. It shows an expanded hypercellular marrow with an increase in the myeloid series, with an excess of early forms.

Leucocyte alkaline phosphatase is low or absent, and the Ph' chromosome can be demonstrated in metaphases in cultured marrow cells. The greatly increased turnover of myeloid cells leads to hyperuricaemia.

Patients who are Ph'-negative usually show more anaemia, a less high WBC, more numerous monocytes in the blood and more abnormal myeloid forms.

Evolution

As the leukaemic mass increases, the spleen enlarges and the patient becomes progressively more anaemic. The WBC doubles every 3–12 months. With treatment (see below) the WBC falls and a stable 'plateau' may then be reached with the patient off treatment. Gradually the 're-missions' become shorter and the recurrences more rapid. Finally, an aggressive disease develops with drug-resistant splenomegaly or rising WBC showing blastic transformation. The clinical picture is now dominated by an acute leukaemia which responds poorly to treatment and with a fatal outcome in a few months.

The transformation is usually accompanied by malaise, splenic enlargement, skin deposits, bone pain which may be localized, and a rising blast count. The median onset of transformation is 44 months. It may be more insidious, the disease showing only a progressive loss of control from chemotherapy and sometimes with features of myelosclerosis.

The transformation is usually into AML, but 20% of cases show transformation into ALL in which the blast cells are Ph'-positive. About 20% of cases of adult ALL are Ph'-positive.

Treatment in chronic phase (Fig. 28.6)

Hydroxyurea is now the drug most widely used for initial treatment [21]. The drug acts on the late progenitor cells. The dose is 1.5–2.0 g by mouth, and the response is more rapid than another widely used drug—busulphan. It has to be given daily to control the WBC. Hydroxyurea appears to confer better survival. Busulphan also appears to confer an additional risk in patients who undergo allogeneic BMT. It is given by mouth at a dose of 0.07 mg/kg (4–5 mg) daily until the WBC falls to about 20×10^9/l. It is important to stop treatment at this point because the myelosuppressive effect of busulphan is delayed so the WBC may fall further, until it begins to rise again later. The rise in count may be very slow and treatment may not need to be restarted for months or even years. Although the WBC usually falls slowly with busulphan, in some pa-

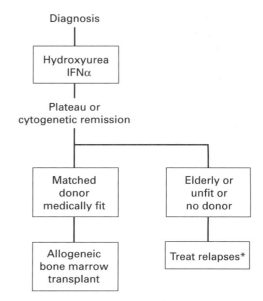

Fig. 28.6 Management of chronic myeloid leukaemia. *Role of ST1571 still to be established.

tients there is a more rapid reduction and they may even become pancytopenic, so careful observation is needed.

Side-effects of busulphan (see Chapter 6) include skin pigmentation and pulmonary fibrosis and azoospermia.

α-Interferon is now widely used. About 80% of patients show blood remission and 20% have a decrease in marrow Ph'-positive cells. The blood counts may remain stable for many months after IFN has been discontinued. Both progression-free survival and overall survival may be improved compared with hydroxyurea and busulphan [22]. With repeated treatments the recovery of the WBC becomes more rapid and the duration of the plateau, or 're-mission', shorter.

Drug treatment produces symptomatic and haematological improvement in almost all patients. The leukaemic mass is reduced with a fall in WBC, reduction in spleen size, improvement in marrow function with a rise in haemoglobin, and a consequent amelioration of symptoms of fatigue and malaise. A dramatic recent innovation has been the introduction of a tyrosine kinase inhibitor STI571 that shows considerable activity in IFN-α resistant disease with 90% remission rates. It appears non-toxic and is likely to radically change management [23].

Treatment of accelerated and transformed chronic granulocytic leukaemia

As the speed of relapse increases the spleen usually starts

to enlarge and marrow failure, due both to the disease and its treatment, becomes apparent. Changing from busulphan to hydroxyurea (1–2 g/day) may produce temporary benefit. If there is massive splenomegaly which is thought to contribute to anaemia and thrombocytopenia, splenectomy may be helpful provided that blastic transformation has not yet occurred. STI 1571 produces responses in some patients.

Blastic transformation is usually to AML and is often treated as such unless the patient is infirm or elderly. In those cases where ALL supervenes, treatment is as for adult ALL. In both cases the prognosis is very bad. Remissions may be obtained but median survival is only 3 months (Fig. 28.6).

Bone marrow transplantation [24]

Allogeneic BMT has been used in both blastic transformation and in chronic phase. The results of BMT in blastic transformation are usually disappointing although occasional patients have had a return of normal Ph'-negative haemopoiesis. Allogeneic BMT is successful when carried out in chronic phase, and sustained remissions have been achieved with Ph'-negative haemopoiesis.

Allogeneic BMT should be carried out in the chronic phase for patients aged less than 50 and who have a matched donor. The earlier in the chronic phase the transplant is carried out the better the outcome. The 5-year relapse-free survival is 75% in such patients. Previous busulphan treatment is an adverse prognostic factor. The high-dose regimen is either cyclophosphamide and TBI, or a chemotherapy regimen containing busulphan. If no matched donor is available a haplotype mismatched marrow might be used, but the graft-versus-host disease is more severe.

Prognosis

Without transplantation less than 5% of patients survive 10 years. The long-term survival of patients undergoing allogeneic BMT in chronic phase remains to be determined.

With transplantation 55% are relapse free at 5 years. After transplantation in accelerated phase the relapse-free survival at 5 years is 25%. The prognosis may improve further with STI571.

Ph'-negative chronic granulocytic leukaemia

These patients differ from Ph'-positive CGL in having a greater degree of splenomegaly at presentation, more profound anaemia and a lower WBC. The blood film reveals more abnormal neutrophils and monocytes, and fewer myelocytes. The disease appears to run a more rapid course than Ph'-positive CGL, with a median survival of only 18 months in some series. Treatment is along the same lines as Ph'-positive CGL.

Eosinophilic leukaemia

This disease is characterized by eosinophilia sometimes accompanied by anaemia, neutropenia and thrombocytopenia. There may be cough associated with transient pulmonary infiltration, and non-bacterial endocarditis occurs, leading to heart failure.

The disease may be difficult to distinguish from other forms of chronic eosinophilia and the diagnosis of leukaemia may be hard to establish. Acute blastic transformation of the disease occurs in some patients and the response to treatment is poor.

Chronic myelomonocytic leukaemia

This is a disease of the elderly. The onset is insidious with bruising or bleeding, fleeting urticarial skin rash, slight splenomegaly and a history of infections. There is a monocytosis with abnormal forms. Bone marrow shows abnormal nuclear morphology of a monocyte type. Chromosome 3 may show karyotypic abnormalities at t(3;16). The clinical course is often slow. Treatment is usually with hydroxyurea but is unsatisfactory and reserved for symptomatic disease.

References

1 Sandler OP. Epidemiology and etiology of leukaemia. *Curr Opin Oncol* 1990; 2: 3–9.
2 Kaldor JM, Day NE, Pettersson F *et al.* Leukaemia following chemotherapy for ovarian cancer. *N Engl J Med* 1990; 322: 1–6. (See also the accompanying paper (*N Engl J Med* 1990; 322: 7–13) describing risk for Hodgkin's disease.)
3 Wintrobe M. *Blood Pure and Eloquent.* McGraw-Hill, 1980: 528.
4 Fialkow PJ, Singer RW, Raskind WH *et al.* Clonal development, stem-cell differentiation and clinical remissions in acute non-lymphocytic leukaemia. *N Engl J Med* 1987; 317: 468–73.
5 Bain BJ. Leukaemia diagnosis. *A Guide to the FAB Classification.* Philadelphia: JB Lippincott, 1990.
6 MIC Study Group. Morphologic immunologic and cytoge-

netic (MIC) working classification of the acute myeloid leukaemias. *Br J Haematol* 1988; 68: 487–94.

7 Chessels JM, Bailey C, Richards SM. Intensification of treatment and survival in all children with lymphoblastic leukaemia: results of MRC trial UK ALL X. *Lancet* 1995; 345: 143–8.

8 Freeman AL *et al.* Comparison of intermediate-dose methotrexate with cranial irradiation for the post-induction treatment of acute lymphocytic leukaemia in children. *N Engl J Med* 1994; 330: 477–84.

9 Barrett AJ, Horowitz MM, Gale RP *et al.* Marrow transplantation for acute lymphoblastic leukaemia; factors affecting relapse and survival. *Blood* 1989; 74: 862–71.

10 Hussein KK, Dahlberg S, Head D *et al.* Treatment of acute lymphoblastic leukaemia in adults with intensive induction, consolidation, and maintenance chemotherapy. *Blood* 1989; 73: 57–63.

11 Czuczman MS, Dodge RK, Stewart CC *et al.* Value of immunophenotype in intensively treated adult acute lymphoblastic leukaemia: CALGB study 8364. *Blood* 1999; 93: 3931–9.

12 Lowenberg B, Downing JR, Burnett A. Acute myeloid leukaemia. *N Engl J Med* 1999; 341: 1051–62.

13 Mayer RJ, Davis RB, Schiffer CA *et al.* Intensive postremission chemotherapy in adults with AML. *N Engl J Med* 1994; 331: 896–903.

14 Zittoun RA, Mandell I, Willemze R *et al.* Autologous or allogeneic bone marrow transplantation compared with intensive chemotherapy in acute myelogenous leukaemia. *N Engl J Med* 1995; 332: 217–23.

15 Burnett AK, Goldstone AH, Stevens RMF *et al.* Randomised comparison of addition of autologous bone-marrow transplantation to intensive chemotherapy for acute myeloid leukaemia in first remission: results of MRC AML 10 trial. *Lancet* 1998; 351: 700–8.

16 Feneaux P *et al.* Effect of all transretinoic acid in newly diagnosed promyelocytic leukaemia. Results of a multicenter randomised trial. *Blood* 1993; 82: 3241–9.

17 Kantarjian HM *et al.* Treatment of therapy related leukaemia and myelodysplastic syndrome. *Haematology/Oncol Clin N Am* 1993; 7: 81–107.

18 Cheson BD, Bennett JM, Grever M *et al.* National Cancer Institute sponsored Working Group guidelines for chronic lymphocyte leukaemia: revised guidelines for diagnosis and treatment. *Blood* 1996; 87: 4990–7.

19 Caligaris-Cappio F. B-chronic lymphocyte leukaemia. a malignancy of anti-self B cells. *Blood* 1995; 87: 2615–20.

20 Lee TC, Piro LD, Saven A. The optimal management of hairy cell leukaemia. *Drugs* 1995; 49: 921–3.

21 Goldman JM *et al.* Choice of pretransplant treatment and timing of transplants for chronic myelogenous leukaemia in chronic phase. *Blood* 1993; 82: 2235–8.

22 Richards SM. Interferon α: results from randomised trials. *Bailliere's Clin Haematol* 1997; 10: 307.

23 Goldman JM. Tyrosine-kinase inhibition in treatment of chronic myeloid leukaemia. *Lancet* 2000; 355: 1031–2.

24 Hansen JA, Gooley TA, Martin PJ *et al.* Bone marrow transplantation from unrelated donors for patients with chronic myeloid leukaemia. *N Engl J Med* 1998; 338: 962–8.

Index

Factors on Provision of care

- Geography
- Lack of Scanners (no MRI)
- MCN's. SCAN
- ↑ agy population
- Children to Glasgow
- dead Cancer group —
- Team from Edinburgh.
- Improving waiting times

- Disadvanged areas.

- travel to Edinburgh

- very good info centre.

Partnerships - working
- Finance.